T0130755

Comprehensive Guide to Supportive and Palliative Care for Patients with Cancer

Comprehensive Guide to Supportive and Palliative Care for Patients with Cancer

—— 4th Edition ——

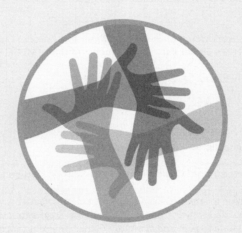

Janet L. Abrahm, MD

With Molly E. Collins, MD, and Bethany-Rose Daubman, MD

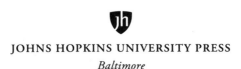

JOHNS HOPKINS UNIVERSITY PRESS

Baltimore

For Stacie

Drug dosage: The author and publisher have made reasonable efforts to determine that the selection and dosage of drugs discussed in this text conform to the practices of the general medical community. The medications described do not necessarily have specific approval by the US Food and Drug Administration for use in the diseases and dosages for which they are recommended. In view of ongoing research, changes in governmental regulations, and the constant flow of information relating to drug therapy and drug reactions, the reader is urged to check the package insert of each drug for any change in indications and dosage and for warnings and precautions. This is particularly important when the recommended agent is a new and/or infrequently used drug.

© 2000, 2005, 2014, 2022 Johns Hopkins University Press
All rights reserved. Published 2022
Printed in the United States of America on acid-free paper
9 8 7 6 5 4 3 2 1

Previous editions of this work were published as *A Physician's Guide to Pain and Symptom Management in Cancer Patients*, by Janet L. Abrahm, MD.

Johns Hopkins University Press
2715 North Charles Street
Baltimore, Maryland 21218-4363
www.press.jhu.edu

Library of Congress Cataloging-in-Publication Data

Names: Abrahm, J. (Janet), author. | Collins, Molly, 1980– author. | Daubman, Bethany-Rose, 1985– author.
Title: Comprehensive guide to supportive and palliative care for patients with cancer / Janet L. Abrahm, MD ; with Molly E. Collins, MD, Bethany-Rose Daubman, MD.
Other titles: Physician's guide to pain and symptom management in cancer patients
Description: Fourth edition. | Baltimore : Johns Hopkins University Press, 2022. | A physician's guide to pain and symptom management in cancer patients / Janet L. Abrahm ; with Amanda Moment and Arden O'Donnell. | Includes bibliographical references and index.
Identifiers: LCCN 2021036802 | ISBN 9781421443980 (hardcover) | ISBN 9781421443904 (ebook)
Subjects: LCSH: Cancer—Palliative treatment. | Pain—Treatment.
Classification: LCC RC271.P33 A27 2022 | DDC 616.99/406—dc23
LC record available at https://lccn.loc.gov/2021036802

A catalog record for this book is available from the British Library.

The enhancements and full bibliography can be found at www.press.jhu.edu.

Special discounts are available for bulk purchases of this book. For more information, please contact Special Sales at specialsales@jh.edu.

Contents

Figures and Tables

Contributors

Janet L. Abrahm, MD
Professor of Medicine, Harvard Medical School

Hermioni L. Amonoo, MD, MPP
Assistant Professor, Psychiatry, Harvard Medical School

Molly E. Collins, MD
Associate Professor, Fox Chase Cancer Center / Lewis Katz School of Medicine at Temple University

Bethany-Rose Daubman, MD
Assistant Professor of Medicine, Harvard Medical School

Amanda Moment, MSW, LICSW
Clinical Social Worker, Intensive Palliative Care Unit, Brigham and Women's Hospital

Arden O'Donnell, MPH, MSW, LICSW, APHSW-C
Adjunct Assistant Professor, Smith College School for Social Work

Rev. Kathleen (Katie) Pakos Rimer, MDiv, EdD, BCC
Palliative Care Chaplain, Boston; and Former Director, Spiritual Care and Education, Beth Israel Deaconess Medical Center of Harvard Medical School

Acknowledgments

As I sit down to write my acknowledgments for the fourth edition, it is the winter of 2021, in the midst of the COVID-19 crisis. I am fortunate to live and work in Massachusetts, one of the safest states. I continue my palliative care inpatient work at Brigham and Women's Hospital, though I spent from March through June 2020 at home, doing virtual consults. But since July, I've been back in person, and I am very grateful to be among the first to be vaccinated.

Palliative care could not be more relevant than it has been this year. I am grateful for the work all my colleagues throughout the country and throughout the world have been doing to ameliorate the suffering of those with COVID-19 and their families and loved ones, as well as the staff taking care of these patients. I cannot be prouder of our field than I am at this moment.

As it has changed many things about how we deliver care, COVID-19 has also changed how we conduct family meetings when families are barred from the bedside. Whether on Zoom, Microsoft Teams, Facetime, Doximity, or other platforms, my colleagues and I try to be sure that the voices of patients and their families are heard and that the clinicians' messages are really understood. Because we couldn't be everywhere we were needed, my colleagues and I prepared numerous palliative care symptom management and communication guides, which we made into pocket cards and put online; we finalized system-wide palliative and comfort care order sets in our electronic health record (Epic) so that clinicians could provide basic comprehensive comfort-focused care when we were not able to consult on all the patients who needed us.

Some things have stayed constant, and for that I'm also very grateful. Mary Cooley, PhD, OCN, CRNP, and I have been working together now for more than 25 years. I have acknowledged and thanked her in each edition of this book. For the first edition, "Mary shared with me her office and her insights into grief, bereavement, and the needs of cancer patients and their families; and for a number of years, she has supported me in my clinical and educational efforts in palliative care, and we continue our close collaboration." Mary continues to be a nationally recognized, award-winning nurse-scientist, my great friend and research mentor, and leader of the innovative projects that we hope will bring the materials contained in this book into the day-to-day care of cancer patients throughout the country, especially where there are no trained palliative care clinicians to provide expert symptom management consultations. We translated our evidence-based treatment suggestions into computable algorithms and just received funding, as part of the government's Moonshot programs, to program them so that palliative care recommendations will be available in the electronic health record for clinicians as they sit with their patients. Oncologists who have no access to palliative care specialists will receive personalized treatment recommendations for patients with pain, nausea, vomiting, constipation, diarrhea, treatment-related skin problems, anxiety, depression, insomnia, and fatigue at each visit. Mary continues to inspire me and challenge me to be more creative and inventive, while remaining practical.

In the eight years since the third edition was completed, I am grateful that I've been able to continue to grow in knowledge and understanding of our field. I owe this growth to the extraordinary generosity of my patients and their families, my colleagues in Boston and throughout the world, my trainees, and the staff with whom I work. I am particularly grateful to Jessica Goldhirsch, LCSW, MSW, MPH, for our work together over the past five years, creating courses with our inpatient and outpatient medical interpreter colleagues that consist of dialogues and role plays. These courses address the challenges the interpreters face when asked to interpret conversations in which bad news is delivered, goals of care and resuscitation options discussed, and in which cultural bumps abound. Jessica and I share these insights and the importance of partnering with interpreters in *Chapter 2, Working with Patients' Families*.

In this edition, I and my coeditors, Drs. Molly E. Collins and Bethany-Rose Daubman, highlight the challenges LGBTQ+ patients and partners face and the impact of systemic racism on the delivery of palliative care. Arden O'Donnell, MPH, MSW, LICSW, APHSW-C, updated *Chapter 2, Working with Patients' Families*, and Amanda Moment, MSW, LICSW, updated *Chapter 4, Sexuality, Intimacy, and Cancer*, with particular attention to addressing these challenges.

There are two other major changes in this edition. *Psychological distress* and *spiritual distress* each have their own chapter, rather than being woven throughout the text. Incorporating relevant material and stories from the third edition, Rev. Katie Pakos Rimer, MDiv, EdD, BCC, wrote *Chapter 3, Spiritual Care in Palliative Care*, and Dr. Hermioni Amonoo wrote *Chapter 9, Psychological Sources of Distress*. I am very grateful to Katie for her insights and sharing her voice with us, and to Hermi for doing something she swore she would never do: write another book chapter!

I would be remiss in not acknowledging the unfailing encouragement and support from those I work with at DFCI and BWH. Dr. Susan Block, professor of Psychiatry and Medicine at Harvard Medical School, is no longer our department chair, but Susan continues to offer her unparalleled expertise weekly as she helps us unravel the difficult psychological and psychosocial challenges our patients present. Dr. James Tulsky, professor of medicine, Harvard Medical School, and chief of the Division of Palliative Medicine at BWH, is also the chair of the Department of Psychosocial Oncology and Palliative Care at DFCI and acting chief of the Adult Palliative Care Division. James encourages my exploration into new arenas and is a champion of the partnership between expert communication and expert symptom assessment and management that is the essence of superb palliative care. My interdisciplinary colleagues on our team and on the staff are now too numerous to mention! Who would have thought that could occur when the first edition of this book was published 20 years ago?

For his love, encouragement, and support, I thank my husband, David R. Slavitt, and for valuable editorial and writing assistance, I thank my coeditors, Drs. Molly E. Collins and Bethany-Rose Daubman.

I (*Molly Collins*) would like to thank Dr. Janet Abrahm for the opportunity to join this project and for her support starting when I was a college student interested in this field. To watch Janet work is to see a master of her craft, and I am delighted that others can learn from the healing language and expertise she demonstrates throughout this book. I thank all my colleagues and the compassionate staff at Fox Chase Cancer Center/Temple Health, especially my team members in the Supportive Oncology and Palliative Care Program. My patients and their families have been my greatest teachers, and I thank them for all that they have shared with me. I wish to thank the supportive village that buoys my family, including my parents, Margaret and Arlen Collins, who taught me that death is a part of life. I thank my children, Reuben and Isadore, who are a renewable source of joy, meaning, and purpose. I courted my husband, Daniel Horton, by encouraging him to sign up for Dr. Susan Block's course, "Living with a Life-Threatening Illness." Though he didn't take the course, I am grateful for his love and support that followed every moment after.

I (*Bethany-Rose Daubman*) extend my deepest thanks to Dr. Janet Abrahm as well. As I write this in the midst of our second COVID surge, it feels like a lifetime ago when we would meet in a small Cambridge coffee shop, huddled together over lattes and scones, dreaming up desired additions to this newest edition. Indeed, I have learned so much in the years since, from both Janet and Molly. To have the privilege of training under Janet is to forever be able to fall back on WWJD?, or What Would Janet Do?, as I and every colleague I know often ask ourselves when faced with a challenging communication issue or pain crisis, pulling out the trusty tools she so patiently taught us.

Many thanks to my colleagues in the Massachusetts General Hospital Division of Palliative Care and Geriatrics for their endless support, for imbuing me with a growth mindset, and for the fact that I never need to worry alone. Special thanks to my chief, Dr. Vicki Jackson, for the space and encouragement to pursue this passion project. Many thanks to my closest colleague and confidante, Dr. Leah Rosenberg, who encourages me to be the best version of my palliative care self each day and is always, always my reality testing. To the newly born Baby Wong, who kindly kept the morning sickness to a minimum during our many early morning editing sessions. To my mother, who has always been my most enthusiastic editor and biggest champion. And last, to my long-suffering husband, Allen Wong, who always knows how to right my world with his perspective and soup dumplings.

Comprehensive Guide to Supportive and
Palliative Care for Patients with Cancer

Introduction

Despite extensive efforts to prevent cancer and find its cure, each year cancer inflicts suffering on another one to two million men and women. Many are cured, but along the way, they may have undergone devastating physical, psychological, and financial injuries. Less fortunate patients whose cancer is resistant to curative therapies may be told, "I'm sorry. There is nothing more we can do for you." But this is not true. Suffering can be prevented or addressed whenever it occurs, whether at diagnosis, during curative therapy, or if the cancer recurs. Patients can find healing even as their disease progresses.

In addition to disease-oriented treatments, cancer patients need attention to themselves as whole persons as well as comprehensive treatment for the physical, psychological, social, spiritual, and existential distress brought on by the disease or by the therapies directed against it. They will benefit from expert clinicians (physicians, nurses, nurse practitioners, physician assistants, clinical pharmacists, chaplains, social workers, psychologists, and psychiatrists) who will make the patient, not the disease, the focus of their attention. Such clinicians can help relieve patients' pain or other troubling symptoms, understand the causes of their suffering and what it would take to make them whole, anticipate hidden concerns, answer unasked questions, and help them deal with their fears.

Several oncology texts focus on the details of disease-oriented treatment. The present volume complements such texts, concentrating on suffering in patients with cancer and offering strategies for real communication and symptom-oriented, patient-focused treatment. Designed for a busy practicing clinician, it is more thorough than a handbook but less comprehensive than a textbook. It is also not simply a fourth edition of *A Physician's Guide to Pain and Symptom Management in Cancer Patients*, the third edition of which was published in 2014. Much of the material for this new book comes from that edition, but this book has been completely updated and enhanced by addressing many additional issues.

A comment on the new title. We wanted to include in our potential audience the many diverse clinicians who care for these patients, and so we changed our title from *A Physician's Guide* to *Comprehensive Guide*. Why did we add *Supportive* to the title? In many parts of the world, the term *supportive care*, or *supportive oncology*, has come to be used for delivering what we would consider palliative care to patients receiving active cancer treatment. In fact, to encourage referrals of patients earlier in their cancer course, some palliative care teams in the United States now call themselves Supportive and Palliative Care teams.

The first edition of the book was largely a guide to symptom management in cancer patients. But from the second edition on, it grew to encompass all domains of palliative care, with equal, if not more, emphasis on the key communication techniques of our field. The sections on relieving non-symptom-related distress also grew, with more discussion of family dynamics, sexuality, spirituality, and existential and psychological distress. To meet the expanded focus and the needs of the broader audience, the fourth edition is the product of three of us: me, Janet Abrahm, who wrote the majority of the material in the book and edited all the contributions by other authors, and my two coeditors, Drs. Molly E. Collins and Bethany-Rose Daubman, both board-certified palliative care physicians, along with four guest authors, each experts in their field. In the text, *I* used to mean just me. But in this edition, *I* can also refer to Molly or Bethany-Rose, or to one of our guest authors. We'll let you know by putting the name of the speaker in italics (e.g., *Molly Collins*).

This edition will be particularly useful to clinicians who wish to enhance their relationships with patients and their families and to expand the focus of their care. Physicians, nurse practitioners, physician assistants, social workers, pharmacists, chaplains, and nurses who work in primary care, general internal medicine, family practice, geriatrics, or oncology (medical, radiation, or surgical) or with hospice or palliative care programs will find information that spans the cancer trajectory. In addition to describing how to assess and manage the most troubling symptoms, we offer help with communication challenges that can occur at any stage, address the issues of most concern to patients and their loved ones, and review how clinicians can provide expert, compassionate care for the dying and their bereaved families.

In writing this book, my colleagues and I relied on the work of experts in the field whose remarkable research and untiring efforts have delineated regimens and approaches that have revolutionized palliative care. The full bibliography is available online at www.press.jhu.edu. We drew also from lessons learned from our patients and their families during our work as teachers and clinicians, as relatives and friends of people who have had cancer, as well as from our students and our colleagues. The clinical stories that appear in the book were crafted from these experiences.

Both superior communication skills and technical expertise are required if we are to succeed in relieving the distress of cancer patients, and the organization of the book reflects these dual requirements. In **Part I, A Team Approach**, we discuss the unique issues that need to be addressed at the beginning of the cancer trajectory (Chapter 1) and those relevant for patients with advancing disease (Chapter 5), offering suggestions for how to address these issues. Part I also includes Arden O'Donnell's work with Jessica Goldhirsch (Chapter 2), which explains how families work and how best to work with them; Katie Pakos Rimer's chapter on spiritual care for these patients and families (Chapter 3); and Amanda Moment's contribution on sexuality and intimacy (Chapter 4). **Part II, Pain Control, Symptom Management, and Psychological Considerations**, complements Part I. It contains detailed presentations of the technical aspects of symptom assessment and management (Chapters 6, 7, 8, and 10) as well as Hermioni Amonoo's discussion of psychological considerations and disorders in cancer patients (Chapter 9). **Part III, End of Life and Bereavement**, deals with communication issues for patients approaching the end (Chapter 11), symptom management in the last days and weeks (Chapter 12), and how to help bereaved families (Chapter 13). In Parts I, II, and III, clinical scenarios illustrate many of the dilemmas presented by patients and their families.

Important practice points are highlighted throughout the text and in numerous tables. There are also audio and video resources that complement the text available on the Johns Hopkins University Press website—such as audios of me doing hypnosis inductions, or videos of interviews describing how to work with patients expecting a miracle. Additional resources include numerous video demonstrations of the communication techniques we describe in the book, such as breaking bad news, the Serious Illness Conversation Guide, or when the disease is far advanced, REMAP. For the full list of resources, and the link where they can be found, see the **Enhancements** section in the back of the book.

PART I. A TEAM APPROACH

"What is wrong with me? Am I dying?"

The questions begin even before the official cancer diagnosis is made, and they continue throughout the course of treatment, whether the patient is cured or enters the cycle of relapse and retreatment that ultimately leads to death. In this way, of course, cancer patients are not unlike any other patients, who deliver the most surprising replies to "What brought you here today?" My father, a general internist who was in private practice for more than 50 years, cautioned me that it is usually more important to listen carefully for what patients don't say than to what they do say.

This is certainly true for patients with cancer, whose concerns often differ in significant ways from those of patients without cancer. The proximity of death and the specter of helplessness, grief, suffering, and loss of dignity demand their attention. Many patients and their families, however, do not openly share with clinicians their fears about the disease, the problems it produces, or the agents used to treat it.

Mrs. Ventimilio*, for example, who had been cured of a small, localized breast cancer for more than ten years, unexpectedly appeared at my oncology office one day for a "full check-up." During the course of the evaluation, she admitted that she had gone to a funeral the previous day and had begun to wonder whether she was really cured or whether the breast cancer was lying undetected inside her.

---

*All names of patients and their clinicians are pseudonyms.

Had I failed to discover that fear, I would not have been able to eliminate it or the stress it was causing.

Another patient, Mr. Ashton, whom I had been treating for metastatic lung cancer, asked me for pills so he could die of suicide "when the time is right." As we discussed his request further, it appeared that he was concerned not for himself but for his elderly wife: he feared that she might ruin her health trying to care for him as he died. As he came to understand about hospice programs and how hospice personnel and his friends and family could work together, he, too, was reassured. In both these cases, the hidden concerns, the unasked questions, were the real source of distress.

Part I addresses how difficult conversations can be conducted in early days (Chapter 1) and as the disease advances (Chapter 5), including the challenges of advance care planning, conducting family meetings, and discussions of prognosis with patients and families. Over the years, either as an oncologist or as a palliative care physician, and in Drs. Collins's and Daubman's careers as palliative care physicians, we have discussed many difficult issues with patients and their families, and some of these talks went much better than others. We include sample dialogues that demonstrate what we have learned about how to communicate concern, elicit useful responses from patients and their families, and satisfy their needs. Part I also includes chapters from palliative care social workers about family dynamics (Chapter 2) and sexuality and intimacy in cancer patients (Chapter 4), as well as from a palliative care chaplain (Chapter 3), who share with us their domains' palliative care expertise.

Chapter 1. Early Days *with Molly E. Collins, MD*

This chapter may be especially helpful for clinicians who are just starting to take responsibility for telling patients bad news, initiating advance care planning, and discussing prognosis. It begins with a review of what makes a conversation difficult; offers techniques to analyze how our own experiences, feelings, and identities contribute to our unease as we prepare for the meeting; and explains how mastering the shared "third conversation" can enhance the outcomes. By understanding what we are bringing to the conversation, we can better address the concerns of patients and their families. A particularly difficult discussion, especially for a beginner, is telling a patient that they have cancer or that cancer has recurred. This chapter includes a review of techniques for breaking bad news and for dealing with the patient's response along with a comprehensive discussion of advance care planning.

Of interest to many may be the discussion of why clinicians can be reluctant to raise the subjects of advance care planning, including discussions of advance directives, resuscitation, or prognosis. We offer methods for presenting these issues to patients and their families, including a presentation of a well-studied effective guide for preparing for the future, the Serious Illness Conversation Guide. We include links to teaching videos in which expert clinicians conduct these conversations. We also review advance care planning documents, Physician/Medical Orders for Life Sustaining Treatment (POLST/MOLST) forms, cultural considerations in discussing prognosis, advice for running family meetings, and the varieties of shared decision-making that clinicians can use in these discussions. Finally, we discuss how to manage conflict, and how ethics consultation teams can partner with the clinical team when a value conflict prevents the teams and the families from reaching consensus.

Chapter 2. Working with Patients' Families
with Arden O'Donnell, MPH, MSW, LICSW, APHSW-C

In this chapter, Arden O'Donnell, MPH, MSW, LICSW, APHSW-C shares her review of the literature and her hard-earned insights as a clinician in her description of the basics of how families function. She first describes family structure, showing us how to identify its elements and why it's important to identify key family members and the role that each family member plays, including our patient's role.

She next gives us tools to assess how the family as a whole functions, which will enhance the success of any family meeting, whether it be about a symptom management regimen or advance care plans. Arden describes how to look at each family as a system and gives us scales on which we can locate the level of family cohesion (on a scale that ranges from "disengaged" to "enmeshed") and the level of family flexibility ("rigid" to "chaotic"). She also helps us assess how much family members communicate with each other, which turns out to be much more variable than we had ever imagined. She ends the assessment section with a discussion of the role of culture.

A new section in this chapter was co-written with Jessica Goldhirsh, LCSW, MSW, MPH, who is both a palliative care social worker and a trainer of medical interpreters. In it we discuss the intricacies of partnering with medical interpreters in palliative care conversations: those that involve breaking bad news, goals of care, prognosis, and advance care planning. We include how to choose an interpreter and how to work together during the *pre-meeting* and the debriefing session after the encounter with the patient, or with the patient and family.

Finally, Arden describes situations in which clinicians really should get expert help from psychiatrists, expert social workers, or psychiatric nurse practitioners: when there is longstanding conflict in the family; when the patient or a family member has a personality disorder, severe mental illness, or substance use disorder; or when there is a history of intimate partner violence.

Chapter 3. Spiritual Care in Palliative Care
with Rev. Katie Pakos Rimer, MDiv, EdD, BCC

Reverend Katie Rimer, MDiv, EdD, BCC brings themes from the previous editions and adds much more to her new chapter, which discusses what she terms "the spiritual landscape in patients with serious illness." As she writes in her introduction,

> Some clinicians can feel tentative about the whole area of spiritual care, not knowing what it is, or what their responsibilities are regarding patients' spiritual and religious lives. *Will my patients ask me about my faith if I open that door with them? How do I ask the question about theirs? And how do I respond to their answer?* In this chapter I hope to help you identify your patients' spiritual needs and show you how to conduct a basic spiritual assessment. I review the ethics of providing spiritual care as a nonchaplain provider, when to bring in a chaplain or the patient's clergy, and common pitfalls to avoid. I consider how religion can affect medical decision-making and offer approaches for working with patients who are waiting for a miracle.

This chapter offers links to interviews with clergy discussing how to approach changing hope for African American patients and how to respond to requests for miracles from patients who hold various beliefs.

Rev. Rimer also explores the differences between religion and spirituality, and between what she terms positive and negative religious coping. At the end of her chapter, she shares why she believes that medicine is a spiritual practice.

Chapter 4. Sexuality, Intimacy, and Cancer
with Amanda Moment, MSW, LICSW

I have had the pleasure and great good fortune to work for years with the author of this chapter, Amanda Moment, MSW, LICSW. She is the social worker on our Intensive Palliative Care Unit team, a respected clinician, and a gifted teacher. In this chapter, Amanda discusses a subject that clinicians often know little about: our patients' concerns about how cancer and its treatment will affect their sexuality and how we can talk with our patients and their partners about this subject.

Amanda first reviews why this subject is important and includes the positive outcomes that can come from our becoming more comfortable with and more expert in these discussions. She describes how cancer and related treatments affect sexuality, and then explores clinician barriers to the discussion and how to approach the subject. She reviews the models and tools available to us and makes practical suggestions for having these much-needed conversations. She ends with a review of special considerations, such as culture, sexual and gender minorities, sexuality across the life cycle, intersectionality, concerns of partners and of single patients, and palliative care, hospice, and sexuality. The enhancements section also includes a link to an interview with a leader in LGBTQ+ innovative web-based health solutions discussing LGBTQ+ palliative care concerns, as well as links to videos discussing how sexuality can be altered by cancer and its treatment.

Chapter 5. Advancing Disease *with Molly E. Collins, MD*

As disease advances, other communication problems surface. In Chapter 5, Dr. Molly E. Collins and I deal with the most common of these. One of the biggest challenges is helping patients whose disease is no longer responsive to treatment, and their families, make a gradual transition in care from a cancer-directed treatment approach to supportive care focused on symptom management and quality of life. We explain how the rigors of the cancer-treatment schedule have caused most patients and their family caregivers to stop being involved in work, their community, and even their family. If the clinical team can encourage patients and their families to reintegrate important activities into their lives, patients are more likely to understand that when you tell them that the burden of another therapy is much greater than the potential benefit, you are not abandoning them. Part of this transition is supporting hope, and we explain how we can both be realistic and support patient and family hope as the nature of hope changes with increasing patient illness.

We readdress the challenges of formulating and discussing prognosis, especially in this era of exceptional responders and targeted cancer therapies. We describe how to move forward if clinicians differ on prognosis. We then discuss how to help patients and families cultivate prognostic awareness and strategies for talking to patients who are reluctant to have this conversation. We provide compassionate language to help patients make the final shift from life-prolonging treatment to fully supportive care, including when and how to readdress resuscitation options. We review REMAP (**r**eframe, **e**xpect emotion, **m**ap out goals, **a**lign, and **p**lan), which is a useful conversation guide that can help patients and families make plans when there are few or no further treatment options. We also offer links to teaching videos of expert clinicians having these conversations. Discussing these issues with children can be challenging, and we end the chapter with a review of principles for doing that from experts in the field.

PART II. PAIN CONTROL, SYMPTOM MANAGEMENT, AND PSYCHOLOGICAL CONSIDERATIONS

Part II is a symptom assessment and management handbook that also discusses psychological disorders and their treatment. Its five chapters review how to assess pain and treat it by pharmacologic and nonpharmacologic means, address psychological sources of distress, and manage distressing problems other than pain.

Chapter 6. Assessing the Patient in Pain

A thorough pain assessment reveals both the cause or causes of the pain and the factors that exacerbate the experience of pain for each patient. It is the foundation on which both pharmacologic and nonpharmacologic therapies rest. Chapter 6 reviews the components of a comprehensive pain assessment, provides examples of several measurement tools available for this purpose, defines the characteristics of the various types of pain, and describes in detail a number of cancer-related pain syndromes that occur only rarely in patients without cancer. We also review the role of culture in determining the meaning of pain and the styles of reporting it to clinicians, both verbal and nonverbal.

Technology is now assisting clinicians and patients in assessing and reporting on pain and other symptoms. We review new ways patients are reporting distress, including smartphones, tablets, or other platforms, and how those reports are being integrated into electronic health records and are alerting clinicians automatically. Natural language processing can identify words in the medical record suggesting patient distress, and these data can supplement patient-reported outcomes (PROs) to improve clinician pain assessment and management. We review the exciting new field of clinical decision support, which can further improve care by integrating these PROs with national consensus guidelines for treatment and present symptom management recommendations to clinicians in the electronic health record during virtual telehealth or office visits with the patient.

At the end of the chapter, we discuss how other dimensions of the patient's experience such as anxiety, depression, delirium, or social or spiritual distress can exacerbate the experience of pain and adversely affect the quality of life of patients and their families. We review how to assess the family's concerns and their cooperation with the management plan, deriving patient-specific goals for comfort and function, and the role of the social worker in helping with social and financial causes of distress that may present as "pain."

Chapter 7. Pharmacologic Management of Cancer Pain

This chapter details pharmacologic therapy, the cornerstone of cancer pain treatment. We discuss the use of nonsteroidal anti-inflammatory drugs and opioids, delivered by the oral, transmucosal, topical, transdermal, rectal, intravenous, subcutaneous, or spinal routes, and how to choose among these agents and routes. Because of the increasing concerns among the public of the misuse of opioids, patients and families have many unasked questions. For clinicians, we include in this chapter a discussion of risk management, with tools to determine a patient's risk for opioid misuse.

Because of the specter of addiction, unless several barriers are overcome, some patients won't take opioid medication and will continue to suffer severe pain. We address the misconceptions of patients and their families about the use of opioids: becoming addicted, having no effective medication later if the pain worsens, becoming constipated or "doped up," or going against the teachings of their religion. We provide examples of patients and families with such concerns, as well as suggestions for anticipating and overcoming them. We also review other impediments to adherence, including patients' reluctance to admit how much pain they are experiencing and the role of hidden agendas in impairing your ability to relieve their pain. Here, we may expect to confront guilt, denial, and anger, all of which we discuss. And we explain how educating colleagues can enhance patients' comfort.

We include how to select an opioid and provide an extensive discussion of using methadone for pain in cancer patients. We also discuss treatment of the common opioid-induced side effects: constipation, nausea, sedation, opioid overdose, opioid neurotoxicity, delirium, and respiratory depression.

We next review adjuvant pain relievers, including adjuvants for nerve pain (such as corticosteroids, anticonvulsants, tricyclic antidepressants, baclofen, clonidine, and ketamine), agents for bone pain (such as NSAIDs, corticosteroids, external beam radiation and radiopharmaceuticals, bisphosphonates, receptor activator of nuclear factor κβ ligand [RANK-L], vertebroplasty and kyphoplasty, and radiofrequency ablation), neuroleptics, and skeletal muscle relaxants. Also included are anesthetic methods, such as topical and oral agents, neural blockade, neuroablation, cingulotomy, and medications infused into the epidural or intrathecal space.

Special mention is made of the considerations needed in selected populations requiring opioids for pain management, including older patients and patients who are cognitively impaired, have active or past histories of substance use disorder, are on methadone or buprenorphine maintenance for substance use disorders, are cancer survivors, or have hematologic malignancies.

Finally, we review common clinical situations you will face, such as managing patients with renal or hepatic impairment, starting patients on opioids, and changing dose, agent, or route of delivery.

Several tables detail the NSAID and opioid drugs available, their formulations, the doses recommended, and caveats about their use; other tables list the same information for laxatives, antiemetics, psychostimulants, agents that treat delirium, adjuvant agents for neuropathic pain, antidepressants, adjuvants for bone pain, and topical and oral anesthetics. We also provide weblinks to our Dana-Farber Cancer Center pain resource book (https://pinkbook.dfci.org).

Chapter 8. Nonpharmacologic Strategies in Palliative Care

This chapter opens with a discussion of integrative and complementary and alternative medicine (CAM) techniques. The National Center for Complementary and Alternative Medicine has defined five domains of complementary and alternative therapies: (1) alternative medical systems, (2) manipulative and body-based methods, (3) mind-body interventions, (4) biologically based therapies, and (5) energy therapies. In this book, we do *not* review the biologically based therapies, which include special diets, herbal treatments, megadose vitamin therapy, or use of particular substances not proved effective by conventional medical studies. We also do not review energy therapies such as qi gong, Therapeutic Touch, Reiki, and healing touch, but we do provide references for those who are interested in these areas.

We discuss those integrative and CAM techniques for which there is the most evidence supporting their effectiveness in relieving pain and other sources of distress in cancer patients. These include acupuncture/acupressure and yoga, two of the alternative medical systems that include philosophies and practices that are completely independent of the usual medical approach.

The majority of the chapter discusses other effective nonpharmacologic techniques for relieving distress. These include manipulative and body-based methods, including cutaneous interventions, massage and vibration, transcutaneous electrical nerve stimulation (TENS), positioning, and exercise. Finally, we review mind-body interventions, including education, cognitive and behavioral interventions such as diversion of attention, relaxation and breathing, guided imagery, mindfulness meditation, mindfulness-based stress reduction (MBSR), and hypnosis, biofeedback, and music and art therapy. Dr. Abrahm is a hypnosis practitioner, and as such she is familiar with the use of hypnosis. She provides a discussion of some misconceptions that have limited its use, along with written and audio sample relaxation exercises that cancer patients may find useful. We also discuss the role of speech and language therapy.

Chapter 9. Psychological Considerations
with Hermioni L. Amonoo, MD, MPP

In this edition, for the first time, information about psychological considerations in palliative care have been centralized into a chapter, written by an experienced psycho-oncologist, Dr. Hermioni Amonoo, assistant professor of psychiatry at Harvard Medical School and a member of the Psychosocial Oncology Division of the Department of Psychosocial Oncology and Palliative Care at Dana-Farber

Cancer Institute and the Department of Psychiatry at Brigham and Women's Hospital. As she states in her introduction to the chapter, "The 2021 [NCCN] guideline documented a surprisingly high cancer-related distress prevalence of 20 to 61 percent." The chapter explores the reasons for this distress and indications for earlier referral.

Dr. Amonoo first reviews the roles of psychological support and counseling and provides questions to help us understand the psychological hurdles newly diagnosed patients must overcome, so that we can target our interventions. She provides practice points for fostering helpful coping skills and, later in the chapter, helps us distinguish adjustment disorder from anxiety and depressive symptoms and offers treatment recommendations. She presents a novel technique for helping ease the suffering of patients with existential distress, a vexing problem of especially our younger patients with advancing cancer.

Dr. Amonoo also demystifies the various personality disorders some cancer patients have that can interfere with our relationships with them and consequently affect the care they receive. After you read the chapter, you will be able to recognize the seven personality disorders that are particularly problematic in medical settings: paranoid, antisocial, narcissistic, borderline, histrionic, dependent, and obsessive-compulsive. The chapter ends with a discussion of recognition and treatment of patients with delirium of several etiologies, including anticholinergic crisis and serotonin syndrome.

Chapter 10. Managing Other Distressing Problems

This chapter concludes the symptom assessment and management guide. The discussion includes oral complications (candida, herpes simplex virus, treatment-induced mucositis, xerostomia); gastrointestinal problems (ascites, constipation, diarrhea, and dysphagia, nausea and vomiting, including treatment-induced nausea and vomiting, and bowel obstruction), with a link to our Dana-Farber Cancer Institute resource for nausea and vomiting in cancer patients (https://pinkbook.dfci.org); respiratory problems (dyspnea, cough, hemoptysis, and hiccups); immunotherapy toxicities; skin disorders (hand-foot syndrome, EGFR-inhibitor-associated skin disorders, fungating skin lesions, pressure sores, and pruritus); insomnia; and hot flashes. We also include the common treatable causes of weakness and fatigue: Lambert-Eaton syndrome, anemia, metabolic abnormalities, anorexia, and malnutrition. Patients and their families commonly believe that enteral or parenteral nutrition will restore patients' strength and prolong their lives. We explain why this is not always the case and why enteral and parenteral feeding are not usually indicated for people with advanced cancer. We also offer coping strategies to help patients suffering from weakness or fatigue modify their activities to maximize what they can achieve despite their diminishing capacity.

The material in the text is supplemented by tables detailing useful drugs and their recommended doses for the problems reviewed.

PART III. END OF LIFE AND BEREAVEMENT

In Part III, we conclude our book by discussing how to communicate with and care for patients in the weeks to months approaching the end of their lives, and in their final days. We also review care for their bereaved families.

Chapter 11. Approaching the End

Here we review the art and science of helping patients as they approach the end. We discuss components of a "good death," the impact of religion and culture on this, and the special concerns of LGBTQ+ patients. We review the tasks of dying, including legacy work and dignity therapy. We also discuss how clinicians can recognize that the priority lists for symptom management of patients and families might differ from each other and from their own, and we suggest how to prioritize which symptoms are amenable to treatment.

Next, we explore the role of hospice programs in ensuring that all the important pieces are in place and describe the services hospice programs provide. We acknowledge that hospice care isn't right for everyone and review the data describing racial and ethnic differences in enrollment. This chapter also covers the utility of Bridge to Hospice programs for some of these patients, and for others, the role of the palliative care team. We detail the benefits of integrating palliative care and oncology care, starting at diagnosis and for patients continuing antineoplastic therapies even when their disease seems refractory.

The chapter ends with a discussion of Medical Aid in Dying, including reasons for the request, ways for clinicians to address those requests, interdisciplinary team challenges after the request, and clinicians' ethical concerns about participating in it.

Chapter 12. The Last Days

Chapter 12 starts with a discussion of care of the dying, including caring for dying physicians. We review how we can let families know when time is short, and when the *transitional phase* is beginning. Clinicians may need to address ethical or religious concerns about pain management hastening death or the burdens and benefits of artificial fluid or nutrition support, issues that can be raised at this time. We revisit the utility of referring the patients to hospice programs, even in the last days or weeks, and of ongoing clarification of wishes about resuscitation. We discuss how to support the inpatient team and families of patients who die in the hospital, and the special challenges posed by COVID-19. The enhancements section also includes a link to a teaching video about how to bring "the Five Things" into the conversation.

Chapter 12 then moves to an outline of the symptom complex of dying patients and treatment recommendations, including a table of pharmacologic therapies for the most common problems: pain, death rattle, terminal restlessness, dyspnea, delirium, dehydration, massive hemoptysis, nausea, vomiting, and myoclonus. We also provide an algorithm for agitation in the last days. Furthermore, the enhancements section includes a link to a teaching video about how to discuss with the family what they can expect in the last days, and how they can continue to comfort their dying loved ones.

Unfortunately, there are rare patients for whom aggressive treatment of symptoms cannot relieve their pain, delirium, or other distress without excessive sedation. Some of these patients will respond to dexmedetomidine (Precedex), but some will require palliative sedation to unconsciousness. This chapter explains how to use Precedex, as well as the differences between sedation as a side effect and palliative sedation to unconsciousness. We offer the procedures we have developed over the years to provide this form of sedation and to support the clinicians administering the sedation and the staff caring for the patient and family.

Because palliative care clinicians can be called upon to assist ICU clinicians when patients require discontinuation of an LVAD, a terminal wean, or an extubation, we discuss the considerations and techniques surrounding these procedures, including communication with the family and the staff, as well as support for them after the patient's death. We end this chapter with a discussion of what our institutions could do for clinicians to help us care for our dying patients.

Chapter 13. Bereavement *with Bethany-Rose Daubman, MD*

Chapter 13 discusses ways we can continue to help the bereaved family and friends. Our colleague Sue Morris, PsyD, was the expert reviewer of this chapter. Dr. Morris is a clinical psychologist and author of several books on bereavement for survivors. She is the program manager of Bereavement Services for the Department of Psychosocial Oncology and Palliative Care at Dana-Farber Cancer Institute. We discuss the manifestations of loss, grief, and mourning, as well as the differentiation between grief and depression.

We also highlight the differences between the *intuitive* and the *instrumental* styles of grieving; intuitive grievers look to us as though they are grieving, but instrumental grievers do not, and we may misunderstand their behavior and not offer the support they need. We describe a typical bereavement program through which we can support survivors and educate them about what they can expect to feel and include the bereavement materials we used before our institution, Dana-Farber, developed an institute-wide bereavement program. We also indicate how to identify those who would benefit from formal counseling, cognitive behavioral techniques, or informal support groups.

An even more troubled group suffers from *prolonged grief disorder*. These survivors delay mourning or may never recover from their losses. We discuss the factors that predispose to this syndrome, provide a screening tool that identifies people at greatest risk, offer suggestions for identifying and providing ongoing support and treatment for them, and describe complicated grief therapy (CGT), which is particularly effective for these patients.

We end this chapter with a section we call "Wounded Healers," which offers suggestions for self-care to prevent and treat the increasing incidence of compassion fatigue and burnout among clinicians. The COVID-19 crisis has only worsened this, subjecting so many to scenes of death and loss as well as patients deprived of loving companionship as they die. We review the manifestations of compassion fatigue and burnout, as well as strategies that have been employed to minimize or reverse it. We end with explaining how talking about our losses with our colleagues during grief rounds or remembrance sessions can be healing.

PART I

A Team Approach

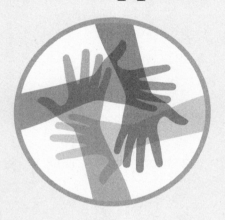

CHAPTER 1

Early Days

with Molly E. Collins, MD

INTRODUCTION

The foundation of your relationships with patients and their families is profoundly affected both by how you first tell them they have cancer and by how you deal with their response to the news. The nonverbal clues you provide during these crucial interactions reveal a great deal about how willing you are to discuss their fears and how certain they can be of your ongoing emotional support.

Patients and their families need to know that you will help them throughout the course of their illness, especially if it eventually causes their death. You must make it clear that you will not abandon them if the medical treatments lose their effectiveness and will use your expertise to help them achieve the best possible quality of life at every stage of their illness.

Part of your responsibility, then, is to communicate clearly your interest in understanding your patients' values, hopes, and goals so that you can choose treatments that best balance burdens and benefits that are meaningful for them. And, should it become necessary, you will then be able to carry out their wishes regarding resuscitation or prolonged support by a ventilator or feeding tube. What do they need to be able to do for life to be worthwhile? Which kinds of disabilities are tolerable, and which not?

In this first chapter, therefore, we review the components of difficult conversations, including how you can most skillfully "break the bad news," and how you can best respond to the reactions of patients and their families. We also consider how to begin discussions of prognosis, preparing for the future, advance care planning, resuscitation and other extraordinary support, and what is known about why such discussions are so difficult to undertake. We include several examples of approaches that work, as well as some examples of conducting family meetings when you can and when you cannot involve the patients themselves. When English is not the patient's or the family's language of choice, or when American Sign Language is being spoken, it is crucial that we partner with a professional medical interpreter for these conversations. We explore that partnership further in Chapter 2.

DIFFICULT CONVERSATIONS: UNDERSTANDING AND MASTERING THEM

To be able to deliver bad news with skill and compassion, you must prepare yourself emotionally for what is likely to be a very difficult conversation and for staying present no matter what happens. In rehearsing what you are going to say, you need to be aware of your own feelings about the impending meeting and to analyze carefully all the elements that make this a "room you would rather not enter." What makes a conversation difficult? Members of the Harvard Negotiation Project (the people who brought us the useful book *Getting to Yes*) lay out the key elements in *Difficult Conversations: How to Discuss What Matters Most*, second edition (Stone, Patton, and Heen 2010). The book is designed for businesspeople, but the principles apply equally well to clinicians, patients, and their families.

Stone and colleagues suggest that within any difficult conversation lie three conversations: (1) the "What Happened?" conversation, (2) the "Feelings" conversation, and (3) the "Identity" conversation.

These conversations can be illustrated by an encounter I (*Janet Abrahm*) had with Yu Hsin and his wife, Jenny, early in my career as a practicing oncologist. Yu Hsin, a 33-year-old man, had non-Hodgkin's lymphoma of the small bowel. He had been married to Jenny for ten years, and they had three children, 8, 6, and 4 years old. Surgical resection of his tumor was not possible. I had tried several chemotherapy regimens, after each of which the tumor had responded. The manifestation of each response, however, was severe gastrointestinal bleeding. I went to visit Yu in the hospital on the day he was going to be transferred to a rehabilitation facility. This had been his third hospitalization for bleeding and near perforation of the intestine because of tumor necrosis. I knew that Yu's bowel would surely perforate if we tried chemotherapy again. The surgeons thought that surgery would not be helpful. As I prepared to enter the room, I steeled myself to tell Yu and Jenny that we could not risk any more treatment.

We chatted for a while about the planned transfer, to which they both looked forward. Jenny asked when Yu would be coming back for his next treatment, and

---

Practice Points: Difficult Conversations

The "What Happened?" conversation
> Given the same set of facts, does your story differ from theirs?
> Can you move from certainty to curiosity?

The "Feelings" conversation
> What are you feeling: Sadness? Anger? Guilt? Frustration?

The "Identity" conversation
> Is your sense of who you are being challenged?
> Have you lost your balance?

The "Third" conversation
> Once you have heard their story and had a chance to share your point of view, create from those a "third conversation" that includes shared goals you both can work on.

(Adapted from Stone, Patton, and Heen 2010)

I replied that, while I wished I had better news, I thought there was nothing more I could do for him, that he would bleed to death or his bowel would perforate if I continued the therapy. Yu took the news stoically, but Jenny asked angrily how I could stop treating him if his lymphoma was responding to the treatment. She accused me of abandoning them and giving up on Yu.

I could barely look at them. I felt numb and distant, as though observing all of us from far away. I reassured Jenny that we would find something to help Yu, hoping that my saying it would make it so. I told Yu that I was glad he was feeling so much better and that we'd talk about next steps when he came to the office. I could not wait to leave.

The "What Happened?" Conversation

I remember clearly how I felt as I left the room. I had given other patients bad news that had elicited anger from both the patients and their families, but rarely had I felt so distraught. I did not understand then what was different about this conversation.

Later, using the framework from *Difficult Conversations*, I was able to understand "what happened." As Stone and colleagues put it, there can be many interpretations of the same facts. So, what were the facts here? As I saw it, I had given Yu state-of-the-art treatment that was placing him in danger of bleeding to death or dying from a bowel perforation. It was unfortunate, but it was certainly not fair for them to blame me for the location of the lymphoma. Jenny, I surmised, was in denial about Yu's true condition and the danger further therapy would bring.

As the authors caution, however, "You only know your own story." In shutting down in response to their anger, I was not able to ask Jenny to tell me more about her reaction to my news. To this day, I don't know why she thought we could continue his treatments. Maybe she thought that the bleeding was a good sign, that the tumor was being flushed out of his system, and the blood transfusions were bringing in clean, safe blood to replace the cancerous tissue.

I would have been much more helpful to them had I explored why she was so angry and learned more about her interpretation of Yu's response to his treatments. How I wish I had at least not said, *"There is nothing more I can do for him,"* even as a part of my explanation of why I wasn't offering ongoing chemotherapy. Was that why she felt I was abandoning her and giving up on Yu? I'll never know.

Stone and colleagues would suggest that instead of my "certainty," I should have allowed my natural "curiosity" about the reasons for her response to emerge. I should have made more of an effort to hear what she was trying to tell me. So why didn't I do that? Why did I withdraw emotionally?

The "Feelings" Conversation

I think the key is in my feelings about Yu, not in Jenny's anger. And that gets us to the "Feelings" conversation, which refers to the emotions that are welling up within us that we don't allow to come to the surface and be named. I am sure I felt very sad, not only for Yu but for Jenny and their children. I think I was also feeling guilty, inadequate, and helpless, and these emotions were contributing to my emotional disconnection from Yu and Jenny.

If, before our meeting, I had reflected on how I was feeling, I could have shared at least my sadness with them, rather than presenting a false cheerfulness. I am sure my body language was giving me away anyway, and the dissociation between what they could see and what I was saying must have contributed to their distrust.

Later, I could have shared my guilt, inadequacy, and helplessness with colleagues. I eventually did seek consolation from a wonderful third-year fellow after he told us of the success he was having with one of his patients. *"Your patients always seem to do so well,"* I said. *"I must be doing something terribly wrong with mine."* He laughed, put an arm around my shoulder, and said, *"Janet, I only talk about the ones who are doing well. There are plenty who don't."* He took me to the cafeteria for coffee, helped me explore my feelings, and gave me some strategies for coping with the emotions raised by the work we both did.

The "Identity" Conversation

I probably could have dealt with my feelings if they were all that was going on. But what shut me down was that Jenny's accusations echoed the doubts I was feeling about myself as a physician. As Stone and colleagues say, "'The Identity Conversation' looks inward: it's all about who we are and how we see ourselves.

How does what happened affect my self-esteem, my self-image, my sense of who I am in the world? What effect will it have on my future? What self-doubts do I harbor? In short: before, during, and after the difficult conversation, the Identity Conversation is about what I am saying to myself about me."

What happened to me, *Difficult Conversations* suggests, was that I lost my "balance." My sense of competence, trustworthiness, loyalty, and professionalism all were under attack. I reeled not from the blows inflicted by Yu's sadness or Jenny's anger, but from doubts of my own competence as an oncologist triggered by her anger and his despair. Unaware as I was of this disequilibrium, I shut down and used only my "executive functions" for the rest of the conversation, going through the motions, and reinforcing Yu and Jenny's sense of abandonment and betrayal. Had I recognized that I was losing my balance, I could have remained present intellectually and emotionally.

Most conversations I had with my patients were much less emotional, even when I had bad news to impart. A discussion of recurrent hypercalcemia, for example, would not have been a "difficult conversation." There is nothing about hypercalcemia that triggers feelings in me of sadness, inadequacy, helplessness, or guilt, and nothing that triggers questions about my competence as a physician. But as a first-year oncology fellow, I was susceptible to all those feelings being triggered in me by the dilemma Yu presented. And that is probably why I dreaded having the conversation in that hospital room.

Now, as a palliative care physician, I'm better at recognizing these loaded conversations ahead of time. I ask patients and their families how they interpret the facts I give them and explore how the case affects my own feelings and my sense of who I am. Now, before the encounter, I can prepare myself by talking over the facts and the feelings with colleagues.

The alternative, it seems to me, is simply to avoid the conversations that are just too painful. Or you might, unconsciously, strictly limit your emotional involvement with your patients. This lack of personal exploration into what makes a conversation difficult for you is likely to contribute to reluctance to share bad prognoses with patients who really need to know them. It is important to recognize how telling patients they have only weeks or months to live affects your emotional equilibrium, and you need to understand how it can challenge your identity as a clinician. Otherwise, the pain you experience at the thought of having these conversations may force you to abandon your patients when they need you most.

Difficult conversations, of course, have a similar effect on patients and their families, who, as we talk with them, also experience the "What Happened?," "Feelings," and "Identity" conversations from their vantage points. As we develop skills for recognizing these conversational triggers in ourselves, we will be able to recognize them in our patients as we guide them through tough times and to offer them more targeted support.

HOW TO BREAK BAD NEWS

Although we can become more skillful in breaking bad news, I don't want to suggest that even the most practiced delivery will diminish the effects on patients and their families; we should continue to anticipate strong emotional responses. As Stone and colleagues (2010, introduction) put it : "There is no such thing as a diplomatic hand grenade." Patients notice our body language, however, and delaying telling them is like "holding it after you've pulled the pin." Patients will notice our distress and may worry about the news, or worse, may worry that they have done something to anger or distress us.

Avoidance, therefore, is not a good strategy. But neither is what I call "truth dumping." I heard a terrible example of this one day as I walked to the cancer center cafeteria for lunch. A new oncology fellow was talking with one of his leukemia patients in the corridor leading to the cafeteria. She had come for blood counts and possibly a transfusion. The fellow knew the results of her recent bone marrow, however, and seeing her in the hallway, he felt compelled to tell her right there, in the entrance to the cafeteria, that her leukemia had relapsed. The poor patient was caught completely by surprise; she had not brought anyone with her because she hadn't expected to need any support. Not surprisingly, she looked shocked, and she burst into tears. That conversation is what I mean by "truth dumping": the fellow dumped his distress at "carrying" the knowledge of the relapse onto the defenseless patient, without thinking of the potential consequences. He hadn't yet been taught how to break bad news, and this was the unfortunate result.

What makes breaking bad news hard to do, in most cases, is how you fear the patients will feel—about the news or about you, especially if you feel at some level that you should have prevented it. But if you can come to accept that what has happened to them is really not your fault, and that your job is to help your patients through this horrible thing that is happening to them, you will be able to tell them and to sit with them in their grief afterward. If you are able to listen for ways you can help them cope with their new status, you will be having what Stone and colleagues call "a learning conversation." They advise, "You may find you no longer have a message to deliver, but rather some information to share and some questions to ask." And that can feel much better.

Remember that "bad news" may be in the eye of the beholder. Most clinicians would frame a new cancer diagnosis as bad news, but so too may be the development of a new metastasis, progression through chemotherapy, or complications like a blood clot or infection. While these scenarios may feel routine and expected to you, they pose an opportunity to use the techniques outlined in this chapter.

When you master the basic components of delivering bad news skillfully—and of these difficult conversations—your patients will not be the only ones to benefit; you will, too. You will start to work within an intellectual framework that allows you to be emotionally open but not vulnerable or unprotected even when you have to break "really bad" news. You will understand the feelings and reactions welling up within you, their origins, and their true meanings. In this book, we encourage clinicians to listen inward, so that we may connect outward. Most important, you will be much less likely to develop compassion fatigue, which commonly afflicts oncology and palliative care professionals. (We discuss how to identify, prevent, and treat burnout and compassion fatigue in Chapter 13.)

When I was a first-year fellow in hematology/oncology, long before I learned how to break bad news, or to have difficult conversations, I had another experience I will never forget: the first time I had to tell someone I'd just met that she had acute leukemia. I was called to the emergency room one evening to see Miss Etta Brown.

"I'm all right, dear. Are you?"

Miss Brown was a 56-year-old woman who presented with a two-week history of profound weakness and the onset that day of a rash. The laboratory called me to review her peripheral blood smear, and I agreed that it contained the blast cells typically seen in patients with acute leukemia. Her rash was petechial, and she had no other symptoms or remarkable physical findings; but analysis of her marrow aspirate confirmed that she had acute myelogenous leukemia.

I was severely shaken by the implications of her diagnosis. But I composed myself, put on what I thought was my most cheerful face, then went into her hospital room and sat on her bed. I took her hand in mine and in my most encouraging manner said, *"I'm sorry, but your bone marrow test shows that you have a cancer in your bloodstream; we call it acute leukemia. It is causing your rash and your weakness. We have good treatment for it, though, and there is every chance you will go into a remission."*

My face must have belied my words, however, because she replied, with evident concern, *"I'm all right, dear. Are you?"*

Miss Brown had been sick for some time, she later told me. She was frightened because she could no longer walk to church without becoming weak and short of breath. When the rash appeared, she was certain she was about to die, but she did not share her fear with me until *after* I had told her about the leukemia. My news actually came as a reprieve from an immediate death sentence, and she was greatly relieved. She now understood what was wrong and could prepare herself to fight it. She felt better that night, she said, than she had felt in a long time.

The reverse situation is probably more common—and more distressing. Mr. Alessio, for example, was a patient who had been admitted for pneumonia. I was called to consult when the team discovered that the infection was caused by an obstructing lung cancer. The reaction I got when I told him of his cancer was disbelief, denial, and intense anger. You may recognize, though, that Mr. Alessio was expressing two of the earliest emotions associated with grief as described by Dr. Elizabeth Kübler Ross in her 1969 classic, *On Death and Dying* (the five emotions are denial, anger, bargaining, depression, and acceptance). The reactions patients have to bad news are, I believe, expressions of their grief, and if we recognize them as such, we'll be better prepared to respond to them.

At the time, I ascribed the difference in the two responses to the personalities of the patients. But subsequently, I found a more likely explanation in the book *How to Break Bad News: A Guide for Health Care Professionals,* by Dr. Robert Buckman, a medical oncologist (Buckman 1992). As he states, "The reactions of patients often depend on the gap between their expectations and what the physicians tell them." Miss Brown's expectations were, if anything, worse than the news I had given her, and she expressed relief. For Mr. Alessio, however, the gap was enormous, and his reaction was commensurate with his shock.

How to Break Bad News, as the title suggests, describes how to convey distressing information to patients and how to cope with their reactions. It delineates the principles that underlie these discussions and includes a step-by-step procedure to ensure that all important elements are detailed.

Dr. Buckman relates that he wrote the book after witnessing the following exchange (which I continue to hope is apocryphal). A urologist stood at the door of a hospital room, talking to two of his patients within. He said that both men could be discharged that day and that the results of their prostate biopsies were available. He told one man that his biopsy showed only inflammation. He then informed the other that his biopsy had shown cancer and suggested that he make an appointment to talk with him about it later that week. Then he left.

I cannot remember ever being quite that callous, but I am sure that there were times when I did not plan the encounter carefully enough to minimize the effects of my news on the patient or his family.

Practice Points: Breaking Bad News

- Make yourself, the patient, and the family comfortable.
- Find out what they know.
- Find out what they want to know.
- Tell them in words they can understand, and in small chunks.
- Appreciate the role of silence.
- Respond to their feelings. Ask how you can help *now.*
- Ask them to summarize what you told them; ask whether they have further questions.
- Tell them the plan; let them know you expect further discussions as time goes on.
- Express your continued support: "I'm here for you."

Assemble the Team

How should we deliver bad news, and whom should we bring to the encounter with us? Suppose the roles were reversed: you just had a colon polyp removed. How would you want to get the pathology report? On the phone? In the office? Who would you want to have there with you? A family member? A trusted friend? Or, let's say you've just had restaging scans after a course of chemotherapy for ovarian cancer. Would you like the infusion nurse who has been giving your chemotherapy to be there when the physician tells you the results? The social worker who has been counseling you and your spouse or partner? Each of us is likely to answer in a different way.

That is why it is so important to be sure the patient has a chance to think about this before the meeting takes place. With a little planning time, patients can usually arrange to have the right people with them. Whenever you or your colleagues schedule tests, you can ask patients to have someone with them in person or online (e.g., in a Zoom meeting) when they learn the results, so that when those results are problematic, patients will have the support they need. If you know the test results are bad, you can ask trusted colleagues to free up time to be there when you meet with the family, both to support you and to counsel the family.

In the inpatient setting, a social worker or other clinician caring for the patient can schedule a meeting at a time convenient for everyone who needs to be there in person or virtually, and to include whomever has been closely involved in the patient's care (e.g., the primary nurse, the chaplain). The person who schedules the meeting should also find a room in which everyone can be seated comfortably, rather than allowing the family and the rest of the team to stand while you and the patient are seated.

For the conversation itself, Dr. Buckman's book contains several useful, often common-sense suggestions, which we review in the sections that follow.*

Make Yourself, the Patient, and the Family Comfortable

With the team, the patient, and the family waiting for you at the meeting place, take a moment before you enter. Rehearse to yourself what you are about to say; try to dispel any feelings of guilt (which are almost always unwarranted), take a deep breath or two, and bring your full focus onto how you can be of most help to this patient and her family. Silence your phone and pager and align the computer screen so that the patient can see and hear those virtually present.

As you begin your encounter, use body language that indicates you have all the time in the world. This I learned from my brother, a gastroenterologist in private practice and a busy guy. When accompanying him on follow-up visits in the

---

*Adapted from Buckman 1992.

hospital, I noticed that he stretched out in a chair near the patient's bed or chair, looking as if he were camped out for the afternoon. He asked the questions he needed to ask, including open-ended ones, let the patients ask all they wanted, examined them, and then left. None of the encounters took more than about ten minutes, but as we left, the patients seemed satisfied with the time my brother had spent with them.

Cancer patients also prefer their clinicians to be sitting when they break bad news. In a randomized controlled trial using a video of a physician who was either standing or sitting while breaking bad news, patients (from a predominantly white U.S. population) considered physicians who were seated to be more compassionate (Bruera et al. 2007).

Find Out What They Know

After you and the family are comfortably settled, and all virtual participants are present, with a box of tissues close by, explore what the patient understands about what is wrong. You may know what the patient has been told by the house staff or by the surgeon who did the operation, but you need to determine what the patient remembers from those discussions and whether he understands the implications. You might say, *"The results of your tests finally came back, and I thought I would let you know what they are and what we're going to do about them. Of course, I will be answering any questions you have. But before I begin, it would help me to know what you already know and what you think is wrong with you."*

Someone has usually told the patient that he has cancer and has explained its type, stage, and location before you, the oncology or palliative care clinician, are asked to see him. Some of these patients, when asked what they think is wrong with them, repeat what they have been told, word for word. They also seem to understand the implications of their diagnosis. Others, given the same information by their own clinicians, have said, *"They told me I have a tumor. You don't think that could be cancer, do you?"* This patient either hasn't understood what he was told (and was too embarrassed to admit this to his clinician) or finds the implications too overwhelming. He may be in a state of denial, unable to accept that he could possibly have cancer. The discussion you have with him will be very different from the one you can have with the first type of patient. For this second type, ask what he thinks a tumor is and what it means to him to have cancer. Follow his lead and try to correct any misconceptions that he reveals. But make it clear that he does have cancer and that you will be there to help him.

I sometimes observe colleagues begin meetings such as these with their explanation of what is occurring medically, rather than allowing patients and their families to share their own understanding. By speaking first instead of listening, we may impose our own agenda. This approach is also less efficient than homing in on what the patient understands, meeting patients where they are, and moving forward together from there. When we hear the words used by our patients, we can later echo these with our own words, to make sure we match their level of understanding. Finally, by giving our patients space to share first, we send a powerful message that we are here to listen.

Find Out What They Want to Know

Dr. Buckman counsels that we should next find out how patients want us to deliver the news and what they want to know. Dr. Diane Meier, FACP, FAAHPM, professor of geriatrics and palliative medicine at the Icahn School of Medicine and Mount Sinai Hospital in New York City, founder and former director of the Center to Advance Palliative Care, suggests we try the following: *"In my experience, I have found that some patients want to know all the details each time I speak with them, while others would rather I described the big picture, leaving them free to ask for more details when they felt they needed them. In general, which would you prefer?"*

Next, having some idea of how broad or fine the strokes should be, find out more about the picture you've been commissioned to paint. Miss Brown, for example, asked me how long she had to live. This sounds like a fairly straightforward question—but so, on the face of it, does a child's question, *"Where do I come from?"* Many parents have responded to this by launching into a discussion of the birds and the bees, only to be met with perplexed looks and the complaint, *"I have to do a report for school on the city I come from. I just need to know if we come from Boston or San Francisco."*

Miss Brown, it turned out, had tickets for a cruise in three months, and she wanted to know whether she was likely to be able to go on that cruise. She did not want to discuss her ultimate outcome. To approach patients' or family members' questions, therefore, ask them to be a little more specific about what they want to know and why they want to know it. You're more likely, that way, to know what question to answer.

Tell Them in Words They Can Understand, and in Small Chunks

Once you have a handle on the question, the next steps are similar to those you would use in any routine form of patient education. If you were explaining a chemotherapy regimen, a colonoscopy, or the fact that someone has an ulcer and needs to take certain medications, you would use words patients could understand and, when appropriate, visual aids.

When you are breaking bad news, however, you need to divide the information into smaller chunks. After the news sinks in that a person has cancer, she is unlikely to remember much else from that first talk. Some oncologists even advise letting patients record that first meeting on their phones, so that they can listen to it later, at their leisure.

HOW TO DEAL WITH THE RESPONSE

The Role of Silence

At this point after you have delivered serious news, stop talking for at least 10 to 20 seconds. (To experience how long that is, slowly count to 20 silently. I think you'll find it takes much longer than you expect it to!) Both the quality of this silence and how you feel during it can vary. For those of you accustomed to silence from your own contemplative practice, you might be interested in enhancing the quality of this time with your patients by learning more about what Dr. Anthony (Tony) Back and his coauthors, all expert spiritual care practitioners, call "compassionate silence" (Back, Bauer-Wu, et al. 2009).

These skilled practitioners use this time in a special way, but for most practitioners, the first minute between when they deliver the news and when the patient or a family member says something can seem endless. As you sit there, if you are lightly touching the patient's hand or arm, be alert to a withdrawal of the limb, since contact may not be welcome then. But your silent presence is very important.

Patients who have just heard bad news are numb and shocked. It can take 30 to 40 seconds for the information to sink in, for patients to replay internally what you've just said and then to voice a thought or a feeling. The longer you let the silence last, the greater the chance that they will have the time they need to process what you've told them.

While you wait for their response, take a moment to assess how you are feeling. If you feel anxious, relax, breathe *mindfully* (i.e., paying attention to each breath, as we discuss in Chapter 8), and check in visually for support from any of the colleagues you brought with you to the meeting.

Since you cannot control your patients' reactions, use the time instead to prepare yourself for their response, the next step in this "difficult conversation," which will often be some expression of grief as discussed above. I use these moments to think of myself as an open vessel, ready to receive whatever arrives next. You have delivered your version of the facts, but prepare to be open to questions from the patient or family, who may have interpreted the same signs and symptoms and even radiology reports very differently from the way you interpreted them. Remind yourself to be curious and to try your best to be sure you ask enough questions so that you understand how they see things. Find out what they know that you don't, instead of assuming you know all you need to know. That will help you to guide them to the reality that you and your team see and will help them move forward in the conversation.

Respond to Their Feelings

As I mentioned above, patients' reactions are likely to reflect the difference between their expectations and what they have just heard. Those who have been very ill or in pain yet have been told there is nothing wrong with them may, like Miss Brown, express relief that the source of their suffering has been identified. It is, naturally, much harder for those who have had no hint about the cancer.

Their first response may be verbal or nonverbal. Some reply with disbelief: *"You must be mistaken. The tests must have been mixed up in the lab. I feel fine. There can't be anything wrong with me."* Others may look up at you in great pain, may cry, or may be totally silent. To the mute-stricken patient, rather than ask, *"How can we help?"* you might say, *"What do you need us to do* right now?" which calls for a more limited response. A patient might reply, *"Schedule the next tests you have to do as soon as possible. I can't wait much longer to find out how far this thing has spread."* Or, *"Call my husband. He said he wanted to come with me, but I was so sure everything would be fine, I told him not to bother."*

When the patient or family member is angry, wait out the storm. Families may express their anger at other clinicians who have "missed the diagnosis," even if it was not apparent at the time of that consultation. Patients can be angry at you, or angry at their families for making them come to the doctor, or at God for allowing this to happen. If they are angry at you, use part of your consciousness to monitor your emotional response to their accusations. You'll be better able to guard against feelings of defensiveness if you have learned to recognize your own personal warning signs that you are in danger of losing your balance. In my case, I learned that I feel a tightness in my chest and dissociation from the situation. It's as though I'm there but not there. Now, when I sense that happening, I slow down or ask my colleagues in the meeting to contribute their thoughts so I can regroup.

Try to determine if the patient or the family member who is yelling at you might be doing that because they have lost their balance—if what you just told them caused such intense feelings or threatened aspects of their identity so profoundly that they cannot hold themselves together. Try to keep the perspective that this really isn't about you or your actions, but is usually about the situation. If you suspect the problem is with the other person's feelings or identity, you don't need to ask about that directly; just give him time and space, and he may find the way to get back to his best self.

Your team members or palliative care consultants may be crucial if either you or the patient and family are overwhelmed by feelings or unbalanced by a threat to identity. When a young patient, Abigail, tearfully pleaded with her oncologist, *"You* can't *give up on me!"* the oncologist was struck dumb. We, as palliative care consultants, were able to help by assuring the patient that he would never give up, but that the burden of further treatment was so great that it was likely to shorten Abigail's life rather than buy the extra time she was asking him for. Her anger turned to a flood of tears, and we all supported them; the physician found his voice and was able to help Abigail and her family move forward.

Some patients bargain with you, and others turn the anger inward and become depressed. They may not seem angry right after you tell them the news, but at later visits they may appear depressed or withdrawn. Some are blaming themselves for sins of omission or commission that they feel caused the cancer or delayed its diagnosis.

Have tissues within reach for the tearful patient and try to offer some form of nonverbal support, such as putting a hand on the patient's arm or shoulder. Speak reassuringly, making no attempt to stop the initial flow of tears, and by making no effort to leave, indicate your willingness to be present no matter how emotional the patient becomes. The tears usually subside quickly, and you'll find you have established trust and a personal bond that will be helpful in the months or years to come.

To provide what Dr. Buckman would call an "empathic response," first identify the emotion, then ask questions that help identify its source, and then respond with nonverbal actions, statements, and further questions that convey your care and curiosity about their experience. Back, Arnold, and Tulsky's NURSE mnemonic, widely taught in palliative care, is a helpful guide here. Our job is not to "fix" or resolve others' painful emotions, but to demonstrate that we can be present with them and that we care.

Jason, a patient with prostate cancer, seemed to be blaming himself for developing the cancer. I said to him, *"I can really feel how angry you are. Why do you think you became ill?"* He responded, *"Well, I smoked, didn't I? And everyone knows that smoking causes cancer."* I was tempted to correct Jason's misconception right away and to reassure him. But if I contradicted him, our conversation would have ended prematurely. Instead, I pursued the questioning, so that I could learn about all his sources of concern: *"And what else do you think contributed to your illness?"*

I did not know what he was going to say. He might tell me he hadn't gone to the doctor for years despite his wife's multiple urgings that he do so. He might report lapses in attendance at church services, failure to eat right, drinking too much alcohol—the list could go on and on. You never know what you're going to hear. As I listened expectantly, Jason said that he had been having an affair and was furious with himself for being unfaithful to his wife, and that his cancer was a just punishment. He finished with, *"I guess that's about it."*

I was totally floored! But I replied, *"As I understand it, you're angry at yourself, and you're angry both because you feel your smoking caused your cancer and because you had an affair, for which you feel you deserve to be punished by getting prostate cancer. Is that right?"* I settled down, as did he. I felt I could now correct his misunderstanding about the relationship between smoking and prostate cancer. But I could also, if I had the time and the comfort level to do so, begin exploring with Jason issues of forgiveness and punishment. If not, I could express my sincere concern for his pain and explore whether he might seek help from a spiritual counselor.

Practice Points for Responding to Emotions: NURSE

- NAME
  - Recognize and name the emotion(s).
  - *Example*: "This must be so shocking to hear."
- UNDERSTAND
  - Acknowledge their emotions and restate your understanding of what you've heard, or you might say, "I cannot imagine," to relay that you can see but not experience the depth of their experience.
  - *Example*: "I can imagine feeling so angry if I were in this situation."
- RESPECT
  - Use words of praise and convey that you respect the patient through your words and nonverbal actions.
  - *Example*: "I am so impressed with the way you have supported your family through all of this."
- SUPPORT
  - Convey a commitment of ongoing support and concern.
  - *Example*: "I may not be able to make this tumor go away, but I will be here for you no matter what."
- EXPLORE
  - Ask additional questions to explore further what they may be feeling.
  - *Example*: "Can you say more about what frightens you most in all this?"

(Adapted from Back, Arnold, et al. 2009)

Tell Them the Plan

Once patients have assimilated both the news and its implications for them (ideally moving on to "acceptance"), had time to react, shared their underlying concerns, and had the opportunity to ask any remaining questions, you can move on to the plan, which usually includes further testing, referrals, a therapeutic regimen (radiation, chemo, hormonal, immune, or targeted therapies) that also addresses sources of distress, or a plan to provide supportive care focused solely on ameliorating their distress if the burdens of therapy outweigh the benefits. Having a plan and a way forward can help lift patients out of despair.

Reassure patients that this is only the first of many discussions, and that your whole team will continue to answer their questions and provide or arrange for the support and counseling they or their family need. I often suggest that patients record all their questions in a notebook or smartphone so that they won't forget to ask them at the next visit. I encourage them to include questions from family or friends who were not at the meeting but who are likely to raise additional concerns.

If patients are unable to shift from the emotional reaction to a problem-focused discussion of the plan, if they get stuck in denial, anger, or bargaining, then you or a colleague who is a mental health professional (e.g., a social worker, psychologist, or psychiatrist) may need to spend more time providing psychological support; see Chapter 9 for further discussion.

Ask Them to Summarize What You Told Them; Ask Whether They Have Further Questions

To bring this meeting to a close, you might say, *"I know we have gone over a lot of ground today. Since I may have used some technical terms that were unclear, it would help me if you would summarize for me what we've discussed."* Patients' answers, like their answers to the first questions about what they knew about their disease, will provide you with important information for your next visit. Despite your best efforts, you will find that some people are still unclear whether they even have cancer!

Most patients understand at least their diagnosis and the need for further tests. Remind them that you are available to answer their questions and those of their family or friends and that you will be talking again later, as new information appears.

While breaking bad news may seem to require a longer session, it usually takes no more than 15 to 20 minutes, though it's good to plan for a 30-minute session. You can use the extra time to debrief with your nurse or social worker, review how they thought it went, and make plans for the next time you see the patient.

Illness as a Threat to Personhood

Although these early conversations in which you discuss serious news may be a routine part of your work, it is important to maintain the perspective that for many patients and their families, you are usually discussing a major turning point in their lives. Keeping this perspective and providing them with support early and often will help you build and sustain rapport and trust.

Cancer can rob some patients and their loved ones of that which they hold most dear: independence, bodily integrity, faith in a fair and just world, relationships, and their core identities. But cancer can also be an impetus to strengthen relationships, find meaning, and provide perspective on what is most important as mortality looms and time becomes more precious. Our job is to listen closely to our patients and meet them where they are. At times we may be "just" a companion and cheerleader as patients and families travel their own journey. At others we may need to draw on a team to help support and guide our patients as their personhood is threatened.

Dr. Eric Cassell described as *suffering* the distress that occurs when the integrity of a person is threatened (Cassell 1999). The relief of suffering is one of the central goals of medicine, and of palliative care in particular. We must be attuned to the experience of illness as more than the biological sum of a patient's medical problems. In his 1999 paper, Dr. Cassell writes:

> Suffering involves some symptom or process that threatens the patient because of fear, the meaning of the symptom, and concerns about the future. The meanings and the fear are personal and individual, so that even if two patients have the same symptoms, their suffering would be different. The complex techniques and methods that physicians usually use to make a diagnosis, however, are aimed at the body rather than the person. The diagnosis of suffering is therefore often missed, even in severe illness and even when it stares physicians in the face. A high index of suspicion must be maintained in the presence of serious disease, and patients must be directly questioned. Concerns over the discomfort of listening to patients' severe distress are usually more than offset by the gratification that follows the intervention. Often, questioning and attentive listening, which take little time, are in themselves ameliorative. (p. 531)

We begin to address suffering when we create space to get to know our patients as individuals beyond their disease and ask questions about how their illness is affecting them. *"How has your illness affected you? What has been the worst part in all of this? What are you no longer able to do?"* Our most powerful tool is to listen attentively, "even when," as Dr. Cassell writes, "the cause of the suffering cannot be removed."

Assess and Strengthen Coping Strategies

We can also reflect back what we hear to dive deeper and try to identify patient strengths and coping strategies. *"I hear clearly that you have always been 'the mom,' and how hard it has been that your cancer has made it difficult to take care of your family. How have you and your kids dealt with this?"* We all use coping strategies to try to regain a sense of control when things feel out of control. Coping is the actions, behaviors, and thoughts we use to manage stress or a threat. There is a deeper discussion of coping in Chapter 9, but here we want to emphasize the importance of assessing and addressing coping early and often.

At early visits I ask, *"How have you coped with difficult times in the past?"* and I ask patients and their caregivers regularly at follow-up visits, *"How are you coping with everything?"* This allows us to identify collaboratively a range of coping strategies, describe and name them for patients who may not be able to see their own strengths, and relay these to the entire team. People may use a variety of coping styles, and certain strategies may work well at some phases of illness but not at others. Our work is to identify and support strengths and help patients reorient to more helpful active coping strategies instead of less helpful, avoidant or self-harming ones. Indeed, there is evidence that early palliative care improves patients' use of active coping strategies (like acceptance and positive reframing), which in turn correlates with better quality of life and mood. Use of denial and self-blame is associated with worse quality of life and mood (Greer et al. 2018; Nipp et al. 2016; Nipp et al. 2017). Patients who lack effective coping strategies may need additional help from social workers, psychologists, psychiatrists, or spiritual counselors.

ADVANCE CARE PLANNING AND PREPARING FOR THE FUTURE

Advance care planning is the process of exploring values and goals to prepare patients for future medical decisions so that they receive care that is consistent with their preferences (Sudore, Lum, et al. 2017). Since fears about the future drive some of the distress and suffering of patients and loved ones, discussions about planning for the future may help alleviate them. Unfortunately, there is a huge chasm between the reality of practice and an ideal in which all patients facing serious illness are supported in advance care planning (Wright et al. 2008).

In this next section, we discuss some of the reasons that clinicians may be reluctant to initiate advance care planning discussions, provide approaches to beginning these conversations early, and provide guidance on creating advance care plans with patients and families. In Chapter 5, we explore patient-related barriers to discussing advance care planning. The communication strategies we discuss below include assessing patients' understanding of their illness, creating a shared model of what the future may hold, eliciting values and goals, and recommending medical care to match patients' preferences.

Ongoing discussions using this framework will help your patients and their families tell you how to provide them with patient-centered care throughout their illness. These conversations are especially important in the final stages, but even in the early days, we can help patients make important choices when cancer and its therapies limit energy and function. When patients and their families practice thinking about the future with you, they will begin to feel prepared along the way.

Why Advance Care Planning Is So Important yet So Difficult for Many Clinicians

Despite the importance of advance care planning, such discussions are by no means routine, either with people beginning intensive chemotherapy or even with those having far-advanced cancer. While there are more data on completion of written advance directives (an easier outcome to measure), the paucity of advance care planning discussions is striking (Brinkman-Stoppelenburg, Rietjens, and van der Heide 2014). A multisite prospective study of patients with advanced cancer and their caregivers found that only 37 percent of these patients reported having an end-of-life discussion at baseline. This study also showed the "cascade" of benefits for those who had these discussions, including less aggressive medical care in the final week of life and earlier hospice enrollment. Those caregivers whose loved ones had less aggressive medical care in turn had lower risk of depression and of experiencing regret (Wright et al. 2008).

Other studies confirm the reluctance to engage in *and* the benefits of advance care planning for cancer patients. When given a vignette that described meeting a new patient who had cancer that carried a four- to six-month prognosis even with treatment, one study found that only 30 percent of oncologists would discuss DNR status with that patient. About 20 percent said that they would discuss DNR only if the patient developed symptoms, and 10 percent would wait until there were no nonpalliative treatments left (Keating et al. 2010). The findings of a large cohort study of more than 2,000 patients with stage IV lung or colorectal cancer showed that while three-quarters of the patients discussed end-of-life care with their oncologists, this discussion happened a median of only one month before they died, usually during a hospitalization. Replicating Wright et al. (2008), those who had these discussions with their physicians were less likely to receive aggressive care and more likely to use hospice services than patients who hadn't had those discussions (Mack, Cronin, Keating, et al. 2012).

You can enhance the chance that your patients will receive care that is in concert with their wishes, whether that be care focused on life prolongation or comfort, if you discuss their hopes, fears, goals, values, and wishes regarding care as illness progresses (Brinkman-Stoppelenburg, Rietjens, and van der Heide 2014; Haines et al. 2019; Mack et al. 2010). If you don't ask them, you may err on the side of providing unwanted, aggressive end-of-life care.

Though I (*Janet Abrahm*) am now more comfortable with discussions about advance care plans, initially I had these discussions only to avoid being in the position of having an intubated patient look up at me accusingly and write on his whiteboard, "*I never wanted to live like this. You told me about the other side effects of the chemotherapy, but you left this one out. Why didn't you ever ask me what I wanted?*"

Luckily, that never actually happened to me. But the question remains: why is it so hard to bring up the subject? What feelings do these difficult conversations evoke? What effect do they have on our sense of self? According to the literature, this reluctance to discuss advance care planning has many components, as discussed in the sections that follow.

> ### Why Are Clinicians Reluctant to Initiate Advance Care Planning Discussions?
>
> - Clinicians are forced to face their own feelings about mortality.
> - Clinicians are loath to cause pain.
> - Clinicians feel guilty or are afraid of being blamed.
> - Clinicians assume they don't need to ask: they know their patients' wishes.
> - Clinicians feel impotent to prevent death and have not grieved their losses. They have unrecognized compassion fatigue.
> - Clinicians are not adequately trained to have these discussions.

Clinicians Are Forced to Face Their Own Feelings about Mortality

Discussions about advance care planning force us to ask ourselves how *we* would answer these questions, and many of us are not ready to face our own mortality. In my own case, I did not complete an advance directive or a document naming my health care proxy until I was in my forties. What prompted me was the combination of frequent travels from Philadelphia to New York City, the perils of the New Jersey Turnpike, and the New York law requiring clear, written documentation of my wishes should I become incapacitated. Since making my own arrangements, however, I noticed that, even when I still practiced as an oncologist, discussing advance care plans with my patients was easier than it had been before.

Clinicians Are Loath to Cause Pain

Clinicians are loath to cause pain, and discussions of mortality are sometimes awkward and, at the worst, terrifying for patients and their families. The stress on the patient and on me, even in my palliative care role, is something for which I still have to brace myself, every time. I can often see the emotional impact of these discussions reflected in pained faces, tears, or resistance. But we should expect emotional reactions to these conversations. We can respond and acknowledge these emotions; they are not a reason to avoid the discussions.

Clinicians Feel Guilty or Are Afraid of Being Blamed

By raising the possibility that a patient might die, you place yourself in what seem to be two contradictory positions—on the one hand, assuring patients that you will try to make them well, and on the other, reminding them that they are, after all, mortal. Patients who don't want to hear this may blame you for their vulnerability to death, and their anger at their disease may be transferred to you as the bearer of bad news. This fear of blame is one of the major impediments, Dr. Buckman says, to clinicians' discussing advance care plans with their patients.

Even when patients don't blame you, you may feel guilty, that it is your fault they are at risk of dying. I would wager that many physicians share with me an experience I had when I entered medical school: we were told that one in three of us would cause someone to come to harm because we had not worked hard enough in medical school and didn't know enough. Our errors of commission or omission might even kill someone. It is not surprising, then, that we are reluctant to bring up the subject of death.

Dr. Jerome Groopman, who cared for many patients dying of AIDS and cancer, states in his book *The Measure of Our Days* a sentiment I fear is shared by many clinicians: "Although I knew that Matt was going to die, that everything had been done for him that could be done, *I still felt a deep sense of failure, of guilt* [italics mine]. We, his doctors, had failed Matt, unable to save his young life" (Groopman 1997, p. 110). Daniel Callahan, who was a bioethicist and cofounder of the Hastings Center for Medical Ethics, explained that, as physicians, we suffer from a delusion: that advances in medical technology will indefinitely postpone death. Any death, in that context, must be one for which we must accept the blame and the guilt (Callahan 1993).

I see this manifest in some trainees—all of them intelligent and compassionate— who suppress their feelings of failure by reducing very sick patients to a list of problems affecting every organ system rather than seeing the suffering human beings under their care. Medicine has taught them to be reductionists, impaired their ability to see the big picture, and made them miss the forest for the trees. If they were taught how to cope with those feelings, they could help their patients and their patients' families to grieve and heal.

Clinicians Assume They Don't Need to Ask; They Know Their Patients' Wishes

Some practitioners may feel the discussion is unnecessary, that they know their patients well enough to be able to act on their wishes or to know the right thing to do on their behalf without ever directly asking them. Studies have indicated, however, that this assumption is incorrect (Downey et al. 2013). Physicians and families could not predict patients' wishes about treatments that would prolong life. Doctors chose for the patient what they would want for themselves, not what the patients, in separate questioning, said they preferred.

Clinicians Feel Impotent to Prevent Death and Have Not Grieved Their Losses

Advance care planning discussions may make clinicians feel impotent; we are admitting that at some point, there will be nothing more we can do to prolong the patient's life. During my first week as an intern, as I vividly recall, I encountered a physician who felt just this way. During sign-out rounds, the resident explained to us that one of the patients was expected to die. If that happened, the intern was to call and inform the family. When the resident left, I heard my colleague, who was on call that night, mutter to himself, *"No one is going to die on my shift!"* And no one did; he kept the patient alive until the next morning, when he would no longer be "responsible."

In my experience, most patients want to be cared for by someone who is knowledgeable, experienced, and confident, but who can also be approached with questions and fears. They want clinicians who know their own and medicine's limitations.

In fact, many patients are disturbed by the knowledge that, in this technological age, they can be kept alive in ways that are not acceptable to them. This knowledge was one of the underlying motivations for the hospice movement and now for legalizing medically aided death, which we discuss in Chapter 11. It is unlikely, then, that patients will lose faith in us or in medicine simply because we ask them to state their preferences for care if they face tradeoffs as disease advances.

Clinicians Have Unrecognized Compassion Fatigue

For some of us, the problem may be unrecognized compassion fatigue or burnout. Compassion fatigue is the detachment and depersonalization that develops in therapists and others who care for people who have experienced extreme suffering (Figley 1995). Clinicians suffering from compassion fatigue may have difficulty bearing the additional pain that always accompanies a discussion of goals of care with a patient who is no longer responding to therapy. In Chapter 13, we discuss the factors that cause oncology and palliative care clinicians, among others, to be susceptible to compassion fatigue and offer strategies for preventing and overcoming it.

Clinicians Are Not Adequately Trained to Have These Discussions

Although evidence-based serious illness communication techniques can improve clinicians' behavior and patient outcomes, "the majority of clinicians now in practice learned to communicate on the job, without a curriculum, explicit role modeling, or learning techniques backed by evidence" (Back, Fromme, and Meier 2019, p. S436). In recognition that most clinicians lack sufficient training in this domain, there is now a national effort to improve and disseminate effective communication training in conducting serious illness conversations (Back, Fromme, and Meier 2019; Gilligan et al. 2017; Institute of Medicine 2014).

WHEN TO INITIATE AN ADVANCE CARE PLANNING DISCUSSION AND WHAT TO SAY

Although you may be ready to have these discussions, when is the best time? And what should you say?

I think of these conversations as occurring on a continuum, and I try to match what we discuss to where the patient is in the trajectory of the cancer course. If my patient is not in a crisis, I focus on getting to know her as an individual. I am curious to hear about the important people in her life; the activities that give her joy, meaning, and purpose; and the narratives she has created about her life and illness that help her make sense of it all.

I use this information as I make choices about treatment recommendations going forward. For instance, a professional violinist may not want to take the risk of developing severe peripheral neuropathy even though a chemotherapy likely to induce that offers the best chance of preventing her cancer from recurring. That side effect is something we'd have to discuss in detail, along with the implications for her if she doesn't include it in her adjuvant therapy. Having built rapport and trust as I demonstrate my care of each patient as a unique individual, it becomes much easier to delve into more challenging conversations about the future when I need to do that.

Medical Power of Attorney / Health Care Proxy

It is appropriate to ask all your patients whether they have an advance directive and whom they want to make medical decisions on their behalf if at any time they're not able to make decisions for themselves. The terminology for this can be confusing. The named person is their health care proxy, agent, or surrogate, and the form used to designate this individual is variably known as a health care proxy/agent/surrogate, durable power of attorney for health care, or medical power of attorney. For consistency we use the term *health care proxy* to designate both this individual and the legal form, but you should use the correct terminology for the state in which your patients live and receive medical care.

Many of your patients will have already thought about this, and some will have already documented their wishes. A recent systematic review found that 37 percent of U.S. adults had completed an advance directive (Yadav et al. 2017).

You might begin the conversation with something like the following:

> *I am very hopeful that you will tolerate your treatment well and that it will be very effective against your cancer. But we both know there can be bumps along the way, that infections or other serious side effects could occur. If they do, and you become very sick and can't speak for yourself, I need to know who you'd like to speak for you, so that your wishes are respected. Have you thought about who you would like to have in that role? . . . We recommend that everyone choose a person they would trust to make decisions for them if it came to that, and to complete a form that lets all their caregivers know who that person is. This is called a "durable power of attorney for health care," or a "health care proxy." . . . If you'd like, I can help you talk to whoever you choose to be your health care proxy. It is important that they hear what an acceptable quality of life looks like to you. Giving your health care proxy this information will be a real gift to them.*

Indeed, research shows that the health care proxy and family are likely to have less distress and feel less burdened if they clearly know the patient's wishes (Wendler and Rid 2011).

Documentation of a health care proxy is particularly critical for some more than others. Legislation in most states outlines who can make decisions in the absence of formal written designation. This is called "next of kin" in many states and typically begins with a patient's spouse, if they have one. As an example of possible complexity, in my (*Molly Collins's*) state of Pennsylvania, if the patient lost capacity before assigning a health care proxy, their spouse would have to share medical decision-making power with the patient's adult children from a different relationship.* Many patients may want to choose a health care proxy other than their next of kin; some avoid potential conflict by designating the one individual they would trust most to act in their own interests using "substituted judgment." A health care proxy that is valid in the patient's state prevents someone else from challenging the patient's choice.

Prior to federal legalization of same-sex marriage through the Supreme Court's 2015 decision in *Obergefell v. Hodges*, documentation of the chosen health care proxy was particularly important for unwed same-sex partners (Acquaviva 2017; Stevens and Abrahm 2019). Providers should seek to identify patients' "chosen family," who may be different from their family of origin (Acquaviva 2017). Indeed, any unmarried partner may not have legal standing to make health care decisions for a partner without designation as the health care proxy. Such documentation is only one of the unique issues seriously ill LGBTQ+ patients may face. We discuss these further in Chapters 4, 11, and 13.

If you normalize this discussion about choosing a health care proxy and explain why you think it is important, I think you will find that this is often "emotionally safe" territory. You are still speaking about a hypothetical time in the future, which helps to make this part of the conversation less threatening. People can usually relate to the importance of choosing someone to speak for them if they cannot make decisions for themselves, and most people can easily decide whom they would want to serve in this role.

Serious Illness Conversation Guide

If when you first meet your patient, they have advanced disease, and you think they are at risk of dying or of having a serious complication soon from the cancer or its treatment, you need to learn more about their wishes than whom they have chosen as their health care proxy. There is no single proven best way to approach these conversations. In a review of 113 advance care planning studies, only 6 were randomized clinical trials, and only 1 looked specifically at cancer patients (Brinkman-Stoppelenburg, Rietjens, and van der Heide 2014). Several

---

*Act of Nov. 29, 2006, P. L. 1484, no. 169, Pennsylvania, https://www.legis.state.pa.us/cfdocs/Legis/LI/uconsCheck.cfm?txtType=HTM&yr=2006&sessInd=0&smthLwInd=0&act=169.

established communication training programs are available, including interactive workshops, classroom presentations, and online tools and modules (Back, Fromme, and Meier 2019). Indeed, we hope our book inspires you to seek further communication training and practice these skills intentionally so that you will have the flexibility you need to deal with the variety of situations with which you're likely to be presented.

To get you started, we will use the case of Jade Markman to demonstrate how to use the Serious Illness Conversation Guide (SICG) (Bernacki and Block 2014; Bernacki et al. 2019; Paladino et al. 2019), one of the free, well-studied communication tools that provides you with specific language for these discussions (Figure 1.1).

Jade Markman was a 30-year-old mother of two with initial stage III triple-negative breast cancer whom I (*Molly Collins*) had been caring for while she underwent a rigorous course of curative-intent surgery, chemotherapy, and radiation. A few months after completing her final chemotherapy, however, she was found to have lung metastases. Jade had to shift from thinking of herself as a survivor to the reality that she would die of her illness and might not even live to watch her children grow up.

Jade was a woman of great faith who hoped that through modern medicine, she would outlive her oncologist's prediction that her prognosis was only a year or two. Even as she developed brain metastases and leptomeningeal disease, she was always clear that she wanted to live as long as possible and have every possible treatment that could help her achieve this. Privately, I worried with her oncologist and social worker that what we knew so far of Jade's wishes could lead to medically aggressive, potentially futile care when the end finally arrived. I envisioned her intubated in the ICU, surrounded by family asking us to prolong her life at all costs, which would be in keeping with her current stated goals. But I knew there were limits to what we would be able to achieve for Jade. I also wanted to expand our discussion beyond her medical care preferences to explore how we could help her accomplish as many of her goals as possible in her foreshortened future.

Over the course of several visits, I used the SICG to deepen our team's understanding of Jade's wishes and goals, and to expand Jade's and her family's understanding of some of the tradeoffs that often come with aggressive care at the end of life. I especially wanted her mother, her health care proxy, to be a part of these conversations.

Jade understood that her disease would take her life and that *"bad things keep happening."* While she wanted to know everything about what the future held for her, she was clear she didn't want to hear a time-based prognosis again, saying, *"The tongue is powerful, and I'm not speaking it into existence."* I used the guide's example of "hope and worry" and said, *"While I'm* hopeful *you can live for a long time, I* worry *that at some point you could get much sicker very quickly, and I want to help you prepare for that possibility."*

Serious Illness Conversation Guide

PATIENT-TESTED LANGUAGE

SET UP

"I'd like to talk about what is ahead with your illness and do some thinking in advance about what is important to you so that I can make sure we provide you with the care you want — **is this okay?**"

ASSESS

"What is **your understanding** now of where you are with your illness?"

"How much **information** about what is likely to be ahead with your illness would you like from me?"

SHARE

"I want to share with you **my understanding** of where things are with your illness..."

Uncertain: "It can be difficult to predict what will happen with your illness. I **hope** you will continue to live well for a long time but I'm **worried** that you could get sick quickly, and I think it is important to prepare for that possibility."
OR
Time: "I **wish** we were not in this situation, but I am **worried** that time may be as short as ___ (express as a range, e.g. days to weeks, weeks to months, months to a year)."
OR
Function: "I **hope** that this is not the case, but I'm **worried** that this may be as strong as you will feel, and things are likely to get more difficult."

EXPLORE

"What are your most important **goals** if your health situation worsens?"

"What are your biggest **fears and worries** about the future with your health?"

"What gives you **strength** as you think about the future with your illness?"

"What **abilities** are so critical to your life that you can't imagine living without them?"

"If you become sicker, **how much are you willing to go through** for the possibility of gaining more time?"

"How much does your **family** know about your priorities and wishes?"

CLOSE

"I've heard you say that ___ is really important to you. Keeping that in mind, and what we know about your illness, I **recommend** that we ___. This will help us make sure that your treatment plans reflect what's important to you."

"How does this plan seem to you?"

"I will do everything I can to help you through this."

© 2015 Ariadne Labs: A Joint Center for Health Systems Innovation (www.ariadnelabs.org) and Dana-Farber Cancer Institute. Revised April 2017. Licensed under the Creative Commons Attribution-NonCommercial-ShareAlike 4.0 International License, http://creativecommons.org/licenses/by-nc-sa/4.0/   SI-CG 2017-04-18

ARIADNE LABS

FIGURE 1.1. Serious Illness Conversation Guide. A free, well-studied communication tool that provides you with specific language for conversations with patients with life-limiting illnesses and their families about goals, hopes, worries, fears, sources of strength, what abilities are critical to their lives having quality, and what they would trade for more time. *Source:* Ariadne Labs; reprinted with permission. https://www.ariadnelabs.org/areas-of-work/serious-illness-care/.

She wanted this too. We also spoke about her goals as her health worsened, what gave her life meaning, her fears, and her sources of strength. Jade's *goals* included spending as much time as possible with her kids and continuing her advocacy work for a cancer support group. Jade had found *meaning* in supporting others, and she could articulate that this would be her lasting legacy after she was gone. I asked about her *fears*, which included being bedbound and losing independence, and I asked about her *sources of strength*, which were her children, family, and God.

When I asked Jade about *abilities that were critical to her life having quality*, she said, *"walking and talking"* but noted that none of that mattered if she could get more treatment for her cancer. I explored this further, using another phrase that the guide suggests: *"How much are you willing to go through for the possibility of gaining more time?"* To this she replied, *"I want to fight until I can no longer get treatment. If I can still get to chemo or radiation, or that is a possibility, I want everything possible done, fight until I flatline."* Jade's mother then shared their experience of watching Jade's grandmother die in an ICU, when *"everything seemed to be falling apart."* Jade told her mother, *"If my doctors don't think I can get to chemo or radiation, then just make me comfortable enough to where my family is not afraid to come into the room to see me or sit with me."*

I knew then that her oncologist was going to play the crucial role in Jade's decision-making going forward. The questions in the SICG revealed what we would need to know to facilitate a gentle landing for Jade rather than, as I feared, a crash. I was able to give Jade a clear recommendation, which I had reviewed first with her oncologist. As long as there was the possibility that Jade could receive treatment for her cancer, we would do everything medically possible to get her there. When the time came that treatment would no longer be safe, however, I would recommend that she enroll in a home hospice program, so that she could spend as much time as possible with her family.

Jade's story reveals an important tenet of palliative care: that we explore values to be able to provide goal-concordant care. We do not pursue our own agendas or what we might want for ourselves or loved ones but work toward what our patients and their families view as their priorities. Many patients like Jade put "the fight" and "leaving no stone unturned" at the top of their priority list. For these patients, aggressive medical care, hospitalizations, and ICU care may be the appropriate outcome at the end of life so long as they are making an informed choice and the alternatives are understood. But we also need to discover whether, if no further treatments remain, patients want to be kept comfortable, surrounded by family. For some, without the resources or caregivers, or whose symptoms are difficult to control, this will still mean dying somewhere other than home, but the goal, wherever that is, will be comfort.

The Serious Illness Care Program

Jade's story illustrates how important these conversations are in guiding and planning care, and how helpful a structured approach can be. To know how to advise Jade, and to help her do useful advance care planning, I needed to know a lot about her. How informed did she want to be about her condition? What did she understand of her prognosis? What was most important in her life? What made her life worth living, and what would be unacceptable to her? If Jade got sicker, which goals were most important to her: longevity at all costs, comfort, independence? How much was she willing to endure for these goals? What did she fear losing, and what level of function would and would not be acceptable? What were her worries about the rest of her family and other aspects of her emotional, social, spiritual, and physical life? How much did her family or her mother, her health care proxy, know about her wishes? Answers to those questions are especially important for patients like Jade, whom you expect to live only months or a year or two.

In Dr. Atul Gawande's book *Being Mortal: Medicine and What Matters in the End* (2014), the surgeon, writer, and public health leader writes of his transformation as he practiced asking these questions of seriously ill patients, friends, and, eventually, his father. He describes learning these vital questions from Dr. Susan Block, professor of psychiatry and medicine at Harvard Medical School and founding chair of the Department of Psychosocial Oncology and Palliative Care at the Dana-Farber Cancer Institute. Drs. Block, Gawande, and other palliative care experts refined these questions into the SICG (see Figure 1.1), which provides clear language for clinicians to elicit patients' values, goals, and priorities as they face the future with their illness.

But they also recognized that without systemic changes in medical care and education, training in the guide alone would be insufficient to transform care for all seriously ill patients. They worked with Dr. Gawande's health systems innovation center, Ariadne Labs, to create the Serious Illness Care Program. "The guide is one element of a multi-component program creating system-level support for clinicians to have these important conversations with their patients . . . The program's goal is for every seriously ill patient to have more, better, and earlier conversations with their clinicians about their goals, values, and priorities that will inform their future care" (Ariadne Labs 2020).

The Serious Illness Care Program was tested in a four-year randomized controlled trial of patients with cancer at the Dana-Farber Cancer Institute, giving us some of the best evidence to date for the value of a structured approach to these conversations backed by systems-level support. The intervention included clinician training in the SICG and systemic changes to address common barriers oncology clinicians face in initiating these discussions. Ninety-one oncologists and advance practice clinicians were randomized to receive training and coaching in use of the SICG, along with triggered reminders to have a conversation with patients at high risk of death and to document these conversations in an accessible template in the electronic health record (EHR). Clinicians were asked to identify patients for the study using the "surprise question": "Would you be surprised if this patient died in the next year?" Clinicians in the control arm provided usual care, and patients of these clinicians were also identified and enrolled in the study using the surprise question (Bernacki et al. 2019; Paladino et al. 2019).

The findings of this trial show that the Serious Illness Care Program accomplished its goal to provide "more, better, and earlier conversations." Nearly all of the 134 patients in the intervention group (96 percent vs. 79 percent in the control arm) had a documented discussion, which occurred a median of 2.4 months earlier than in the control group. Conversations in the intervention group were more comprehensive, with greater focus on values, goals, and patients' prognoses or illness understanding and life-sustaining treatment preferences (Paladino et al. 2019). Patients in the intervention group had less anxiety and depression, and the anxiety reduction was sustained at 24 weeks. Fewer than the expected number of patients died during the study (64), which may have contributed to the lack of difference between the intervention and control groups in the primary outcomes of the study, which were goal-concordant care and peacefulness at the end of life (Bernacki et al. 2019).

These are remarkable results, which may inspire clinicians to overcome their discomfort in having these discussions. We may worry that we are causing the distressing emotions that arise in our patients and their families as we talk about their future and mortality. But these emotions are already present. Families, patients, and clinicians may tiptoe around one another hoping to avoid these painful discussions, but by having them, you can validate their emotions and enable patients and their families to explore the future. You can help patients begin to plan and gain a sense of control over what often feels like an uncontrollable situation.

More on the Timing of Advance Care Planning

We should aim to have these advance care planning talks and conversations about the future with all patients who have a limited prognosis. This goal is aspirational, and it is one of our goals to help our colleagues change not only their own practices but also how our medical culture approaches care for those with life-limiting illness.

While a systematic review of advance care planning studies showed that advance directives alone had mixed results on outcomes aside from increased enrollment in hospice and use of comfort plans, more complex interventions that looked at a *process* of communication were more effective at increasing compliance with patients' end-of-life wishes, satisfaction with care, and decreasing aggressive end-of-life care (such as hospitalizations and deaths in the ICU and in the hospital; Brinkman-Stoppelenburg, Rietjens, and van der Heide 2014). As stated above, what matters most in advance care planning is not admission to hospice or comfort care, but the concordance of care with patients' goals. We are yet far away from measuring this accurately or having clear data for interventions that support this outcome.

We can all be alert to opportunities that hospitalizations provide to initiate or revisit the topic. Hospitalizations can be used as "near miss" events to heighten the importance and timeliness of having a conversation about advance care plans with patients and their families. Patients may bring up wishes about the future or share the illness experiences of loved ones who have died, both of which can be seen as invitations into these conversations. Of course, evidence of progressive disease with limited treatment options should prompt these discussions if they have not begun already. We discuss this further in Chapter 5, along with some of the challenges associated with prognostication.

Practice Points: Discussing Advance Care Planning

- Initiate the discussion with patients early in the relationship.
- Discover whom they want to have with them when you have the discussion, ideally their health care proxy.
- Anticipate and address unasked questions.
- Find out what makes the patients' lives worthwhile, as well as what would be completely unacceptable, what they are hoping for, and what they fear.
- Find out what the patients are willing to go through for the possibility of more time.
- Reassure patients that having this discussion does not mean that you think the treatment will not work.
- Encourage patients to continue these discussions with you again at later visits, and when their clinical situation changes.

BARRIERS TO DISCUSSING PROGNOSIS

Your patients cannot really engage in a meaningful discussion about the future or participate in shared decision-making until they understand their prognosis. Patients and families make different treatment decisions when they believe time is short and the cancer incurable (Mack et al. 2015; Weeks et al. 1998). Prognosis, however, is shrouded in uncertainty, and the natural tendency when confronted with uncertainty about such an important subject is to avoid the discussion altogether (Levy 1999).

Resistance to discussing prognosis can come from clinicians, patients, or their families. In Chapter 5, we discuss helping patients and families "cultivate prognostic awareness" when they may be reluctant to prepare for the future and their eventual death (Jackson et al. 2013; Jacobsen et al. 2018). Here, we discuss the barriers clinicians face and what happens when they aren't able to overcome them.

The cultural "norms" of medicine dictate that we be optimistic rather than accurate (Christakis 1999). Of 700 oncologists (64 percent of the 1,100 ASCO members initially queried) who completed a self-report survey, more than 98 percent replied that they told their terminally ill patients that they would die. But almost half (48 percent) said that they did so only when patients specifically asked for information about their prognosis. Fifty-seven percent said they "sometimes, rarely, or never" gave an actual estimate of how much time the patient was likely to survive (Daugherty and Hlubocky 2008).

In a separate study, 60 percent of medical oncologists reported that they would rather not talk about advance directives, code status, or hospice until no more effective treatments remained (Keating et al. 2010). The outcome of this reluctance should not be surprising: studies have documented discordance between patients' and their oncologists' beliefs about the curability of their cancer or estimated survival (Loh et al. 2019). A study of more than 1,000 patients with newly diagnosed stage IV lung or colorectal cancer revealed that 69 percent of patients with lung cancer and 81 percent of patients with colorectal cancer "did not report understanding that the chemotherapy was not at all likely to cure their cancer" (Weeks et al. 2012). A study of 236 patients with advanced cancer and their 38 oncologists showed that 68 percent of patient-oncologist pairs were discordant regarding the probability of surviving two years, and discordance was much higher in nonwhite compared to white patients (95 percent vs. 65 percent) (Gramling et al. 2016). Nearly all the patients with discordance (96 percent) were more optimistic than their oncologists.

This inaccuracy seems to be true worldwide: a survey of 1,390 patients receiving palliative care in 11 countries showed that 68 percent of patients with advanced cancer believed that the goal of their therapy was "to get rid of their cancer" (Yennurajalingam et al. 2018, p. 501). When patients or their families seem unrealistic about the prognosis, it is our responsibility to integrate information about their prognosis into the discussion about advance care planning, with compassion and sensitivity to the emotional distress that this can cause.

You might assume that patients who want to know their prognosis will ask you about it, but patients are known to withhold concerns from their oncology providers because they want to be "good patients" and "fighters," not "quitters" (Derry, Carrington Reid, and Prigerson 2019). As we discuss in Chapter 6, patients often don't tell you about their unrelieved pain, and only about 15 percent of them volunteer the information that they have completed an advance directive (Lamont and Siegler 2000), thereby saving us the pain of this talk altogether.

As more studies have examined patients' prognostic understanding or "awareness," one important question is whether patients' lack of understanding is a result of what is communicated by their clinicians, how it is communicated, or what patients are able to hear and process (Derry, Carrington Reid, and Prigerson 2019). It is common for us to hear from one of our oncology colleagues, "But I *told* her she had stage IV incurable cancer! How could she and her family be surprised that she is dying of this?"

We think the surprise we often see when patients and their families finally register the patient's poor prognosis is due to a combination of complex factors. The language we may use (e.g., "our goal is to control your cancer," or "you have metastatic cancer") can be unintentionally misunderstood, and emotional states such as distress and anxiety can impair patients' ability to understand the prognostic information (Derry, Carrington Reid, and Prigerson 2019). Health literacy also clearly plays a role here.

Regardless, all these data and studies point to the need to revisit our reluctance to have discussions about prognosis with our patients and their loved ones (Gilligan et al. 2017). Delaying this discussion for too long robs them of opportunities to make choices about how to spend the limited time that remains, and the sicker patients may be less able to participate fully in the discussion or in decision-making. Executive function, which involves planning, insight, abstraction, and judgment, is impaired in patients with serious chronic medical illnesses like hypertension, COPD, and diabetes (Schillerstrom, Horton, and Royall 2005) and is therefore likely to be impaired in patients with advanced cancer. If you need to check formally for decision-making capacity in such a patient, several instruments are available (Palmer and Harmell 2016).

Clearly, discussing prognosis does not fit easily into a standard office visit and requires skills that your medical training was unlikely to develop (Yuen, Reid, and Fetters 2011). Only when I (*Janet Abrahm*) began to practice palliative medicine did I learn the skills I would have needed to discuss prognosis well with my patients and their families, such as how to run a family meeting, counsel patients in psychological distress, and help people cope with their grief and anger (Tulsky, Chesny, and Lo 1995; von Gunten, Ferris, and Emanuel 2000; Back, Arnold, et al. 2009). Those of you who have not been adequately prepared for these tasks may decide not to mention prognosis for fear of harming patients or family members through lack of expertise.

Why else might we resist having the discussion? Drs. Jenny Mack and Thomas Smith, both oncologists, identified four more possible concerns:

1. Patients get depressed.

2. The truth kills hope.

3. Hospice or palliative care reduces survival.

4. This discussion is not culturally appropriate.

But the data don't support these concerns (Mack and Smith 2012). Patients don't get more depressed. Data actually indicate that patients who reported having end-of-life discussions did not have a higher rate of depression and anxiety (Emanuel et al. 2004; Enzinger et al. 2015). In fact, almost 90 percent of 988 patients who were thought by their physicians to have six months or less to live, who were interviewed about death, dying, and bereavement, reported no stress at all after the interview; only about 2 percent reported experiencing a great deal of stress (Emanuel et al. 2004). Their caregivers reported similar remarkably low levels of stress, and about half of each group found the conversation helpful.

Not having the discussion, however, is likely to lead to worse outcomes for the bereaved family. Patients who don't have those discussions are more likely to have more aggressive care at the end of life, and their bereaved caregivers are more depressed (Wright et al. 2008). A small majority of advance care planning studies showed that psychosocial measures such as satisfaction, stress, depression, and anxiety were positively affected by advance care planning. Notably *none* showed adverse psychosocial effects (Brinkman-Stoppelenburg, Rietjens, and van der Heide 2014). As noted previously, in the randomized trial assessing the Serious Illness Care Program, patients in the intervention arm had less depression and anxiety (Bernacki et al. 2019).

The truth doesn't kill hope. Patients and the parents of pediatric patients maintained hope even when they were told of a poor prognosis, low likelihood of response to treatment, or no chance of a cure (Mack and Smith 2012). In a small study of adult cancer patients, hope (as measured by the Herth Hope Index) did not change when patients were given truthful information by their oncologists about a bad prognosis (Smith et al. 2010). A study of adolescent and young adult cancer patients showed that those who reported more prognostic disclosure had higher odds of trust in the oncologist, peace of mind, and hope related to physician communication (Mack, Fasciano, and Block 2018). And 93 percent of surrogate decision-makers for critically ill ventilated patients also agreed that they would not want to avoid discussions of prognosis just to maintain hope. Rather, they wanted accurate estimates of how long the patient was likely to live so that they could support the patient and prepare themselves for what lay ahead (Apatira et al. 2008).

Neither hospice nor palliative care decreases survival. Patients in a hospice program do not have reduced survival rates (Connor et al. 2007), and in two studies of patients with advanced lung cancer about to begin chemotherapy for it, palliative care actually increased survival (Temel et al. 2010). Furthermore, those patients with poor-prognosis cancer that enroll in hospice have lower rates of hospitalization, ICU stays, and invasive procedures, as well as lower costs in the last year of life compared with those not in hospice (Obermeyer et al. 2014). Since Temel's landmark 2010 study, other studies have confirmed that palliative care for cancer patients either improves or does not decrease survival (Bakitas et al. 2015; Ferrell et al. 2015; Grudzen et al. 2016). As we discuss further in Chapter 6, carefully monitoring patients' symptoms may lead to improved survival (Basch et al. 2016), which many of us who practice palliative care believe may account for the observation that hospice and palliative care may improve, not decrease, survival.

Cultural Considerations

The prognostic discussion should be invited across cultures. The cultural background of your patients and their families informs their views about information preferences, decision-making, preferences for care, and documentation of advance care planning (Cain et al. 2018; Jia et al. 2020). Our own cultural backgrounds as providers, acculturated to medicine, also affects how we approach these discussions. Although cultural and ethnic variations can be observed in outcomes relevant to palliative care, these are the result of many complex factors that include preferences as well as structural "social, historical, and political circumstances" (Cain et al. 2018).

While there are differences between groups in observed outcomes, disparities, and preferences relevant to palliative care, we must aim to avoid stereotyping and instead build awareness of our own biases. We discuss cultural humility and the role of systemic racism in perpetuating disparities in greater depth in Chapter 2. There is no "one size fits all" discussion for each person, and care should be individualized. Gilligan, Bohlke, and Baile's 2018 ASCO Consensus Guideline summary on patient-clinician communication recommends we enter encounters "with a sense of curiosity, aware that any patient and family, regardless of their background, may have beliefs, experiences, understandings, and expectations that are different from the clinician's" (Gilligan, Bohlke, and Baile 2018, p. 45). We need to explore the ideas of each individual patient and his or her family system without making assumptions. All patients should be asked whether they or their family would like to hear prognostic information, and how their family typically makes medical decisions.

A medical interpreter should be part of the discussion for patients for whom English is not their language of choice, or who use American Sign Language (Gilligan et al. 2017). Interpreters do not simply translate words; they are cultural mediators. They can explore whether the patient and family align with the usual cultural norms of their ethnic and cultural group, advise the team what those norms are, and alert them when a relevant cultural belief is likely to affect the discussion (Cain et al. 2018). We discuss this further in Chapter 2.

Here, we provide a few examples of between-group variation but want to emphasize that these differences are not fixed, nor true of all individuals in a given cultural group. Some patients prefer not to acknowledge terminal illness openly, whereas others prefer prognostic disclosure. For example, discussing death among some Native American communities may be considered taboo (Colclough 2017), and Hispanic patients are less likely to want prognostic disclosure than white patients, or to acknowledge terminal illness (Smith et al. 2008). Some patients may prefer family-centered decision-making, whereas others prioritize individual autonomy in decision-making. Asian and Hispanic patients are more likely to rely on family to help with decisions, whereas Black and white Americans express a preference for autonomy in decision-making on the whole (Blackhall et al. 1995; Hobbs et al. 2015). Some patients are less likely to discuss and document their wishes regarding advance care planning, whereas non-Hispanic white patients are more likely to document preferences (Clark et al. 2018; Sanders, Robinson, and Block 2016; Smith et al. 2008). On the whole, studies have shown that Black and Hispanic patients in the United States are more likely to prefer aggressive life-prolonging care than white patients (Smith et al. 2008; Modes et al. 2019).

A study of adults living outside China and Taiwan who identify themselves as ethnically Chinese (the Chinese diaspora) reported that they were willing to engage in advance care planning. They preferred it to be initiated by clinicians and community councils, for the communication strategies used to be "indirect and depersonalized," and for "harmony, the desire to avoid tensions, upsets, and turmoil for the self, family and others" (p. 11) to be central to the discussions (Jia et al. 2020). A mixed-method systematic review of studies (from mostly high-income Asian countries) of the preferences of Asian patients in southern, southeastern, and eastern Asia regarding their views of advance care planning similarly revealed that their willingness to engage in the process was affected by the perception of its advantages and disadvantages; whether it was in accord with their faith, or their or their family's wishes; their understanding of their prognosis; and the presence or absence of barriers within their communities or connection and trust with their health care provider or health care system (Martina et al. 2021).

We include the examples above to illustrate that we "must understand culture as a source of meaning" (Cain et al. 2018, p. 1413), which affects all of us as we grapple with serious illness and death. A recent study of audiotaped palliative care encounters found that clinicians discussed prognosis less often with Black and Latinx patients with advanced cancer than they did with white patients (Ingersoll et al. 2019). We need to explore this subject with every patient with a life-limiting illness, and when discussing preferences for care at the end of life, not assume that they share the statistical preference of their "group" or "groups" as reported in a small number of studies. We discuss clinician barriers to these discussions more fully in Chapter 5, but a full discussion of the effects of culture on communication is beyond the scope of this book. For those readers who wish to pursue this subject in greater detail, we recommend the work of Marjorie Kagawa-Singer and Shaheen Kassim-Lakha (2003), who have written extensively on the role of cultural differences in health care. The effect of culture on pain assessment is reviewed in Chapter 6.

DISCUSSING RESUSCITATION, INTUBATION, AND LIFE-SUSTAINING TREATMENTS

As you would anticipate, patients will make different choices about resuscitation if they know what you know, in terms of both their prognosis and the likely functional or cognitive impairment resulting from resuscitation (Modes et al. 2019; Shen, Trevino, and Prigerson 2018). Patients who reported that they knew their disease was terminal (or who had a discussion about end-of-life issues with their physicians) were much less likely to want life-extending care than were others (Wright et al. 2010). The data overwhelmingly suggest that resuscitation of patients with cancer usually has a terrible outcome. Overall survival to discharge in patients with cancer is 6–7 percent (Bruckel et al. 2017; Reisfield et al. 2006). Bruckel et al. (2017) compared resuscitation outcomes in patients with and without advanced cancer in a large national cohort following in-hospital cardiac arrest. While 58 percent of patients with advanced cancer had return of spontaneous circulation, only *1 in 13 of them survived to discharge*. Sharing this information with patients is likely to help them make more informed decisions about being resuscitated, especially if their idea of what is likely to happen to them if they're resuscitated is based on what they have seen on television (Diem, Lantos, and Tulsky 1996).

Looking at it another way, patients may elect to be resuscitated unless they think their disease is so far advanced that they have a very small chance of surviving a year. The Coping with Cancer studies (two multi-institutional, longitudinal cohort studies of patients with advanced cancer and their informal caregivers) showed that when both patients and their caregivers understood the patient's prognosis to be ≤12 months, 70.7 percent had a completed DNR order compared to 31.6–38.9 percent of patients when only they or only their caregivers believed they had this limited a prognosis (Shen, Trevino, and Prigerson 2018).

Patients who have been resuscitated for an uncomplicated cardiac arrhythmia in the past and have gone home with no sequelae, or who have a close relative or friend who has been successfully resuscitated without serious sequelae, are particularly likely to want resuscitation. It is much harder for them to understand that having metastatic cancer greatly reduces their chances of being successfully resuscitated and being able to return home from the hospital after a cardiac arrest.

When you begin a discussion about resuscitation preferences in a patient like this, you might say something like the following, stopping to address the patient's comments as they occur:

> *As we discussed before, your cancer has spread. We will be doing everything we can to help you maintain an active and fulfilling life for as long as possible. As we go along, you'll decide, as you always have, which treatments are worth the side effects. And I will let you know, as I always have, what the chances are that the treatment will be of benefit to you.*

At some point, I will need you to tell me how you feel about some extreme treatments we would use only if you died, like restarting your heart should it stop. Or, if you couldn't breathe on your own, how would you feel about us keeping you alive on a breathing machine? I feel fairly confident that you or your family have thought about this a little already; you might even have discussed it among yourselves—or you may have been afraid to bring it up because you didn't want to hurt each other.

It's important for you to take into account, while you're making your decision, what the outcome is likely to be if you die and we do resuscitate you. I would imagine that you're thinking, "Well, if I die in the hospital, of course I want to be resuscitated so that I can go back home." *Unfortunately, while there is a good chance we could restart your heart, there is really almost no chance that you would get well enough to go home and go on living as you are right now. I know that seems hard to believe, but it's true, and I thought you would want to know this to help you decide.*

More than half the patients I (*Janet Abrahm*) talk to about this in my role as palliative care consultant have an answer ready the first time I ask them. Others often stop me before I get far into the discussion, saying that if their time has come, they want to be left in peace, or that they never want to be "a vegetable living on machines," or, like Jade, that they want to fight "until I flatline." In fact, patients seem much less reticent to discuss these issues with me than I had ever imagined.

It is important to clarify patients' wishes about being intubated, not as part of a resuscitation but to prevent them from dying. Many people who do not want to be resuscitated if they die would be willing to receive respiratory support for a time to allow them to recover from a reversible process. I therefore include a discussion such as this:

I also need to understand how you feel about being kept alive on a breathing machine. The treatments are likely to decrease your resistance to infection, and you could develop a serious pneumonia. While you are recovering, in order to survive, you might need a breathing tube and a machine called a respirator to help you breathe. You wouldn't be able to eat or to talk, and you may not be able to communicate with us initially. Would that be OK with you?

Because many patients are worried about having their lives prolonged by these machines, I also add, "*We would never use a breathing machine to prolong your suffering, though. If it looked as if you were so seriously ill that the respirator was no longer helping you achieve any of your goals and was merely keeping you alive, we would help you to die naturally and peacefully.*"

I don't think it makes sense to list for patients all the procedures we can perform, even if we explain them in terms that patients and their families can understand. Dr. Steven Pantilat* shared with me a useful analogy that illustrates the problems with that approach.

He asked me to imagine that I was going to buy a computer for the first time, and that I encountered two different salespeople. He asked me to decide which person was more likely to be able to help me buy the computer that would best fit my needs.

> Salesperson 1: *"How many Gigabytes of memory and how much RAM do you need? What kind of processor do you want? How big do you want the hard drive to be?"*
>
> Salesperson 2: *"What do you want to use the computer for? Do you make presentations for talks and use videos or materials from other documents in the talks? Do you make your own videos? Do you need a lot of room for photographs?"*

Clearly, I hope we would all resemble Salesperson 2.

We, too, have specialized knowledge and experiences that our patients are unlikely to share. And we hope to have the advantage of knowing our patients over time, so that we can factor in their goals. Knowing the answers to questions about their priorities will help you advise your patients on the burdens and benefits to them, personally, of cardiopulmonary resuscitation (CPR) and life-sustaining treatments when they die or become critically ill. A recommendation framed by earlier conversations about your patients' values, goals, and tradeoffs might sound like this:

> *You've told me that your quality of life is most important to you right now, and that if you get sicker, you want the focus to be on spending time with your family. Given this, I would recommend we continue treating your cancer as long as the side effects of treatment are not too bad and the cancer is responding. This is our plan A, and I hope this lasts as long as possible. But I also want to help you prepare for a plan B, since it's my responsibility to help my patients prepare for when things worsen. If we had no more treatments for the cancer, and you were to get so sick that you would otherwise require intensive care unit (ICU) care or CPR, that would be a sign that you were dying. In this situation, I recommend we*

---

*Dr. Steven Pantilat is a clinical professor of medicine, the Alan M. Kates and John M. Burnard Endowed Chair in Palliative Care, director of the Palliative Care Leadership Center, and founding director of the palliative care program in the Department of Medicine at the University of California, San Francisco.

allow you to die peacefully, not put you through CPR when you die, focus on keeping you comfortable, and support your family. What do you think?

When you make a recommendation, it is important to give patients the space to respond, express their emotions, or disagree.

Following up on the recommendation that Jade, her mother, and I (*Molly Collins*) had previously discussed was helpful for them. Jade continued to have progressive neurological deficits as the leptomeningeal disease worsened. After a course of radiation, there was nothing left for her oncologist to try against the cancer.

I sat down with Jade, her mother, and her oncologist, Dr. Mehta. Dr. Mehta carefully explained each treatment they had tried up to this point, and why Jade was experiencing so many different physical symptoms. I watched Jade and her mother trying to absorb the details and waiting for what she always heard from Dr. Mehta—the next plan. I picked up Jade's hand and said simply, *"This is bad news."* Usually so stoic, she began to cry, and her mother put her arm around her. After a few minutes of silence together, I said, *"Jade, unfortunately this means you are facing the final chapter."* She turned to us asking, *"So what do we do now?"*

I replied, *"You told us that as long as there was the possibility of more treatment for your cancer, you wanted whatever we could give you. Now we're in a different place, and there isn't anything else we can do to fight the cancer. But there's still a lot we can do to take care of you and your family. When this time came, you said you wanted us to make sure you could be comfortable enough to spend time with your family. A hospice program would help support you and your family at home, and Dr. Mehta and I will always be just a phone call away."*

Jade agreed, saying comfort was most important to her right now. She was also clear she hoped to transfer to a hospice facility at the very end of her life so that her young children would not have the memory of her dying at home. She asked her mother if focusing on comfort was OK with her, because she didn't want to let

---

Practice Points: Discussing Resuscitation and Intubation

- Clarify the difference between taking measures to prevent death and taking measures to restart and sustain life once a cardiac or respiratory arrest has occurred.
- Ask specifically about patients' wishes regarding resuscitation when they die, and the expectations about what life would be like after the resuscitation attempt.
- Correct unrealistic expectations and misconceptions about the process and likely sequelae of resuscitation and about the experience of being kept alive by a respirator.
- Encourage patients who are undecided at the initial encounter to discuss the subject with you again at later visits.

her down. Her mother hugged Jade again, reassured her that she could never let her down, and asked us how soon she could be discharged home and enrolled in a hospice program. They both agreed she did not want resuscitation attempted when she died and asked us to put those orders in her chart and to send her home with documentation of that decision.

Over the next day, with our support, Jade and her mother shared the news with her family. Before she left the hospital, I recommended that she complete advance care planning documentation, which we had been encouraging her to do for months. Jade had already completed a health care proxy, but now she and her mother together completed *Five Wishes*, which documented her wishes for medical treatment, what would make her comfortable as she approached the end of her life, how she wanted to be remembered, and her funeral plan.

Jade wrote her treatment wishes simply as *"I, Jade Markman, want to stay home on hospice care as long as I can do for myself. Once self-care is not possible, I would like to be transferred to the hospice facility. In the event I am unable to speak for myself, my doctors know to do as much as they can and then just keep me comfortable."* When she was discharged, we sent her home with a completed Physician Orders for Life-Sustaining Treatment (POLST) form, which we discuss further later in the chapter. Jade documented her DNR/DNI wishes, and I signed an out-of-hospital DNR order ensuring that she would not be resuscitated if she died at home and that she would be rehospitalized only for comfort. Jade's story continues in Chapter 5.

DOCUMENTING ADVANCE CARE PLANS: ADVANCE DIRECTIVES

While advance care planning is the process of preparing patients for future medical decisions, advance directives are legal documents that record guidance about treatment preferences and appoint a health care proxy (Sudore, Lum, et al. 2017). Once you and your patient have defined the advance care plan, it's vital to document your discussions, especially when your patient's wishes evolve over time.

Ideally, you would be able to record the advance care plan somewhere that is accessible not only to all colleagues in your practice but also to Emergency Department and inpatient clinicians in your usual referral hospitals, and to rehabilitation and nursing home personnel, when that's relevant. The EHR EPIC, for example, includes an Advance Care Planning Module and accessible links in its standard package. It would be helpful if all EHRs had similar features.

POLST and Out-of-Hospital DNR Forms

The POLST, which may have a different name in your state (e.g., MOLST, Medical Orders for Life-Sustaining Treatment), and out-of-hospital DNR forms are portable documents that are *legal medical orders* to limit treatment. If you have a patient with a life expectancy of a year or two who wants to limit life-sustaining therapies, completing a POLST is a clear way to communicate this choice to all caregivers and health care personnel (Institute of Medicine 2014) (Figure 1.2). If emergency medical personnel in your state do not yet recognize POLST, you may need to complete an out-of-hospital DNR form for patients who wish to be protected from all resuscitative efforts.

POLST forms are not designed to replace health care proxy forms or living wills; rather, each is a two-page set of *legal medical orders* signed by the patient's physician, nurse practitioner, or physician assistant. These orders specify the patient's choices for CPR and medical interventions (directed at comfort, at full treatment, or at limited treatment), when or if the patient wishes to be transferred to a hospital or to an intensive care unit, and when or if the patient wishes to receive antibiotics, artificial nutrition, or hydration.

POLST forms are legally valid for care *across all settings*, including the home, nursing homes, and acute care hospitals (Institute of Medicine 2014). The Institute of Medicine's report *Dying in America* recommends that all states implement a POLST program. The POLST was used first in 1994 in Oregon. As of 2020, "The POLST Paradigm exists at some level in 50 states and Washington DC: *Existing* is a spectrum from just having legislation passed, to implementing the POLST Paradigm with regional pilots, to having implemented the POLST Paradigm so it is standard of care within that state" (National POLST 2020).

I urge those of you who work in states in which the forms are recognized to become familiar with them, keep a stack in your office, and complete them as you have these discussions with your patients and their families. Copies are as valid as the original, so you can keep the original in your files or scan it into your EHR and give copies to patients to keep with them in the car and at home on the refrigerator, where they can be easily seen by emergency medical service personnel.

Other Advance Directive Forms

For some patients, no written advance directive, other than naming a health care proxy, is acceptable (Sudore, Lum, et al. 2017). These patients rely on their family members to make decisions for them when needed, based on what they know the patient would have wanted in that situation. But other patients wish to complete portable written advance directives (other than the POLST-type forms) to guide clinical decisions and urgent conversations about aggressive, often life-sustaining treatments. Patients who have had an end-of-life discussion with their clinicians and completed an advance care plan are more likely to have their preferences honored (Brinkman-Stoppelenburg, Rietjens, and van der Heide 2014; Silveira, Kim, and Langa 2010; Detering et al. 2010).

Advance care planning documents, unfortunately, differ from state to state. In some states, only the health care proxy and the POLST are legal documents; in those states, all other documents, like living wills, inform clinicians but are not legally binding. Your institution likely has a standard state-specific form or its own version(s) available. Complete sets of state-specific advance directives can be found on the National Hospice and Palliative Care Organization website (www.nhpco.org).

SEND FORM WITH PERSON WHENEVER TRANSFERRED OR DISCHARGED
To follow these orders, an EMS provider must have an order from his/her medical command physician

pennsylvania DEPARTMENT OF HEALTH

Pennsylvania Orders for Life-Sustaining Treatment (POLST)

Last Name

First/Middle Initial

Date of Birth

FIRST follow these orders, **THEN** contact physician, certified registered nurse practitioner or physician assistant. This is an Order Sheet based on the person's medical condition and wishes at the time the orders were issued. Everyone shall be treated with dignity and respect.

A Check One

CARDIOPULMONARY RESUSCITATION (CPR): Person has no pulse and is not breathing.

☐ CPR/Attempt Resuscitation ☐ DNR/Do Not Attempt Resuscitation (Allow Natural Death)

When not in cardiopulmonary arrest, follow orders in **B**, **C** and **D**.

B Check One

MEDICAL INTERVENTIONS: Person has pulse and/or is breathing.

☐ **COMFORT MEASURES ONLY** Use medication by any route, positioning, wound care and other measures to relieve pain and suffering. Use oxygen, oral suction and manual treatment of airway obstruction as needed for comfort. ***Do not transfer*** *to hospital for life-sustaining treatment.* ***Transfer*** *if comfort needs cannot be met in current location.*

☐ **LIMITED ADDITIONAL INTERVENTIONS** Includes care described above. Use medical treatment, IV fluids and cardiac monitor as indicated. Do not use intubation, advanced airway interventions, or mechanical ventilation.

Transfer *to hospital if indicated. Avoid intensive care if possible.*

☐ **FULL TREATMENT** Includes care described above. Use intubation, advanced airway interventions, mechanical ventilation, and cardioversion as indicated.

Transfer *to hospital if indicated. Includes intensive care.*

Additional Orders ______________________________

C Check One

ANTIBIOTICS:

☐ No antibiotics. Use other measures to relieve symptoms.

☐ Determine use or limitation of antibiotics when infection occurs, with comfort as goal

☐ Use antibiotics if life can be prolonged

Additional Orders

D Check One

ARTIFICIALLY ADMINISTERED HYDRATION / NUTRITION:
Always offer food and liquids by mouth if feasible

☐ No hydration and artificial nutrition by tube.

☐ Trial period of artificial hydration and nutrition by tube.

☐ Long-term artificial hydration and nutrition by tube.

Additional Orders

E Check One

SUMMARY OF GOALS, MEDICAL CONDITION AND SIGNATURES:

Discussed with
☐ Patient
☐ Parent of Minor
☐ Health Care Agent
☐ Health Care Representative
☐ Court-Appointed Guardian
☐ Other:

Patient Goals/Medical Condition:

By signing this form, I acknowledge that this request regarding resuscitative measures is consistent with the known desires of, and in the best interest of, the individual who is the subject of the form.

Physician /PA/CRNP Printed Name:	**Physician /PA/CRNP Phone Number**
Physician/PA/CRNP Signature (Required):	**DATE**

Signature of Patient or Surrogate

Signature (required)	**Name (print)**	**Relationship (write "self" if patient)**

PaDOH version 06-28-2021 1 of 2

FIGURE 1.2. Sample POLST Form, Used in Pennsylvania (Pennsylvania Orders for Life-Sustaining Treatment). *Source:* UPMC, April 30, 2018, https://cdn.upmc.com/-/media/upmc/services/seniors/resources-for-caregivers/documents/polst-form.pdf. Reprinted with permission of the Pennsylvania Department of Health. (*continued*)

SEND FORM WITH PERSON WHENEVER TRANSFERRED OR DISCHARGED		

Other Contact Information

Surrogate	Relationship	Phone Number	
Health Care Professional Preparing Form	Preparer Title	Phone Number	Date Prepared

Directions for Healthcare Professionals

Any individual for whom a Pennsylvania Order for Life-Sustaining Treatment form is completed should ideally have an advance health care directive that provides instructions for the individual's health care and appoints an agent to make medical decisions whenever the patient is unable to make or communicate a healthcare decision. If the patient wants a DNR Order issued in section "A", the physician/PA/CRNP should discuss the issuance of an Out-of-Hospital DNR order, if the individual is eligible, to assure that an EMS provider can honor his/her wishes. Contact the Pennsylvania Department of Aging for information about sample forms for advance health care directives. Contact the Pennsylvania Department of Health, Bureau of EMS, for information about Out-of-Hospital Do-Not-Resuscitate orders, bracelets and necklaces. POLST forms may be obtained online from the Pennsylvania Department of Health. www.health.pa.gov or www.papolst.org

Completing POLST

Must be completed by a health care professional based on patient preferences and medical indications or decisions by the patient or a surrogate. This document refers to the person for whom the orders are issued as the "individual" or "patient" and refers to any other person authorized to make healthcare decisions for the patient covered by this document as the "surrogate."

At the time a POLST is completed, any current advance directive, if available, must be reviewed.

Must be signed by a physician/PA/CRNP and patient/surrogate to be valid. Verbal orders are acceptable with follow-up signature by physician/PA/CRNP in accordance with facility/community policy. A person designated by the patient or surrogate may document the patient's or surrogate's agreement. Use of original form is strongly encouraged. Photocopies and Faxes of signed POLST forms should be respected where necessary

Using POLST

If a person's condition changes and time permits, the patient or surrogate must be contacted to assure that the POLST is updated as appropriate.

If any section is not completed, then the healthcare provider should follow other appropriate methods to determine treatment.

An automated external defibrillator (AED) should not be used on a person who has chosen "Do Not Attempt Resuscitation"

Oral fluids and nutrition must always be offered if medically feasible.

When comfort cannot be achieved in the current setting, the person, including someone with "comfort measures only," should be transferred to a setting able to provide comfort (e.g., treatment of a hip fracture).

A person who chooses either "comfort measures only" or "limited additional interventions" may not require transfer or referral to a facility with a higher level of care.

An IV medication to enhance comfort may be appropriate for a person who has chosen "Comfort Measures Only."

Treatment of dehydration is a measure which may prolong life. A person who desires IV fluids should indicate "Limited Additional Interventions" or "Full Treatment."

A patient with or without capacity or the surrogate who gave consent to this order or who is otherwise specifically authorized to do so, can revoke consent to any part of this order providing for the withholding or withdrawal of life-sustaining treatment, at any time, and request alternative treatment.

Review

This form should be reviewed periodically (consider at least annually) and a new form completed if necessary when:
  (1) The person is transferred from one care setting or care level to another, or
  (2) There is a substantial change in the person's health status, or
  (3) The person's treatment preferences change.

Revoking POLST

If the POLST becomes invalid or is replaced by an updated version, draw a line through sections A through E of the invalid POLST, write "VOID" in large letters across the form, and sign and date the form.

FIGURE 1.2. (cont.)

Many advance directives and advance care planning aids do not include what we now consider to be an essential part of advance care planning: elicitation and clarification of *values* (Bridges et al. 2018). For patients who desire this more comprehensive documentation of their wishes, one common form is the one Jade used, *Five Wishes*. It is available online from Aging with Dignity, at $5 per copy (Five Wishes 2020). Aging with Dignity has also developed a special form for adolescents and young adults titled *Voicing My Choices: A Planning Guide for Adolescents and Young Adults*. These are useful in facilitating discussions among patients and their families, who can then share their decisions with you.

Two other programs that have been studied deserve mention here, PREPARE and Respecting Choices. PREPARE for your care (https://prepareforyourcare.org) is a patient-centered website that walks patients and families through the steps of comprehensive advance care planning. Compared to an easy-to-read advance directive alone, access to PREPARE increased documentation of advance care planning from 25 percent to 35 percent in 414 veterans (Sudore, Boscardin, et al. 2017) and from 33 percent to 43 percent in a diverse primary care population (Sudore et al. 2018). Respecting Choices includes a licensed "stepped-approach" to advance care planning based on current health state and "in-depth counseling by trained non-physician facilitators" (MacKenzie et al. 2018).

If you think your patient might want to complete a living will, you might introduce the idea by saying:

> You and I have had a long conversation about what's important to you if your health worsens. I have written this down so, if needed, all the caregivers at our hospital can see the decisions we've made. As long as your medical team can get your input about medical decisions, we will. But if you are admitted to another hospital and are too sick to share your wishes, the clinicians there will need guidance.
>
> Would you like more information on how to fill out a document that would instruct others in your wishes if you are no longer able to make decisions for yourself, and the clinicians caring for you have to ask your family or loved ones what you would have wanted? Although you might think having this conversation feels tough, it can be a gift to family members to tell them your wishes ahead of time, so they don't feel burdened by not knowing what you would have wanted.

I (*Molly Collins*) learned more about the complexities of advance care planning through personal experience. Even after years as a palliative care physician promoting advance directives to others, it took a nudge to help my parents complete one. We'd talked about their wishes here and there for years, and I felt I had a pretty good sense of their values and what they'd want as they faced serious illness. When my father, a physician, was diagnosed with stage I melanoma requiring a series of operations, we all agreed it was time to for a full discussion. On a Saturday morning, my husband took my small children out of the house, and I settled in with a cup of coffee to FaceTime with my parents, halfway across the country.

My mother came prepared with her "mission statement," which appeared simple at first glance: *"If I'm at a time in my life that without intervention I could die, and if that illness prevents me from leading a quality life, stop everything."* I delved, *"So how do you define a quality life, Mom?"* It didn't take long to home in on cognitive capacity, ability to interact with family, and freedom from significant pain as key quality-of-life indicators for my mother. She could imagine finding quality of life in a debilitated state: *"I can imagine a state when I couldn't do anything physically but could have a 'zest for life' if I could interact with others."* My father wanted more: *"A languishing existence with occasional visits from family wouldn't be enough . . . I'd need to have some enjoyment and stimulation from the outside world."*

It quickly became clear that if either of my parents were suffering from a declining terminal illness such as cancer or dementia, quality of life would be the priority over life prolongation. We then spent a long time exploring what we labeled "the gray scenarios." These included sudden catastrophic events with an uncertain prognosis for recovery, such as a massive stroke or accident. We thought of people who'd been through similar situations, including my mother's friend who survived a debilitating stroke, my husband's 93-year-old grandmother with multiple life-threatening injuries following a car accident, and famous individuals like Christopher Reeve and the writer Jean-Dominique Bauby, who wrote a magnificent book, *The Diving Bell and the Butterfly*, after a stroke that left him locked in.

After an hour of discussing their wishes, values, how much they were willing to go through for the possibility of more time, and how they defined quality of life, we felt ready to put pen to paper. I encouraged them to use the PREPARE website to record their wishes, in part because I was curious to see how this interface could help support individuals to complete advance care planning documentation outside of a clinician's office.

It took us another hour to walk through the PREPARE site for one parent. There were many explanatory videos that could have been helpful to someone who needed more information about each advance care planning step the site walked through. As a self-labeled "techno-poop," my mother found the site overwhelming and said, *"I would never do this on my own; too many questions and some are confusing."* My father was more charitable: *"This is just a tool, and people need tools like this. It's well-thought out."* When we were done walking through each step of the site, it produced a summary of my father's wishes and an "action plan" but was unable to convert this to an official Texas advance directive, although he could convert it (with additional steps) to some other states' official forms.

At the end of our two-hour advance care planning marathon, my chattering children returned, along with the demands of the day. While I found myself exhausted, I'd learned several important lessons walking through this exercise with my parents. First, and most important, I understood my parents' wishes and heard some clarification on several issues. The second lesson was just how much time, effort, and careful guidance it took to arrive at a full understanding.

I am sure that my own clinical experiences directed where our conversation traveled, having watched decline and death manifest in so many different ways.

And it was evident that two hours and one conversation wasn't enough. Advance care planning is a process; it is iterative and evolving. Once and done is rarely enough.

In my own practice, I aim to document ongoing conversations about values and goals with all my patients as their illness progresses. I encourage everyone to document a health care proxy along with the values and goals that should guide others in decision-making. For any patient who wants specific treatment limitations (e.g., no attempts at resuscitation, feeding tubes, or prolonged ventilation), I offer to provide a legal medical order (such as a POLST or out-of-hospital DNR), and I encourage them to document their wishes in a version of a living will.

FAMILY MEETINGS: HOW TO DISCUSS ADVANCE CARE PLANNING WITH THE PATIENT'S FAMILY

We have discussed how to talk with patients' families about advance care planning when the patient can participate. Even more difficult situations can arise with patients who lose decision-making capacity and who have not told you or their family their advance care plans, have not given you any advance directive forms, and have not discussed with you their wishes about artificial life support or resuscitation. You are then forced to discuss these issues with family members or loved ones whom you may or may not have met. The experiences I (*Janet Abrahm*) had with the families of Mr. Madison and Mr. Jordan illustrate many of the problems that arise in such situations, as well as the techniques for addressing them. The advice on holding family meetings in these situations, which was offered in the book *Mastering Communication with Seriously Ill Patients* (Back, Arnold, et al. 2009), based in part on *How to Break Bad News* (Buckman 1992), was key. The steps we included were:

1. Hold a pre-meeting with all the patient's health care providers to establish consensus on best choices and identify family decision-maker(s). When there is disagreement about prognosis among providers, seek to find consensus on the best case / worst case / most likely case (Taylor et al. 2017). Ensure that key personnel can be present for the meeting, including someone who knows the current medical details and, ideally, someone from the outpatient team who has a longitudinal relationship with the patient and family.

2. Find a site and a seat for all participants and have tissues available.

3. Ask participants to introduce themselves and their roles.

4. Ask the family to review with you how they think the patient is doing and what they see as the problems.

5. Ask the family what they think is likely to happen.

6. Ask the family what they hope and fear will happen.

7. Let each person who wishes to speak do so.

8. Validate the family's understanding, or if needed, further clarify the patient's current medical condition in global terms first, using lay language.

9. Discuss the current prognosis; a frame of best case/worst case/most likely case can work well to discuss prognosis (Taylor et al. 2017).

10. Answer questions about the medical condition, using lay language; check for understanding frequently.

11. Ask the family again, in light of this new information, what they hope and fear will happen.

12. Delineate any key differences in priorities among the patient, health care proxy, and medical care team.

13. Explain to the family what is possible and what is likely.

14. Work to achieve consensus.

15. Address, provide space for, and validate emotions as they arise.

16. Document the personnel present, key information gained, and next steps.

(Back, Arnold, et al. 2009; Buckman 1992)

The Role of the Pre-Meeting

A pre-meeting was the key to resolving the dilemma of how to proceed with the care of John Madison, a patient I had cared for over several weeks before his admission to the ICU. A pre-meeting helped the care team come to a consensus and decide how to communicate their concerns to Mr. Madison's wife, Alana.

John Madison was a 56-year-old man with refractory progressive pancreatic cancer. He had spent six weeks recuperating from a series of infectious complications related to his chemotherapy and was stable enough for discharge to a rehabilitation facility when he developed a pulmonary embolus and was intubated. His wife had brought him more than a thousand miles from their home in Barbados, hoping that he was eligible for an experimental treatment. He had made her promise, however, that she would not let him die in this strange city, that she would bring him home if he got worse.

We had met the Madisons weeks before the intubation, when we were asked to help with his pain management. We had spent many hours talking with Alana. During these talks, Alana described John as the love of her life and the man who had rescued her from terrible social and financial circumstances (the details of which she declined to share).

The ICU attending physician, Dr. Bush, and the social worker, Nancy Lopez, asked us to participate in a family meeting that was being held because Alana was distraught. John could communicate with her by writing her notes, and he repeatedly begged her to take him home. Alana was asking everyone she could find to help her locate and pay for a medical flight so that John could die at home, as she had promised him. Our palliative care team asked Dr. Bush, Nancy, and John's nurses to have a short (15-minute) pre-meeting with us before we all met with Alana.

A pre-meeting ideally includes the attending physician, key consultants, and the social worker, nurses, and chaplain who know the family well. It should also include a representative of the outpatient team who has a long-term relationship with the patient and family and an interpreter for patients or family members with limited English proficiency or who use American Sign Language. During this meeting, the group members review what they know about the patient's medical condition and likely prognosis, how much and how the family and patient want to be involved in making decisions, and what they know of his values and goals, either from direct communications with him or from his family. They also discuss what they know about his family's goals and values, especially those of his health care proxy, and determine whether there are key differences between these values and the patient's. If there is no health care proxy, they try to identify the best surrogate decision-maker for the patient.

Finally, at the pre-meeting the team members discuss their own agendas and how they match the priorities of the patient and his family. The group then determines what information is missing that the patient's family can supply. If the group members feel they know enough, they can come to a consensus on a draft of a plan of care or medically reasonable options to offer during the family meeting.

The "Third Story"

In our pre-meeting, though, it became clear that the ICU team members did *not* agree on what the meeting with Alana should accomplish, and it wasn't clear why. As the palliative care consultant, I realized that I might need to bring more to the group than what Alana and John had shared with us prior to his ICU admission.

I thought I might need to use a strategy I learned from Stone and colleagues (2010), who advise that we "Move from certainty to curiosity . . . to understand the other person's story." To paraphrase: *What could they know or believe that will help you make sense of what they're saying?* I realized that I needed to understand the "story" of each member of the medical team, and to share with them any differences I found among their stories. If necessary, I was prepared to create for them what Stone and coauthors call the "Third Story." The Third Story accommodates all the facts in the first two stories and offers a different interpretation that allows for different conclusions. I find that in my role as palliative care consultant, the Third Story is often what breaks up the logjams; it releases the two sides from their dug-in positions and enables them to adopt a solution they can both agree on.

Understanding each of the ICU team members' stories was the first step. I asked what each of them thought was most important to Mr. Madison's care. It turned out that Nancy's priority was Alana and John's relationship and the work that needed to be done before he died. She wanted to focus on the futility of Alana's quest and on counseling her to use the time they had left discussing the things they needed to say to each other. Mr. Madison's nurses, however, wanted most for the team to respect John's wishes by supporting Alana's efforts to get them home. Dr. Bush surprised everyone. He revealed for the first time to all of us that what made him unwilling to even consider sending John home was his concern that he would not be able to find a hospital in Barbados that could deliver care comparable to the care John was receiving in our ICU, and that he would be condemning John to a terrible death.

In this case, I did not need to create a Third Story. Once they understood Dr. Bush's concern, everyone agreed that should be a main focus of the family meeting. And Dr. Bush realized that he had found the words that would convey to Alana how seriously he took his obligation to John. We all decided that Nancy would first offer her thoughts to Alana, and then Dr. Bush would explain why he needed to transfer John to a comparable facility in his home country.

We were now ready to meet with Alana. Alana listened to Nancy's concerns but told her that their "good time" had occurred when John was recuperating; what was happening now was a nightmare. Alana repeated her request that we help her take John home by financing the plane ride and contacting the appropriate home services.

Only when Dr. Bush talked to Alana about their shared ideas of duty to Mr. Madison was Alana finally able to understand our reluctance to send him home.

> *Alana, you have very eloquently explained to us the duty you owe John. You promised you would not let him die here, and you are doing everything you can to keep that promise. But I have a duty to him, too. I cannot send him somewhere that cannot give him the level of comfort we can give him here. If you can find a physician back home who agrees to accept him for care in a local ICU, and I satisfy myself that John can get the care he needs there, I would be happy to help him get a flight home.*

For the first time since Mr. Madison had been admitted to the ICU, Alana seemed to sense the team's compassion for her and her husband. She understood the concern that prompted Dr. Bush's resistance to the transfer and agreed that she wouldn't take John home unless it could be to an ICU.

When You Have Never Met the Family

Although our palliative care team had known Alana and John Madison for some time before his admission to the ICU, we had never met Mr. Jordan's family. They did not even know that Mr. Jordan had cancer and had been undergoing chemotherapy treatments. Weissman and colleagues provide tools for these discussions in two Fast Facts titled "Helping Surrogates Make Decisions" and "The Family Meeting: End-of-Life Goal Setting and Future Planning" (Weissman, Quill, and Arnold 2010a, 2010b).

Mr. Jordan had just begun treatment for an aggressive large-cell lymphoma. He was the 70-year-old patriarch of a large family, with many children, grandchildren, and great-grandchildren. His oncologist told us that Mr. Jordan wouldn't let her speak with any of his family members. He said that he had not wanted his family to treat him any differently because of his illness, and he felt that this would inevitably occur if she spoke with his wife or anyone in his family. He had also not given clear answers to questions about resuscitation or being maintained by artificial means.

Practice Points: Advance Care Planning with Families When the Patient Cannot Participate

- When you don't know the patient's wishes, consider consulting the palliative care team to help you hold a family meeting. Ask the family to help you determine what the patient would have wanted. Consider asking, "What would your mom say if she were here with us?"
- When you know the patient's wishes, share these with the family and ask the family whether the patient told them the same information. If all are in agreement, assure the family members that you will honor these wishes. Do not ask families, "What do you want me to do?"
- If the family disagrees with what you know to be the stated wishes of the patient, consider consulting palliative care to work with the treatment team (including the chaplain, social worker, and nurses) and family to resolve the disagreement. Some situations require serial family meetings to come to a consensus.
- If it cannot be resolved in this way, or if there is a disagreement among the treatment team members, obtain an ethics consultation.

Now, Mr. Jordan was intubated, suffering from neutropenic sepsis and pneumonia. His family members were the only ones who might be able to help the ICU team determine what he would have wanted, and our palliative care team was called to assist them. When I first met the Jordans, they were having an anguished family meeting with the chaplain, trying to decide what they should tell the doctors to do. After I introduced myself to the family, I explained that despite what the intern had asked them, they did not have to be the ones to make the decisions, that their ICU team was perfectly prepared and willing to make them, but we needed to know *"What* Mr. Jordan *would have wanted."*

By asking *what the patient would have wanted*, we maintain the ethical principles of Autonomy and Beneficence. *Autonomy* affirms that patients have an absolute right to refuse or accept any offered treatment. If family members can discern the patient's wishes, they will be acting as a *surrogate* for the patient, expressing these wishes since their loved one no longer can. *Beneficence* means that we should act in the best interest of the patient. We exercise beneficence when we use our knowledge of both the long-term and short-term complications and the prognosis to advise the family what we expect the medical outcomes to be.

Families are the experts on the patients as persons: their goals, hopes, fears, and what functional outcomes would not be acceptable to them. Recommendations that clinicians make with all that information in mind do not interfere with patient autonomy; they enhance it (Quill and Brody 1996). For some patients, their family is the locus of their "autonomy." They would never make a serious decision without consultation with them, especially with the respected elders in their family. Nathan Cherny, MBBS, FRACP, FRCP, an internationally known oncologist and palliative care and ethics expert, has developed the concept of relational autonomy to help us work with these patients and their families. He introduces the concepts of voluntary diminished autonomy as well as "soft" and "hard" paternalism (Cherny 2012) that can inform our thinking and serve as an alternative ethical framework for decision-making that is just as valid as the autonomy we are accustomed to.

Shared Decision-Making

Clinicians actually rarely rely solely on the autonomous decisions of the patient. Sharing decision-making is now a critical part of patient-centered care. Shared decision-making can be defined as "a collaborative process that allows patients, or their surrogates, and clinicians to make healthcare decisions together, taking into account the best scientific evidence available, as well as the patient's values, goals, and preferences" (Kon et al. 2016, p. 190). The American College of Critical Care Medicine and the American Thoracic Society Ethics Committee published consensus recommendations for shared decision-making. They suggest that to help patients and surrogates make the best decisions, and to minimize the burden that this responsibility places especially on surrogates, our conversations with families should not only provide medical information and elicit patient values and preferences, but also explore the family's preferred role in decision-making and deliberation (Kon et al. 2016).

Providing Medical Information and Eliciting Preferences

You can enhance this information sharing by setting up a private place for discussion; spending time *listening* rather than talking; acknowledging and addressing their emotions; concentrating on what the patient's values and treatment preferences are; explaining what it means to be the surrogate decision-maker, checking for understanding, and supporting family decisions; reassuring them that you won't allow their loved one to suffer; and making sure that the communication is consistent, no matter which team member is delivering it.

Role in Deliberation and Decision-Making

Families differ in how they want to participate in deliberation and decision-making. For a family suddenly facing such a serious loss, who have never discussed these issues with the patient, the question of what *they* want done can be overwhelming. Some families want us to make all the decisions, some hope to drive the train themselves, but most fall somewhere in between (Kon et al. 2016). Family members who serve in the role of surrogate decision-makers are under enormous stress, and a third of surrogates experience significant anxiety or other psychological problems from the emotional burden. The effects of playing this role usually last for months and may last much longer (Wendler and Rid 2011). Surrogates who served this role in the ICU setting "frequently used terms such as 'difficult,' 'intense,' 'painful,' 'overwhelming,' 'devastating,' and 'traumatic'" (p. 342) and are at risk for developing post-traumatic stress disorder (PTSD).

For a moment, let down your guard and imagine yourself in the position of a family member being asked, *"Do you want us to take your mother off the ventilator?"* It's overwhelming, as though I just threw you a 30-pound bowling ball. You can also understand the answers that families give to clinicians who ask such a question: *"I can't take the responsibility of turning off the machines"*; or *"We can't decide right now. We have to wait until [so-and-so] comes and we discuss it with [him]."*

It became clear as we all worked with Mr. Jordan's family that they wanted the clinical team to make the decisions; it was too much responsibility for any one of them, or even for them collectively to let us know *"What Mr. Jordan would have wanted."* And the team agreed to do that, thereby decreasing the chance that his family would later suffer from PTSD or depression.

Ask-Tell-Ask

In these types of family meetings, you can use the VALUE mnemonic (below) (Shanawani et al. 2008, p. 780) and ask-tell-ask to good effect.

Ask. After introductions of everyone present, address each family member in turn and *ask* how they think the patient is doing and what they think the likely outcome will be. Ask them what is of most concern to them, and what questions they have.

Tell. Only after you have heard from everyone should you begin to *tell*, to answer questions, correct misconceptions, and provide what you think are realistic goals of care. To begin a discussion about prolonging the patient's life using extraordinary measures, you might say:

> *Unfortunately, your [parent, child, spouse, partner, sibling, etc.] never told me directly what she wanted done if the only way she could be kept alive was by being connected to these machines. She never told me what to do if she died—whether the doctors should try to prolong her life at all costs or whether she wanted to be left in peace. As her [physician/NP/PA], carrying out her wishes is an important part of my responsibility to her, which I am happy to do. And I need your help to determine what she would have wanted.*
>
> *If she were sitting here with us in this room, what do you think she would say? Did she ever let any of you know how she felt, possibly while watching a medical TV show? Did she ever comment on relatives or friends who were resuscitated or needed machines to keep them alive? Sometimes people say things like, "I would never want to be kept alive if I had a disease that couldn't be made better," or "If I go, just let me be. At least I'd have my dignity, not like [so-and-so], who was on those machines for months before he finally died." Other people say they want any chance at living as long as possible no matter what the quality may be.*

Practice Point: The VALUE Mnemonic

V = Value statements made by family members.
A = Acknowledge emotions.
L = Listen to family members.
U = Understand who the patient is as a person.
E = Elicit questions from family members.

Ask. At this point, you can *ask* again. Ask what they're taking away from the discussion so far. This may feel like the right time to begin to explore how they want to be involved in the deliberations and decision-making. Ask how their family typically makes big decisions. Ensure that you have answered all their questions, paraphrase what you heard them say, and ask for corrections or any additional material. And ask what you can do for them now.

You can offer a visit with a chaplain or determine whether they simply want to be left alone to talk as a family. After the group breaks up, one of the palliative care team, often the social worker, can stay with the family to help them with practical issues and continue the exploration of their preferences about shared decision-making.

Conflict

Conflicts between family members, between the family as a whole and the medical team, or between medical team members are common, especially when withdrawal of life support is being considered. One study found that either the physician or surrogate identified conflict in 63 percent of ICU cases (Schuster et al. 2014). Moral distress can also result from asking critical care providers to continue aggressive care that they feel is futile, and moral distress is associated with burnout (Fumis et al. 2017). We discuss burnout further in Chapter 13.

Practice Points for a Family Meeting

- Pre-meeting
  - Hold a pre-meeting with all the patient's health care providers to establish consensus on best choices and to identify family decision-makers. Ensure that key personnel can be present for the meeting, including someone who knows the current medical details and, ideally, someone from the outpatient team who has had a longitudinal relationship with the patient and family. Find a site and seats (or room for the bed) for all participants, including the patient if the patient wants to be present. Introduce everyone present. During the meeting, let each person in the family who wishes to speak do so.
- ASK
  - Ask the family to review with you how they think the patient is doing and what they see as the problems.
  - Ask the family what they think is likely to happen.
  - Ask the family what they hope for and what they fear will happen.
- TELL
  - Explain the patient's current medical condition in global terms first, using lay language, and clarify the current prognosis.
  - Answer questions about the medical condition, using lay language; check for understanding frequently.
- ASK
  - Ask the family again, in light of this new information, what they hope and what they fear will happen.
  - Delineate any key differences in priorities among the patient, health care proxy, and medical care team.
  - Explain to the family what is possible and what is likely.
- Work to achieve consensus.
- Document the personnel present, key information gained, results, and next steps in the electronic medical record as well as in the written chart.
- If the patient has asked not to be present, choose someone or a group to inform the patient about the results of the meeting.

Carefully run meetings among the staff or between the staff and family members can resolve these conflicts. Stone and colleagues (2010, pp. 145–46 and 206.) provide helpful suggestions for approaching meetings in which we know there will be conflict. They suggest that we have three purposes in the meeting (pp. 145–46): "Learning their story; expressing your views and feelings; problem-solving together." They advise us again to move toward a learning conversation: "You can't move the conversation in a more positive direction until the other person feels heard and understood" (p. 206).

Practice Points: Learning Conversations

- You no longer have a message to deliver, but rather have some information to share and some questions to ask.
- Arguing without understanding is never persuasive.
- People almost never change without first feeling understood.
- We have to understand the other person's story well enough to see how their conclusions make sense within it.

(Adapted from Stone, Patton, and Heen 2010)

Back, Arnold, and Tulsky (2009) advise much as Stone and coauthors do (and in fact quote Stone et al., as you'll see below), that if we recognize there is a conflict, we should try to be curious: why is their answer to the same problem so different from ours? Stone would say, "What else do I need to know for that to make more sense?" or "I wonder how I can understand the world in such a way that that would make sense?"

As Back, Arnold, and Tulsky write (p. 95): "Ask yourself: why is this otherwise well-meaning person wanting something different in this situation than what I want? The well-meaning attribution is important . . . You will not be successful if the other person feels dismissed." Stone and coauthors offer: "It's always the right time to listen." Reframing may work, but if there's emotion, your best tools are listening, questioning, and trying to understand, not defend.

Here is the "Roadmap" that Back, Arnold, and Tulsky offer for dealing with meetings when there's conflict (pp. 95–98):

1. Notice there is a disagreement . . . You may notice that you feel irritated, or "bored" ("This again?") or exasperated—your internal signals may be the most useful sensors for noticing conflict.

2. Find a nonjudgmental starting point . . . Why is this otherwise well-meaning person wanting something different in this situation than what I want?

3. Listen to and acknowledge the other person's story/concern/viewpoint . . . Douglas Stone describes three things to listen for: (1) their story about what has happened; (2) the emotions (theirs and yours) generated by what happened; and (3) their view of their identity—how does it shape their views. They add: "If the block to their listening is that they don't feel heard, then the way to remove that block is by helping them feel heard—by bending over backwards to listen to what they have to say, and perhaps most important, by demonstrating that you understand what they are saying and how they are feeling . . . unexpressed feelings can block the ability to listen."

4. Identify what the conflict is about and try to articulate it as shared.

5. Brainstorm options that address the shared concern.

6. Look for options that recognize the interests of everyone involved.

7. Remember that not every conflict can be resolved.

Of course, sometimes a family tells the medical team that they don't care if the patient did not want life support, they want everything done anyway. In fact, that's not an uncommon reason for calling a palliative care consult. The family members may cite religious beliefs that mandate doing everything to stay alive, hopes for a miracle, or a belief that no matter what the patient told the health care team, they know what the patient really wanted. Some may be simply unable to imagine life without their loved one.

Engaging social workers and other counselors; asking clergy to provide spiritual support and a forum for voicing religious beliefs and values; and having a proactive approach to medical decision-making may all provide support for these families (Widera et al. 2011). These colleagues can both support the family and help you unravel unspoken concerns so that you eventually reach a mutually agreeable plan. Spiritual concerns are addressed further in Chapter 3.

Ongoing attention to the patient's comfort, frequent check-ins with the family to see how they are doing, and exploration of new concerns as they arise help the family during their anticipatory grieving process, promote trust in clinicians, and can lead to the family seeing that the hoped-for recovery is not going to take place. We discuss in Chapter 3 how to help the families who are hoping for a miracle.

ETHICS CONSULTATIONS

If conflict persists after all attempts to improve communication, then consider asking for an ethics consult (Kon et al. 2016). Many hospitals have an ethics committee that develops guidelines (that are then approved by all clinical services) in such areas as advance care directives, withholding or withdrawing life-sustaining treatment, consent from patients with limited decision-making capacity, medical futility in care at the end of life, and disclosure of adverse events. Some hospitals also have individuals specially trained in medical ethics who are able to provide consultation services to help the dissenting parties come to a consensus about the path to take.

The ethics consultant (who can be a physician, nurse, social worker, chaplain, or nonclinician specializing in medical ethics) first interviews the medical caregivers (including all members of the medical team) and then the patient and family. He or she clarifies the medical history and hospital course of the patient, the facts of the situation in dispute, the values that are in conflict, the medical options that are available, and the reasons for the disagreement. If the dispute is between groups of caregivers (e.g., the nursing staff versus the doctors), the consultant will interview each group separately. If the conflict is between the caregivers and the patient or family, the consultant will interview all the caregivers together.

After the caregiver interviews, the ethics consultant interviews the patient and family, including the health care proxy, first to review the history leading up to the present conflict, and then to determine what they understand to be the facts, what they feel their options are, what they hope and fear will happen, what they feel would be the patient's wishes and values as they apply to this situation, and what they believe are the reasons for the disagreement with the caregivers.

After concluding these meetings, the consultant often discovers misunderstandings that can be clarified, or heretofore unidentified common ground that can lead to a solution. The consultant then facilitates a meeting between the two groups with this information in mind, working to reach a consensus between warring parties. References in the online bibliography provide more information about ethics consultations.

SUMMARY

As this chapter illustrates, the early days after a diagnosis of a serious illness hold many challenges for patients and their clinicians. You must learn to recognize which conversations are likely to be difficult and why. You need to prepare yourself to tell patients bad news and then do so, clearly and compassionately, accepting whatever reaction ensues, be it despair, anger, or silence. There is no better way to demonstrate at the outset your commitment to being there to help.

As you begin to understand why you might be reluctant to raise the subject of advance care planning and prognosis, you will be better able to initiate conversations about the future early, and to discuss a prognosis that may be limited. Knowing patients' priorities and goals, you can conduct effective meetings using well-established techniques, particularly supporting families to honor patients' wishes when they are no longer able to communicate their choices. When you don't know, you can employ shared decision-making and the ask-tell-ask methods to elucidate them. When goals differ, palliative care and ethics consultation teams can help create a path forward.

Innovative programs that train all practitioners who care for patients with cancer in these communication skills should create providers who are as well prepared to conduct these tough discussions as they are to give chemotherapy and treat its side effects. Such preparation, and the ability to grieve their losses, may protect oncology and palliative care practitioners from compassion fatigue, and help them have long, productive careers.

CHAPTER 2

Working with Patients' Families

with Arden O'Donnell, MPH, MSW, LICSW, APHSW-C

A cancer diagnosis transforms patients, but it also alters the lives of their families and friends. Our patients are members of much larger family systems that both influence our patients and are influenced by them. As people get sicker, the importance and influence of family increases, usually reaching an apex when patients can no longer make decisions for themselves. Oncology and palliative care teams naturally include care for the family as a unit, but broadening our focus to the issues presented by some families can feel more complex than treating the patient. We will always have the expertise of our social work, chaplain, and psychiatry colleagues to help us care for the most challenging families, but it is surprising how much physicians, nurse practitioners, and physician assistants can do on our own if we understand the basics of how families function and the important roles we play during times of transition and terminal illness.

Drawing from the field of social work and research on family therapy, this chapter provides tools, case examples, and insights to help you and your team navigate family dynamics and optimize communication with all families. We discuss family assessment tools and present a model you can use to assess family dynamics and to increase the overall effectiveness of your interactions and meetings with family members. We provide a section describing the various ways families seem "difficult" for us to work with and highlight the need for expert help when families struggle with a history of mental illness, substance use disorder, or family violence. The primary author of this chapter, Arden O'Donnell, MPH, MSW, LICSW, APHSW-C, adds her personal insights and recommendations throughout, and our colleague Jessica Goldhirsch, LCSW, MSW, MPH, contributed to the discussion of partnering with interpreters.

FAMILY STRUCTURE

Identifying Key Family Members

In today's world, *family* comes in different forms and can be defined in many ways. The best way to find out whom patients consider "family" is to ask them directly who the important people in their life are. Knowing whom they consider family, and which of these people should be involved in decision-making, is essential. Many times, a social worker or nurse will be able to provide you with a good assessment of family structure, dynamics, and overall functioning. If this is not the case, you can collect a reasonable amount of information through a few questions and with careful observation. Asking some open-ended questions during the assessment can gather a good amount of information. Always ask questions in the broadest way, such as *"Tell me about who you consider your family"* or *"Who are the most important people in your life that will support you through this?"* Asking if someone has a "partner or significant other" can also broaden the answers you receive and quickly indicate you are open to nontraditional ways of thinking of family. This type of questioning allows for inclusion of the LBGTQ community and also invites individuals to tell you about a significant relationship that is not a spouse.

We can also gather information from observing the dynamics in the room, even in a short interaction. As a social worker, as soon as I (*Arden O'Donnell*) walk into a room, I begin to gather information about the family system. Who is in the room? Who is referenced but missing? Whom does the patient look to for leadership? Is there tension in the room? Does this family speak to each other with respect? Are there significant pictures or cultural or religious objects in the room?

I do this because I know the consequences of not considering the patient as a part of a dynamic family system. We have all been in situations when we have spent a significant amount of time and energy with a patient and then a key family player arrived, or a belief surfaced, and we had to start all over again. I also know that an important part of a patient's end-of-life work requires mending

---

Practice Points: Key Areas to Explore about Each Family

- Who is in the family? Who are the key players and who needs to be involved in information sharing and decision-making?
- What are the significant relationships and dynamics in the family? What role does this patient play? What are the key family stories around illness and death?
- What is the family's basic level of functioning?
- What are the spiritual and cultural beliefs of the family and how do these influence decisions about treatment and goals of care?

and honoring past relationships (personal and spiritual), and that estrangements, conflicts, and guilt can influence end-of-life decision-making.

I remember working with Mrs. Simone, a 76-year-old woman with ovarian cancer, who was making decisions about the placement of a G-tube. When her husband and son were visiting, she presented as upbeat and positive, but as soon as they left, she was tearful and anxious. After several days, I uncovered Mrs. Simone's family secret: she had another son, who was estranged and living in California. Although she could not tell her family, Mrs. Simone longed to see or speak to her son one last time; she needed help to work through her feelings about the past estrangement, perhaps to forgive him or herself, to prepare for the end of her life.

The Family as a System

This chapter provides tools to help you quickly assess significant family dynamics and common family roles. Yet, clinicians also need some familiarity with how whole families work. Not all clinicians are expected to be therapists, of course, but understanding the underlying principles of family systems theory will enable you to identify a family's strengths and areas of difficulty, which can in turn help you understand why patients make the choices they make.

Bowen's family system theory views the family as an emotional unit that functions as a system (Kerr 2000; Bowen Center, www.thebowencenter.org). Members of a family seek attention, approval, and support from each other while also reacting to each other's pain, anger, and expectations. This connection and reactivity contributes to a family's interdependence on one another. Additionally, the family system is balanced like a scale. As stress or problems arise, the system can become unbalanced, which can disrupt family roles, routines, and expectations, causing chaos. For example, if one person's anxiety increases, the other family members react. While some may try to fix the situation, others may move away; either way the entire system is affected. Although we cannot concern ourselves with every emotional shift in the family system, it is important to remember that the patient is an individual who is also deeply interconnected to a dynamic family unit. The best outcomes can be achieved when our care, communication interventions, and support are directed both at individual patients and to the family as a group (Northouse et al. 2010; Steele and Davies 2015).

Family Roles

A *role* is a collection of behaviors, attitudes, responsibilities, and *expectations* related to a particular niche a person fills and is important to family functioning (Epstein et al. 1993; Radina 2018). These roles can be associated with a relationship, such as spouse or daughter, but can also be associated with function, such as caregiver (Quinn 2012). Social role theory argues that people's behavior is affected by social expectations, group interactions, and the anticipation of rewards and punishments. Families, cultures, and society have certain relationships based on role expectations. While each family is unique and may not fit every category, members of families do play roles. And having a sense of the role of the patient and key family members can greatly help you navigate family meetings and assist and support a family through decision-making processes (Mynatt and Mowery 2013; Quinn 2012). Below are some common roles you are likely to find people playing. Look for them as you get to know your patients' families.

Patriarch or Matriarch

Some families have one member who is the dominant decision-maker and is seen by everyone as the person in control. When the patriarch or matriarch is the patient and they are unable to make decisions, you can expect the family to struggle with decision-making. That was the case with Olive's family.

Olive was a 75-year-old woman who had run her family of five children for 50 years. Her attending physician called us in, saying, *"I've held three family meetings in the last two days, and each time, family members argued and contradicted each other. After all that, we still couldn't make any decisions."*

I held an informal family meeting and asked about what was happening. I learned that despite the delirium their mother was experiencing, she was barking orders, and they were jumping to meet her needs and fighting over who was doing the most. I asked them, *"Can someone tell me what role your mom played in the family?"* and they all shouted out *"Boss!" "Leader!" "President!"* The siblings said their father was passive and unable to make family decisions. This was clearly a pack that had lost its leader and that had yet to establish who would take over.

Once this was brought to light, the care team could support the family's transition into new family leadership. The team reinforced that Olive had named Maureen, her eldest daughter, as her health care proxy because Olive trusted her daughter to do what her mother would have wanted. So if they allowed Maureen to represent them, they would be fulfilling Olive's wishes, as Maureen expressed them. In this way, I hoped that the family would accept the transition of leadership for the time they were in the hospital. The family discussed this among themselves and agreed that no one knew better than Maureen what Olive's wishes were, and that therefore she could speak for the family. The team's consistent reliance on Maureen during family meetings helped the family move the leadership role to her, and the family meetings became much less chaotic.

Family Spokesperson / Peacekeeper

Some families have one person who serves as the central communicator. This individual helps maintain connections among all members of the family and manages conflict or difficult relationships when they arise. When this mediator is sick, families often struggle with how to talk to one another. I once met with a family

in the ICU who was struggling with withdrawing the ventilator from their wife/
mother. At one point, the woman's daughter said, *"We don't know what we will do
without her; she is like the hub of our family. She keeps us all connected to each other.
I wouldn't know what was going on with anyone if it was not for Mom!"*

After reflecting back to her that it sounded like she was afraid the family would
stop communicating if her mother were gone, we discussed thinking about how
communication could continue if the patient were not here. As the family began
to volunteer ideas of how they could each take a piece of this role, they began to
shift from fear of losing her to strategies of how they could keep her alive in spirit
by honoring her commitment and keeping the family connected.

Teams who see that the family has lost a peacekeeper or communicator can
help them by working to make it possible for all members of the family who
should be present to attend family meetings. It is also helpful to have someone,
often a social worker, talk with individual family members prior to meetings so
that they can articulate their questions and feelings, feel prepared to ask their
questions, and have all of them answered. The social worker can take the family
spokesperson/peacekeeper role temporarily and help family members to assume
pieces of the role.

Caretaker/Protector

The caretaker often takes responsibility for the emotional well-being of the family
and may serve as a protector, working tirelessly to shield family members from
unnecessary pain or discomfort. They may also be the primary caregiver to the
patient, and they are looked to for issues surrounding quality of life. When the
caretaker is the one who is sick, it is often difficult for her to accept help. Caretak-
ers may also have a desire to die quickly to relieve the family of financial or caregiving burdens. One patient lamented, *"I can't get another procedure; it is too much
for my husband. He can't take care of me—I have always taken care of him. Sometimes
I feel like I should just stop all of this. I can't bear being a burden to my family."* You
will need to encourage these patients to accept caregiving from family, and you
will need to support and teach the newly identified family caregivers how best to
care for the patient.

Sibling Positions

Other key family roles can be linked to the sibling position (Kerr 2000). While
these can vary, the idea is that people who grow up in certain sibling positions
have common characteristics. Oldest siblings, sometimes characterized as "the
heroes," tend to hold leadership positions. These children usually assumed the
parental role when the parent was not present in childhood and are looked to for
support in decision-making (Kerr 2000). The eldest are often health care proxies.
When you recognize this person in a family, it can be helpful in discussions of
care goals to ask, respectfully, that the other siblings be allowed to offer their

opinions. It may be the only way they feel able to express a contrary view. I once asked a woman what she thought about the decision not to turn off her mother's implantable cardioverter defibrillator (ICD) and she said, referring to the "hero," *"I don't agree, but my sister gets to decide, just like she always has."*

The youngest children tend to be more willing followers and can play the role of "the comics." Those in this helpful role can make a joke or comment that can ease family tension during a conflict or provide an outlet for emotional pain. Most of the time, the comics are great to have in a family meeting because they can bring in humor to lighten the mood, which can also open space for further conversations. Middle children play different roles depending on the characteristics of the other children and have varying degrees of authority.

Sometimes you will find a child in the role of the "lost child." A *lost child* is a sibling who may have been "lost" to substance use disorder or mental illness, but they are still loved. Though they hold little authority within the family, they are people the family feel they need to protect. In one family, our failure to recognize the lost child led to repeated bouts of family chaos. She spent the night with her father every night, and we thought she was the person the family looked to for updates from us. So, each morning the team would come in and give her the updates. After two mornings of post-rounds family chaos, we realized that this sweet daughter had a history of an anxiety disorder and would call the family after the team came in and give them anxiety-driven misinformation. The family, of course, would rush to the hospital and demand a team meeting. Things calmed down when we realized that and began to round on the patient only after other family members had arrived.

Other informal roles that have been identified in the health care setting are the medical expert, the patient wishes expert, the primary caregiver, and the out-of-towner (Quinn et al. 2012). While there is not space to detail every potential role, the identification and understanding of the function of these roles can guide how to support the family discussions and decision-making (Quinn et al. 2012)

Practice Points: Questions Related to Family Roles

- Identify the role that the patient plays in the family: *"Can you help me understand more about who your mother was in the family and to each of you?"* (Back et al. 2007)
- How is the patient affected by [his or her partner/parent/child]'s role in the family?
- How will this family function without this patient? Who will step into the role they played?
- Whose role is missing from family meetings? Consider assigning a family spokesperson if this person appears to be absent.

Using a Genogram to Map Relationships among Family Members

Information about a family can be gathered in many ways, but one useful information-gathering technique is to construct a genogram. Although few clinicians take the time to draw out a genogram, an understanding of the concept and what questions one would ask to create one can give you a conceptual reference for how and how well the family works, what challenges it is facing, and what unfinished business it has. Answers to all these questions will help you care for your patient as a part of that family.

Genograms are schematic diagrams by which you can represent family members and their relationships to one another, usually spanning three generations (Figure 2.1). Men are represented by squares and women by circles, with their age in the middle of the shape; the patient is indicated by a double circle or double square. You can also include dates of marriages and deaths. What makes the genogram dynamic and helpful, especially for family meetings when the patient's disease is far advanced, is that the diagram shows who is close to whom, who is cut off from whom and how long ago, and where there are areas of conflict. It can detail relevant family illnesses and deaths and the family members' previous experiences with these, where the family members are living now, and even the coping mechanisms of the patient and family (McGoldrick, Gerson, and Petry 2008).

Genograms can be helpful in working with families who seem to be stuck, as you'll see in Matt and Sally's case. Matt was a 62-year-old man with refractory

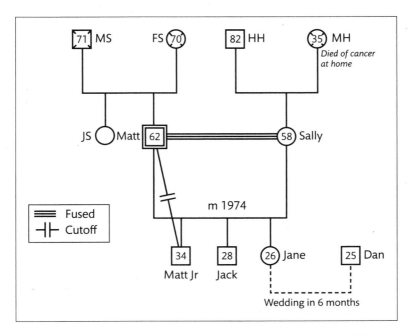

FIGURE 2.1. Sample Genogram. A diagram documenting family relationships

lung cancer. He had been admitted for pain control, and this had been achieved with the help of our palliative care team. The physician on our team asked me (*Arden O'Donnell*) to meet with this family because she thought they were very anxious and that Matt's wife, Sally, always seemed to have a reason to delay Matt's discharge. Even Matt's children, Jane and Jack, could not understand what the problem was; they thought he was ready for discharge home with hospice care.

To help me solve this riddle, I needed to know more about this family, so I created the genogram shown in Figure 2.1. To begin it, I drew the patient, 62-year-old Matt, as a double square near the center of the diagram. Matt had one sister, JS (one could add sibling family and details if there were significant connections or disconnections, but that was not the case here). He and Sally were married in 1974 and had three children. So I drew two vertical lines from Matt and Sally's icons and connected them with a horizontal line with this date above it and then drew vertical lines dropping down from that horizontal line, to add Matt and Sally's children below them: 26-year-old Jane is the daughter (I drew a circle with her age in it), 28-year-old Jack is the middle son (same process, but with a square), and Matt Jr. is the elder son.

As I sketched out the genogram with Sally and Matt, the first thing it revealed was the existence of their older son, Matt Jr., whom they had not mentioned before. Matt became tearful speaking about Matt Jr., sharing that they'd had a falling out two years ago, around the time of his diagnosis. When I learned that, I marked the line connecting Matt to Matt Jr. with slash marks to denote this ruptured relationship. I was able to provide education in the moment to Sally and Matt about the importance of revisiting difficult situations that had occurred in the past and reinforced how healing this can be. Matt also shared that the upcoming marriage of his daughter (which I designated with a dotted line to her fiancé, Dan) was an important family event. Throughout the interview and in the nursing assessment, it was clear that Sally and Matt were close, showing signs of *enmeshment*, discussed later in this chapter. I added three parallel lines directly between their icons on the diagram, to indicate an intensely close bond, a so-called fused relationship.

As the conversation progressed, Sally revealed that her mother had died of cancer at 35, when Sally was only 16 years old, which gave me an opportunity to ask her directly about that experience for her (never discussed before). Sally tearfully told me that her mother had died at home, but glancing at Matt in bed, she quickly brushed off her tears, saying, "I was very young when that happened." Her father was 82 and still living, though both of Matt's parents had died. I placed their initials next to squares or circles containing X's, which represent their deaths, and added their ages when they had died.

Armed with the information I now had, I simply needed to follow the clear roadmap they had given me during our conversation, a roadmap that highlighted where they needed help. First, I sought out Sally alone and revisited the death of her mother. She revealed tearfully the story of her mother's death at home, one that Sally felt was filled with suffering, along with Sally's own feelings of helplessness trying to care for her. Sally said that she has never even been able to reenter the room in which her mother had died. She was sure that if she took her husband home, he, too, would suffer, and she would be helpless to prevent that. While she was feeling guilty for not wanting to take him home, she felt she could not tell him or their children the reasons. It is no wonder that she repeatedly "blocked discharge."

Next, I was able to revisit with Matt his relationship with his oldest son and help him and his family navigate the complexities of helping to repair this ruptured bond. After this conversation, the nurse noticed a decrease in Matt's anxiety.

The genogram also helped the team with decision planning. When Sally and Jane asked whether a feeding tube would make Matt stronger, rather than discuss the benefits and burdens of a feeding tube in a vacuum, the team was able to ask them directly whether what they hoped for was that the feedings would help Matt be strong enough to attend Jane's upcoming wedding. They agreed that that was, in fact, the underlying question, since Matt had never expressed any hunger or desire for the tube. We explained that it was unlikely that a feeding tube would achieve that goal and then supported the family during the difficult conversation that followed, which centered on ways to include Matt in the wedding even if he could not be there in person.

Later in the week, with Sally's permission, I helped her share with her family what she told me about her experience with her mother's dying at home. Both Matt and the children immediately understood, as did the medical team. Since Matt was not yet in his last weeks, Sally wanted to take him home and felt relieved that she had her family's support in making a plan that would include a transfer to an inpatient hospice facility for his last days.

The construction of a genogram is not needed in most situations, but I have found that with complex families or families like Matt and Sally who appear to be "stuck," it provides a graphic roadmap indicating places that would benefit from an intervention. I have also found that the graphic depiction uncovers family patterns and dynamics that don't come to light in a verbal family history.

Practice Points: Things to Listen for as You Complete a Genogram

- Who is listed on the genogram but not present?
- Are there any major conflicts, cut-offs, or estrangements?
- Are there any strong bonds in the family?
- Are there any significant deaths? If so, how does the patient feel about them? How might these feelings affect views on the current situation?

ASSESSING FAMILY FUNCTIONING

What Is Normal?

In times of transition and crisis, even the most functional families can buckle. It is a rare family that doesn't benefit from some sort of additional support during times of extreme stress, but we all know that regardless of the level of stress, some families fare better than others. Can we predict which families will need the most support? Not always, but understanding the basic level of family functioning can help us set realistic expectations for the time and effort each family will need.

Before we head into assessing family functioning, let's consider broadly the types of families we work with. Kissane and colleagues use the Family Environment Scale to measure a family's self-perception of their own cohesiveness, expressiveness, and capacity to deal with conflict (Kissane et al. 2006; Zaider and Kissane 2009). Through this, they classify families into three broad classes (well-functioning, intermediate, and dysfunctional) to help identify which families are at high risk of having an especially difficult bereavement. Data suggest that if we provide basic communication, leadership, and support, more than one-quarter of our patients' families will be able to navigate end-of-life decisions and fare well with minimal additional support from our teams. These well-functioning families are not perfect, but we can assume that they show appropriate affect and attachment to each other (and to us), are capable problem solvers and likely understand our treatment suggestions. These are the families we consider resilient.

Just under half of our patients' families will demonstrate intermediate functioning. They will need some additional support to deal with the complexities of advanced illness, to understand and accept troubling medical information, to navigate the changing roles of family members, or to be successful in their struggles with anticipatory grieving. With the support of regular communication and family meetings as well as short-term intensive support from social workers, psychiatrists, or psychologists around any particularly problematic issues, these families will be able to come together and support the patient.

The remaining 20 percent to 35 percent of our families struggle with family conflicts, or in some cases significant psychological morbidity; these families need additional support (Kramer et al. 2009; Meyer and Block 2011; Zaider and Kissane 2009). Struggling families appear to create crisis even in the most reasonable situations. They "split" (pitting one family member against another, or the physicians against the nurses); they argue; they disagree. Overall, these families have difficulty communicating with each other and, many times, with us (Schuler et al. 2014). They display what we commonly view as irrational and irritating behavior throughout the course of the patient's illness. These families are often viewed as unrealistic and at times hostile, and they may never develop a working alliance with the caregiving team. These are the families who take up the most of our time and leave us feeling exhausted or frustrated or questioning ourselves. These are the families with whom we need to set clear boundaries and expectations. And these are the families for whom we should call in reinforcements—palliative care teams, social workers, or other psychosocial clinicians.

My intent is not to pathologize but rather to acknowledge that a significant percentage of our families need more help than one or two clinicians can give. These families need a social worker or at times a psychiatrist to help the family or the team serving them. Palliative care social workers have expertise in helping families navigate the stresses of end-of-life decisions amid complex family dynamics or larger stressors, such as mental illness, substance use disorder, or trauma histories. Just as you would call in a radiation oncologist when radiation therapy might be needed, when you realize a family might fall into the "dysfunctional" category, you should call in a social worker or, if none is available in your setting, another mental health professional. The next section provides some tools to help you identify these families early in your relationship with them.

Using the Circumplex Model to Assess Family Functioning

We need to have a sense of the family's level of functioning because it can influence a patient's plan of care and even determine how we should interact with family members. The Circumplex Model can help. It is a systems-based theory that focuses on a family's level of (1) *cohesion*, (2) *flexibility*, and (3) *communication* and has served many clinicians as a guide to understanding overall family functioning (Olson, Russell, and Sprenkle 2014). More than 700 studies have been published using this evidenced-based model and the associated Family Adaptability and Cohesion Evaluation Scale (FACES) self-report family assessment tool (Olson 2011).

We learned from these studies that families who score as "balanced" on the scales of cohesion and flexibility are higher functioning than those who are unbalanced (i.e., have very high or very low cohesion or flexibility). Once you learn how to place families in the right position on these scales of functioning, you'll know how best to use the meetings that you and your staff have with them to improve the family's ability to function and to care for the patient during this stressful time.

Level of Family Cohesion

Olson defines family cohesion as "the emotional bonding that family members have towards each other" (Olson 2000, p. 145). Key dimensions of family cohesion are the family's level of *emotional bonding*, how family members balance *togetherness* and *separateness*, standards of *acceptable family boundaries*, and *group decision-making capacity*. Families range from disengaged (very low cohesion), separated (low to medium cohesion), connected (medium to high cohesion), to enmeshed (very high cohesion) (Figure 2.2). The families that work the best are those who are in the middle of the spectrum (i.e., "separated" or "connected").

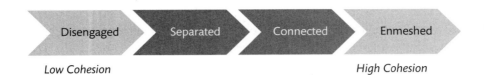

Low Cohesion   *High Cohesion*

FIGURE 2.2. Cohesion: The emotional bonding between members

Disengaged Families

The lack of family cohesion in *disengaged* families can create significant frustration for our teams as we try to talk with them. Members assume rigid roles, and individuals seem separate rather than being attached or committed to each other (Olson, Russell, and Sprenkle 2014). Members of disengaged families have a great deal of personal independence; they tend to grow even more distant to avoid conflict, and they are usually unable to turn to one another for problem solving or support (Olson and Gorall 2003). We see these family members sitting in separate areas of the waiting room and visiting at separate times, and we can be baffled at the lack of information sharing that seems to occur.

When working with one disengaged family, for example, the team had mistakenly assumed that Eileen, the patient's health care proxy, had asked her sisters to attend each of three scheduled family meetings. The team showed up each time, but no one else but Eileen was present. When I asked Eileen if she had called her sisters, I was shocked by her answer: *"I can't. I don't have their numbers."*

With disengaged families, therefore, you should not assume that information shared with one family member will be conveyed to another. Make sure all family meetings involve all the key members of the patient's stated family. You will need to be clear and provide consistent information about the patient's illness and consider encouraging them to find a way to come together, if only temporarily, for the good of the patient. Your social worker can help provide a safe structure in which that can happen.

When they do come together, these families need support, because they minimize interaction with each other to avoid conflict. They don't know how to communicate with each other in good times, and this is a crisis. Your staff or a palliative care social worker may need to help each individual feel safe contributing to the conversation, rather than struggling through disagreement after disagreement or long periods of silence.

Separated Families or Connected Families

Separated and *connected* families are the most "balanced" families, falling in the middle range of the cohesion scale, with good levels of attachment to each other and defined but flexible roles. Though they may disagree with each other, they are generally able to draw on a foundation of trust and caring during times of crisis. Often these families are drawn temporarily closer during an illness. They need some, but not extensive, support from you or your staff.

Enmeshed Families

Enmeshed families are also difficult. They have high levels of cohesion with an extreme amount of emotional closeness with each other. Enmeshed families have diffuse boundaries and seem overly dependent and intrusively involved with each other. Loyalty to the family is demanded and independence strongly discouraged; many times, these families have no clear leadership.

Suspect that you're dealing with an enmeshed family when all family members attend every appointment, when family members speak for each other, and when they use *we* when *I* is more appropriate. These families cannot tolerate disagreement, so they will at times prevent you from starting conversations, such as those about moving to comfort care, that could reveal different opinions. Enmeshed family members seem unable to envision life without any one of their family members, and this can greatly influence the end-of-life decisions of both the patient and the health care proxy.

When working with enmeshed families, social workers understand how difficult it is for one member to share concerns that she feels will not be welcome within the group, and so they will privately seek out the opinions of individuals. Social workers may use the health care team as a model of a functioning group, each of whose members has a definite role, and help families define appropriate roles for each member. Within the family meeting, we need to support everyone's right to speak up, saying something like, *"It is very normal that each of you will have some differing opinions about this, and I would like to hear from each of you."*

These families also tend to protect each other; not only will the patient tell you not to tell his family how sick he is, but his family will forbid you from telling the patient how sick he is!

Practice Points: Questions that Will Lead to Insight into Family Cohesion

- *How close is your family? Are there people in the family the patient is closest to?*
- *How is information shared in your family? When and how did you find out about this illness?*
- *How does your family typically resolve conflict?*

One word of caution: don't mistake frequent checking in with each other, or presence of a large number of family members at the key family meeting with you, as being diagnostic of an enmeshed family. When assessing for level of cohesion, look for patterns of emotional closeness precrisis and be aware of the family's cultural norms. Many families will draw closer emotionally to each other during a crisis, and various cultures have differing levels of closeness. For example, in

general, more White non-Hispanic Americans seem to have high levels of autonomy and independence, while Hispanic families may be more connected, though
they are not necessarily enmeshed.

Level of Family Flexibility

The second guidepost in assessing family function in the Circumplex Model is
family flexibility. Flexibility is measured by how the family can balance *stability*
and *change* (Olson, Russell, and Sprenkle 2014, p. 57). Key elements of this guidepost include family leadership, family negotiation style, relationship rules, and
role relationships. Families range from *rigid* (those with very low flexibility), *structured* (low to medium flexibility), *flexible* (medium to high flexibility), to *chaotic*
(very high flexibility) (Figure 2.3). Here, too, the groups in the middle of the spectrum (*structured* and *flexible*) function the best.

Functional families have good levels of flexibility and are able to interchange
roles based on personal strengths or necessity. For example, if the traditional caregiver of the family is not present, another family member can temporarily shift
into that role. When a patient is dying, however, the family system must adjust
to the loss of the patient in that caregiver role. Depending on the flexibility of the
family and the role the patient held, there is often distress and there can be, at
least temporarily, chaos as the system adjusts even in these healthy families.

Similarly, functional families can adapt to situations that are not stable, by
being flexible and integrating the changes that need to occur. They trust that the
new configuration they will achieve will be a beneficial one and will provide as
much stability as their former configuration. There are likely to be more problems,
however, in families with less or too much flexibility.

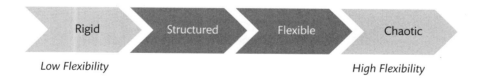

Low Flexibility   High Flexibility

FIGURE 2.3. Flexibility: The ability to balance change

Rigid Families

Families with very low levels of flexibility (*rigid*) are ones that have strict and un-
changing roles; one family member is in charge. Decision-makers are highly controlling; they make most of the decisions, and they are never questioned. These
families have strict rules and boundaries about who does what and when, and
who speaks and when.

If the family decision-maker is the patient, the family can become paralyzed.
For these families, we should make strong recommendations or suggest they
imagine that the patient is still making decisions, using questions like *"If your*

father were sitting here now, what would he say?" If the family decision-maker is the health care proxy, you should not expect other family members to volunteer opinions or for there to be much family discussion; you may need to ask directly what each of the other individuals thinks, and this may not be received well by the decision-maker. You or the social worker should investigate whether there have been family estrangements and whether the social worker is aware of how the family members dealt with other family conflicts.

Often you will discover family alliances or covert strategies they have used to balance their rigidity. This happened with Julia, a 68-year-old woman who was speaking with me before she had a high-risk procedure. I asked if she had ever thought about her advance care directives and whether she would like any limits on her care. *"Oh yes, I have those; in fact, I signed one of those living wills that says I don't want to live on machines. But I never told my husband about it!"*

She went on to explain his role as the decision-maker in their family and their disagreements about her views about code status. She could not stand up to him overtly, but she revealed that in a medical situation, her sister would come forth with the living will. After much work with her, she finally agreed to tell her wishes to her husband in a structured and supported family meeting and allowed us to put her living will in the medical chart.

Structured/Flexible Families

The most balanced families fall into the moderate level of flexibility, either being *structured*, which is characterized by democratic leadership and some sharing of roles, or *flexible*, characterized by a more egalitarian leadership and fluid sharing of roles when needed. These families are viewed as adaptable and able to make decisions, share leadership roles, and see others' points of view.

Chaotic Families

Chaotic families have excessively high levels of flexibility. They are characterized by unclear family roles, limited leadership, and erratic decision-making. These families appear impulsive, and decisions do not seem well thought out. They frustrate us greatly, agreeing to one treatment or home care option one day and completely changing their minds the next. Remember Olive, the matriarch of her family, whom we met in the "Family Roles" section above? She had a chaotic family. In addition to help in redefining roles, they benefited from high levels of structure and clear and consistent information and recommendations from us. Chaotic families benefit from pre-meetings with a social worker to help them sort through questions and thoughts before the team expects them to make decisions. At times these families will even need us to assign roles, such as "spokesperson" or "caretaker," to members.

> ### Practice Points: Questions that Will Lead to Insight into Family Flexibility
>
> - *How does your family usually make decisions?*
> - *Do you generally get along? Does your family have a main caregiver? Decision-maker?* (King and Quill 2006)
> - *How has your family dealt with other major transitions in life?*

Level of Family Communication

The level of communication among family members is the third key marker in this model, both because of its role in assessment of family function and because this is where we can help families achieve greater levels of functioning. Good communication can support families as they try to establish or reestablish their balance and create a functioning system that can support the patient.

The level of communication in a family is a significant factor in its ability to adapt to the crisis of the patient's serious illness. Clinicians can measure communication levels by assessing the family as a whole. Families with good communication skills are able to listen to each other with empathy, express themselves clearly, respect other views, and share personal feelings about the situation. Good communication skills also include the ability to follow the conversation and problem solve without changing the subject.

For disengaged, enmeshed, rigid, and chaotic families, increased communication is usually the best and easiest intervention.

> ### Practice Points: Questions that Will Tell You More about a Family's Communication Skills
>
> - *How would you describe the level of communication in your family?*
> - *How does the family usually make big decisions?* (King and Quill 2006)
> - *Has your family ever been a part of making decisions for someone who was very sick? What was that like for the family?*
> - *All families have disagreements, and with difficult decisions, this can feel even harder. How are disagreements usually handled in your family?*
> - *What are your family's worries and fears?*
> - *What is the hardest part of this for your family?* (Back et al. 2007)
> - *What is most important to you now?*

Communication as an Intervention

Using skillful communication, we can help families move toward the center, to a balanced place, on both the cohesion and the flexibility scales. Good communication not only improves a patient's adjustment to illness, adherence to medications, and pain and physical symptoms. It can also make a family meeting successful and greatly improve the family's satisfaction with care (Langer, Brown, and Syrjala 2009; Zaider et al. 2020).

Palliative care practitioners, social workers, clinical psychologists, and psychiatrists are skilled in communication, an integral part of which are listening, ability to regulate what we say even when we are feeling a strong emotion, and awareness of our internal reactions to others. When we are facilitating a family meeting, we will often share our internal emotional reactions, which helps family members understand that their internal emotional reactions are normal and often enhances communication among the family members present at the meeting. These families may simply have little experience in discussing difficult emotional issues; inviting family members to do this can shift family dynamics and create empathy for others in the family. Team members may be able to increase family communication by aligning with those of the patient's family members who may be reluctant to focus on their own needs (Zaider et al. 2019).

Remember Matt and Sally? Sally appeared to be blocking Matt's discharge home, and his children did not know why. But the social worker did and asked Sally's permission to share this with her family. Later, during a family meeting, the social worker, with Sally's prior consent, asked Sally directly about the death of her own mother and how she had felt as her mother had died at home. As she spoke, her adult children understood for the first time that their father dying at home would be difficult for their mother and helped her make a plan to ensure that he would die in a hospice house, where Sally was sure he'd get the best of care.

While many families can be stabilized by our focused interventions, some also benefit from referrals to an outside therapist or need more specific interventions that can be performed by our social work or psychiatry colleagues. One therapy that has shown to increase family communication and cohesiveness in oncology patients is family-focused grief therapy. Families who have low communication skills may benefit from this manualized intervention (Zaider and Kissane 2009).

Most families, the ones Kissane would label as "well-functioning" or "ordinary," are able to adapt and to cope with the stresses of terminal illness but simply don't have any experience with how to discuss the emotional or taboo subjects that arise when a loved one is dying. As we take the lead in these conversations, we help the family access its own strengths.

Questions that help families move toward a greater state of balance focus on increasing each member's ability to understand another's thoughts and feelings. Once these are understood, family members have a greater capacity to problem solve and support one another.

THE ROLE OF CULTURE

The last key component in assessing a family is to understand any cultural, religious, or spiritual beliefs that influence the patient and her family system. *Culture* is the behaviors and beliefs characteristic of a particular group, be it a social group, ethnic group, or even age group. With an increasingly diverse patient population, greater attention has been paid to the vital role that culture has on the experience of living and dying (National Consensus Project 2018). Although each individual's perspectives are influenced by his or her personality, education level, and gender, cultural influences fundamentally shape patients' perceptions of illness, suffering, and death, as well as the decisions they make during advanced illness. The National Consensus Project for Quality Care's clinical practice guidelines define the "Cultural Aspects of Care" as one of the eight core domains for quality palliative care (National Consensus Project 2018). The goal is to strive for skilled attention to culture and language to provide appropriate and relevant care to our patients and families.

Cultural Competency versus Cultural Humility

Palliative care teams care for patients of many racial and ethnic backgrounds, diverse gender identities and sexual orientations, and across every socioeconomic status. Disparities have been documented in the care provided because of lack of cultural competency in the organizations in which the providers work, stemming from a lack of awareness and training (Periyakoil 2020). Periyakoil reviews the components of culturally competent care for seriously ill patients that should take place on the organizational level. She notes that organizations will find themselves in one of six stages but can strive to advance to cultural proficiency. The Practice Points box below lists the key characteristics of each stage; a full description can be found in Periyakoil (2020).

Cultural competence is also included in many of the professional mandates across health professions and is associated with skills, proficiency, and expertise. Cultural competence implies, however, that a person can gather information about a particular group's characteristics and values and assume it is mastered. This "mastery" is usually limited to generalizations about a culture's dominant privileges, group values, or norms, such as in the Tran et al. (2019) review of care for seriously ill Vietnamese Americans or in the Lin et al. (2019) report of the 2019 Taipei Declaration on Advance Care Planning. An excellent online resource for general cultural information is the Stanford School of Medicine Ethno Med site (http://geriatrics.stanford.edu/ethnomed). The site is organized by ethnic group and gives clinicians a quick overall view of each group, including their medical vulnerabilities, spiritual beliefs, and common cultural themes.

While the above resources can help prepare us with general knowledge, key

Practice Points: Stages of Organizational Cultural Competence

Stage	Key characteristics
1. Cultural destructiveness	Demonstrates and condones disrespect and biased treatment of persons from minority and disadvantaged backgrounds.
2. Cultural incapacity	Fears or ignores the unique needs of persons from minority and disadvantaged backgrounds; exhibits discrimination in policies and hiring practices.
3. Cultural blindness	Functions with the belief that color or culture makes no difference.
4. Cultural precompetence	Realizes its weaknesses in serving persons from minority groups and those from disadvantaged backgrounds.
5. Cultural competence	Expects, accepts, and respects individual differences.
6. Cultural proficiency	Conducts ongoing research and implements and evaluates new approaches.

values, and cultural beliefs of different groups, it is important to remember that patients' cultural backgrounds are also influenced by their individual life history and experiences. Makoff (2020) reminds us, for example, of the racial trauma experienced by many of our Black patients. Similarly, practitioners who care for sexual and gender minority individuals should be aware of the many negative experiences they have had with oncology care and learn to address their unique health needs. The palliative care of sexual and gender minority patients is discussed in Chapter 4 and reviewed in Kimberly Acquaviva's excellent book, *LGBTQ-Inclusive Hospice and Palliative Care* (Acquaviva 2017). Although certain beliefs may be more common in individuals with particular cultural backgrounds, or sexual or gender identities, making assumptions without speaking to the patient and family about their cultural beliefs can be not only unhelpful but damaging.

The concept of *cultural humility* is therefore an important adjunct to cultural competence. Cultural humility is never mastered but is, rather, a process of self-reflection, curiosity, and openness (Fahlberg, Bishop, and Ryan 2016). It involves developing partnerships to address power imbalances, an other-oriented stance, and curiosity when new cultural information arises (Mosher et al. 2017).

While you can use references such as the Stanford School of Medicine Ethno Med site to understand how to begin discussions with families about common cultural practices or concerns that you see in your patient population, asking questions and presenting a sincere curiosity about the spiritual and cultural beliefs of each patient or family is best.

Asking questions that reveal the family's story of the illness (their "narrative") and the influences of their culture on how they think the patient should be cared for can greatly enhance families' perceptions of being heard and understood. These influences range from the single-family level, apparent when someone says, *"Our family does not talk about feelings,"* to the broader influences affecting those who come from cultures that have experienced longstanding inequities, societal oppression, or abuse. It is also important to be curious about the differing cultural beliefs across generations; for example, it is not unusual for children born in the United States to have different views from their parents who immigrated later in life. Exploring these differences during an assessment can allow for easier decision-making in the end.

Cultural Determinants of Communicating Information, Truth Telling, and the Role of the Physician

Key areas that have been strongly linked to culture include views on sharing and communicating difficult information; the locus of decision-making; and the role of the physician (Coolen 2012). In Peek et al.'s 2009 study, African Americans generally wanted to be informed about the diagnosis and prognosis of their illness but were less likely than Caucasian Americans to feel included in the decision-making. Knowing this, you will want to spend time ensuring that all your patients feel that they are contributing to the decisions being made. Patients who grew up in other countries, however, may have significantly different views from those born in the United States surrounding the open disclosure of prognosis.

Although informed consent and truth telling about the diagnosis is a major tenet of the U.S. health care system, many other cultures find it appropriate to withhold from patients the knowledge that they have serious medical conditions. In many parts of Asia, Eastern Europe, Central and South America, and the Middle East, withholding information is felt to be more humane (Gysels et al. 2012; Kagawa-Singer and Blackhall 2001). Physicians in these cultures might avoid speaking of the potential terminal condition by using terminology that obscures the diagnosis, speaking of the "mass" or "growth" rather than talking about the "cancer" (Kagawa-Singer and Blackhall 2001). Although this may not be something you are comfortable doing, an understanding of the cultural norms and expectations of families can allow for a discussion about informed consent and can preserve patient autonomy while respecting cultural norms. As we discuss below, ask the medical interpreters to advise you about relevant cultural norms when the patient or family members have limited English proficiency.

Who should make medical decisions can also vary greatly from culture to culture. Although the U.S. medical system places emphasis on patient autonomy and self-determination, many communities hold the values of collectivism. In a collective decision process, family members expect to receive medical information and make decisions without the patient's input. Asian, Mexican, and Mexican American patients may be more likely to want family members included as they make decisions or to delegate the decision-making to them (Coolen 2012). In Asian cultures, filial piety, the expectation that children will care for their parents as a form of honoring them, can greatly influence decision-making. When speaking about hospice to families who prioritize filial piety, be sure to emphasize the major role the family will continue to play as caregivers, because they may reject hospice services if they feel that another person will be caring for their parents (Kagawa-Singer and Blackhall 2001).

The degree of authority, respect, and deference given to physicians can also be tightly linked to culture (Coolen 2012) and can interfere with communication between the family and the physicians. A family who had come from China to seek treatment for their son seemed to listen and understand when the team told them that we had no new treatments to offer him. But later, the team was

---

Practice Points: Questions to Assist in Cultural Assessment

Kagawa-Singer and Blackhall (2001) developed a cultural assessment model to help avoid stereotyping and to improve communication, including around cultural issues. Some key questions from the ABCD cultural assessment are outlined below.

Attitude (general)

- What are the patient and family beliefs around truth telling with regard to diagnosis and prognosis?

Beliefs

- *"Spiritual or religious strength sustain many people in times of distress. What is important for me to know about your faith or spiritual needs?"*

Context

- *"What language are you most comfortable using when talking about your health care?"*
- *"What other important times in your life might help us better understand your situation?"*

Decision-Making Style

- *"How are decisions about health care made in your family?"*
- *"Is there anyone else I should talk to in your family about your condition?"*

Environment

- *"What resources and support systems are available to support you and your family?"*

(Full assessment available via PDF at EthnoMed, "End-of-Life Care Cultural Assessment Models with Sample Scripts," May 1, 2012, https://ethnomed.org/wp-content/uploads/2020/01/EndOfLifeCareCulturalAssessment Models.pdf.)

dismayed to discover that the family was seeking care at another institution. Our misunderstanding may have come from not recognizing that, in their deference to authority, his family did not feel comfortable verbalizing doubts in front of the doctors; that would have been disrespectful. Other families with similar beliefs may find it easier just to not follow our treatment instructions; without having visiting nurses or other eyes and ears in the patient's home, we might not understand why our intervention hasn't been helpful.

The final area in which views of illness are tightly linked to culture is the role of religion and faith. Religion and faith can influence the narratives and causes that patients and families associate with illness, the meaning of specific symptoms, the importance of rituals, the sense of divine intervention, and how they perceive, interpret, and articulate pain and suffering (Coolen 2012; Steinberg 2011). This is discussed further in Chapter 3.

Although it is impossible to have a thorough knowledge of the many possible cultures of your patients, combining basic knowledge with a genuine interest in a family's cultural, spiritual, and religious beliefs is likely to enable you to provide culturally sensitive care with an understanding of the patient's health care preferences. You are also more likely to find common ground between your beliefs and those of your patients and their families.

PARTNERING WITH MEDICAL INTERPRETERS
with Jessica Goldhirsch, LCSW, MSW, MPH

Clear communication of medical information, treatment options, and patient priorities is a foundational component of patient- and family-centered care and essential for shared decision-making. Care for patients and families from other cultures, or with limited English proficiency, or those who are deaf or hard of hearing or communicate using American Sign Language, must include medical interpreters who are integrated into the team because of the health care outcome disparities that still exist (Green and Nze 2017) even at the end of life (Kirby et al. 2018). Racial and ethnic disparities in palliative care delivery are well documented (Johnson 2013). Among patients with limited English proficiency such disparities have resulted in lawsuits stemming from serious medical errors when professional medical interpreters were not engaged (Silva et al. 2016). As we discuss in Chapter 1, the often emotionally laden nature of palliative care encounters requires carefully constructed conversations with carefully chosen words. These conversations are all the more difficult across language and cultural differences, heightening the need for quality linguistic interpretation and cultural mediation (Kirby et al. 2016). This section focuses on how we clinicians can best partner with medical interpreters, each of whom is a communication professional, to provide culturally respectful and sensitive care for these patient and families.

Choosing an Interpreter

While working with an in-person professional medical interpreter is a best practice and available in many larger institutions, this service is logistically or financially impossible for others. Video or telephonic interpreter services, however, are available around the clock (e.g., LanguageLine Solutions, http://languageline.com; CyraCom, http://www.cyracom.com; or Stratus Video, stratusvideo.com). Patients and families should be told that all interpreter services, in person, video, or telephonic, are being offered free of charge.

Even if you or a staff member speak the patient's language, providing a medical interpretation in the patient's or family member's language is not the same as being bilingual or being able to treat patients in their language, and it is not the same as engaging in interpretation. Interpretation is a skill requiring training and practice, and medical interpretation is nuanced and complex, regulated by a strict code of ethics, and requires a distinct set of skills that differ significantly from skills required for conversational facility in that language. In the United States, clinicians who speak a second language and who wish to treat patients in that language are given screening examinations by their institutions to ensure that their skills meet a standard level for providing health care. Even clinicians qualified to practice in a second language should not both provide care and attempt to serve as the medical interpreter in the conversation. The Joint Commission (TJC) and federal law require that we employ qualified interpreters for the latter challenging task.

Asking family members to try to render information in the patient's preferred language can be fraught with problems. At a basic level, it is a violation of hospital policy and is not supported by TJC or federal law, and often it is not in the best interest of the patient or family. Family members and patients may feel uncomfortable or ashamed interpreting questions and answers around sensitive issues (Hadziabdic and Hjelm 2013). Family members may not be familiar with medical terms or procedures, which may result in patient misunderstandings. Additionally, family members may have personal agendas about what patients should be told, may not interpret all information, or may provide unsolicited advice or opinions (Juckett and Unger 2014).

And there are cultural implications. Asking an English-speaking granddaughter to render information for a monolingual grandparent who is the patient can be disrespectful. It creates a role reversal, may rob the patient of her seniority in the family, denies the patient both privacy and confidentiality, and puts undue stress on the younger person who fears making a mistake. That family member cannot offer support to the patient if she becomes focused on the linguistic challenge, rather than taking in the emotional impact of the message, and possibly grieving or thinking about how to support her loved one.

Steps for Partnering with Medical Interpreters in Clinical Encounters

Keeping all the above concerns in mind, you can take several steps to make the most of partnering with a medical interpreter.

Pre-meeting

Pre-meeting with the face-to-face or virtual interpreter before meeting with the patient or family can greatly enhance the experience for you, the patient, and the interpreter. In this meeting you can build rapport as a team and provide relevant medical information. In many clinical settings, professional interpreters do not have access to the medical record, and therefore, to prepare for the encounter, they require a briefing from you about the medical background as well as a general overview of the planned discussion and any decisions you are hoping the patient or family will be asked to make.

During the pre-meeting, you can also discover whether the interpreter has worked with the patient before and has important information for you about the patient or family. If you are working with a virtual interpreter, that person can instruct you in how best to position a speaker phone or where to place a video screen and how best to communicate on that specific platform.

Additionally, it is important to consider the characteristics of the interpreter that may affect the interpretation for that patient's specific cultural norms. Are there going to be discussions surrounding sexuality or reproduction that may be most appropriate for someone of the same gender? Ask the interpreter during the pre-meeting; he or she can serve as a cultural broker or mediator.

If the interpreter shares the same culture as the patient, not just the same language, he or she can help the clinician understand the cultural beliefs surrounding the illness or care plan. A Spanish speaker from Spain, however, would not necessarily be a useful cultural broker for a Spanish-speaking family from Guatemala (Juckett and Unger 2014). As a cultural mediator, an interpreter may suggest that there is a barrier to effective communication and that learning more about a patient's cultural norms may be helpful. The interpreter can then assist the clinician in asking the patient to share more about her beliefs surrounding her illness and treatment.

Acknowledge that you are aware of this important facet of the interpreter's role and welcome him or her to keep you informed about the meaning of the illness for the patient or any concerns regarding your goals for the encounter. If interpreters require a clarification themselves during the meeting, they will alert you by stating, "This is the interpreter speaking; I am concerned that . . ." (Juckett and Unger 2014). There may also be times when interpreters cannot interpret in words the emotional or nonverbal reactions of the patient; encourage them to tell you if this happens.

Palliative care family meetings held to break bad news or to establish goals of care pose unique ethical and cultural challenges for interpreters. Family members may ask the interpreters not to tell the whole truth—to try to protect their loved ones. A Western-trained clinician is usually direct in communicating bad news, for example, to a patient and family, while the interpreter may know that the patient and family are from a culture that is accustomed to a "softer" delivery. Interpreters are often put in the position of having to render terms like "palliative care" and "hospice" into a patient's language that may not have an equivalent, while an anxious family is holding its breath at the harm such direct communication may be having on their loved one (Kirby et al. 2016). Ask interpreters to alert you should they be concerned about the style of the delivery.

Finally, although professional interpreters engage in professional distancing and other measures to protect themselves emotionally from challenging encounters, a pre-encounter chat or huddle, especially before a family meeting in which, for example, disease progression or the lack of further treatment options will be discussed, offers them an opportunity to prepare themselves emotionally for the encounter (Kirby et al. 2016) and can help facilitate the interpretation.

During the Meeting

Explain the ground rules. Begin by asking the interpreter to introduce him- or herself to you and the patient and any others present in the room; interpreters must share their name, role, that they will be interpreting in the first person, and that they will interpret everything that is said during the encounter, including "side bar" comments from the clinician, between the clinician and family member, or between the patient and the family member. Remind interpreters to reassure patients and family that everything said will remain confidential; they will not be sharing information outside the room.

Position yourself so that you are looking directly at the patient or the family member who needs the interpreter and so that you can also see the interpreter. If the interpreter is sitting beside or slightly behind the patient or that family member, it will be easier to speak directly to both of them. Keep your attention on the patient and use first-person statements (I), speaking directly to the patient rather than using the third person ("tell her . . .").

Remember, the interpreter is working to render your words as accurately as possible into the patient's language, so you need to speak slowly, in short sentences (Schenker et al. 2012). Medical interpreters abide by a code of ethics that guides them toward fidelity to the intended meaning/message of our statements. When we speak in long-winded or complicated sentences without pause, we make it difficult for them to meet the level or quality of accurate communication they are striving for. Their standards of practice guide them to avoid paraphrasing except in unique circumstances, such as with patients who are unable to pause (e.g., thought-disordered patients). In trying to render the *message* of what you are intending with your words, they must do much more than simply "translate" them. Don't be surprised if a short statement by you requires several sentences to convey your meaning in the language of the patient or family.

Avoid medical jargon or specialist terminology and complex and lengthy explanations that could be difficult to interpret and difficult for a patient to comprehend. In complex conversations, choose two to three points to convey. Before moving to the next decision point, check for understanding by doing a *teach back*, that is, asking the patient to share with you what was just discussed, rather than asking, "Do you understand?" Ask interpreters to alert you if they suspect that the patient or family member is not fully grasping your intended message. No interpreter really knows whether a patient understands what you said. Interpreters can suspect confusion sometimes and should be invited to alert you to this, but only in a teach back can you learn whether the patient understood your message.

The interpreter's suspicion is particularly important for patients who come from cultures where it is unheard of to ask a physician to explain or clarify what was said, or to question it. The latter can be seen as disrespectful, and a patient would rather leave an appointment or conclude a bedside consult confused than be offensive. If the interpreter alerts you that the patient may not have understood your message, you can provide a clearer explanation without the patient having to request one.

Family Meetings

Family meetings can be especially challenging for interpreters, whether the meeting takes place in a conference room or at the bedside. Meetings usually include multiple clinicians, who may be chatting among themselves while the clinician leading the meeting is communicating with an English-speaking family member and the interpreter is trying to interpret everything said to the patient. You, as the leader, need to partner with the interpreter by keeping everyone present in one conversation. Then, the interpreter can "manage the flow" of the conversation, as he or she has been trained to do, and provide accurate and complete interpretations of everything said to the patient.

Not only should all clinicians avoid speaking in English with bilingual family members during the family meeting, but, if necessary, you should remind them to please keep side bars to a minimum, since the interpreter must interpret to the patient and family all conversations occurring in the room. Be sensitive to patient and family reactions to emotionally laden information. As the leader, assure family members that you are available for further discussion with the family after you convey the key information. Ask them to speak one at a time, rather than all at once, to give the interpreter time to interpret all their comments. All conversations, whether directly with the patient or with family members, should be slow enough that the interpreter can provide effective interpretation.

Post-meeting Debrief

The interpreter may be running off to the next appointment, and a debrief may need to be scheduled for later; or you may need to take the speaker phone or video unit out of the patient's room or conference room for a private debrief after informing the interpreter of what you are doing so that he or she does not sign off. But if the interpreter (in person or on video or phone) is not booked directly after the meeting, debrief with him or her.

The interpreter may be able to explain cultural nuances or provide insight into the emotions or nonverbal cues the patient or family members were sending but not saying. Ask directly, *"Do you have any concerns about the patient's understanding?"* (Schenker et al. 2012). Allow the interpreter to ask any questions surrounding the session; his or her questions could give you insight into potential misunderstandings.

Practice Points: Partnering with Medical Interpreters In Person, Video, or Phone

Pre-meeting

- Introduce yourself to the interpreter.
- Explain the relevant medical information and the purpose of the meeting.
- Encourage the interpreter to ask questions for clarification if needed for accuracy.
- Review with the interpreter any nontranslated forms requiring site translation during the session.

During the Meeting

- Allow interpreters to introduce themselves to the patient and family, explain their role, position themselves to promote direct eye contact between the provider and the patient, and explain the ground rules.
- Speak slowly and clearly with patients and family in the first person, using simple language (rather than medical jargon) and speaking in a normal tone and speed.
- Speak a complete thought and then pause for interpretation, asking only one question at a time, and ensure that only one person is speaking at a time.
- Lead the family meeting, avoiding side bars with either colleagues or family members, enabling the interpreter to interpret everything said.
- Respect the interpreter's judgment about what is culturally appropriate to discuss in the meeting.

Debrief

- Thank the interpreter.
- Discuss with the interpreter issues that could not be addressed during the meeting and debrief about any emotionally charged or contentious issues that arose.

(Hadziabdic and Hjelm 2013; Juckett and Unger 2014; Schenker et al. 2012; Scamman 2018; IMIA 2020)

It is also important to consider the emotional impact that difficult discussions can have on interpreters, and to allow them to speak about the effects on them if needed. I will never forget one session with a family that had arrived from China to see their son, who was at college in the United States, when he was diagnosed with a terminal cancer. The first family meeting was delivering serious news. The mother was emotional and desperate to save her son. After the session, we found the interpreter in the hall, crying. He expressed that he was reminded of his own mother, and he had not been prepared to give such bad news.

FAMILIES THAT REQUIRE ADDITIONAL SUPPORT

We hope that we have introduced you to basic tools that you can use to assess, characterize, and navigate family dynamics. But there are situations in which you should always get help. Families with longstanding histories of conflict among their members; families that have a member suffering from a personality disorder, severe mental illness, or substance use disorder; or families in which there is domestic violence usually have extreme imbalances in flexibility and cohesion, and their patterns of communication are rooted in dysfunction. These families will need referrals to psychiatry, social work, chaplaincy, addiction specialists, or domestic violence specialists. It is also important for you to set realistic expectations and to understand that you will be working in crisis-control mode with them.

Longstanding Conflicts

A family's history of conflict is the strongest predictor of end-of-life conflict (Kramer et al. 2009). Some families will display a high level of conflict in and between members. You may sense this in a meeting or by comments family members make. Usually, these conflicts are longstanding with complexities on all sides (Kissane et al. 2006; Kramer et al. 2009). It is key to identify these families early and set expectations for yourself and others around communication and behavior in family meetings and in decision-making situations. This is especially relevant for families in which you identify that one of the members was disowned, there is no contact with children, or some members are isolated from other family members.

A deeper assessment of families you suspect may be conflictual can help. Assessing family functioning and relationships with several family members will give the broadest perspective of the situation. Ask questions surrounding prior experiences with death or how the family has dealt with conflict in the past (Kramer et al. 2009). Although there is no association between conflict and socioeconomic status, financial and resource constraints can cause conflict in all situations. Assessing the family's resources in relation to the demands that will likely arise will allow the team to anticipate constraints that may cause conflict in the future. Regular family meetings can help build trust and increase communication between family members, as well as setting the stage for greater shared decision-making when decisions are necessary. Finally, have a social worker with you as often as you can when you meet with these families. If there is clear conflict in the room, the social worker can acknowledge it directly and set clear boundaries with a statement such as *"I can see that you all have disagreements on a number of issues, but I am wondering if we can put those aside so we can focus on what is going on with your father?"* (Back et al. 2007). In many cases, however, the social worker will need to set up a more concrete plan to contain the disagreements.

Practice Points: Strategies to Use with Conflictual Families in Family Meetings

- Set modest expectations about what level of collaborative decision-making is possible.
- Choose one clinician to lead and set ground rules for communication.
- Encourage family members to speak to you directly about issues rather than directing accusations at members.
- Remain neutral.
- Increase communication between providers to avoid mixed messages.

(From King and Quill 2006 and Kramer et al. 2009)

Personality Disorders or Severe Mental Illnesses

Families who have members with personality disorders or other mental illness are likely to fall into Kissane's "dysfunctional" groupings and to be considered "difficult" (Meyer and Block 2011). These difficult patients likely function at chaotic levels of flexibility and with little cohesion. Unfortunately, we are rarely told that history either by the medical record or by a family member, but if we pay attention to the emotions patients evoke in us, we can identify the problem and get help.

If you find yourself feeling anger, guilt, or frustration when you're working with a patient, you have difficulty forming alliances with her, she doesn't come to appointments on time or adhere to your recommendations, or she's calling your staff repeatedly throughout the week (or throughout a day!), you are likely dealing with one of these challenging patients (Meyer and Block 2011). We cannot address this topic fully here, but we suggest you read the Meyer and Block (2011) article "Personality Disorders in the Oncology Setting" or the discussion of patients with personality disorders in Chapter 9. If you are like us, you will have many "Aha!" moments.

Even if you are not able to "contain" difficult behaviors, you will be better able to identify these patients, understand their otherwise puzzling behavior, and work quickly to find a clinician who is expert in this area (or refer the patient to another physician who has access to such help). Specialists will advise you to be vigilant about giving clear and consistent information about the illness and any care options, because any mixed or conflicting messages the patient hears from you or your staff will cause the patient to "split" the members of your staff ("But she told me X when you told me Y") and fuel distrust. One patient like this is enough to disrupt an entire practice if not contained.

Tools for Working with Patients with Personality Disorders

- Focus on building and maintaining a therapeutic alliance.
- Acknowledge and empathize with the real stresses in the patient's situation.
- Set consistent, appropriate expectations, limits, and boundaries.
- Evaluate patients for suicidality and homicidality.
- Hold ongoing personal and team meetings reflecting on the effect this patient is having on the team.
- Refer to another physician if you are not able to identify a psychiatrist or social worker who can work with your staff as they care for these patients.

(From Meyer and Block 2011)

Substance Use Disorder

It is crucial to know whether a family's history includes aberrant use of alcohol or other substances. Chapter 7 reviews the medical and physical concerns around treating a patient with substance use disorder, while this section focuses on the effect on the family system.

When substance use disorder is present (or was present historically) in a family, many issues can come up at the end of life that make the situation more complex. Key issues that can affect the family system revolve around access to resources, stigma, shame, and fear (Bushfield and DeFord 2009). One concern that can affect the family surrounds access to services. Depending on the type of substance use disorder, patients may be denied placement at facilities, creating greater burden on the family. Families members may also have fears surrounding the administration of pain medication to patients who are in recovery or express concerns about tolerance. Family members may need additional education or equipment to feel comfortable if caring for a patient at home.

These families may also need additional emotional support. Many times, an individual's substance use disorder has been a family secret or not discussed; as the end of life draws near, discussion of this may be necessary but difficult. Feelings of shame and guilt can arise in patients or family members, especially if the illness could be linked to or exacerbated by the substance use disorder. Emotions such as anger and guilt are common in family members, who often feel they should have stopped the behavior or who blame the patient. A social worker can help families talk about and work through these emotions, which can complicate decision-making as well as bereavement in these families. Additionally, those with a history of substance use disorder commonly have ruptures in primary relationships. These individuals may need additional support to make amends or repair connections with friends and family they have cut off or hurt while their substance use disorder was active. While it is not our job to address every family issue, these patients and families commonly have large emotional and spiritual needs at the end of life and benefit from additional psychosocial support.

Intimate Partner Violence / Domestic Violence

One in every four women is a victim of domestic violence across their lifetimes, and a much larger percentage of women are in relationships that involve extreme imbalances of power. Men can also be victims, as can the elderly. These imbalances affect family dynamics and an individual's decision-making. We should therefore be alert to any hints of a history of domestic violence or other emotionally controlling behavior when we are asking patients and families to make decisions about discharge placements or location of care at the end of life (Fischer 2003; Wygant, Bruera, and Hui 2014).

If you suspect or know there was a history of domestic violence, if one member of the family or the partner seems to exert extreme power over the patient, or if there seems to be a lot of conflict or personal violence in a relationship, these are immediate red flags to involve a social worker or mental health professional. In situations when the batterer is ill, the victim may be unable to take on the role of decision-maker. When the batterer is the caregiver, it is essential that the team set clear boundaries around decision-making and consider including a domestic violence specialist and or an ethics consultant.

A complex ICU case may be illustrative of this dangerous and painful dynamic. The palliative care team was called to help with symptom management of a 65-year-old woman with multiple nonhealing postoperative wounds. Her husband exhibited extremely controlling behaviors that escalated as his wife got sicker. Nurses were afraid to work with him, and many clinicians felt that the team was being bullied into providing medical interventions based on his coercion and legal threats. He repeatedly accused the team of trying to "kill his wife."

Whenever she was alone with the ICU team, the patient would beg the doctors and the nurses to make her "do not resuscitate or intubate" (DNR/DNI) and allow her to die, but when her husband was in the room, she agreed with him when he yelled, "You want to live, don't you? You must, and you do!" At one point the patient changed her health care proxy to her daughter and asked her to allow her to die, but after two days, her daughter revoked the proxy and would not talk openly about the reason. In this complicated case, it was necessary to involve specialists in domestic violence, psychiatry, and ethics to help the team navigate the complexities of the family dynamic. In the end, the medical team acted on behalf of the wife and set boundaries that the husband could not be in the room alone with her. She was made DNR and died peacefully there.

Practice Points: Signs that You Need to Get Help from Psychiatry or Social Work

- History of conflict or violence in the family
- Signs of a major mental illness or personality disorder in the patient or health care proxy
- History of substance use disorder
- History or suspicion of domestic/intimate partner violence, elder abuse, or extreme power discrepancies

---

SUMMARY

We hope that the tools we describe in this chapter will help you identify the patient's role in the family, the general level of family functioning, and the areas of family dysfunction. Understanding the three fundamental dimensions of a family—*cohesion*, *flexibility*, and *communication ability*—enables you to set realistic objectives for what you can achieve with them as well as helping you begin to think how best to approach different types of families. Families that are balanced usually have the resources and skills to adapt the family system in a way that can deal with stress or a crisis; unbalanced families lack these resources and will need more time, assistance, and resources. To be most effective with them, you and your team will need to increase your level of communication, structure, and consistency in proportion to the level of instability in the family system.

Understanding the cultural beliefs of your patients is also essential to helping them and their families smoothly navigate decisions regarding therapy and those that arise at the end of life. A patient's culture is a foundational piece of who he is and influences how he views illness and death. Medical interpreters can serve as key partners in helping clinicians understand the cultures of patients with limited English proficiency and their families and discuss issues that arise in those with advanced illness and who are nearing the end of life.

With families that have longstanding histories of conflict, past or present domestic/intimate partner violence, mental illness, or substance use disorder, you should call in a specialist. Always be realistic in your goals and remember, it is not your job to change these patterns. Try your best to work within them to achieve the best quality of life for your patients.

CHAPTER 3

Spiritual Care in Palliative Care

with Rev. Katie Pakos Rimer, MDiv, EdD, BCC

What then does one seek? Not a hidden power, but a source of kinship for mature persons. And also the assurance that it is not totally absurd to have suffered.

—Emmanuel Levinas

INTRODUCTION

Caring for patients living and dying with cancer has been a tremendous privilege for me as a chaplain, priest, and psychologist. In my (*Katie Rimer's*) experience, tender attention to a patient's spirit, when offered carefully and well, enhances all elements of good palliative care: the treatment of symptoms, conversations about medical decision-making and goals of care, and support for family, caregivers, and friends.

Some clinicians can feel tentative about the whole area of spiritual care, not knowing what it is, or what their responsibilities are regarding patients' spiritual and religious lives. *Will my patients ask me about* my *faith if I open that door with them? How do I ask the question about theirs? And how do I respond to their answer?* In this chapter I hope to help you identify your patients' spiritual needs and show you how to conduct a basic spiritual assessment. I review the ethics of providing spiritual care as a nonchaplain provider, when to bring in a chaplain or the patient's clergy, and common pitfalls to avoid. I consider how religion can affect medical decision-making and offer approaches for working with patients who are waiting for a miracle. But first, meet Rex.

Rex was a lovable, angry patient. Diagnosed with a rare sarcoma, he was losing his life before the age of 50, leaving behind a wife and three teenage daughters, one of whom was in and out of juvenile jail, another with autism, and four brothers, all as big and feisty as Rex. The brothers worked together at their family's auto repair shop in a gritty suburb of Boston. Rex's wife, Jill, was devoted and overwhelmed. Whenever Rex's oncologist shared news that a treatment had failed, Rex got angry. At important appointments his brothers joined him and lined the wall in the exam room like bouncers at a club, wearing thick chains and impressive tattoos. Yelling was common.

My colleagues and I steeled ourselves when we saw Rex's name on the clinic schedule. We expected conflict and ensured that no provider saw him alone.

During one appointment I asked Rex what he liked to do when he wasn't feeling crummy, working in the shop, or busy with his kids. To my surprise, he shared that he raised pigeons: he had several pairs, had built a coop for them with a heater in the winter, and ordered a special seed mix from a distributor in North Carolina. Rex's delight in raising these birds stood in sharp contrast to his intimidating demeanor and hot temper, and that delight showed me a side of Rex that was playful and caring. At each subsequent visit he shared updates about the birds' well-being, imitated how the pigeons cooed, and told me their names. I enjoyed learning about raising pigeons, and Rex enjoyed being my teacher. A spiritual care relationship was born.

Rex's disease was unrelenting. Until his last visits to the clinic, despite increasing weakness and debilitation, Rex still flexed his muscles when he arrived, a playful reminder of his intimidating "strongman" persona. Over time we talked about his Catholic faith, his concern for his daughters and wife, and his fears about dying. We prayed together. Tough to the end, Rex became more accessible, less reactive. With trust established, the palliative care team could lean in and care well for Rex in all domains: his symptoms were managed, he eventually transitioned to a hospice facility (though we heard later that a brawl had broken out there between his brothers, which did not surprise us), and I provided bereavement support for Jill after Rex died. Pigeons were at the heart of my spiritual care of Rex and opened a door to better palliative care.

I tell this story of Rex for two reasons. First, because it illustrates what I consider to be the *charism** of spiritual care: the capacity to see deeply and respect what makes a person unique and support him in that. Spiritual care is attention to one's intimate, unique personhood. It is care for the soul. By always welcoming Rex to the clinic, by responding to his bravado and anger with equanimity, and by prodding gently to know him better, we found a fuller, more complex picture of this initially intimidating man. I believe Rex felt seen, known, and respected by us, and because of that, he let us care for him compassionately until his death.

Second, I hope Rex's story illustrates that sensitive, patient-centered care *is* spiritual care. These conversations need not be heavily religious, but they *are* intimate. As you can see from this story about Rex, within the context of a trusting and respectful patient-provider relationship, spiritual topics (in Rex's case, his love for his pigeons and his family, his Catholic faith, his fears about dying) can manifest naturally. I believe this is as true for clinicians as it is for chaplains. Chances are, you are already practicing spiritual care. I hope this chapter equips you to do so more confidently.

RELIGION, SPIRITUALITY, AND SPIRITUAL CARE

What, really, is spirituality, and how does it relate to religion? A consensus conference held in 2009 to explore the role of spirituality in palliative care (Puchalski et al. 2009, p. 887) came to this definition of spirituality: "The aspect of humanity that refers to the way individuals seek and express meaning and purpose and the way they experience their connectedness to the moment, to self, to others, to nature, and to the significant or sacred." A physician who participated in spiritual care training suggests this definition: "Spirituality is my being; my inner person. It is who I am—unique and alive. It is my body, my thinking, my feelings, my judgments, and my creativity . . . Through my spirituality I give and receive love; I respond to and appreciate God, other people, a sunset, a symphony and spring. I am driven forward . . . I am a person because of my spirituality" (Tarumi, Taube, and Watanabe 2003, p. 30–31).† With this generous understanding of spirituality, one could say even atheists have a spirituality, an essence, a center of connection out of which they live their lives. All patients can be recipients of spiritual care, as spirituality is an aspect of personhood (Cassell 1982, 2014). Religion is but one expression of spirituality. I enjoy this analogy: religion is to spirituality as music or poetry is to the arts.

---

*The word *charism* (from the Greek χάρισμα, "a gift of grace") originated in ancient Greek texts and denotes a spiritual gift or talent given by God to an individual or community intended for the good of others. In Christian religious circles, a person's charism is their unique and precious style or strength in ministering to others (Cross and Livingstone 1997).

†See also A. Stroll, *The Essence of Spirituality: Spiritual Dimensions of Nursing Practice* (Philadelphia, PA: Saunders, 1989), pp. 4–23.

THE SPIRITUAL LANDSCAPE IN PATIENTS WITH SERIOUS ILLNESS

Despite a rapidly growing group of "religious nones" (those unaffiliated with any specific faith tradition or community), America is a very religious country. The vast majority of American adults report they believe in God: of those who reported they belonged to any of these groups, the Pew Religious Landscape Study (2014) indicates that 61 percent of white Americans are absolutely certain God exists, compared with 83 percent of Black Americans, 44 percent of Asian Americans, and 59 percent of Latinx Americans (Figure 3.1). Over 50% of Americans say that religion is very important in their lives (Figure 3.2).

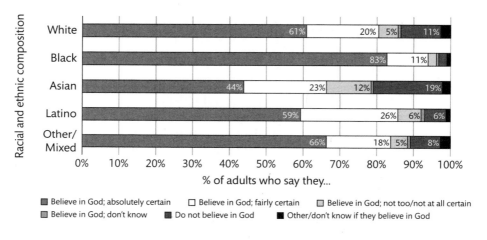

FIGURE 3.1. Belief in God by Race/Ethnicity. *Source:* Pew Research Center.

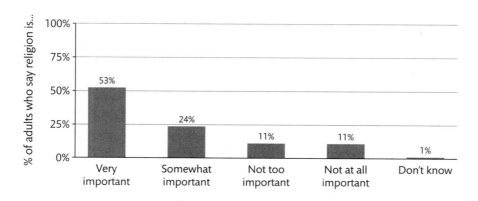

FIGURE 3.2. Importance of Religion in One's Life. *Source:* Pew Research Center.

Data also suggest that religiousness and spirituality increase with the onset of life-threatening illness (Balboni et al. 2007), and my experience as a chaplain confirms this. A cancer diagnosis can create a rupture in the narrative of one's life and challenge one's implicit assumptions about oneself, God, and the predictability of life: *"I am a healthy person," "If I'm a good person, God will reward me,"* or, *"Everything happens for a reason."* Most patients—even those who under normal circumstances would not describe themselves as religious—bring their shock and dismay upon a cancer diagnosis to some conceptual understanding of God. *"Oh my God!" "Why is God doing this to me?" "Please God, give me strength,"* or the common adage, *"God doesn't give you more than you can handle."* A Buddhist may think about karmic retribution; a Jew may wonder if her plight is related to her lack of observance. This intimate and urgent reckoning is for many patients at the heart of their illness experience. Furthermore, we know religion and spirituality are important factors that influence medical decision-making in the event of a terminal illness, especially in nonwhite populations (Balboni et al. 2007; Ehman et al. 1999; Koenig 1998; McClain et al. 2003). If clinicians acknowledge and engage with this aspect of their patients' lives, all dimensions of care are enhanced.

POSITIVE AND NEGATIVE RELIGIOUS COPING

A patient's religious coping can be positive and protective, or negative and harmful. Studies indicate that religion and spirituality can be important sources of hope and coping for patients at the end of life, and that spirituality "preserves patients' quality of life despite severe physical symptoms, supports prognostic acceptance, and protects against hopelessness and despair near death" (Phelps et al. 2012, p. 2538). Religious service attendance is a powerful predictor for several health outcomes in healthy populations, and if service attendance wanes with increasing age and disability associated with illness, there is a corresponding increase in private spiritual activities (Balboni and Balboni 2018). In one study of Black patients with cancer pain, positive spiritual coping was associated with decreased pain and lower symptom burden and may have served as a protective factor against diminished overall quality of life, specifically in the social, emotional, and functional domains (Bai et al. 2018). Patients' surrogate decision-makers use spiritual and religious coping frequently to deal with the stress of decision-making for their loved ones (Maiko et al. 2019); they endorsed personal prayer and trusting in God for guidance or to be in charge, along with other sources of support such as family, friends, and coworkers.

At the same time, *negative* manifestations of spirituality may be associated with poorer health outcomes. Religious struggle and spiritual distress have been associated with increased mortality in elderly patients, as well as with more severe depression and desire for hastened death in patients at the end of life (Pargament

2001; McClain et al. 2003; Rodin et al. 2009). Spiritual distress might have a potentially harmful effect on patients' prognosis and quality of life (Monod et al. 2007).

Determining whether a patient's faith is fortifying him or compounding his suffering is one of the first things I do in a spiritual assessment. Two patients I worked with in our immunotherapy oncology clinic illustrate this difference.

I had followed Robert and Joe during the previous year. Both described themselves as very religious, and when I saw them on the same afternoon in back-to-back appointments, it was clear that both were declining quickly with debilitating symptoms of metastatic renal cell cancer. Robert, 69, arrived for his appointment in a wheelchair, pushed by his wife, Michelle. This Black couple lived in Rhode Island, and the burden of Robert's disease had taken a physical, emotional, and financial toll on the family. I knew they had a supportive church community back home (they were nondenominational Christians), and community members had collected money to help them pay their monthly bills now that Robert couldn't work in his machine shop.

The biweekly trips to Boston for medical appointments had cast an unwelcome rhythm into this family's life: grueling traffic, long waits in the clinic, and usually, bad news about the failure of treatment after treatment. This particular day, crippling back pain was Robert's most acute symptom, and he spent time with my physician colleague discussing options to minimize the pain.

When my colleague left, I asked the couple gently how they were doing spiritually, given this new intensity of symptoms. *"Is your faith a support?"* I asked. Robert's answer stays with me still. The couple held hands as Robert answered, *"You know, it's been really tough. But isn't this what a life of faith prepares you for? We are walking in the valley of the shadow.* Sometimes we read the Psalms together, or Lamentations. The church community has been great, supporting Michelle and making sure we're not alone. The pastor says we can call him anytime, any hour. This isn't easy, but we do feel God is with us."* Michelle nodded, with tears in her eyes.

The next patient I saw that afternoon was Joe. Joe, 71, always entered the clinic with a certain gusto, energetically greeting the front desk staff and the nursing assistants, shouting out, "Hey Doc!" to anyone in a white coat. Joe came to clinic with his supportive wife, Pearl, who was diminutive and always chuckled at Joe's antics. Joe wore a prominent gold crucifix and a medal of his patron saint. He was a white Italian Catholic and had worked in car dealerships for years. He attended mass throughout his life but told me he had been attending church less often in recent months. Like Robert, Joe had been living with metastatic renal cell cancer for a few years. He had done reasonably well but was now facing more debilitating symptoms and increasingly limited treatment options. The couple had two supportive daughters who sometimes joined the appointments, and it struck me

---

*A reference to Psalm 23:4: "Yea though I walk through the shadow of the valley of death, I will fear no evil, for Thou art with me; thy rod and thy staff comfort me."

that Joe was used to "holding court" with the women in his life, who clearly adored him. Lately, pain had been preventing Joe from sleeping, and he described trying to sleep in a reclining chair, managing his sleep apnea, and his difficulty making it to the bathroom at night. It sounded miserable. I asked Joe about his faith, and whether it was a support to him during this difficult time. Joe stopped and looked at me searchingly: *"You know, Katie, I have lived a good, clean life. Why is God doing this to me? They say God won't give you more than you can handle, but why would God give this to me in the first place? It's like He forgot about me or something! Or He's punishing me for something I did? But I am praying for a miracle. I know I'll be cured yet. Right, Pearlie?" "That's right, Joe,"* Pearl answered.

The difference between these two men's responses was striking. Both were men of the same age, both had listed religion as very important to them when we did the initial intake screening, and both had metastatic renal cell cancer. But Robert was finding consolation and strength from his faith, while Joe was in considerable spiritual distress. Joe's spiritual distress, hidden behind his extroverted presentation, was compounding his suffering considerably. If I had not asked the question, I would have missed the chance to do important work with Joe and Pearl before he died a few months later.

Psychologist Kenneth Pargament and others developed the framework of positive and negative religious coping (Pargament, Feuille, and Burdzy 2011), which I find to be a useful tool during an initial assessment. Examples are listed in the Practice Point box below.

Practice Points: Positive and Negative Religious Coping

Positive Religious Coping

Patients may . . .

- Feel a sense of God's presence, consolation.
- Seek to understand how God might be trying to strengthen or guide them in their illness.
- Feel connected to a tradition.
- Find solace in ritual (e.g., prayer).
- See one's story in the narrative of the faith.
- Trust a larger meaning-making framework as they move toward death.

Negative Religious Coping

Patients may . . .

- Feel abandoned by God, desolation.
- Feel punished by God.
- Question God's love for them.
- Feel abandoned by religious community.
- Believe the devil caused the affliction.
- Feel crippling shame for past decisions or actions.

(Adapted from Pargament, Feuille, and Burdzy 2011)

Once I have determined whether a patient's religious or spiritual coping is positive or negative, I adapt my intervention accordingly. In Robert's case, for example, I affirmed his and Michelle's faith, we read Psalms together, discussed what they might need from their church community in the weeks ahead, and explored the ways they felt God moving in their lives.

In Joe's case, by contrast, I explored any real regrets or feelings of guilt he had that informed his sense of being punished. I offered alternative ways of conceiving of God using scripture and sacred stories; I tried to embody a merciful and loving God (rather than a punitive one); and with Joe's permission I reached out to his parish priest to arrange for sacramental care for Joe, which I suspected could lead to important healing and reconciliation.

SPIRITUAL NEEDS

What are spiritual needs? Considering a definition of spirituality that includes but also extends beyond religious practice, all human beings have spiritual needs. These needs typically relate to transcendence of the self and to connections to things greater than ourselves. Spiritual needs include the need to give and receive love, to belong, to have hope, to be able to express ourselves creatively, to contribute, and to have meaning and purpose in our lives (Highfield and Cason 1983; Jacobs 2008).

> **Practice Point: Spiritual Needs**
>
> - Give and receive love
> - Belong
> - Have hope
> - Express ourselves creatively
> - Contribute
> - Have meaning and purpose in life

When we face our mortality, we consider those from whom we have been estranged and seek reconciliation (Attig 2003). We may feel guilt or shame about decisions made or things left undone (Fitchett and Canada 2010). Some research suggests that among patients with advanced illness, being at peace with God is ranked, along with freedom from pain, as one of the most important elements of a good death (Steinhauser et al. 2000).

Chaplain researcher George Fitchett (2020) developed an evidence-based spiritual assessment model specifically for use by palliative care chaplains, the PC-7. Fitchett and his colleagues identified common spiritual concerns of patients living with advanced cancer. These themes, based on literature in the field and their own extensive clinical experience, include:

- The need for meaning in the face of suffering
- The need for integrity, a legacy, generativity
- Concerns about relationships, family and/or significant others
- Concern or fear about dying or death
- Issues related to making decisions about treatment
- Religious or spiritual struggle
- Other

The researchers identify indicators for each theme and instruct chaplains to generate a score based on their assessment of the patient's level of unmet need for each. With this tool chaplains can identify the prevalence and intensity of unmet religious and spiritual needs and develop interventions for each (Fitchett et al. 2020).

Marvin Delgado Guay and physician colleagues (2011) at MD Anderson study *spiritual pain* in advanced cancer patients. Using Mako's (2006) definition of spiritual pain as "a pain deep in your soul (being) that is not physical," Delgado Guay found that approximately half of the 100 advanced cancer patients they asked reported spiritual pain to be present. Similarly, Mako (2006) found that 96 percent of advanced cancer patients had experienced spiritual pain some time in their lives, and 61 percent reported experiencing it at the time of the interview, with a mean intensity of 4.7 on a 0 to 10 scale. In Delgado Guay's study, patients who reported spiritual pain were significantly more likely to feel that spiritual pain made their physical (6 vs. 0, $p < 0.001$) and emotional (6 vs. 0, $p < 0.001$) symptoms worse. Delgado Guay concludes that it is important to consider routine spiritual assessments to identify patients' needs, particularly in those with refractory symptoms. His findings suggest that patients who report refractory symptoms might have spiritual pain as a contributor, and that unmet spiritual concerns and needs may be a contributing factor to spiritual pain (Delgado Guay et al. 2011; Mako 2006).

SPIRITUAL ASSESSMENT

The aim of a spiritual assessment is to identify the unique spiritual needs of a patient to create interventions that can address those needs; spiritual care is never "one size fits all." If you, as a clinician, identify that a patient like Joe is coping negatively, I recommend you make a referral to a professional chaplain. Intensive spiritual care for patients who have serious spiritual distress or whose faith is compounding their suffering is beyond the scope of your work as a provider. If you do not have access to a professional chaplain,* you can encourage the patient to reach out to their own clergy person, or see if, with the patient's permission, you or a colleague can reach out on her behalf.

CLINICIANS PROVIDING SPIRITUAL CARE

But what *is* within the scope of your role as a provider regarding your patients' religious and spiritual needs? Studies suggest that patients do want their providers to consider these needs. They show that when doctors engage in spiritual discussion, patients find it promotes the provision of holistic care, strengthens the doctor-patient relationship, and allows the doctor to accommodate religious beliefs in the management of their illness (Best, Butow, and Olver 2016c).

Patients typically do not expect their clinicians to ask about religious or spiritual concerns in order to provide spiritual guidance or counseling; rather, they understand the inquiry as cementing the relationship between provider and patient to receive more comprehensive and supportive care (Best, Butow, and Olver 2016). Patients expect their providers to refer them to chaplains if serious spiritual concerns exist, and chaplains, as the spiritual care specialists, expect the same.

Prospective studies have found associations between medical team spiritual support and (1) improved patient quality of life near death, (2) increased hospice utilization, and (3) among highly religious patients, decreased aggressive care at the end of life (Balboni et al. 2010). Terminally ill cancer patients who report not receiving spiritual care by the medical team have high medical costs at the end of life. This is particularly true for highly religious patients and patients who are not white (Balboni et al. 2011). The degree to which staff address the spiritual needs of patients is related to overall patient satisfaction and likelihood to recommend the hospital (Marin et al. 2015; Astrow et al. 2007).

Barriers

The Religion and Spirituality in Cancer Care Study, a multi-institutional, quantitative and qualitative study of 75 patients with advanced cancer and 339 cancer physicians and nurses, found that patients reported being provided with spiritual care only 25 percent of the time, although 77 percent of patients, 72 percent of

---

*In 2020 there were approximately 11,000 board-certified chaplains in the United States. As such it is possible you will not be able to find a trained chaplain at your institution, in which case you may want to urge those of your patients who have good relationships with clergy to seek increased support from them. There are also some online chaplaincy resources; if patients and families search for online support, encourage them to ensure that the chaplain is board certified by one of the three main certifying bodies: the Association of Professional Chaplains (APC), the National Association of Catholic Chaplains (NACC), or Nashema, the Association of Jewish Chaplains.

physicians, and 85 percent of nurses thought it would be beneficial. In the setting of terminal illness, 41 to 94 percent of patients want their physicians to include attention to patients' religious and spiritual needs, and such attention is included in national palliative care guidelines. Yet despite patients' desire for their medical teams to care for their spiritual needs, and recommendations by the World Health Organization, the National Consensus Project on Quality Palliative Care, and the Joint Commission, most providers do not provide spiritual care (Balboni et al. 2014). Why not?

Physicians and nurses report several barriers to providing spiritual care. Predictors of not providing such care include lack of training, a felt sense that inquiring about religion or spirituality is not within the purview of the physician's professional role, and concern about power inequity with the patient (fear of being perceived as proselytizing, violating a boundary, or making a patient uncomfortable). These are all important concerns (Best, Butow, and Olver 2016c).

Nurses also desire to provide spiritual care for their patients with terminal illness, but 40 percent of them report that they provide such care less often than they would like to. Like their physician colleagues, nurses identify lack of training as a primary barrier to providing spiritual care, along with a lack of privacy for patient conversations.

There are data suggesting an association between insufficient confidence in some psychological aspects of end-of-life care and clinician burnout. Some scholars, me included, speculate that teaching clinicians to engage with their patients about religion and spirituality at the end of life could mitigate burnout and even promote the clinicians' personal growth (Penderell and Brazil 2010). Discovering a patient's deep well of spiritual resources reassures a provider that the patient is coping well and points to meaning beyond a cure. Training that introduces the broader definition of spirituality (centered in meaning making and a connection to something greater than oneself) makes the topic more accessible to providers who are skeptical of religion or not religious themselves.

My palliative care physician colleague and I cared for a patient named Frank who was of special concern for the oncology team. By exploring Frank's spiritual resources, we were able to reassure the team that he was, in fact, coping as well as possible. Our looking "under the hood" with this patient and family reassured the team, and they continued to follow the patient's wishes and provide good care until his death.

Frank was a 38-year-old musician-accountant whose metastatic melanoma raged through his body faster than any treatment could contain for long. With several pathological fractures and crippling fatigue, Frank and his wife, Alejandra, came to the clinic one Wednesday; the team was especially concerned. Frank's nurse practitioner and attending oncologist waved us over. *"His scan looks terrible. We think Frank and Alejandra are in denial. We don't think they realize how serious this is; Frank's disease is advancing on this last line of treatment, and we need to talk with them about hospice. They still don't have any nursing help at home, and Frank is declining quickly. Can you explore what they know, and how they are* actually *doing?"*

Such a charge to the palliative care team is not unusual in the oncology clinic, and in this case, it was not surprising. Frank and Alejandra had been cared for by this particular team for three years. They had been newly married when Frank was first diagnosed. Aware of Frank's diagnosis and likely prognosis, the couple had decided to conceive a child, and by the time I met them, their curious, quick-to-smile 6-month-old son, Frank Jr., sometimes joined them in the clinic. The care team had rallied around the pregnancy and birth, selected Frank and Alejandra to be recipients of the department's toy and diaper collection for Christmas and were fully invested in the care of this young family. Frank's disease was a tragedy of the first order. Everyone, clinicians included, preferred to focus on the baby, the weather, Frank's favorite baseball team, *anything* but the fact that Frank was dying.

My palliative care physician colleague Mary and I steeled ourselves and went to talk with the couple. As usual, we admired pictures of Frank Jr. and heard about his latest antics and milestones. Then the tone of the conversation shifted when Mary asked what Frank understood about the current state of his illness. Frank explained what he understood from his oncologist: *"The scan results are 'mixed': the cancer in the 'dangerous places' [organs] is shrinking, but the cancer in the bones is growing."* This was somehow comforting to Frank, he explained, because *"at least it's growing in the less dangerous places."* Mary gently mentioned the fact that he had fallen recently, and Frank agreed that could have been serious. We said we wanted to talk with them about setting up some more support at home *"just in case,"* and ideally before they really needed it, before there was a crisis.

A bit of a pall came over the conversation, and Mary continued, *"Have you thought about your preferences, in case things don't go well?"* Frank answered, *"I want to live. If there's a reasonable chance that something will help me live longer, I want to try it."* We discussed what a reasonable chance might look like, and how to make those decisions. And then Frank said, *"I've been afraid of dying since I was a teenager."*

"Are you afraid of the dying process, or of being dead?" I asked.

"Being dead. Being nothing. It just freaks me out. But then I think, I won't know I'm dead, so why worry about it?"

Knowing Frank is Catholic, I ask, *"Does your faith help you at all?"*

"A little."

I offered, *"You could call a priest you know, or I can connect you with one, and you could talk with him about what the Church teaches about death. The Catholic Church has a deep theology about death and dying, and some beautiful rituals; there are a lot of resources there."*

With a glimmer in his eye, Frank said, *"I could . . . but what if the priest and the Church are wrong?"*

"No easy answers for you, I see," I respond, playing along. We discussed some books written by scientists who had near-death experiences; Frank was only slightly curious. And then we talked about courage, and the Ultimate Voyage, and how none of us knows what it will be like to die. I assured Frank we would do all we could to ensure he feels safe, and these conversations, though hard, were a part of that. We discussed Frank Jr.'s birth: I asked about their experience with birth, and with other loved ones who have died. *"It's all such a mystery,"* Frank said, shaking his head, and pulling up a picture of Frank Jr. on his phone.

My colleague Mary continued the conversation about Frank's wishes for the end of his life and explained how having these conversations before there's a crisis can be a gift to one's health care proxy and family members, so they're not left guessing. At that point Alejandra chimed in and said they really have discussed these matters, she knows what Frank wants, that they have talked at length, and she feels OK. *"We just don't like to focus on it; we try to enjoy each day."* The couple agreed to talk with the case manager about bridge to hospice, and we planned to see each other again in two weeks.

When Mary and I returned to the work room, our oncology colleagues asked us expectantly, *"So how are they, really?"*

And how *were* Frank and Alejandra, spiritually speaking, as they faced Frank's impending death? If spiritual wellness relates to being connected, to self, to others, to something larger than oneself, our conversation with Frank and Alejandra told me they were spiritually equipped. They were sad, they were grieving, but they were well resourced. They were not in denial. They were hoping for the best but preparing for the worst. Frank's connection to Alejandra, Frank Jr., and his music did sustain him, and he knew the end of his life was approaching.

In this case, the oncology team's affection for this young family added to their worry and distress. By asking the palliative care team to ask the harder questions, and hearing that the couple was, in fact, spiritually preparing and well resourced, the oncology team was reassured and continued their good care of this family. In my opinion, our conversation with Frank and Alejandra was an intervention to address both the family and the oncology team's spiritual distress, and that is palliative care at its best.

Frank and Alejandra never did contact visiting nursing or hospice. Before Frank died, his musician friends held a benefit concert for the family, which Frank was able to attend, even playing one song on the keyboard. Frank died at home a couple months after our conversation, cared for by Alejandra and their extended family and friends.

I wonder whether an oncology team with basic training in spiritual care would have been able to look "under the hood" with Frank and Alejandra themselves. If chaplains are spiritual care specialists, other clinicians can be trained to be spiritual care generalists (Bandini et al. 2019; Robinson, Thiel, and Shirkey 2016). Educational offerings exist in many settings to provide nonchaplain clinicians with the tools and resources they need to provide the basics of spiritual care. Data suggest that teaching clinicians basic spiritual assessment skills can have a positive impact on clinician confidence, comfort, and ability to provide generalist spiritual care (Zollfrank et al. 2015; Bandini et al. 2019).

Further benefits for doctors who discuss religion and spirituality with patients are enhanced provision of patient-centered care and increased personal spiritual growth. One hospice agency reported that by training their providers in spiritual care, they had created a culture change in their organization that lead to higher overall satisfaction scores for both patients and staff (Daudt, d'Archangelo, and Duquette 2018). It is worth noting that 29 percent of nurses and 49 percent of physicians in one study did not desire training in the provision of spiritual care; those less likely to desire this training not surprisingly reported lower self-ratings of spirituality (Balboni et al. 2014).

The goal of most spiritual care curricula is to train providers to be comfortable identifying and talking about religious and spiritual issues, to model hospitality for all religious traditions and spiritual practices, to learn a basic spiritual screening tool, to understand the ethics involved in being a spiritual care generalist, and to know when to refer to a spiritual care specialist (a chaplain or clergy in the community).

SPIRITUAL CARE SCREENING TOOLS

Some core spiritual screening questions include *Do you consider yourself spiritual or religious?*; *What is your faith or belief?*; *Is faith important in your life?*; *Are you part of a spiritual or religious community?* If exploring religious and spiritual histories is new for you, you may find it helpful to have a framework or mnemonic. FICA and HOPE are two commonly used screening tools.

FICA

The FICA© tool, a series of questions developed by Dr. Christina Puchalski, is based upon a broad definition of spirituality that is focused on how a person seeks meaning, purpose, and transcendence and how they experience a relationship to the significant or sacred as they understand it, whether through religious, spiritual, secular, or humanistic perspectives (Borneman, Ferrell, and Puchalski 2010).

Faith, Belief, Meaning: *"Do you consider yourself to be spiritual? Is spirituality something important to you?"*; *"Do you have spiritual beliefs, practices, or values that help you to cope with stress, difficult times, or what you are going through right now? (Contextualize to visit)"*; *"What gives your life meaning?"*

Importance and Influence: *"What importance does spirituality have in your life?"*; *"Has your spirituality influenced how you take care of yourself, particularly regarding your health?"*; *"Does your spirituality affect your healthcare decision making?"*

> **Practice Point: FICA© Spiritual Assessment Tool**
>
> **F**aith, Belief, Meaning
>
> **I**mportance
>
> **C**ommunity
>
> **A**ddress/Action in Care
>
> *(Borneman, Ferrell, and Puchalski 2010)*

Community: *"Are you part of a spiritual community?"*; *"Is your community of support to you and how?"*; "For people who don't identify with a community consider asking, *Is there a group of people you really love or who are important to you?"*

Address/Action in Care: *"How would you like me, as your healthcare provider, to address spiritual issues in your healthcare?* (A also refers to the *Assessment and Plan* for patient spiritual distress, needs, and/or resources within a treatment or care plan.)"

HOPE

HOPE questions similarly provide a framework for spiritual assessment. Examples of questions using the HOPE framework can be found in Anandarajah and Hight (2001).

> **Practice Point: HOPE Spiritual Assessment Tool**
>
> Hope (H): Sources of hope, meaning, comfort, strength, peace, love, and connection
>
> Organized (O): Organized religion
>
> Personal spirituality/practice (P): Personal spirituality and practice
>
> Effects (E): Effects on medical care and end-of-life issues
>
> *(Adapted from Anandarajah and Hight 2001, p. 86.)*

Taking a Spiritual History

The spiritual history itself can be incorporated into the social history, which normalizes the inquiry so that it is less likely to raise suspicion (*"Are you asking me about religion because I'm dying?"*). As a chaplain, sometimes my very presence causes patients to worry that I've been sent by a doctor because "bad news" is coming. Putting people at ease and reassuring them that I am simply "making my rounds" is an important part of what I do each day. The more we can help patients feel this is a routine screening that simply helps the provider take good care of the patient, the better. Asking these questions early in the patient-provider relationship, during the time when the provider and patient are getting acquainted and before there is a crisis, is key.

Some clinicians I work with admit that they do not know how to respond to their patients' answers to their questions about religion and spirituality, or they worry patients will ask them about their own religion; for that reason, some of them avoid asking the questions at all. It is important to remember that simply asking the question is experienced by many patients as being supportive enough. Staying in one's primary role as provider (not spiritual counselor) is essential. Don't try to answer the "big" questions (*"Why is this happening to me?"*); typically, these are rhetorical questions anyway, or merit a referral to a chaplain. It is often enough to respond, *"I hear you asking important questions about the meaning of this experience for you. I don't have answers, but you might find it helpful to talk with others in your faith about this."*

If a patient asks you about your religious affiliation, remember you do not have to answer. (Try saying something like *"What I really care about are your beliefs, and how I can support you in those while I'm caring for you medically."*) If you do answer, keep it succinct and refocus the question back to the patient: *"I am Jewish, but my focus here is what is important to you—how the rest of the team and I can best support you and your family."*

If a patient asks you to pray with or for them, be authentic. Leading a prayer with a patient in the room, though, is beyond the scope of your role and is more complex than it seems. It is acceptable, however, to maintain a respectful silence while a patient herself prays, or to refer the patient to a chaplain. One palliative care fellow I worked with was nonplussed when a patient, at the end of her appointment, asked him to pray for her. This physician does not believe in God and does not pray, but he wanted to respond in a way that felt supportive to the patient and authentic to himself. For this fellow, that meant carving out a bit of time in his day to call this patient to mind and think of her. That was his way of "praying" for her, and he felt he was honoring her request while also being authentic to himself.

Ethical Concerns

From an ethical perspective, it is crucial you know your limitations and the boundaries around your role as provider. You should never "sell" your own spiritual, religious, or secular beliefs to a patient. (This applies to chaplains as well: our professional organizations and certifying bodies prohibit chaplains from proselytizing or bringing a religious agenda to patient encounters.) Always keep in mind the relationship imbalance between you and the patient, as well as the ethical risk of coercion. Never try to "fix" or "adjust" the beliefs of a patient in your care; doing so can cause harm (Robinson, Thiel, and Meyer 2007; personal communication with Mary Martha Thiel during joint curriculum development, Spring 2021).

One misstep I made years ago illustrates this point. I was called to support the wife of a man in his sixties who had fallen from a ladder while cleaning leaves off his roof. The man, a professor at a nearby college, survived but suffered a devastating spinal cord injury. Just days after the accident, the family was reeling. They were Episcopalians, active in their church. The wife said to me, *"You know nothing like this has ever happened to me before; I have had such an easy, blessed life. Maybe all that time God was preparing me for this because He knew Tom was going to have this accident."* I do not remember exactly what I said, but somehow in my response, I refuted her. *"I don't believe God works that way; I think things just happen, and God is with us as we try to find our way through."*

Of course, I was trying to be helpful. But I could see in the expression on the woman's face that my comment was not, in fact, helpful. She was in shock and casting about for some meaning in this accident. In her conception, God was a kind God who had protected her all those years to ready her to cope with this event, a benevolent God in control of her life. This was positive religious coping, a fragile step toward meaning making that seemed to be propping her up in a time of need. She was in no state to consider alternate theological understandings of "how God works," and I risked toppling the fragile meaning-making structure she was building. Mine was not an egregious error, and I worked to correct it and maintain our alliance, but it was a lazy mistake, and more self-centered than patient centered. While it is vital for us as providers to reflect on our own meaning making around illness and trauma, we have to do it in a way that does not risk harming the patients in our care.

It is important to remember that every patient is a culture of one; there are no two Muslims who are exactly alike, no two Jews or Christians. Early in my career I worked hard to learn as much as I could about diverse religious traditions. One day I had a patient who was a Zoroastrian from India. I called a mentor and quizzed her, *"What do you know about Indian Zoroastrianism? What should I do?"* My mentor warmly reminded me, *"Ask this patient what you should do, how you can be helpful. Be hospitable, curious, and kind; the rest will follow."* We should all aim to be culturally and religiously competent, and humility and curiosity are important parts of that competence.

THE ROLE OF RELIGION IN MEDICAL DECISION-MAKING

When disease progression leads to discussions about goals of care, many patients turn toward their faith for guidance and strength. Sometimes you will discover your patients hold a deep faith in a loving God who is expected to "take them home." These patients are typically more comfortable accepting care that focuses primarily on their comfort, not cure. Others, however, hold tenets that make the transition more difficult.

Some patients, for example, feel that their religion prohibits them from accepting any course of treatment that might shorten their life. While there is controversy especially among the Evangelical and Pentecostal Christians and Orthodox Jewish and Islamic clerics, most Christian, Jewish (Rosenberg et al. 2020), and Islamic teachings support the right of the patient to refuse futile and excessively burdensome treatments and to accept pain relief even if they risk an earlier death; in my experience, however, many patients need reassurance from their clergy that this is so. The Catholic Church, for example, expresses its understanding that people who are dying are not expected to accept extreme measures to prolong their lives (Bradley 2009). Refusing to be resuscitated or to be kept alive by artificial means is acceptable to the Church; it is not a sin and is not considered suicide. This has been true in the Catholic Church since 1957. As written again in the new edition of the Catechism, "Discontinuing medical procedures that are burdensome, dangerous, extraordinary, or disproportionate to the expected outcome can be legitimate; it is the refusal of 'overzealous' treatment. Here one does not will to cause death; one's inability to impede it is merely accepted" (*Catechism of the Catholic Church* 1997, Respect for Human Life, 2278, 2279). Copies of this Catechism are commonly kept in hospital chaplains' offices, and much of the work of priest-chaplains is to reassure patients that their decisions are in keeping with the teachings of the Church.

In fact, the teachings of most Christian, Muslim, Jewish, and Hindu traditions affirm the same principle: people with terminal illnesses are not required to endure unrelieved pain or suffering or to allow their lives to be prolonged by technological means. For Buddhists, the question hinges more on the quality of the dying than on the death itself: for some, the mind must be alert to do the work that needs to be done to prepare the soul for death and eventual rebirth. For others, compassion for persons dictates that comfort is paramount, even if sedation is the result. Judaism teaches that if possible, dying people should purify themselves by saying the Vidui, a final confession. Commentaries suggest that "if one cannot say the Vidui audibly, one can say it in their heart... someone near the person can lead them in the Vidui, they can say it, and the dying person can repeat it (Shulchan Aruch Y.D. 338:1, [Yachter 2007]). Even if the patient is comatose, the rabbi can lead the patient in the Vidui, as one can hope that the patient is saying it in his heart. In Islam, too, the ability to recite the Shahaadah, or declaration of faith, before one loses consciousness is valued, but in neither case is the transition toward a natural death refuted or prevented (Chakraborty et al. 2017).

Some Orthodox rabbis and some Evangelical and Pentecostal Christian sects take the premise that all God-given life is sacred and precious to mean that nothing that would shorten it by even a moment is acceptable. Some patients of those faiths might feel that accepting a transition away from aggressive care and toward comfort care is tantamount to admitting that they no longer have faith in God. These patients and their families can be challenging for providers and staff to care for. I have attended countless family meetings in the ICU setting in which providers try to steer families toward letting their loved ones die a natural death, only to have families refuse and insist that God will perform a miracle. A Haitian-Creole medical interpreter taught me during our work together with a particular family that asking this family to agree to compassionate extubation was akin to asking them to sin against their God, and they would never agree. In my hospital, an Orthodox Jewish patient's family insisted on all measures to maintain their loved one's life, even while their loved one suffered visibly and faced little to no chance of meaningful recovery. The nursing staff felt they were inflicting pain on the patient and had strong feelings about the family's decision. Much of the Jewish chaplain's job in this case was to reassure the team that these medical decisions were in keeping with the patient's faith, encouraging them to support her morally and emotionally as they bore witness to what was, in their minds, "senseless" suffering.

If you find yourself in a situation like this, consult with a professional chaplain, or consider conferring with the family together with their clergy or spiritual leader. I often provide moral support to my oncology and palliative care colleagues who watch patients die highly technical deaths in pursuit of life at any cost. If a patient's decisions have integrity according to their belief system, if the option of a particular treatment is still on the table, and if the patient or family understands the consequences, we need to honor those decisions. At the same time, having a physician state clearly that a particular treatment is no longer helpful or medically indicated, and will not achieve the patient's goals, can take the burden of medical decision-making off patients and families who feel they would be committing a sin or demonstrating lack of faith if they chose not to pursue it. These are complex issues; do not hesitate to reach out to chaplaincy and ethics for support.

Patients' beliefs about the nature of an afterlife and the effects of their past activities on it can also enhance or inhibit the acceptance of death and consequently can affect patients' ability to accept moving to a focus on comfort measures. Religious Christians or Muslims who expect to be judged and sent to heaven or hell based on their actions, or Buddhists, who believe that the sum of the worth of their deeds (karma) will determine the nature of their reincarnation, may fear death if they judge themselves to have led a life that will be found morally wanting. They may seek any treatment to defer a death that is terrifying to them.

Again, if you discover religious ideas are negatively affecting your patient's coping or decision-making process, call in the professional chaplain or offer to connect with the patient's religious leader.

"I'M WAITING FOR A MIRACLE!"

Some patients hold fervently to a belief that God will perform a miracle and declare this belief deep into their illness even as they continue to decline physically, like Joe. I am accustomed to receiving referrals from physician and social work colleagues who are concerned the "miracle language" means that the patients are in denial or that the provider has somehow failed to help them understand how grave the situation is. Alicia was one such patient, a young mother and Seventh-Day Adventist. Alicia clung so tightly to her faith as she became sicker with gastric cancer that she refused to talk with anyone who brought up the possibility of her death. *"These people who come in my hospital room,"* she told me, *"they are bad for my spirit! I rebuke them! I know this illness came from God, and God will heal it completely. I need to get out of this hospital."*

I heard a psychiatrist once say that when faced with loss, patients tend to intensify their attachment behaviors, not loosen them. Desperate hope for a miracle is a natural manifestation of this fear of impending loss. In my experience of working with patients who talk about hoping for a miracle, the vast majority have what I call a "double consciousness." They do, in fact, hear what their physicians are saying, and they know themselves to be increasingly unwell. They are also, sincerely and deeply, praying for God to bring a complete healing. This dynamic inconsistency indicates an urgent reckoning but usually does not flag denial. If your patient is talking about a miracle, remember she is in the midst of a process, and her desperate hope for a miracle is not static. Your job as a provider is to maintain your alliance in the meantime.

Chaplain Brenda Cooper, along with nurse and physician colleagues, developed a mnemonic for working with patients who are hoping for a miracle, called, suitably, the AMEN protocol. Cooper explains that the goal of the protocol is to help providers remain engaged with patients and families during challenging conversations that involve patients' religious beliefs, particularly in response to a poor prognosis (Cooper et al. 2014). The aim is not necessarily to change patients' minds but to align with them while staying in one's primary role as medical provider.

The AMEN protocol is a communication tool that enables you as a provider to bear witness to and shore up a patient's meaning making. The disease will continue to declare itself, but with AMEN, conversations are more likely to be collaborative rather than confrontational. Cooper explains it this way:

In the midst of these challenging conversations that are daily occurrences in medical professions, success cannot simply be equated with a perfectionistic expectation that everyone is on the same page, apart from acknowledging the hopes—and fears—of those receiving care. When the provider claims the role of an incrementalist, joining with and/or actively engaging the patient and family can be the best possible outcome. Continued conversational engagement between provider and the patient and family may well be the best measure of successful communication. (Cooper et al. 2014, p. e195)

I found I needed to reach out to Alicia's pastor for help. I became involved when Alicia and her family were in crisis, their alliance with her medical team was frayed, she was becoming increasingly ill, and her team was concerned she would have a serious gastric bleed and die quickly. I knew she needed the cultural and theological authority of her own pastor for the hard days to come.

Practice Points: AMEN Protocol

- **A**ffirm patients' beliefs. Validate their position: *"Ms. X, I admire your strength and your faith,"* or, *"I also have hope."*
- **M**eet patients and family members where they are: *"I join you in hoping (or praying) for a miracle/a better outcome/a change in how things are."*
- **E**ducate from your role as a medical provider: *"I want to speak to you about some medical issues."* It is important here not to use the word *but*. *But* can feel dismissive to a patient. Cooper suggests, "It is God's role to bring the miracle, and it is my role as your physician (or nurse) to bring you some important information that may help us in our decision making." In this way, hope can become the common ground for provider, patient, and family (Cooper et al. 2014, p. e192).
- **N**o matter what, assure the patient and family that you are committed to them: *"No matter what happens, I/the team will be with you every step of the way."*

Fortunately, Alicia's Seventh-Day Adventist pastor was receptive to my call. He came to the hospital and counseled her. He told me he studied a Bible passage with her, Luke 22:42, in which Jesus pleads with God to be spared his suffering and ultimately surrenders to God's will. I supported the staff in their moral distress. I encouraged the team to stop discussing with Alicia the fact that she was dying (she and her husband had assured me that they understood what the doctors had been saying), which they did. Some members of the team still desperately hoped she would accept hospice care, go home, and be with her young daughter, but Alicia's disease was progressing faster than Alicia's emotional and spiritual process.

Alicia did die in the ICU, from a gastric bleed. By the time she died, some trust in the medical team had been reestablished, and the ICU team felt able to care for her as she died. After she died, her husband expressed gratitude for the good care she received. I regret spiritual care was not called in earlier. I could have helped the team understand Alicia's spirituality earlier in her course, how it supported her, and how her pastor could also provide support. We could have avoided the breakdown of communication that added to her and her family's distress for a good portion of her hospital stay.

MEDICINE AS SPIRITUAL PRACTICE

As a clinician you may or may not work closely with a board-certified chaplain. We chaplains and clergy are here to support you, to show up when you discover a patient's religious coping is compounding their suffering or affecting medical decision-making in important ways, or if you need help understanding a religious worldview that is very different from yours. But I am sure you already provide spiritual care. If you tend sensitively to patients and families, if you spend time listening and not only "fixing," if you acknowledge patients' spiritual needs to belong, to love, to hope, to find meaning, to reconcile, to contribute . . . you are delivering spiritual care. Whether or not you are religious, I invite you to consider your careful tending of patients' bodies, minds, and emotions as a spiritual practice, as a means of connecting with something greater than yourself, a way of finding your place, as the poet Mary Oliver says, in the larger "family of things."*

---

*"Wild Geese" from *Dream Work* by Mary Oliver. Copyright © 1986 by Mary Oliver. Used by permission of Grove/Atlantic, Inc.

You do not have to be good.
You do not have to walk on your knees
for a hundred miles through the desert, repenting.
You only have to let the soft animal of your body
    love what it loves.
Tell me about despair, yours, and I will tell you mine.
Meanwhile the world goes on.
Meanwhile the sun and the clear pebbles of the rain
are moving across the landscapes,
over the prairies and the deep trees,
the mountains and the rivers.
Meanwhile the wild geese, high in the clean blue air,
are heading home again.
Whoever you are, no matter how lonely,
the world offers itself to your imagination,
calls to you like the wild geese, harsh and exciting—
over and over announcing your place
in the family of things.

CHAPTER 4

Sexuality, Intimacy, and Cancer

with Amanda Moment, MSW, LICSW

Next to conversations about the end of life, the hardest topic for most of us to broach with patients may be sexuality. It can feel just too intimate, with its minefield of cultural pitfalls and awkward moments. No wonder most of us would prefer to avoid it. In this chapter, Amanda Moment, MSW, LICSW, my colleague and an expert in the palliative care needs of cancer patients, helps us explore why sexuality is important, what barriers we face, what patients really want from us, and how to improve our practice, and it will be her voice that is speaking as I.

Many studies show that patients want to know about the effect of cancer and cancer-related treatment on their sex lives, and that we clinicians are notoriously poor at helping them anticipate and navigate these concerns. This chapter includes a review of the literature about sexuality and cancer. Those of you already familiar with this information may want to skip ahead to the sections called "How to Approach the Subject" and "Practice Suggestions." Tables appear near the end of the chapter.

WHY IS THIS SUBJECT IMPORTANT?

Sexuality and Quality of Life

Even in the midst of treatment, people with cancer can think beyond fears of mortality to aspects of life that enrich them or highlight loss. Life is not solely defined by surviving, and grief is not simply related to the idea of death but to all the other losses that come with change. The World Health Organization (2020) recognizes that sexuality and intimacy are important contributors to quality of life.

Sexuality can mean various things depending on a person's age, gender, culture, religion, education, sexual orientation, and personal history. It includes our relationship to another person, such as how we think about our ability to have sex with a partner, and it includes a connection to the self, such as a woman's sense of identity before and after a mastectomy or a man's sense of masculinity after androgen-deprivation therapy. Our patients are each likely to have unique views of their own sexuality and concerns about changes that treatment will bring. Often the great issues of identity, engagement in life, sexuality, and intimacy are related, and if one diminishes, so can the others (Hawkins et al. 2009; Navon and Morag 2003).

Sexuality and Cancer: Impact and Prevalence

Given the importance of sexuality and intimacy for a patient's sense of self, the changes brought about by cancer and its related treatments are significant. With more than 15 million people living with current or prior cancers and more than 1.7 million new cases in 2019, large numbers of people are moving beyond the initial goal of survival and wondering how to live as well as they can with their diseases (ACS 2019). A patient once said to me, *"My doctors were so focused on helping me survive, that none of us stopped to think about what it would be like to live with the aftermath of treatment."* She was grateful to be alive but working to orient herself to her new body and new reality.

Estimates of sexual dysfunction after various cancer treatments range from 40 percent to 100 percent, with the most common problems in women being dyspareunia (pain with intercourse), vaginal dryness, and low desire, and for men, erectile dysfunction and loss of desire (National Cancer Institute 2020). Sexual problems often become more apparent or distressing during the first months after completing active treatment (Schover 1999).

One couple I met with, in which the husband was battling renal cancer, talked about the medical interventions that slowed and then stopped their sexual life altogether. They were both tired from balancing the many demands of the illness, and sometimes he would be in too much pain to be touched. Once the treatments were over, they both found themselves avoiding a sexual reconnection. He had a hard time looking in the mirror because of all his scars, and in a desire to be supportive, she had not wanted to push him. While they wanted to bridge the gap between them, they didn't know how to approach a conversation about these changes. Before I met with them, no one had explored this area of their lives with them. They were both grateful that I asked about it.

Stigma

Though we may not realize it, patients are often faced with the "dual stigmatiza-tion" of cancer and sexual dysfunction (Navon and Morag 2003, p. 1379). Some unaddressed sexual issues or concerns may interfere with patient compliance with treatments, such as hormone therapy (Schover 1999), and may even affect the decision to undergo potentially life-saving procedures (Bober et al. 2013). Un-fortunately, clinician attitudes can contribute to this sense of stigma. MacElveen and McCorkle (1985) say that when we treat patients as asexual beings because of their age or how ill we think they may be, we can unwittingly hurt people whose sexuality is already traumatized and vulnerable. Because of the power we hold as clinicians, our patients often feel they need our permission to discuss issues of sexuality and intimacy, and they are likely to be grateful for reassurances that what they are experiencing is normal (Hawkins et al. 2009).

Mrs. A was a cancer survivor who told me, "*It is amazing how quickly you become invisible to those taking care of you. Sometimes it feels like they could treat the disease without ever having to really look at you. No one ever asked me about the impact on my sexuality, and yet it was there. I didn't feel that it was acceptable to bring that up.*"

Are We Talking?

Despite the importance of this issue, often neither we nor our patients have the language to begin the discussion. As a couples therapist, I can attest that people often struggle to talk about sex and intimacy even in good physical health. Wei-jmar Schultz and Van de Wiel (2003) noted that when cancer enters the picture, "suddenly, words need to be found to discuss and express wishes, desires, options, and impossibilities" (p. 121). The data suggest that we are missing the mark. Al-though significant research shows that patients want health professionals to bring up issues of sexuality and intimacy (Ananth et al. 2003; Hordern and Currow 2003; Mutsch et al. 2019; Price 2010), health care professionals believe patients will bring these issues up if they are important to them (Carr 2007; Price 2010; Saunamaki, Andersson, and Engstrom 2010), and therefore the number of us who initiate this conversation is low (Hawkins et al. 2009; Hendren et al. 2005). We are more likely to talk about sexuality and intimacy with patients whose cancer or its treatment directly affects sexual function (Schover 1999; Shell 2007), ignore the emotional effects, and talk only about the physical implications, such as erections, menopause, and fertility (Hordern and Street 2007).

Whose Responsibility Is It?

Because of the natural power differential between our patients and us, and because they look to us to guide all the rest of their symptomatic support during treatment, it is our responsibility to bring up the topic of sexuality and to incorporate sexuality screens into our practice. Patients may believe that raising the subject, which is already fraught with stigmas, shame, and uncertainty, is a waste of our time. Sharon Bober and colleagues note that when clinicians do not address issues of sexuality, patients may "wrongly assume that little or nothing can be done to manage the sexual side-effects of cancer and cancer treatments" (2016, p. 45) and that sexual dysfunction is just "collateral damage that must be endured" (Bober and Varela 2012, p. 3715).

Research shows that patients prefer to receive sexual health information from providers who initiate the conversation, who are knowledgeable, and who seem comfortable addressing sexual concerns (Wittenberg and Gerber 2009). Thus, we need to practice making ourselves more comfortable with discussions of sexuality. This chapter offers some guidance.

Positive Outcomes

What can we hope for if we discuss these issues? Ideally, we can hope to hit on a topic that is meaningful for our patients, allay a sense of isolation, provide avenues for support and resources, and improve quality of life.

Mr. D, a 29-year-old single man who had been undergoing treatment for testicular cancer, said that it had been really useful for his oncologist to open up the topic of sexuality with him. He had been casually dating prior to his diagnosis but felt that he had no outlet for discussing with anyone he knew how his health and his romantic life now intersected. *"I hadn't realized that this was a subject I could talk about with my doctor, but once he asked if I had any questions about how it was affecting intimacy in my life, I realized I wasn't alone with it."*

Even if patients don't have specific questions about sexuality or intimacy, an open and curious approach lets them know that you are interested in all the ways cancer affects their lives. You can show that you provide care for the whole person and increase your patients' ability to make informed decisions about all aspects of their treatment.

HOW DO CANCER AND RELATED TREATMENTS AFFECT SEXUALITY?

According to Weijmar Schultz and Van de Wiel (2003, p. 122), "sexual problems are nearly always caused by a complex combination of physical, psychological, and social problems" and often are influenced by people's sexual functioning before they became ill. The authors add that "disease extent, magnitude of treatment, and location of disease are all important determinants of risk" (p. 122). A Macmillan Cancer Support survey offers a helpful categorization of the aspects of sexuality that change when someone becomes a cancer patient: (1) physical ability to give and receive sexual pleasure; (2) thoughts about one's body or body image; (3) feelings, including fear, sadness, anger, and joy; and (4) roles and relationships (Davis 2009). Below is broad overview that may add to your understanding about each of these aspects.

Physical Changes

A list of the changes that affect sexuality is found at the end of this chapter (Table 4.1).

Much of the information in this table is a highly condensed version of sexuality information available at the National Cancer Institute's website, with specific articles listed at the end of this chapter, under Resources.

Sense of Self and Emotional Changes

Mrs. B was a 56-year-old woman with ovarian cancer who had an ileostomy, colostomy, and a venting G-tube due to cancer-related complications. One day she confided in me that she didn't want to see herself naked anymore. The landscape of her body and self-concept had changed so much that it no longer felt like her own. She echoed a theme I often hear from patients about feeling as though they have been betrayed by their bodies and are unable to feel at home in them.

Disruption of sexual identity is only one of the changes that cancer and its treatment can bring. Others include emotional disturbances like anxiety and depression, general malaise, apathy, and loss of self-confidence (Weijmar Schultz and Van de Wiel 2003), as well as broader feelings of asexuality or undesirability (Navon and Morag 2003). Patients often bring up feelings of uncertainty about who they are now and report a surreal sense of being out-of-body. Those whose ability to have sexual activity has decreased may mourn this loss and experience feelings of self-blame, rejection, lack of fulfillment, frustration, and obligation (Hawkins et al. 2009).

Social and Interpersonal Changes

Experiencing cancer can affect peoples' desire and ability to interact with their world. Patients may prefer the safety and protection of being around only their immediate family or even being entirely alone over activities that involve a larger social circle, such as a book club or a bowling league. Mr. M, a retired accountant, used to meet up with friends every week at a restaurant, but he says he now avoids this once important ritual for fear that his colostomy will leak or smell. Treatment may also limit a person's ability and energy to socialize. A study by Bergmark and colleagues (1999), for example, found that women who had cervical cancer were more likely than controls to be single. And in Navon and Morag's (2003) study of men receiving hormone therapy for prostate cancer, they found that men avoided places where they would be expected to wear fewer clothes, like beaches and locker rooms. They deliberately demonstrated "masculine" tendencies, to distract others from their body feminization, declined social invitations so that they could avoid conversations about sex, and avoided any courtship of women that might be interpreted as having "serious intentions."

According to Judith Butler, many people think of coitus as the only "real sex" (Hawkins et al. 2009). Hawkins and colleagues conclude that when sexual inter-course ceases due to illness, patients and their partners also stop having other forms of physical contact because they can no longer experience the intercourse that used to be the pleasurable outcome of that foreplay. Patients therefore experience the loss of not only the pleasures of intercourse, but also those of mutual masturbation and other kinds of physical affection and support, losses that can impair their recovery.

Tanya was a 30-year-old woman with breast cancer who was stunning in her floral head scarf and came to her appointment without her boyfriend. She said that during her treatment, they had not been able to have sex, and the most devastating part was that it had been their only form of intimacy. With that gone, she felt removed from him and hurt that he was unable to express love for her in any other physical form. His association between sex and intimacy was limiting their relationship, and she wondered whether the relationship could survive her illness.

These changes in sexuality and intimacy are shared by the caregivers and partners of people with cancer. In a survey of 122 caregiver-partners of people with a wide variety of cancer diagnoses, Hawkins and colleagues (2009) found that 28 percent of men and 47 percent of women caregivers reported that their role led to a "repositioning of the person with cancer as a patient, non-sexual, or a child" (p. 275). Several male caregivers reported that they felt sex was inappropriate with their ill partners because they had become accustomed to seeing their partners as children in need of care.

Fertility and Reproduction

Women and men undergoing treatment for cancer may have serious concerns about the effect of the treatment on their fertility and reproductive abilities. It is therefore crucial to give them and their partners specific information about the effects of their cancer treatment on fertility, along with possible fertility preservation options, resources for support and decision-making, and if appropriate, referral to a reproductive endocrinologist, urologist, obstetrician-gynecologist, or fertility center. You should offer this information regardless of the patient's age, sexual identity, relationship status, or the status of the disease.

Positive Changes

Some research shows that people's sexuality and intimacy changes for the better during or after they discover they have cancer. Some women with gynecological cancer reported less painful intercourse after surgery and, choosing to look on the bright side, were relieved that they no longer had to worry about birth control (Bourgeois-Law and Lotocki 1999). Some patients and partners felt increased understanding, acceptance, affection, devotion, and closeness or described becoming more considerate and better companions (Hawkins et al. 2009; Navon and Morag 2003). Paul, a 58-year-old man with prostate cancer who was on hormone therapy joked about his "manopause" and said, *"Now I finally understand what my wife was going through when she had her hot flashes and mood swings."*

Mary, a 67-year-old woman with gastric cancer, always welcomed the team with a warm smile and quick wit in the mornings. When speaking with me alone about her 35-year marriage she reported, *"Who knew that getting cancer would be one of the best things to happen to my marriage?! We had been living side by side for years and had really come to take one another for granted. Now, every day we make sure to say, 'I love you,' and cuddle together whenever we can."*

CLINICIAN BARRIERS

Given the significance of sexuality in patients' lives, why is it that we as clinicians rarely include sexual issues in our assessments? We may believe that, since they have a life-threatening disease, these patients find sexuality of less importance, or that they are simply too sick to be interested in sexual activities (Saunamaki, Andersson, and Engstrom 2010). As mentioned earlier, many of us believe that patients would raise the subject themselves if it mattered to them, and we assume erroneously that silence indicates that it doesn't.

Our challenges are multifactorial. Some of us may want to discuss these issues with our patients but feel we are not able to because of time constraints (Dizon, Suzin, and McIlvenna 2014; Wiggins et al. 2007). With all the important issues to cover and a limited amount of time in which to meet with patients, not every subject can get robust attention. Additionally, longer-term survivors may be transitioned to community primary care providers who may be less familiar with cancer and treatment-related sequelae (Schover 1999; Zhou, Nekhlyudov, and Bober 2015). In inpatient settings, patients rarely see the same clinician over

---

Assumptions and Hesitations about Cancer and Sexuality: Self-Assessment

- *I do not feel adequately educated in this area.*
- *The concept is complex, and I wonder how far discussions could or should extend.*
- *My upbringing has taught me that it is impolite to inquire about sexuality.*
- *Sexuality is not routinely discussed in relation to health, so I feel as though I am prying.*
- *I am not sure what cues the patient might use to signal a readiness to discuss sexuality.*
- *I am worried about what the patient might ask. What if they confide things that seem strange, abhorrent, or even illegal?*
- *It's difficult to find a private place for discussion, and I fear embarrassment.*
- *If I draw on my life beliefs, this might upset the patient.*
- *I don't believe it is as important to discuss sexuality if the patient is not in a relationship.*
- *I think that discussion of sexuality is dependent on the age or illness stage of patients.*
- *Other:*

---

time, and concerns and interventions may not be passed on from one to the next (MacElveen and McCorkle 1985).

Another problem is that current educational curricula often don't adequately prepare us for discussing sexuality and intimacy with our patients. A survey (by Mosher in 2005) of U.S. and Canadian medical schools revealed that more than half of the 101 responding schools provided only between three and ten hours of sexual medicine training, and just a third provided more than 11 hours (Shindel et al. 2010); physician assistant education held a median of 12 hours of sexual health training (Seaborne, Prince, and Kushner 2015). One study found that sexuality education in U.S. nursing programs is "lacking consistent and adequate information," and that only 16 percent of nurse educators believe that their students are "prepared to deal with sexuality issues" (Aaberg 2016). Students agree; only 37 percent of medical students feel adequately trained to address or treat sexual concerns, though they feel they are important (Wittenberg and Gerber 2009), and nursing students feel their faculty does not model the importance of a sexual assessment (Dattilo and Brewer 2005).

Another barrier is concern about how our patients will perceive us if we attempt to bring up this subject; will we be seen as disrespectful, insensitive, intrusive, or flirtatious (Schover 1999)? These concerns are particularly strong when we take care of patients of the opposite sex, in an age group different from our own, or from a different cultural background (Dattilo and Brewer 2005; Price 2010). Some of us may worry about where the conversation might go once it has begun or how we might end the conversation (Price 2010). Some simply may not feel equipped with answers or the right language.

Though the prevailing message in research is that current undergraduate medical education is not adequate (Dattilo and Brewer 2005; Shindel et al. 2016), there are models for best practices (Bayer et al. 2017; Rubin et al. 2018; Shindel et al. 2016). Additionally, clinical exposure to care for transgender patients while in medical school improves clinician comfort and knowledge (Park and Safer 2018).

Finally, we may be personally uncomfortable with discussing sexuality, and our own experience may become a barrier in our professional work. Unlike typical medical training, in my field of social work, we are asked to spend a great deal of time reflecting on our own beliefs, prejudices, upbringing, and biopsychosocial makeup and how these things may bias our work with patients. This *countertransference awareness* encourages us to face the assumptions we bring into clinical encounters and to work on balancing those beliefs with the needs before us. It helps us to open our minds and provide more comprehensive care.

If you haven't had a chance to reflect on these subjects, you can use the list above (adapted from Price 2010) to test some of your own assumptions and hesitations around the subject of sexuality and its effects on your work. Add any other thoughts of your own.

In a post–#MeToo world, it would also be natural to wonder if raising the issue of sexuality would be perceived as entering the territory of harassment or conveying/inviting sexually inappropriate communication. I am hopeful that my suggestions in this chapter will mitigate some of these concerns.

If you want to try a more open-ended exploration of your comfort level and attitude about sexuality, consider some of these questions adapted from Shell 2007.

Deeper Exploration of Attitudes toward Sexuality in Cancer Patients

Level of Comfort

1. How comfortable do you feel discussing sexual matters?
2. Notice physical tension, body position, eye contact, and facial expression when listening to specific sexual content. What makes you feel uneasy?
3. What sexual terms can you comfortably use to describe sexual fantasies, interest, arousal, orgasm, and behaviors?

Attitudes

1. List three values you have about sexual behaviors.
2. How would these values affect the way you would work with clients/patients whose problems reflect a conflict with your values?
3. List any areas regarding sexuality that are unacceptable to you.
4. What could you do to compensate for your attitudes if a patient presented something in one of these areas?

· HOW TO APPROACH THE SUBJECT

Mutual Explorer

We can view our role in discussing sexuality and intimacy issues through many frameworks, but one of my favorites is offered by Bob Price in his 2010 article "Sexuality: Raising the Issue with Patients." He invites us to accept the role of "mutual explorer" and states that "expertise develops . . . with facilitation of discussion rather than the sharing of knowledge" (p. 35). This approach allows us to learn as we go, admit when we don't know something, and keep our patients' needs at the forefront of the conversation. We don't need to be experts, especially if we don't have ready answers. Instead, we can help our patients explore or express their own needs. If you wait until you feel expert enough to answer every question, you're likely to find yourself continuing to avoid the subject altogether (Clifford 1998).

Here's an example of what a typical conversation might sound like if you raised the subject early in your relationship with the patient:

You: *Many people who are dealing with cancer or going through treatment notice some changes to their sexuality or their ability to be intimate. Is this something you have noticed or are worried about?*

Patient: *Well, I'm not sure. But I know my wife and I haven't really been able to be intimate since this back pain started about three months ago.*

You: *Is that different from before the pain started?*

Patient: *Yes. Before my back, we would be intimate at least once a week.*

You: *Is this change something you have been able to talk about together?*

Patient: *Um, not really. We've been focused on other things and haven't stopped to discuss this. Will we be able to resume our previous level of activity together?*

You: *As your pain gets better, it is likely that you will be able to. Most people are able to resume sexual activity given time, though sometimes they need to learn how to adapt to the changes brought about by the cancer or its treatment. As you know, we plan to start chemotherapy after your radiation therapy is done, and that could affect your sexual relationship in other ways. I will let you know about the aspects I am familiar with (particularly before beginning any treatment), but I also want to know what changes you notice as the treatment proceeds. If there are answers I don't have, I will try to find them or connect you to colleagues and resources that can provide you with the information and support you need.*

Notice that you don't need to promise that you know all the answers, just that you are committed to supporting the patient and to providing access to other sources of information.

Timing

Though sexuality or intimacy are important subjects to raise at the start of your relationship, questions may not come up the first time you approach the topics with patients. Early on in your relationship with them, patients may be so afraid of dying, or may have such high anxiety about treatment, that the subject of sexuality fades into the background. Often it is merely enough to let patients know that we are open to discussing issues of sexuality at any time.

A brief discussion over one or two visits is all most patients and partners may need. Because sexual problems often become more apparent or distressing during the first months after finishing active treatment, incorporate these questions into your routine follow-up appointments (Schover 1999). For a patient who may not be finishing treatment and will remain on chronic therapy, make sure to incorporate assessment of the impact on identity or sexual function into routine visits. For people who may be coping with advanced disease, see the section on "Palliative Care, Hospice, and Sexuality."

Humor

How about using humor? Sexuality can be one of the most inherently awkward and therefore most amusing subjects within the cancer experience. But we need to walk a delicate line if we use humor, being careful not to minimize a patient's experience inadvertently or introduce any lewd or inappropriate suggestions while still remaining open to the humor of the situation. Using our "mutual explorer" model, we can inquire about whether our patients or their partners have been able to use humor to cope and tap into their resilience.

One young patient opened his wallet and revealed that he carried around a playing card with a big C on it, reporting that he "played the cancer card" often. *"You need help moving? Nope sorry, I got this here cancer." "Your unattractive cousin needs a blind date? Wish I could, but I've got cancer; see my card?"*

TOOLS, EDUCATIONAL MATERIALS, AND WRITTEN SURVEYS

If you're the kind of person who likes an acronym to guide your practice, two of the most popular models for providers addressing sexuality and intimacy are PLISSIT (Permission, Limited Information, Specific Suggestions, Intensive Therapy), created by J. S. Annon in 1976, and BETTER (Bring up the topic, Explain, Tell, Time, Educate, Record) developed by Mick, Hughes, and Cohen in 2003. For more detail on each model, see Tables 4.2 and 4.3 or read the articles in the online bibliography by Cagle and Bolte (2009), Katz (2005), and Shell (2007).

To help better inform your patients about resources available to address sexuality and intimacy, you can easily get literature on sexuality and cancer for your waiting rooms, including the American Cancer Society booklets for men and women on sexuality, Springboard Beyond Cancer's Action Cards for male and female sexuality, and/or information sheets with links to the National Cancer Institute or Livestrong's sexuality pages, just to name a few. As part of the information sheets you provide to patients and their families before they start treatment, include the side effects that could affect their sexuality so that they are informed well before they have to make a treatment decision (MacElveen and McCorkle 1985). Giving information in this way improves sexual outcomes (Carr 2007).

Additionally, self-assessment screening tools may help your patients efficiently identify areas for concern that you can then address with them during your visit. Table 4.4 lists some valid assessment tools and surveys related to sexuality that are easy to interpret and that your patients can complete while they wait to see you. Furthermore, some programs have used electronic survey tools (Hill-Kayser et al. 2011) to assess sexual side effects in survivorship with relative success.

PRACTICE SUGGESTIONS

Language, Practice, and Setting

You are likely asking, *"But how do I actually do this? When I am sitting across from my patient, what do I say that won't make us both feel awkward?"* In the sections below, using the guidelines in the Practice Points box, I offer specific language (*in italics*) and suggestions for how to conduct the interview. I have drawn from several sources (ARHP 2008; Bober and Varela 2012; Cort, Monroe, and Oliviere 2004; Davis 2009; Hordern and Currow 2003; Katz 2005; National Coalition for Sexual Health 2016; Shell 2007; Shell and Smith 1994; Spaulding 2006) including my own practice experience.

Practice Points: How to Approach the Conversation

- Ensure privacy from other patients and confidentiality during the conversation.
- Introduce routine sexuality discussions early and throughout treatment.
- Stay patient centered and use neutral language.
- Do not use medical jargon.
- Refer patients with complex problems.
- Listen for entry points to areas of concern.
- You do not need to fix everything, just provide support.

Privacy and Confidentiality

Make sure to close doors or pull curtains and minimize interruptions. A private room is ideal when possible. Try to find time to talk with the patient without family present (sometimes this is most easily done before or after a physical exam) to assess the patient's perceptions of safety in a relationship. *If you are a male clinician with a female patient, you can welcome a female colleague to join you or vice versa if you are a female clinician with a male patient.* For more information on how to assess for safety, see the article by Dicola and Sparr (2016). If patients raise concerns of violence or coercion, offer your support and your appreciation for them in sharing this difficult matter. Then offer them resources for a mental health professional in your practice, or if you don't have one available, refer out to a local mental health professional or agency with experience in intimate partner violence. Do not try to handle it on your own.

Once you've assessed for safety, raise the question of sexuality/intimacy and ask permission to include the partner in the conversation. *"Along with everything else I will be discussing with you, I would like to address any questions you may have about how your cancer treatment may affect your body, your experience of intimacy, and your sex life. I'm happy to discuss that with you individually or with a partner."*

If the patient declines to have the partner join, ask permission to continue the conversation in private. Even if the patient reports feeling safe it is important to ask things like:

> *"Do you have particular concerns about discussing issues of sexuality in front of your partner?"*
> *"Would you like us to include your partner in these conversations? Would you feel comfortable if [X] joined us?"*
> *"Is there anything you would like to discuss before your partner rejoins us?"*

There are many potential benefits to including a partner if the patient feels safe doing so. First, in the role as caregiver, the partner may be experiencing changes in their sexual relationship and have no other outlet for exploring these issues or other opportunities to be educated. Second, having both partners in the discussion with you encourages and models more open communication between them. Finally, two sets of ears are better than one for remembering what you've told them.

Introduce and Normalize Issues of Sexuality Early and throughout Treatment

Here are examples of language you can use to introduce or address the topic of sexuality:

- *"Many people find that aspects of their sexuality and intimacy change as a result of cancer or cancer treatments. Some of these changes can affect relationships with others and some affect how patients view themselves. These* changes can be just as distressing as pain or nausea, and during our work together I'll welcome you to share if you're experiencing any problems in this area that you want to discuss with me or members of our team."

- "Some people who are going through an illness like yours have been concerned about how it affects their sexuality, so I ask everyone: Is this something on your mind? I want you to feel comfortable discussing these matters with me at any point, even if you do not have any questions or concerns now."

- "Women undergoing this procedure often have questions about how this may change their intimacy with a partner. Are there any concerns you would like to talk about?"

- "Do you feel that your sexuality or your sense of your identity has changed since your diagnosis?"

- "People who are single or dating often describe some worries about how to cope with the issue of cancer when meeting new partners. Has this happened for you?"

- "Some men taking this medication have problems getting or maintaining an erection. What questions can I answer about how your medication will affect your sex life?"

- "Since your [surgery / diagnosis / chemotherapy / radiation therapy], do you feel any different [as a man / as a woman / in your gender identity]?"

- "Some people find that their sexual feelings, or their desire for sex, change when they go through this treatment. What about you?"

- "Other women who have been given this treatment have experienced some pain during intercourse. There are things we can try to help with this if that is an experience you have."

- "I want to be able to address all aspects of your recovery process. Have there been any sexual changes you have experienced since the [procedure/ intervention]?"

Stay Patient Centered and Use Neutral Language

It is critical that we avoid making assumptions about gender identity, partner status, or sexual orientation based on visual cues. Inquire about and use patients' expressed pronouns and names regardless of what their physical chart says (and work to reflect these in your electronic records). Use the term *partner* or *significant other* instead of *husband/wife/girlfriend/boyfriend* until you know what terminology they feel most comfortable with. Also, do not assume that your patient is exclusively with one partner even if married or that single patients don't have concerns about sexuality. It is important to remain nonjudgmental and avoid overreaction when a patient communicates preferences. This helps communicate that they are safe and that you are open to discussions of this kind.

- *"Are you sexually active?"*
- *"Do you have sex with men, women, or both?"*
- *"How has your illness affected your close relationships?"*
- *"Do you and your partner have any questions for me about how your intimacy is changing because of the cancer/treatments?"*

Avoid Medical Jargon

Try not to use acronyms or technical terms. Instead of p.r.n., say "as needed"; instead of "libido" say "sex drive." Additionally, be mindful that some of our medical terms are confusing: when we say a test is *positive*, that may sound hopeful to a nonmedical person but actually indicates a bad result. Be direct and simple when educating or giving suggestions.

- *"While you should not have vaginal sex until six weeks after your surgery, it is fine to kiss and cuddle with your partner."*
- *"Because you have been experiencing some pain from your cancer, you may want to time your "as needed" pain medication about 30 minutes before you have sex, so it has the opportunity to kick in before you get active."*

Refer for Complex Problems

When patients present complex problems, do not try to handle them on your own. It is always important to offer your concern for the person's experience, stress nonabandonment, and offer appreciation for them being willing to share this difficult information with you, but be honest about your limitations. Any mention of sexual abuse, violence, control, fear, suicidal ideation, or substance use, for example, are important times for referrals to a social worker or other mental health provider who specializes in these issues. A sexual therapist is also the right person to handle any issues that connect to longstanding sexual problems.

- *"It sounds to me like the sexual abuse you describe has had long-lasting effects on you. I'm sorry you've had to go through this. I'm really glad that you were able to share this with me. I want to make sure you have access to someone who is a specialist in these issues. If you are open, I would like to refer you to our social worker [X], who is an expert in this area and could get you help in dealing with these issues."*
- *"I can hear that the sexual concerns you had with your wife prior to your cancer diagnosis have only magnified since then. It is so helpful to know how things were before we started treatment so that we can track changes. Would it be OK with you if I got you the names of some counselors who specialize in helping couples with these issues?"*

Listen for Entry Points

Even if patients say no to initial questions about sexual concerns, they may provide cues to the contrary during their visits with you. Often, there are "entry points that provide openings to conversation and give clues to areas of concern such as 'He just doesn't seem to love me anymore' or 'I just look so ugly'" (Cort, Monroe, and Oliviere 2004, p. 351). We may feel tempted to retreat and reassure them or to change the subject to avoid our own discomfort (*"I'm sure he still loves you"; "Oh no, you're not ugly"*). Resist that temptation, and explore further:

- *"What makes you feel like he doesn't love you anymore?"*
- *"Are there ways in which your relationship has changed since the cancer?"*
- *"Tell me what makes you feel ugly."*

You Don't Need to Fix Everything

Although patients may want information, sometimes they simply want to be heard. If you reflect back what they just said, they're more likely to feel understood; then ask follow-up questions to help you assess how problematic these issues are for them.

- *"It sounds like your level of fatigue has really caused some challenges for your and your girlfriend's sex life.* [Pause.] *Is this something that it would be helpful for us to brainstorm about?"*
- *"I can hear how strange it is for you to look down and see that scar. Is this something that might affect your thoughts about dating?"* If yes: *"Do you think you would like to talk further with someone about this?"*

Many providers fear opening these conversations because of limited time or worry that they won't know how to help. Remember, you don't have to have answers, nor spend hours discussing the issue. Just a few minutes of listening can make a difference. Then you can recap, normalize (often by bringing in other patients' experiences), voice appreciation for what the person has shared, be candid about any limitations you may have, and offer continued support:

> *"It sounds like the ways your body has changed have affected your feelings of being a man. Many patients have similar feelings when they undergo treatments like this one. I'm glad you were able to tell me about this, and while I may not always have an easy answer for you, as your provider, it is important for us to explore all the impacts from your cancer and treatment. We may not have time to talk about this more today since we still need to talk about your next treatment, but I think it is an important topic and would like to keep an eye on it together. And if it's OK with you, I would like to set you up with a member of my team who can talk more with you about how to manage these feelings/experiences."*

Suggestions to Address Sexual Concerns

Whether still in the midst of treatment or beyond it, patients are often anxious about engaging in or resuming sexual activities (Schover 1999). You may wonder what kinds of suggestions you should offer to your patients once you have identified and explored their sexual concerns. Many researchers (Bober and Varela 2012; Cagle and Bolte 2009; Cort, Monroe, and Oliviere 2004; Gianotten 2007; Hordern 2000; Hughes 2000; MacElveen and McCorkle 1985; Schover 1999) offer helpful suggestions that I have grouped into what I hope are useful categories in Table 4.5.

Wrapping Up

Wrapping up this discussion of sexuality and intimacy can be as simple as saying thank you, summarizing, emphasizing your presence, being candid about time limitations during this visit, offering the support of other team members, or setting expectations for duration of symptoms.

- *"Thank you very much for sharing these things with me. It is important that I understand all the ways in which this treatment is affecting you so that we can work on them together."*

- *"So, it sounds like the nausea has made it difficult to be as intimate with your wife as you would like. Let's try the antinausea medication that I suggested and follow up during our next visit to see whether it has made a difference."*

- *"I can hear how isolating it has felt for you to be going through this experience. I want you to know that [I/our team] will continue to be available to support you through this illness."*

- *"I am aware of the time and want to make sure that we have a chance to talk about your pain management too. Can we plan to continue this discussion at our next visit?"*

- *"I wish we had more time to discuss this right now, but your infusion is in ten minutes, and we still need to review this paperwork. Would it be OK if we asked another member of our team to follow up with you about this later in your appointment today?"*

- *"It seems like the pain from surgery has continued to make intimacy difficult for you and your partner. I know this time can be so hard, but I also want you to know that it won't always feel this way. The pain should subside within [X time], and you will begin to feel better. Most patients report being able to return to their daily activities within a few weeks, and that includes sexual activities."*

SPECIAL CONSIDERATIONS

Although stereotyping a patient's sexual experiences by culture, race, age, or severity of disease can be problematic, being informed in general about how these aspects might influence attitudes toward intimacy and sexuality can be helpful. Below, I offer some abbreviated thoughts about special considerations and populations. Readers interested in learning more about any of these topics can use the resources listed in the online bibliography.

Culture

Culture encompasses a broad scope of social characteristics, beyond ethnicity or race, including socioeconomic status, education, religious beliefs, community norms, geographic identities, and family communication. Individual families have cultures, as do smaller communities and nations. Sometimes we are lucky enough to have cultural brokers such as medical interpreters, spiritual care providers, or social workers who may be able to let us know if a question is "off-tone" for a specific community, or if a certain word or concept has different meaning. Often, though, we are working through things on our own. Awareness of culture, especially one different from our own, may make us more wary of addressing issues of sexuality, but with a respectful curiosity and open-ended questions, we can cautiously assess issues of sexuality and look for cues to a patient's level of engagement in these issues.

Similarly, the "culture" of medicine may differ across practice setting, discipline training, and geography. This chapter is written by a white female American social worker and edited by a white female American physician. We practice with our colleagues in a large academic hospital in Boston, and our suggestions are likely not universally applicable to every medical environment or context. We count on you to adapt our suggestions to serve the patients and their partners and families for whom you care. If you serve a large amount of one population, it is useful to strive to understand generalities about how sexuality is understood in that group, while remaining open to individual differences.

I would also caution you not to assume that if you share the same cultural background as a patient, you automatically know what they need or how they will communicate. I once worked with a physician fellow who shared the same ethnic background as the patient we were seeing. After our visit he reflected with awe that, being from the same background, he would have assumed the patient would not be open to our discussion and therefore would not have approached it with her, but now that he saw how much she needed and appreciated the support, it caused him to question his assumptions.

The literature on culture and sexuality in oncology is relatively thin and tends to focus predominantly on certain diseases, like breast cancer. What we do know is that there are health disparities in cancer patients for members of minority racial and ethnic groups (National Cancer Institute 2020). We see these disparities across issues of sexuality and treatment as well. In one study, Asian and Latinx women were more likely to receive mastectomies, and Black breast cancer survivors were least likely to receive adjuvant therapies (Ashing-Giwa et al. 2004); in another, Latinx women breast cancer survivors were found to have lower quality of life than white survivors (Graves et al. 2012); a third (Namiki et al. 2011) found significant interethnic variations among what the study termed "Caucasian, Japanese, and Japanese American" men with prostate cancer in terms of their "sexual profiles," including sexual desire and erection ability.

Some research is looking at the utility of group-specific screening and counseling interventions for issues of sexuality or sexual health care (Schover et al. 2011) and the efficacy of translating evidence-based programs for use with a specific population (Nápoles et al. 2015). Religion, another aspect of culture, "may provide a moral code of conduct or a sexual compass as to sexual norms and behaviors," and Kellogg Spadt et al. (2014, p. 1607) offer a helpful primer on several major religions and their relationship to sex and sexual mores. And while most of the literature has been derived from studies of white patients or does not specify racial/ethnic/cultural information at all, Shell (2007) offers us a brief summary of cultural considerations about sexuality in Black, Asian American, and Hispanic cultures that may influence the lives of our patients and help guide our questions.

Because some cultural groups may be less open to discussions of sexuality or intimacy, simply raising the subject may be enough. If you sense discomfort at the subject, or get pushback, simply normalize the fact that many patients have these questions and that you are open to discussion at any time if it becomes relevant to them. You can also reinforce that any member of your team is open to providing this support, in case they would feel more comfortable raising the topic with someone else.

Sexual and Gender Minorities

Lesbian, gay, bisexual, transgender, and queer people (LGBTQ+), otherwise identified as sexual and gender minorities (SGM), face daily concerns about stigma and inequality even before they get a cancer diagnosis (Acquaviva 2017). According to a 2017 Gallup poll, about 10 million adults now identify as LGBTQ+, though there are no comprehensive numbers about the incidence of cancer in this group. While same-sex couples can now be married across the United States, there are still many legal, local, social, and policy challenges that often intersect with medical concerns. In a review of LGBTQ+ disparities in cancer, factors including lower income, barriers to health insurance coverage, confidentiality concerns, later access of medical care, higher incidence of smoking, increased existence of comorbidities such as HPV or HIV, reduced pregnancy rates, and increased obesity all create higher risk of developing cancer (Quinn et al. 2015).

Representatives from the National LGBT Cancer Network, Malecare, and the National LGBT Cancer Project report that invisibility and lack of disclosure are some of the most crucial challenges (Adams 2017) in navigating medical systems. They report that some SGM people with cancer may not feel comfortable disclosing their sexuality or sexual practices with us for fear of judgment, or that small moments of provider surprise during disclosures were enough to cause avoidance of medical care in the future. Additionally, they note that some people worry that because of provider bias, they risk getting worse care if they bring same-sex partners to medical appointments or correct misgendered pronouns. Sarah, a 55-year-old transgender patient, told me that she was wary of correcting providers who called her *"he"* on the basis of her assigned gender at birth, saying, *"They hold my life in their hands,"* and she didn't want to *"get on their bad side."* She felt she had to choose between her medical care and her identity.

Judith Butler asserts that our culture typically places all sexual discourse in the "heterosexual matrix" (Hawkins et al. 2009). This essentially equates penetrative sex between a man and a woman with "normal" healthy functioning sex and anything else as abnormal. If we also adopt this stance, or worse, are unaware that we hold this bias, we are likely to alienate any patients who do not live this way (Hawkins et al. 2009). When we use nonneutral language or make heterosexist assumptions about sexual orientation, marital status, or gender identity, we may be amplifying these fears and making it impossible for our patients to share their concerns about sexuality with us. Also, imagine how many providers a cancer patient comes into contact with during a hospitalization, or even a routine clinic visit. Imagine having to decide whether to disclose sexual orientation or gender identity not just to one person, but to multiple providers who casually or formally ask about a presumed heterosexual partner or address you with the wrong pronoun, again and again. If clinics and electronic medical records have a way to record this information for those who choose to report, it reduces some of the anxiety about disclosing multiple times (Adams 2017).

Daryl Mitteldorf from Malecare notes an important clinician misunderstanding that "treating all patients equally" means providing good care. Given all the disparities listed at the start of this section, "equal" treatment typically means treating "straight, middle-class people." He recommends, instead, treating patients as individuals and "contextualizing discussions about sex within the actual sexual practice of their patients" (Adams 2017).

Generally, we tend to inflate our ability to provide culturally curious care. In a nationwide survey of oncologists at the National Cancer Institute, providers showed an initial high degree of confidence about and comfort with caring for LGBTQ+ patients (Schabath et al. 2019). After completing a survey about aspects of LGBTQ+ patient care, however, they reported a decrease in confidence, likely revealing a "developed awareness of lack of knowledge." More than half of the respondents indicated that their intake forms did not inquire about sexual orientation, sex at birth, or gender identity, and only a small number of providers felt that knowing their patients' sexual orientation was important.

This survey highlights what the National Institute of Health and National Academy of Medicine (formerly known as the Institute of Medicine) have identified as the importance of capturing sexual orientation and gender identity (SOGI) data (Cahil and Makadon 2014). Not only does collecting SOGI matter for awareness, funding, and institutional decisions about interventions, but it also contributes to patients feeling "seen" by their medical system. Other ways to help address feelings of invisibility or hesitations about disclosure are to create safe spaces (Griggs et al. 2017). Clinics should have visual aids or language that shows support for SGM patients (posters or pamphlets showing same-sex partners, or rainbow stickers on ID cards), use gender- or family-neutral language such as *partner*, and ask what pronouns patients use and who is in their support system (Adams 2017).

People in LGBTQ+ relationships may feel compelled to love in secret and thus may not receive the same degree of support that their heterosexual counterparts do (Hordern 2000; Srinivasan et al. 2019). Imagine the impact of not having your primary loved one present or "legitimized" at your most vulnerable times.

Gay and lesbian patients have also reported experiencing higher stress associated with diagnosis and treatment of illness, lower satisfaction with care provided by physicians, and lower satisfaction with emotional support from health care providers (Katz 2009). Additionally, some in the gay male community may be concerned that society will misinterpret the manifestations of their cancer as arising instead from HIV/AIDS (Katz 2009) and cast judgment.

Older gay and lesbian people who live in communities that do not support gay rights can often remain hidden from one another and feel isolated (Horsley and Anike via Hordern 2000). We can help by making available to them the names and contact information of gay-friendly or gay-identified counselors, support groups, and online supports (Katz 2009).

Stevens and Abrahm (2019) highlight a case in which a transgender patient, though legally married at the federal level, lived in a state that did not recognize his marriage and thus his wife was not eligible to take time away from work under the Family and Medical Leave Act. His family, with whom he had not been in contact for years, was not aware of his gender identity but was now present as he neared the end of his life. Luckily, this patient had a compassionate medical team that worked hard to use his correct pronouns and limit sensitive medical information to just the patient and his wife, and the outcome was peaceful and goal concordant. This experience could have been profoundly different with providers who were not attuned to these needs, and it is difficult to think of how fragile outcomes are when systems are not in place to protect them. Stevens and Abrahm

(2019) also synthesize recommendations for older LGBTQ+ patients needing hospice and palliative care, including the importance of documenting surrogate decision-makers, assessing preferences for discontinuation of hormone therapy, and exploring a person's family of choice.

Not surprisingly, studies show that gay and lesbian cancer patients, just like their heterosexual counterparts, also experience changes to their sexuality during treatment. Indeed, one study found that four of six lesbian partners of patients with cancer reported complete cessation of sex after the diagnosis (Hawkins et al. 2009).

Several entities have put out policies or position statements on standards of care for SGM patients, including the American Medical Association, the Joint Commission, the Centers for Medicare and Medicaid Services, and the American Society of Clinical Oncology (Quinn et al. 2020), that you can look to for further information. These include recommendations for

- Patient education and support
- Proper health insurance coverage
- Referrals to LGBTQ+-friendly providers and facilities that meet compliance for LGBTQ+ equity and safety
- Workforce development and representation
- Improvement in policies that reduce disparities
- Increased population data in intake forms, medical records, and clinical trials
- Improved funding for research into LGBTQ+ demographics and risk factors

It is particularly important to be aware of your own assumptions and biases around SGM, and how these may affect the patients you care for.

Sexuality across the Life Cycle

If cancer and sexuality are awkward for practitioners to discuss, having those discussions with significantly older or younger patients who could be our grand/parents or grand/children can create a perfect trifecta of discomfort. Since more than half of all cancer diagnoses occur in people over 65 years of age (with some estimates that by 2030, as many as one-fifth of people living in the United States will be over 65; Browner 2020), and 70,000 young people (ages 15–39) are diagnosed each year (National Cancer Institute 2013), we'd better get busy working through our discomfort.

Though sexuality remains important for many older people, issues such as embarrassment, perceived disinterest by health professionals, and dissatisfaction with treatment can all be barriers to discussion (Bauer, Haesler, and

Fetherstonhaugh 2016). One in five older adults report recent sexual activity (March 2018), so it is important for us to know that this is a subject that matters to them.

Mr. R was a 73-year-old man who was hospitalized with complications of prostate cancer and whose wife was consistently at his bedside. One day after a long conversation, I told them that I would leave and give them some alone time. He smirked and said that I *"had better do that since he and his wife hadn't had the chance to have their daily conjugal yet."* He quickly followed by saying he was joking, but that *"people assume that just because we have wrinkles, we don't still take pleasure in one another . . . but we do."*

Shell and Smith offer a detailed list of suggestions and interventions that we and our teams can incorporate into our practice with elderly patients (1994, p. 557). These include screening for depression and anxiety, which can decrease their ability to feel sexual; assessing their precancer sexual functioning; and reassuring them that we understand that sexuality can be an important component of their relationship. Changing positions and locations for sexual activity can be a way to cater to aging bodies and monotony. Shell and Smith (1994) agree that we should broaden the definition of sexuality to indicate sharing, intimacy, and communication, as well as endorsing good nutrition, sleep, exercise, and self-care.

On the other end of the spectrum are adolescents and young adults (AYA, 18–35 years old) and adult survivors of childhood cancers. Young adults with cancer often tell me about being out of step with their peer group, with cancer pausing their lives at a time when their cohort may be meeting new people, partnering, or building families, and they often raise a special interest in fertility planning. Ellen was a 30-year-old woman with sarcoma who said, *"I feel more lonely when I go out with my girlfriends now. They discuss who they are dating or engaged to, and my only news is my next line of chemo. It's easier to just say no when they ask me to go out with them."*

Literature shows that AYA with cancer experience detrimental sexual effects on erection, ejaculation, orgasm for men, and desire for females (Stanton, Handy, and Meston 2018) and that sexual changes exist for AYA with all types of cancers, not just in those with reproductive cancers (Mutsch et al. 2019).

Sarah was a 26-year-old breast cancer survivor who said that, even though her cancer was many years in the past, she still could not imagine a partner being able to love her with all her physical and emotional scars. She reported feeling uncomfortable with how to approach the subject in dating situations, so she avoided these situations. Additionally, she felt that her cancer experience, while remote, remained intense and relevant in her current life, and she worried that new partners would minimize or fail to understand the power of this history.

Research supports Sarah's experience and has found that seeking new relationships can cause stress for cancer patients, particularly around the idea of when to disclose their history of cancer to new potential partners (Hordern 2000).

You might encourage these patients to talk to some of their friends about their feelings and to find new friends, including other young adults with cancer, or to seek out others who have had similar experiences via websites and blogs.

There is conflicting evidence of the impact of childhood cancers on sexuality. One study (Olsson et al. 2018) found that adolescent and young adult survivors felt less satisfied with their sexuality, while another showed some positive findings that "long-term childhood cancer survivors are comparable to healthy peers regarding relationship status, body image, body dissociation, sexual experiences, and sexual and status satisfaction" (Lehmann et al. 2015, p. 214), though they urge specific attention be paid to survivors of brain tumors and those who received amputations, both of whom may have more complicated experiences of sexuality or body image. These studies and others (Mutsch et al. 2019) show that this population is concerned about issues of sexuality and wants to speak with their providers about it.

Intersectionality

It is important through all these special considerations to keep in mind the concept of intersectionality, which identifies the interconnected nature of social categories (Crenshaw 1989). If there are challenges to being a Mexican woman in a white-majority city, there are increased challenges in being an older lesbian Mexican woman in the same place, which create many layers of richness but also additional experiences of discrimination. With each aspect of intersectionality, people have fewer opportunities to see themselves represented or normalized. The awareness of intersectionality is important for providers to bring to meetings with patients who may face multiple minority statuses.

Partners

There is often little formal acknowledgment of the sacrifices partners make or the ways in which their lives change to accommodate the needs of the patient—even less so of the ways in which their sexual needs are altered. Medical providers, literature (such as brochures), hospital systems, and even patients themselves can ignore the experience of loved ones. Even if partners provide support lovingly and willingly, they may still struggle with what the illness takes away from them. In the same way that patients can lose sight of the wholeness of their identity while sitting in a hospital bed, a partner can feel distilled down to the role of caregiver. One man I worked with said, *"I love my wife, but I miss being her husband."*

One study (Hawkins et al. 2009) looked at the ways in which companions experience change, finding self-blame, rejection, sadness, anger, and lack of sexual fulfillment. They cite the primary causes as exhaustion from caregiving and a repositioning of their loved one from a sexual partner to a patient.

In an older study (1998), Kuyper and Wester found that partners could no longer structure their daily lives based on their previous interests or social activities as a couple, which included, of course, their sexuality and intimacy. Moreover, partners often "had no contact at all with the treating doctor," were "insufficiently informed about the possibilities they have of supporting the patient during examination and admission in the hospital," and subsequently experienced feelings of "fear and of powerlessness" (p. 246). Partners can feel worried that they are being selfish if they tend to their own issues or desires and can struggle if both the patient and partner pay attention only to the patient's needs and concerns.

Partners also face new and unaccustomed tasks, such as being the sole wage earner or insurance carrier, which can lead to significant financial losses; what time remains in the day may now be filled with parental duties and caregiving. Partners can easily find themselves developing stress, burnout, and fatigue, as well as feelings such as loss, frustration, isolation, and resentment; communication between couples can become strained. It is not hard to imagine the effect this could have on a person's feelings of warmth, intimacy, and sexual desire toward a partner.

One middle-aged caregiver I worked with said, *"I try to prioritize all the needs of our household and spend my day raising our children, going to work, doing the bills, picking up prescriptions, and the minute I walk in the door, she jumps on the things I haven't done yet. It is driving a wedge between us."*

When a loved one has a terminal illness, partners must confront the fact that their partnership is ending (Taylor 2014). And when they most need support, the bulk of attention is usually focused on their sick partner. Even their own friends and family may fail to recognize that they have their own needs outside a partner's illness and may unreasonably expect that they constantly be at the patient's bedside and never take time for themselves. The distress, anger, and sadness caregivers may feel can all affect sexual functioning and their desire to be intimate with their partner.

One woman whose husband had colorectal cancer told me angrily, *"You really find out who your friends are when you go through something like this. Friendships I thought were solid have just disappeared. I no longer have people to talk to, and it makes me feel bitter and alone. Sometimes it makes me resent my husband because he is the focus of everything. Sometimes I just pull away from him because I don't know what to do with all of these feelings."*

Having the opportunity for the caregiver to explore these feelings with a social worker or other mental health or spiritual counselor is likely to benefit both the partner and the relationship as a whole and to encourage positive changes such as increased closeness and intimacy.

After one session, a couple who had been experiencing frustration and difficulty communicating told me they felt relieved that they could finally voice their opinions. During our talk, the patient became aware of how centered their lives had become around his illness and ways in which his husband would benefit from more balance. His husband acknowledged that he needed to communicate his frustrations more often rather than keeping them bottled inside or assuming that the patient should read his mind. The energy between them shifted from tense and distant to more open and compassionate. The session had started out with them on opposite ends of the couch; it ended with them clasping fingers and moving closer.

Palliative Care, Hospice, and Sexuality

There is a myth that patients who have advanced cancer or who are experiencing distressing symptoms are not interested in or capable of intimacy or sexual expression. Accordingly, within palliative care and hospice settings, patients are "rarely given an opportunity to share sexually-related issues with their health care providers" (Cagle and Bolte 2009, p. 224; Cagle et al. 2017). This situation is only amplified by the misconception that we discussed earlier, that elderly adults, who are high palliative care utilizers, are no longer sexually active or interested in intimacy issues (Hordern 2000).

Loving relationships, intimacy, and sexual contact are still important to patients and their loved ones during terminal illness, and sexuality can be an important aspect even in the last weeks and days of life (Gianotten 2007; Hordern 2008). But as you might expect, the form that sexuality takes at that time shifts somewhat, often becoming centered on "emotional connectedness" and "intimacy through close body contact, hugging, touching, kissing, hand holding, and eye contact" (Lemieux et al. 2004, p. 634).

In comparison with other cancer patients, elderly patients reported "the greatest difficulty with sexual function" (Ananth et al. 2003, p. 203), including poor or changed body image, altered sexual functioning as a result of anxiety and depression, fear of rejection, poor communication, loss and grief, bereaved partners coping with loss of interdependence, and changes in family roles (Cort, Monroe, and Oliviere 2004). For some, "memories from the past can pop up," either "unfinished business like missed sexual opportunities, or jealousy regarding real or supposed extramarital relations," and "in some couples the sexual future of the surviving partner" becomes a focus (Gianotten 2007, p. 302). For many patients with advanced cancer, however, continuing sexual connection can provide "energy, physical and emotional relaxation, pain-relief, better sleep, togetherness, consolation, comfort, self-esteem, or better coping with heavy emotions" (p. 302).

Mr. B was a 55-year-old patient with gastric cancer. He and his wife had asked me to educate them about home hospice supports. They had mentioned needing a hospital bed for the living room when his wife said tearfully, *"That's the worst part, not being able to sleep together at the time when we need each other most."* We brainstormed ways for them to still sleep near or with one another, and to prioritize hugging, kissing, and cuddling, which they both reported missing during the last months of his illness.

The Inpatient Setting

In my role as an inpatient palliative care social worker, I have found that for several reasons, the inpatient setting makes it difficult to bring up the topics of sexuality and intimacy with my patients. Often, the issues that bring cancer patients into the hospital are acute enough that the initial part of their visit is focused on treating their pain, nausea, dyspnea, and so forth. The idea of asking a patient in those circumstances to reflect on how her sexuality has changed as a result of her cancer can seem insensitive, ill-timed, and inappropriate. When, as sometimes happens, our patients have to share a room with another patient, privacy is limited, and other providers are frequently visiting for care. Also, the realities of today's medical care are such that as soon as patients begin to feel better, they are discharged. For all these reasons, the outpatient setting might appear to be better suited to conversations about sexuality and intimacy.

As with other sensitive topics, however, no matter the setting, I try to invite patients to let me know if these issues are important to them. They might arise as patients try to decide whether or not to have an intervention (for example, a G-tube or an epidural catheter) that could affect their ability to be intimate or to experience pleasurable sensations. If a procedure such as a nerve block might cause numbness or decreased sensation in sexual organs, that important potential side effect can easily be included in the discussion of the risks, burdens, and benefits.

Physical touch and intimacy can be extremely therapeutic and can be encouraged even in the inpatient setting. Remarkably, even in the sterile, chaotic environment of the hospital, patients often still need intimacy or sexual fulfillment. We can give permission for partners to lie in bed with their loved ones or for patients and their partners to close their doors or be "undisturbed" for a period (Cagle and Bolte 2009).

INTERDISCIPLINARY PRACTICE AND REFERRAL LIST

Ideally, one of the members of your office or practice will be a reliable source of information on issues of sexuality (Schover 1999). A provider or combination of providers on your team should be able to discuss the effects of illness on sexual functioning; suggestions on resuming sex comfortably and improving sexual communication; advice on how to mitigate the effects of physical changes—such as having an ostomy—on sexuality; self-help strategies to overcome specific sexual problems, such as pain with intercourse or loss of sexual desire; counseling regarding fertility, hormone replacement therapy, high-risk obstetrics for pregnant cancer patients, and support around the emotional impact of changes to self or relationships.

Smaller cancer centers that do not have the funding to offer all the needed specialists on staff should build a referral network that includes experts in the areas described below. Wiggins et al. (2007) notes the "importance of establishing systems where patients can refer themselves for both advice and management options," though only "63 percent of physicians felt they had access to local resources for referral of patients with sexual problems" (p. 66).

Leslie Schover, who has written extensively about cancer and sexuality (1999), and Sharon Bober et al. (2016) provide suggestions for the resources and professional team members needed for comprehensive cancer care:

- *Mental health professionals* trained as sex therapists, familiar with cancer and treatment issues as well as being sensitive to LGBTQ+, age, and cultural issues, and available for emotional support in coping with identity changes
- *Gynecologists* well versed in issues of female sexual dysfunction, pelvic pain after treatment, fertility, and hormone treatment
- *Urologist or internist* who specializes in male health and is familiar with medical and surgical options for male sexual dysfunction
- *Palliative care clinician* who specializes in pain and symptom management to optimize daily functioning and energy, as well as in communication and eliciting goals of care that can be shared with the oncology team
- *Rehabilitation specialist* to help patients resume physical activity despite handicaps, including pelvic floor exercises
- *Enterostomal therapist* to assist patients who may have concerns about ostomy appliances being intrusive or perceived as unattractive
- *Respiratory therapist* to suggest sexual positions for patients who are connected to respirators
- *Physical therapist* to advise on issues such as whether to wear a prosthetic limb during sex or best positions for sexual contact after a hemipelvectomy
- *Reproductive endocrinologist* to help with fertility concerns

If you are not certain what is available at your own facility, the clinical nurse educators, mental health professionals, patient navigators, or resource specialists are likely to know. In addition to staff, it is important to have availability of, or referrals for, places to procure sexual aids such as vaginal dilators, moisturizers, or vacuum erection devices, since Bober et al. (2016) found that more than 70 percent of leading cancer centers did not offer sexual aids on site (Fisher 2018), as they did wigs or other cancer aids.

SUMMARY

Sexuality and cancer is an area of medicine that, more than most areas, requires us to explore our own assumptions, biases, and areas of discomfort before we are likely to become comfortable or confident in having these discussions with our patients. We will be much better equipped to pick up subtle cues of concerns about intimacy and sexuality, and more helpful to our patients and their partners, once we have acquired this self-awareness. We can improve our practice if we increase our general knowledge about how cancer and its treatments can affect sexuality for patients and their loved ones and provide this information routinely as we do with the other risks and burdens of the therapies we offer. Providing a safe space for discussion, education, and access to resources, as well as being vulnerable and saying "I don't know" if something is outside our experience, go a long way. Remember that you don't have to be an expert, or even fix everything, but showing you care makes a difference. Let's work to feel more comfortable as we search for answers along with our patients and make a serious effort to help them improve this aspect of their quality of life.

Tables

TABLE 4.1 Changes That Affect Sexuality and Intimacy

Causes	Changes
Cancer itself	Pain
	Fever
	Incontinence
	Nausea/vomiting
	Weakness
Surgical interventions	Anatomical changes, such as loss of genitalia and other body parts (breasts, testicles, ovaries)
	Pain
	Wounds/scars
	Ostomy or catheter placements
	Loss of sensitivity
	Penile or vaginal shortening
	CNS damage
	Incontinence

TABLE 4.1 (*cont.*)

Causes	Changes
Chemotherapy and radiation therapy	Fatigue
	Nausea/vomiting
	Loss of sexual desire
	Decreased frequency of intercourse
	Pain
	Erectile dysfunction
	Changes to bowel motility
	Vaginal pain for patients or irritation for partners
	Hair loss (on head and body, sometimes causing feelings of being childlike)
	Premature menopause
Hormone therapy	Reduced androgens that promote sexual desire
	Hot flashes
	Night sweats
	Vaginal discharge
	Breast development and weight gain in men
	Loss of erotic dreams and fantasies
	Decreased libido
Medications used to treat pain, depression, and anxiety	Decreased libido
	Fatigue
	Suicidal ideation

TABLE 4.2 PLISSIT Model for Addressing Sexuality and Intimacy with Patients

P	Permission	Help patients and partners understand that you think their sexual health is important, that sexual concerns are legitimate, and that comprehensive cancer care includes addressing this issue. Let patients know that you will routinely screen for this issue and ask open-ended questions.
LI	Limited Information	Educate patients about the ways in which their sexuality might be affected by the cancer or related treatments, how long these disturbances might last, and whether there are red flags to watch for. Include written materials addressing these issues when they are available. Address any questions that patients broach.
SS	Specific Suggestions	Depending on your proficiency in this area, you or a member of the interdisciplinary team might offer specific suggestions, including likely side effects of a patient's particular cancer course and practical suggestions for addressing them.
IT	Intensive Therapy	If no one on your team is able to address a patient's questions adequately, or the patient's experience appears to require more extensive conversation, this would be the time to make a referral. (Check the resource list for useful referrals.) One study by Derogatis and Kourlesis in 1981 estimated that only 30 percent of the cancer population will need this last level of intervention (Cagle and Bolte 2009).

TABLE 4.3 BETTER Model for Discussing Sexuality and Intimacy with Patients

B	Bring up the topic	Let patients and partners know that you want to talk with them about the ways in which their cancer might affect their sexuality and intimacy.
E	Explain	Help patients understand that sexuality is a part of living well and that sexual concerns are an important part of comprehensive cancer care.
T	Tell	Let patients know that you will help them find resources and clinicians who can address any concerns that may arise.
T	Time	Let them know that they may bring up issues of sexuality at any time.
E	Educate	Educate patients about the ways in which their sexuality will be affected by their cancer or related treatment.
R	Record	Include this discussion in the patient's record so that others will know it has happened.

TABLE 4.4 Sexuality Assessment Tools and Surveys

CARES	Cancer Rehabilitation and Evaluation System	P. A. Ganz, C.A.C. Schag, J. J. Lee, and M. S. Sim, 1992, "The CARES: A generic measure of health-related quality of life for patients with cancer," *Quality of Life Research* 1:19–29.
FSFI	Female Sexual Function Index (19-item index)	R. Rosen, C. Brown, and J. Heiman, et al., 2000, "The Female Sexual Function Index: A multidimensional self-report instrument for the assessment of female sexual function," *J Sex Marital Ther* 26:191–208.
FSFI a	Female Sexual Function Index validated for use in lesbian populations	J. K. Tracy and J. Junginger, 2007, "Correlates of lesbian sexual functioning," *J Womens Health (Larchmt)* 16:499–509.
IIEF	International Index of Erectile Function (15-item index)	R. C. Rosen, A. Riley, G. Wagner, et al., 1997, "The International Index of Erectile Function: A multidimensional scale for assessment of erectile dysfunction," *Urology* 49:822–30.
IIEF a	International Index of Erectile Function validated for use in homosexual, HIV-positive men	K. Coyne, S. Mandalia, S. McCullough, et al., 2010, "The International Index of Erectile Function: Development of an adapted tool for use in HIV-positive men who have sex with men," *J Sex Med* 7:769–74.
ISL	Index of Sexual Life (11-item instrument)	M. Chevret, E. Jaudinot, K. Sullivan, et al., 2004, "Quality of sexual life and satisfaction in female partners of men with ED: Psychometric validation of the Index of Sexual Life (ISL) questionnaire," *J Sex Marital Ther* 30:141–55.
PEDT	Premature Ejaculation Diagnostic Tool (5-item index)	T. Symonds, M. A. Perelman, S. Althof, et al., 2007, "Development and validation of a premature ejaculation diagnostic tool," *Eur Urol* 52:565–73.

TABLE 4.5 Suggestions to Address Sexual Concerns

Safety concerns	• Reassure them that cancer cannot be spread through sex.
	• Let them know which sexual acts may come with risk for pain; e.g., during recovery from surgery, intercourse may irritate the surgical cut.
	• If they are immune deficient:
	    — Avoid intercourse if the white blood counts are dangerously low.
	    — Clear tracheotomies of mucus and cover them lightly during sexual activity.
	• The first 48 hours after chemo, couples should use condoms to protect against cytoxic waste that is present in blood and bodily fluids.
	• Reassure them that external beam radiation does not leave the body radioactive, nor do radiation implants once they are removed from the body.

Cosmetic interventions	• Aromatherapy minimizes odors (eucalyptus, peppermint, or coffee grounds). • Specialists in salon care, makeup, wigs, ostomy pouches or prosthetics, penile or breast implants may help improve patient appearance. • Wearing camisoles or scarves during sex can help cover stomas or scars.
Treatments/ complementary therapies	• If sexual side effects are causing distress, review all medications and alter if possible. • Consider recommending Reiki, massage (except in patients with coagulopathies), exercise, aromatherapy, relaxation, meditation, yoga, and warm baths for comfort, mood enhancement, energy, or decompression. • Refer to mind-body work for connecting emotionally with changed physical landscape or self-concept. • For dryness, prescribe lubricants that are water based and estrogen- and perfume-free. • Kegel exercises may decrease incontinence in women. • Evaluate for need of antidepressants for mood or energy.
Sexual expression	• Encourage exploring alternative methods of sexual expression (such as masturbation, reading erotica) and reciprocation (such as fantasy, anal penetration, oral or manual stimulation). • Discuss different sexual positions or use of pillows to facilitate comfort. • Have partners show each other physically what they want. • Ask them to try removing penetrative intercourse from options initially and encourage couples to "do anything but." • Discuss acts of intimacy and sensuality, such as washing, hair brushing, touch or massage with oils. • Encourage them to strengthen the often blurry divide between dual roles of caregiver/lover and patient/lover by establishing a romantic environment: candlelight, music, wine, and dressing for the occasion.
Recalibrating expectations	• Help to align their expectations within the reality of the disease. • Let them know they may need to plan sexual activities like any other exertion, for example, if they need to take pain meds 30 minutes prior. • Help patients find a time of day when they have good energy. • Ask them to regard sex as time to share pleasure not to perform. • Urge partners and patients to discuss whether one may need to withdraw from the physical part of the relationship and give them "permission" to do that. • Ask them to resume sex gradually by looking at/touching changed parts of the body; nonsexual touching, massage, cuddling; then starting with manual or oral contact. • Acknowledge that it may take time to learn to love one's new body and to change past foreplay patterns or sexual positions, and that first attempts may be disappointing. • Encourage intimacy regardless of ability or desire to engage in sex. • Help people weigh the potential side effects of medications or interventions for sexual issues (getting implants may come with its own risks).

(continued)

TABLE 4.5 (*cont.*)

Communication	• Encourage more open communication between partners about sexual needs, either with a counselor or alone. • Have the couple establish ground rules and private time to talk. • Suggest that they review what has changed, what hurts, what excites. • Advise that they make specific, positive requests for change rather than criticizing current practices. • Encourage single people to rehearse a comfortable approach or explanation for any sexual issues that arise when dating and beginning sexual activity with new partners.
Referral	• When necessary, refer for the following: pharmaceutical interventions (vaginal lubricants, oral medications, contraceptive options); surgical interventions (penile or breast implants, injections, reconstructive surgery); hormone therapy; physical rehabilitation for major physical handicaps; therapy (psychosexual, intimate partner violence).

Resources

If you want to educate yourself further, consult colleagues who incorporate sexual assessment into their practices, such as mental health counselors or sex therapists, and attend seminars or workshops designed to assist you in examining your attitudes, values, and beliefs about sex. Go online or contact your profession's national organizations for any current continuing education offerings on sexual health training.

The American Cancer Society (ACS) has several resources on sexuality and intimacy. ACS's comprehensive list of resources for patients and clinicians includes national websites, books, pamphlets, LGBTQ+ information, fertility resources, cancer- and treatment-specific guides, information on sexuality at different ages, and resources for sexual health professionals. To access these resources, go to www.cancer.org and search "sexuality." The National Cancer Institute also has a vast array of information for health professionals and patients about cancer and sexuality in their Sexual and Reproductive Issues (PDQ) section.

Patient Resources

AARP.org: multiple articles on sex over 50.

ACS, "How Cancer and Cancer Treatment Can Affect Sexuality," http://www
.cancer.org/Treatment/TreatmentsandSideEffects/PhysicalSideEffects
/DealingwithSymptomsatHome/caring-for-the-patient-with-cancer-at
-home-sexuality

ACS, "Sex and the Adult Female with Cancer" (also available in Spanish and
in pamphlet form), http://www.cancer.org/Treatment/Treatmentsand
SideEffects/PhysicalSideEffects/SexualSideEffectsinWomen/Sexualityfor
theWomanindex

ACS, "Sex and the Adult Male with Cancer" (also available in Spanish and in pamphlet form), http://www.cancer.org/Treatment/TreatmentsandSide Effects/PhysicalSideEffects/SexualSideEffectsinMen/SexualityfortheMan /index

Livestrong, https://www.Livestrong.org

National LGBT Cancer Network, https://www.Cancer-network.org

OncoLink, https://www.oncolink.org

Provider Resources

To conduct a sexual assessment: National Coalition for Sexual Health, "Sexual Health and Your Patients: A Provider's Guide," https://national coalitionforsexualhealth.org/tools/for-healthcare-providers/document /ProviderGuide.pdf

To conduct an intimate partner violence screen: D. Dicola and E. Spaar, "Intimate Partner Violence," *American Family Physician*, https:// www.aafp.org/afp/2016/1015/p646.pdf

For cultural recommendations in cancer care and a list of resources, see Y. Colón, 2007, "Ethnic Diversity and Cultural Competency in Cancer Care," *Oncology Issues* 22(5):28–31.

CHAPTER 5

Advancing Disease

with Molly E. Collins, MD

In this chapter, we focus on the communication skills that we can use to help prepare our patients who have advancing disease and their families to look toward and plan for death. For most people, this is an ongoing process that we can support with compassionate, honest information and wise medical guidance. We need to provide prognostic information, knowing that prognostication is inherently imprecise, help prepare patients and families for the range of possible illness trajectories, and help them tolerate the inherent uncertainty.

There are unique challenges in formulating and discussing prognosis in the age of targeted treatments and immunotherapy. But we can foster *prognostic awareness* throughout the trajectory of a terminal illness and help patients who are reluctant to talk about the future. As disease advances, we need to consider carefully how to balance the potential life-prolonging benefits of intensive medical care and cancer-directed therapies with their burdens, using each patient's priorities and values as the north star.

This chapter focuses on communication because many of the challenges that arise in the terminal phases of illness are due to problems in communication—between you and the patient, between you and the family, and between the patient and her family and friends. Some of these difficulties may arise because each of us (clinician, patient, family member, friend) has a different view of the patient's illness, estimated prognosis, and the remaining options for care. Others are unintended consequences of family members' efforts to protect one another from distressing information and strong emotions. Sometimes misunderstandings occur because the true source of distress is not clearly communicated. At other times, we clinicians are responsible, because the words we use when we attempt to explain why fully supportive care focused on quality of life is the only remaining option can suggest to families that we are withdrawing care. We discuss each of these communication issues in the pages that follow.

THE SPECTRUM OF RESPONSES TO TERMINAL CANCER

My (*Janet Abrahm's*) uncle John visited his neurologist because he was having difficulty speaking and new right-sided weakness, and he was found to have numerous brain metastases. Despite an extensive search, no primary cancer was found. He received palliative cranial irradiation, which led to some improvement.

His doctors asked me to coordinate communication between them and our family. I explained to our family that Uncle John was getting appropriate care but that his chances for prolonged survival, or even survival beyond six months, were small. His general internist, medical oncologist, radiation oncologist, neurologist, and I all agreed that there was no indication for further antineoplastic treatments, that symptom management should be our goal, and that his internist was in the best position to manage this. My husband and I, visiting my uncle, had found him to be comfortable but mildly confused and exhausted by minor exertions, such as going out to eat.

John's main source of distress, however, was the feeling that he ought to be doing something to fight the cancer—that was his interpretation of the advice he had been getting from friends and other members of the family. Some had suggested he go immediately to a nearby university-affiliated cancer center and sign up for experimental therapy. Others insisted that the NIH in Bethesda, Maryland, was the only place to be. Still others sent Uncle John alternative-medicine pamphlets and catalogs, extolling "natural products" and diet regimens they were sure would be effective.

Uncle John expressed to me his dismay at all this: "*I am so confused. I trust my doctors, and they tell me that there is no treatment that will make me live longer or better. But our family and my friends keep telling me that I should be doing something, and each one has a different idea of exactly what that should be. What do you think I should be doing?*" Although I explained to him many times that they could not cure his cancer or delay its progression, he continued to ask me repeatedly, "*But shouldn't I be doing something?*"

At first I could not understand why Uncle John was dismissing the unanimous advice of all his physicians, and I was furious at our family and his friends for supporting his "delusions." What was causing this breakdown in communication?

The answer, I later realized, could be found by analyzing our family's behavior using the framework of the emotional stages cancer patients often experience after they are told they have a terminal illness. Dr. Elisabeth Kübler-Ross first described these stages in her seminal 1969 book *On Death and Dying*: they include *denial, anger, bargaining, depression,* and *acceptance.* In this first book, Dr. Kübler-Ross cautioned that some patients do not experience all stages and that some experience them in a different order, or even simultaneously (e.g., anger and bargaining). She later expanded her conception of the emotional processes that occur as a person faces death, but this first formulation still provides a useful framework for understanding the spectrum of patients' feelings.

I began to notice that our family members and friends were going through these same emotional stages, but we were each going through them at a different rate. Our problems of communication arose because we were almost never in the same stage of the process at the same time. (I suspect that some of us who care for patients with far-advanced disease also go through these stages to some degree, and a similar mismatch in stages may compromise our ability to understand patient and family goals.)

In fact, my uncle was not *denying* that he had cancer (*What do you mean I have cancer? I just came here for a check-up and now you tell me I'm going to die!*); he was denying the grimness of the prognosis. Despite his symptoms and debility, he simply could not accept that he might not get entirely better after radiation therapy, could not be cured, and was likely to die.

John's *anger* manifested later. Anger can be directed at God, at the doctor, at the patient himself (*Why didn't I get that colonoscopy?*), or, in Uncle John's case, at my husband, Fred (not his real name), who was unlucky enough to be the one to tell him something he really did not want to hear. During a phone call, Uncle John repeatedly asked Fred to tell him his prognosis. So Fred finally did. "Fred," Uncle John bellowed, "*What are you telling me? That I'm not going to make it to Christmas?! That's only six months away! Who died and made you king? You're not even a doctor! How dare you tell me such a thing!*" And he slammed the phone down.

We are all familiar with what is likely to happen to the bearer of bad news, and thus I might have expected this response from my uncle. But I did not expect it from the family, too. As we soon discovered, they were also in denial—less than he was, perhaps, but more so than we were—about Uncle John's prognosis. They were furious that we had presumed to tell him that he might die of his illness in a relatively short time. There were several suggestions that my husband was an unfeeling brute who had recklessly taken away whatever hope my uncle might have had left.

Unlike the other relatives, my husband and I had already worked through three reactions to a terminal prognosis: *denial, anger,* and *bargaining (if he goes through all his treatments and is a good patient, the cancer will miraculously disappear).* We were now experiencing a little *depression* and *acceptance.* Because we had accepted Uncle John's grim prognosis and had begun grieving, my husband and I were focused on making his remaining days as comfortable and rewarding as possible. And we wanted to be sure he knew time was short, so he could have the choice to do the things many people do when they're dying while he could still think relatively clearly, fulfilling as many of his goals as possible. The rest of the family were still in a bit of denial and were not ready to talk about such matters. They were still focused on fighting his disease and were urging him to seek treatments that might at least delay the disease's progression.

My uncle, though still not sure about his ultimate prognosis, had accepted that his tumor was unlikely to respond to any antineoplastic chemotherapy. By insisting otherwise, family members were denying him an important avenue of support. Instead of letting him share with them his daily progress in overcoming the side effects of radiation and dexamethasone, they were making him feel worse by implying that he wasn't doing everything possible to treat his cancer.

Once I understood what was underlying our various positions, I was able to explain to other family members why their efforts were counterproductive and to convince them to stop hounding my uncle to seek out a miracle cure. His anxiety decreased when they stopped raising questions that he thought had already been answered satisfactorily. He sought psychological counseling to help him deal with his overwhelming situation and focused on the remaining goals he wished to achieve before he died.

Isolation: An Unintended Consequence of Protection

As it becomes clearer that the final months are approaching, patients and their families often seek to protect each other from the impending loss.

The Case of the Disappearing Walls

One morning I had to tell Simon Babar, a patient with colon cancer and extensive metastases to his liver, that the chemotherapy no longer appeared to be working—the metastases in his liver had become larger. I added that no other therapies were likely to stop the tumor from growing and that I felt he was likely to die within the next few months. Simon said that he was not really surprised, because he had been feeling weaker and had almost no appetite. He said he was OK with the news but asked me not to share this information with his family. Similarly, when I had to inform a family of bad news before I'd been able to talk with the patient, some asked me not to share the information with the patient, going so far as threatening to sue me if I did.

Whether it is understood as such, in both types of situations, the underlying motivation is to protect loved ones. Patients and families are often unaware of this protective instinct; they are worried that if the truth were known, either the family would decompensate from grief, or the patient would "give up" and die precipitously.

Rather than betray Simon's trust, I tried to help him understand that he would be hurting his wife and children more by keeping the grim prognosis from them than by telling them. I said something along the following lines:

> I realize that you want your wife and children to be spared the pain that you're now feeling. And I can certainly understand that impulse. But your family is pretty smart and must have a sense of what has been going on. Your weight loss, your increased pain, and your profound weakness are hard to ignore. By pretending they're not happening, you make it impossible for your family to talk with you about what they're feeling. They are unlikely to initiate the conversation because they want to protect your feelings as much as you want to protect theirs.
>
> By shielding them, you are isolating them from you, leaving them to face their fears and grief alone. They want to comfort you, to help you set and reach goals for the time you have left. There may be things they want to say to you, and you to them, that have been hard to say before but would be easier to say now.
>
> When you don't talk to them about something as important as the fact that you're dying, it's as though you are building a room around them without doors or windows. But when you tell them how serious things are, you are letting them know that it's OK to talk with you about it. You create a door in one of the walls through which they can come out and join you. Then, instead of being isolated from your family, you can share your love and concern and can comfort each other.

Simon thought over what I'd said, then asked me to be present when he shared the information with his family, who were waiting outside his room. He said that he hadn't wanted me to tell them because, somehow, if he did not talk about it, nothing would change. He did not want his family feeling sorry for him, treating him differently, or being sad because he was dying. But he now realized that they probably did know that his illness had gotten much worse, and he welcomed the chance to get everything out into the open. Before I let in his wife and children, he joked, "Go ahead and open the door, doc. I'm ready to blow down all four of those lousy walls!"

Avoiding Patient Abandonment

Sometimes a clinician can unwittingly be the source of unnecessary distress to a patient with far-advanced cancer. Clinicians have their own ways of coping with the mortality of their patients, and some may have difficulty transitioning their role from one focused on treating the cancer to one focused on treating the patient *with* cancer, no matter what. The Smiths' story is a sad example of how good intentions can be subverted by poor communication skills.

Abandonment

Mr. Smith was treated for several years by his local oncologist, Dr. Verna, for metastatic prostate cancer. When it stopped responding to the standard therapies, Dr. Verna referred him to Dr. O'Brian, an oncologist at an academic cancer center one hour away who specialized in experimental therapies for prostate cancer. Mr. Smith underwent several trials at the cancer center but had not been back to see Dr. Verna for more than a year when he and his wife reappeared, crestfallen.

They told Dr. Verna about their last visit with Dr. O'Brian and repeated what she had said, "word for word": *"Mr. Smith, your last bone scan showed progressive disease,"* she had told them. *"I'm sorry, but there's nothing more I can do for you. I think it would be better if, in the future, you went back to Dr. Verna for your care."*

It is likely that Dr. O'Brian thought she was doing the Smiths a favor by sending them back to their local oncologist and not forcing them to make the hour trip each way to the cancer center. But *the way* she told them upset them very much.

The Smiths told Dr. Verna that they had been crushed by that last visit: not only was the cancer progressing, but there was "nothing more to be done." Think how much better Mr. Smith would have felt if Dr. O'Brian had at least thanked them for their help in advancing the field by participating in the cutting-edge clinical trials and offered to call Dr. Verna for them to ensure there would not be anything missed during the transition. That would have made her reasons for referring him back much clearer and would have spared their feelings.

Dr. Verna reassured the Smiths that he was delighted to resume Mr. Smith's care and that he could do a great deal for them. He suggested that although Dr. O'Brian was an expert in the aggressive treatment of the cancer, he could offer therapy that was just as aggressive to control any cancer-related symptoms that arose at this stage of the disease. He also encouraged them to tell him more about how they had felt when asked to leave the cancer center.

The Smiths admitted that they had felt abandoned, worthless, and hopeless. By continuing to show sensitivity to his patients' feelings and by meticulous attention to his medical as well as their psychosocial and spiritual concerns, Dr. Verna helped them regain feelings of worth and hope. Your patients might reveal anxiety or similar signs or symptoms of depression. If these are severe, you may need to refer them to a psychologist, psychiatrist, pastoral counselor, or social worker with psychological training.

SHIFTING THE FOCUS OF CARE

Many patients go through a gradual transition in care from a cancer-directed treatment approach focused on life prolongation to fully supportive care focused on symptom management and quality of life. It's critical to prepare patients for this shift along the way rather than waiting until the last moment, as difficult as that can be for clinicians to do.

Before the final transition, there comes a time when the burdens of antineoplastic treatment need to be carefully weighed against the potential benefits. Even when the treatment itself has few side effects, the frequent trips for therapy or the constant monitoring of blood counts and renal and hepatic function can become a drain on precious energy reserves. The burden/benefit ratio will vary depending on the patient's goals and values, her mental and physical condition, whether the problem is likely to be reversible, and how far the underlying disease has advanced. Maintaining a focus on treatment without letting patients know clearly that "good time" is limited is likely to result in their not using this precious time to complete personal and professional goals.

As you would expect, these burden/benefit dilemmas become more frequent as the disease progresses. For some patients with shortness of breath from a pleural effusion, an indwelling catheter is the answer. For others, oxygen and morphine given at home provide more appropriate palliation. Two patients, one with newly diagnosed non–small cell lung cancer and the other bedridden with widely metastatic, refractory breast cancer, might have the same cancerous invasion and pathologic fracture of the T10 vertebra, with epidural extension of tumor but no compression of the spinal cord. Neither has been irradiated in that area, and thus both are candidates for surgery and radiation therapy or radiation alone. For the patient who has no other complications from lung cancer and has an active life and no other sources of pain or disability, the choice is clear—the spinal metastasis should be treated aggressively (i.e., fractionated radiation therapy or surgery followed by fractionated radiation therapy) to prevent the spinal cord compression that is otherwise likely to follow. But for the patient riddled with multiple painful bone metastases from refractory breast cancer, pain medication alone or combined with a single treatment of radiation therapy may be preferable.

How can patients and their providers begin shifting the focus of care without risking their relationship? Sara Bloom's story is illustrative of the dilemma.

Beginning the Transition

Sara was a 53-year-old widow with a PhD in psychology. She had been diagnosed with colon cancer five years before, received adjuvant chemotherapy, and for the last three years had received treatment for metastatic colon cancer. Her tumor had slowly progressed despite a series of agents, and she was now on a daily oral regimen that required monitoring of her blood counts and renal function. Her bimonthly taps of ascites were now needed every two weeks, and her fatigue was increasing despite red blood cell transfusions about every six weeks. Sara was also quite sensitive to the cognitive effects of the opioids she needed for pain control. Dr. Olinsky, her oncologist, asked our palliative care team to work with Sara to identify a regimen that would be less sedating. Sara had three adult children, one of whom always accompanied her to her office visits.

During a follow-up visit with all of us, Dr. Olinsky told Sara that her recent CT scan showed slight progression. Dr. Olinsky added that he thought Sara should stop her current therapy and take a break for a while to "regain her strength," after which they could consider adding something new. Sara was very upset. She angrily accused Dr. Olinsky of abandoning her now that she was no longer eligible for experimental therapy trials. She directed her daughter to wheel her "out of here" and, glaring at Dr. Olinsky and me, said, *"What do you all expect me to do now . . . just sit by the window waiting to die?"*

The work of Schou and Hewison (1999) can help us understand Sara's reaction. These sociologists studied patients receiving radiation therapy as well as their families. These families were negotiating care systems for the first time, and Schou and Hewison tried to determine which elements of the experience contributed to or detracted from the patients' quality of life. Their insights are equally applicable to patients like Sara, who are undergoing other antineoplastic regimens.

Before they begin treatment, patients usually have various plans for the future. Schou and Hewison suggest that to understand what is happening, we think in terms of calendars by which patients and families run their lives: the *sociocultural calendar*, which includes holidays like Diwali, Thanksgiving, Christmas, Kwanzaa, the Moon Festival, and Passover; the *personal and private calendar*, which includes birthdays, anniversaries, weddings, and graduations; and the *life calendar*, with church, soccer practice, and social gatherings. In addition to these events of daily living, the life calendar also includes plans for achieving goals in the realms of work and relationships.

Once treatment starts, Schou and Hewison argue, all these calendars are superseded by the *illness calendar* and the *treatment calendar*. The *illness calendar* begins during diagnosis and continues as long as the patient requires medical check-ups. Of more immediate concern to patients and families, however, are the *treatment calendars*, which they create each time a patient begins a new therapy. Patients and their families vest the current treatment calendar with the power to bring about a dramatic improvement in their cancer or cure. Any disruption in that calendar is therefore distressing: many strive to complete the treatments "on time" so that all will be well. When white blood cell or platelet counts are too low, patients see the nutritionist and ask what they can do to "get back on schedule."

You may know that the schedule is not so important for palliative treatment regimens, but patients do not know this, and they rarely ask to delay a treatment to feel better for an important event. For example, offers to delay chemotherapy until after Thanksgiving may be met by patients with a puzzled refusal. It is as though you were thoughtlessly jeopardizing the patient's future.

Dr. Olinsky and his team needed a plan for when they resumed Sara's treatment. To prevent a recurrence of her feeling of abandonment, they needed to encourage her to reintegrate into her daily life the activities that were meaningful before treatment began; the things that filled up her *personal and private* calendars. Sara and her family could work with his team to schedule treatment sessions to accommodate important family events or holiday celebrations. When he reinitiated treatment, Dr. Olinsky reassured Sara and her children that minor alterations in the schedule would not affect the efficacy of the treatment. In this way, Dr. Olinsky was able to help Sara rebuild her *personal calendar*, and as that calendar filled up, to help her begin to adjust to the knowledge that for whatever time she had remaining, he could accommodate her schedules.

In the meantime, we encouraged Sara to use the energy she had during this break to think about which important events she would like to be a part of, and how to create her legacy. Some patients hope they can participate in a child's graduation or be present for the birth of a grandchild. For Sara, the event was her daughter's wedding, planned for four months hence, although the odds were that she would not survive that long, or if she did, would not have the energy to enjoy it. We therefore urged Sara to make use of her time before the next treatment started to ensure that she would have some presence at the wedding, in case it could not be the presence she wanted. We helped her children make videos with her, including one in which she narrated the family scrapbooks and other photos and videos as part of her wedding gift.

Our palliative care team often suggests that patients with children or grandchildren consider writing letters to them for events far into the future or create or purchase gifts that will embody their love and ensure that they will be there in spirit. Another gift we suggest for small children is a stuffed animal with a recording of the patient's voice. For patients who assure us that they will be there in person, we reply that if all goes as they hope, the children will simply have extra gifts to enjoy, knowing they were in the patient's thoughts even when things looked darkest.

As disease progresses despite ongoing treatment, patients who, like Sara, have begun to reengage in non-treatment-related activities and have developed a broader relationship with their oncology team are more likely to understand later that you are not abandoning them when you tell them that the burden of another therapy is much greater than the potential benefit. When Dr. Olinsky next proposes that therapy be discontinued, Sara will be less likely to say that for her, stopping treatment was "waiting around to die," because she will have found other activities to fill her days.

SUPPORTING HOPE

In the Greek myth, Pandora's curiosity led to the release of the many evils that plague humanity, but she slammed the lid shut before hope, too, could escape (D'Aulaire and D'Aulaire 1962). Hope remained to sustain us through dark times. Emily Dickinson (Franklin 1999) also wrote of the persistence and compassion of hope:

> "Hope" is the thing with feathers –
> That perches in the soul –
> And sings the tune without the words –
> And never stops – at all –
> And sweetest – in the Gale – is heard –
> And sore must be the storm –
> That could abash the little Bird
> That kept so many warm –
> I've heard it in the chillest land –
> And on the strangest Sea –
> Yet – never – in Extremity,
> It asked a crumb – of me.

Hope is the elusive backdrop to the world (and business) of cancer care. Reimbursement to our hospitals and clinics allows clinicians to offer "nth line" treatments, and hope drives our patients and their families to *keep going*. Hope enables those of us who practice palliative care to accompany our patients through their journeys even as cancer advances to claim life itself. I (*Molly Collins*) routinely make bereavement calls after my patients have died. I often hear hope amid great sorrow. Hope for the new grandchild, hope to live a life as the deceased would have wanted, and hope to keep memories alive in the hearts of those who remain.

Hope is subjective and essential. It can be future and goal oriented, or expansive and evolving. In a deeply reflective article, Dr. Brad Stuart and colleagues (2019) discuss how clinicians can provide support as patients transition from "focused hope" centering on a cure or recovery, to "intrinsic hope" focused on domains such as quality of life, connection, and meaning. Dr. Gloria White-Hammond, a pediatrician and pastor, explains that for many, and especially for Black patients, hope is derived from their faith, the hope preached in the often more than 20,000 hours spent celebrating in their church's religious, educational, and service activities (personal communication, "God Is Able: The Significance of Belief in Miracles for African American Patients with Serious Illness," 2021; Elk et al. 2020). With our help and that of their pastor, she says, as patients' cancers advance, they may transition from "I know God has healed me," through "I trust that God will heal me" and "I hope that God will heal me," to "God's grace is sufficient for me," coming at last to acceptance with "Not my will but thine be done."

Even patients who say, "I know God has healed me," are not in denial of their medical condition. They are simply restating their spiritual orientation and their confidence in God as a healer. We need to affirm to our spiritual patients our commitment to see and respect their foundation of faith as we support their transition. The Practice Points box below includes Pastor Gloria's prayer for parishioners and a version that Dr. Gloria adapted that clinicians can use with their patients.

Practice Points: Conversation with Spiritual Patients

Pastor Gloria's Prayer	Dr. Gloria's conversation
Pray for God's grace	Express gratitude for the patient
Acknowledge emotions	Acknowledge emotions
Affirm trust in God	Affirm the patient's faith
Ask for healing	Affirm the hope for healing, and "I worry . . ."
Ask for strength to endure	Commit to support *all* the way
Pray for the wisdom of clinicians	Appreciate thoughts and prayers for clinicians
Express, however, ultimate confidence in God	Affirm the patient's faith
Gratitude for God's grace	Express gratitude for the patient

(Personal communication, Gloria White-Hammond, MD, MDiv, 2019)

With all our patients, we need to use honest communication about prognosis, compassionate presence, assistance creating concrete plans for the end of life, and patience as people move through grief to "find life on the other side of despair" (Stuart et al. 2019, p. 684). Formulating and communicating prognosis, as we discuss in depth below, is key to this process, and to the reframing, rather than the taking away, of hope.

THE CHALLENGE OF PROGNOSTICATION

One of the fundamental difficulties of caring for patients with advanced cancer is accurate prognostication. Even after we overcome the barriers to making and discussing prognoses (discussed in Chapter 1), when we are caring for someone with advanced disease, we must both share the inherent uncertainty of prognostication and try to paint a rough picture of the patient's future for ourselves, our colleagues, and our patients and their families. We can paint this prognostic picture in several different ways: using time, function, and illness trajectory (Taylor et al. 2017).

Time-based prognoses. Survival length is difficult to determine in patients with a new diagnosis of metastatic solid tumors. With current therapies, many patients will have responsive or stable disease for months to many years; a small number of exceptional responders may even have no evidence of cancer for many years (Hui, Maxwell, and Paiva 2019). Unlucky patients will either not respond or have a fatal complication even before their treatment has time to work.

Oncologists are the best resource for treatment-specific prognostic information and an estimate of the best- and worst-case scenario. Palliative care clinicians rely on their oncologic colleagues for the latest trials, as well as disease- and treatment-specific survival information. Oncologists can tell their palliative care colleagues what and how many additional lines of treatment are available and the expectations of response and burden, including who is likely to derive significant benefit from treatment, gaining years, or even a cure. To be most helpful to our patients, palliative care and oncology clinicians need to learn whether, despite potential toxicity, the outcome of treatment is likely to be one most concordant with the patient's goals.

At the time of diagnosis, oncologists usually use cancer site, stage, pathologic tumor characteristics (e.g., grade), and biomarkers such as mutation and PD-L1 expression status to estimate prognosis of patients with solid tumors (Hui 2015). Clinicians have population-level and group-specific estimates of survival, including data from cancer registries (such as those collected in the National Cancer Institute's SEER program), the *AJCC Cancer Staging Manual* (Amin et al. 2017), and clinical trial data, in which the effect of treatment on survival can be assessed.

Giving a time-based prognosis for patients with hematologic malignancies is particularly challenging. They may still be cured despite refractory and relapsed disease (Gray, Temel, and El-Jawahri 2020). "Moreover, the rapid and unpredictable trajectory of decline at the end of life leads to an absence of a clear transition between the curative and palliative phase of treatment" (Gray, Temel, and El-Jawahri 2020, p. 4).

Time-based prognoses that estimate median survival time, percentage survival to certain end points (e.g., 24 and 60 months), or progression-free survival may aid prognostication, but these statistics may be hard to interpret for the patient who asks us, "How much time, doc?" While there are many models that stratify patients into groups that correlate with differences in survival, the "rate of accuracy is below 80% for a vast majority of prognostic tools" (Hui 2015, p. 495). They are especially limited in guiding prognostication for patients with advanced cancer (Hui 2015; Hui, Maxwell, and Paiva 2019).

Despite this lack of precision, these tools can be helpful if they "facilitate clinical decision making by providing approximated time frames (months, weeks, or days)" (Hui 2015, p. 489). Rather than share the statistics, therefore, palliative care and oncology clinicians can share likely time ranges, such as "hours to days," "days to weeks," "weeks to months," "months to years," or "a number of years," which are easily understood. Or prognosis could be framed as the likelihood of a patient reaching a certain goal or event, such as an upcoming wedding or the winter holidays.

Functional status-driven prognoses. When disease advances and the likely range shortens to a small number of months or less, population and trial data become less helpful than individual, patient-specific factors (Hui 2015). Declining functional status is the single most important indicator that a patient's prognosis may be as short as weeks to months. A functional prognosis, such as that the patient is unlikely to regain strength, but rather likely to weaken and require more help in the coming weeks to months, can help patients and families with essential planning.

The most useful tools have been studied and validated in various settings and typically rely on functional status as a core factor (Simmons et al. 2017). These include the Palliative Performance Scale, Palliative Prognostic Score, Palliative Prognostic Index, Objective Prognostic Score, Eastern Cooperative Oncology Group (ECOG) Performance Scale, Karnofsky Performance Scale, and Glasgow Prognostic Score (Hui 2015; Hui, Maxwell, and Paiva 2019; Simmons et al. 2017).

Other than the ECOG, most of these tools have not been integrated into routine care (Hui, Maxwell, and Paiva 2019). Several websites guide clinicians to prognostic calculators and their interpretation, including ePrognosis (https://eprognosis .ucsf.edu/) and Dr. David Hui's site, developed with Dr. John Maxwell, Predict Survival.com. Perhaps in the future, novel prognostic models using machine learning will be integrated into the electronic health record to help guide our predictions (Hui, Maxwell, and Paiva 2019; Parikh et al. 2019).

Illness trajectory. Patients with solid cancers most often have a "terminal illness" trajectory (Figure 5.1), unless they become exceptional responders, as discussed below. In this trajectory, patients have a steep decline in function after a period of slower decline or relative stability (Hui 2015; Lunney, Lynn, and Hogan 2002). Patients typically lose ~70–80 percent of their function in the final few months of life (Weissman 2003; Lunney et al. 2003). They spend more time resting or in bed and have decreased energy, weight loss, less interest or ability to eat, and diminished independence in activities of daily living/instrumental activities of daily living (ADLs/iADLs). If we have not already started discussions about their care choices at the end of life, we need to now.

Patients with hematologic malignancies (especially patients with hematologic malignancies undergoing transplant or CAR T-cell therapy) follow a trajectory that looks more like the "organ failure" model (Figure 5.1), in which patients have a fluctuating course characterized by acute declines in function that may be completely or partially reversed with management of each illness episode, or with initiation of a novel therapy, which can "reset" their function back to a higher level, even cure, or end in death (Gray, Temel, and El-Jawahri 2020).

Rarely, cancer patients have a more gradual but inexorable decline consistent with the "frailty" model (Figure 5.1). Knowledge of these different trajectories—and sharing the most likely with each of your patients—can be particularly helpful for them.

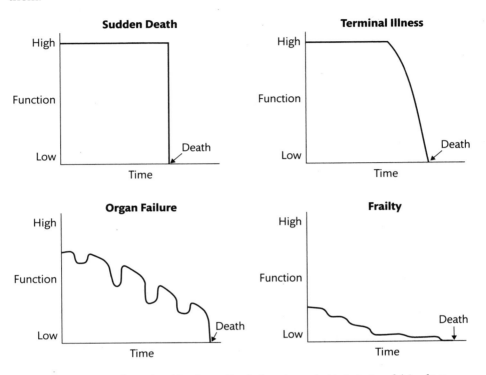

FIGURE 5.1. Trajectories of Functional Decline to Death. Four theoretical trajectories of dying from different types of illnesses. *Source:* Reproduced with permission from J. R. Lunney, J. Lynn, and C. Hogan, "Profiles of Older Medicare Decedents," *J Am Geriatr Soc* 50: 1109, 2002.

Practice Points: Principles of Prognostication

- Oncologists are the best resource for treatment-specific prognostic information and an estimate of the best- and worst-case scenario.
- Tools can help but have significant limitations.
- Functional status predicts prognosis in the last weeks to months.
- Prognosis can be formulated and expressed in several ways:
  - Time, in a range of "hours to days," "days to weeks," "weeks to months," "months to years," or "a number of years"; or likelihood of reaching a goal or event
  - Function
  - Illness trajectory
- Prognostication is an evolving process, not an event.

Prognostication is an evolving process, not an event (Hui 2015). The skill and art of prognostication includes acknowledging our uncertainty, communicating what we do know when that is helpful, and conveying the range of possibilities as the clinical situation evolves.

DISCUSSING PROGNOSIS WHEN TIME IS SHORTER THAN HOPED

In Chapter 1, we review the barriers to discussing prognosis with patients with newly diagnosed disease. When patients are first being offered therapy, prognostic discussions are crucial to the process of beginning advance care planning because they inform choices patients and families make. These early prognostic discussions usually center on whether the disease is curable, how long the patient is likely to live if the disease does or does not respond to therapy, and whether antineoplastic therapy will improve or shorten the patient's life.

But for patients presenting with advanced disease or those who are no longer responding to the usual therapies, clinicians have a harder task (Back 2020). Patients are known to be much more optimistic than their oncologists about their likelihood of response or cure (LeBlanc, Temel, and Helft 2018; Temel et al. 2018) and choose therapies based on those misunderstandings. In one study of leukemia patients over 60, for example, 74 percent thought they had a ≥50 percent chance of cure, but 89 percent of their physicians thought that chance was ≤10 percent (Sekeres et al. 2004). Most patients want to know their prognoses and options for care, and when they are told these by their oncology clinicians, they have better quality care as they die. Those patients who reported they knew they had a small chance of cure were less likely to choose aggressive therapies at the end of their lives (LeBlanc, Temel, and Helft 2018). Some patients rely on family and clergy for support and even prognostic information, and prognostic conversations should include them when that is the case (LeBlanc et al. 2019).

It is not enough to say, "I don't have a crystal ball" or "I just don't know," because you are uncertain about a precise prognosis. Much of the time, the clinician knows whether the prognosis is likely to be days, weeks, months, or years, and even that broad an estimate can be helpful to patients and their families, who may be under the mistaken assumption that as we manage advanced cancer "like a chronic disease," they may potentially have decades left to live. The difference between a patient's estimate of 10–20 years' survival and a clinician's of "a small number of years" is quite discrepant and important to unearth. When clinicians have even *some* idea, they can let patients and families know the true chance of a clinically meaningful response, how long that would take to occur, and what the likelihood of side effects are.

Oncologists need to be explicit. Conveying simply that the disease is incurable, and that they will work to "control" it as long as they can, is not the same as telling a patient he has "weeks to months" or "months to years" to live. Palliative care clinicians can help oncologists share this difficult information. Tom Walsh, for example, was clear that he did not want to discuss the future, but he gave us permission to speak to his wife, Janelle, a nurse, who wanted prognostic information so that she could plan for what lay ahead. Tom had metastatic tonsillar cancer and several comorbidities, including severe peripheral vascular disease and osteomyelitis. Tom was eating less and spent most of his day resting or seated, but he was still (stubbornly) independent in his ADLs. His oncologist, Dr. Puri, offered immunotherapy, which Tom declined because of the low likelihood of improvement and the risk of side effects.

Dr. Puri gave me (*Molly Collins*) his permission to discuss prognosis with Janelle, which he and I both thought was weeks to as many as six months. Janelle told me that she was hoping to hear how much time Tom had, and whether he would make it to Christmas in two months. I replied, *"Dr. Puri and I are worried that his time is most likely in the range of weeks to months. He might make it as long as six months, but that's much less likely. We think there's a decent chance he will make it to Christmas, but he may not make it that long. We'll know that time is short if we see that he's needing help with everyday activities, like getting dressed, bathing, and getting out of bed, when he's sleeping much of the day and not interested in eating or able to eat. But Janelle, you need to know that something sudden could happen like an infection, difficulty breathing, confusion, or bleeding, and Tom could die before Christmas."* Janelle voiced her understanding, and we then turned to the practicalities of how we could best support Tom and Janelle, which, in their case, was with home hospice care.

As we discuss in Chapter 1, it can be difficult for oncology clinicians to have these discussions. A 2014 review showed that 75 percent of patients with advanced cancer were unaware of their prognoses (Applebaum et al. 2014). In another study of oncologists and reports of their patients and the nurses who work with them, a quarter to a third never told their patients about the possibility of death, even when the patient specifically asked for prognostic information (LeBlanc, Temel, and Helft 2018).

Oncology clinicians face several barriers to having these discussions, as we review in Chapter 1, and they have a wide range of comfort and skill in this kind of communication (LeBlanc, Temel, and Helft 2018; Temel et al. 2018; Back 2020). Many clinicians are poorly trained to address the emotional responses of patients and families, although emotions are a predictable and unavoidable aspect of caring for patients, especially at the end of life (Geerse et al. 2019). Addressing emotions appropriately can become one of the most rewarding elements of providing care for any patient, but it can require support to feel competent and to do it well.

Oncologists often walk a tightrope. On the one hand, they want to convey as accurate a prognosis as they can and encourage and support their patients in choosing therapies that may help in the long run, either by extending life or improving quality of life. But sometimes the chances of achieving a good outcome are small, and in the short run, the treatments are likely to cause significant side effects. I (*Molly Collins*) have seen this tension manifest in a discrepancy between the words that are conveyed (e.g., a limited prognosis, incurability, or low likelihood of treatment benefit) and the oncologist's too-casual body language and nonverbal communication that suggest instead that there is "nothing to worry about here." Unfortunately, even with an intention to convey support and foster hope, the patient may be misled into underestimating the risks and overestimating the benefits of the proposed treatment.

Fortunately, there are skills that can overcome these common pitfalls (Back 2020) and validated training programs that can improve clinicians' comfort and skill in such discussions, such as the Serious Illness Care Program that we reviewed in detail in Chapter 1 (Paladino et al. 2019). The VitalTalk technique REMAP, which we review below, and NURSE mnemonic to respond to emotion (reviewed in Chapter 1) are helpful here. Palliative care clinicians can conduct skills training for those interested, partner with their oncology colleagues to have the needed discussions in the inpatient or outpatient setting, and support oncology clinicians in this difficult aspect of their work. In Chapter 11 we discuss the role of the palliative care team in depth.

Discussing Prognosis in the Age of Exceptional Responders

By creating "exceptional responders," genome-targeted therapies and immunotherapies have made prognostic certainty, and therefore this discussion, even more difficult. More than half of patients with melanoma, for example, respond to combination immunotherapy with significantly improved survival, and the response rate in a trial of patients with non–small cell lung cancer eligible for first-line treatment with pembrolizumab was 44.8 percent (Temel et al. 2018).

Overall, however, as of 2021 only a minority of patients will become exceptional responders. There is no definite way to know who will respond, or to predict who will develop severe toxicities (Temel et al. 2018). The lack of clarity about what they are giving up if they don't try genome-targeted or immunotherapy may prevent patients who would otherwise qualify for hospice care from ever enrolling. Rates of grade 3 to 4 autoimmune toxicities range from 10 to 60 percent (Temel et al. 2018) and can lead to hospitalizations and the devastating news that the patient must stop what had been an effective therapy. Immunotoxicity may affect the skin, lungs, liver, kidney, endocrine system, joints, GI tract, and brain and may not reverse off therapy.

As we have emphasized, prognostication is inherently uncertain. We can help our patients prepare for the possible range by "hoping for the best, while preparing for the worst," or initiating a "plan A/plan B" discussion (Temel et al. 2018). We call this communication strategy "walking both roads" with the patient (Collins and Abrahm 2019). Clinicians can—and should— acknowledge prognostic uncertainty, but they owe it to their patients and families to provide best case/worst case estimates in those receiving targeted or immunotherapies.

Finding a Way Forward When Clinicians Differ on Prognosis

In some cases, clinicians of different specialties see patients' prognoses from quite disparate perspectives, which can present substantial barriers to moving discussions of goals and plans of care forward. Since prognosis is inherently uncertain, no one "owns" the truth. When there is conflict about the prognosis between the oncology clinician and the hospital team, or the oncology clinician and the patient and family, palliative care clinicians need to resist taking a side, instead attempting "shuttle diplomacy" (Collins and Abrahm 2019).

Palliative care specialists can seek to understand what facts and feelings form part of the decisions on each side. These often include emotional barriers, such as feelings of grief and personal failure not yet realized by some clinicians themselves. NURSE statements may unearth these, offering colleagues empathic support: for example, *"I can't imagine how it must feel to try your best to treat someone who has a curable cancer, and then have all these medical complications make her so very ill."* Or, using the R in REMAP, we can help them reframe with *"When you started treating her, she looked so much better. But it seems that we are in a different place now"* (Childers et al. 2017).

We may need to help our colleagues grieve and see other ways to show their care (Meier 2014). If they are basing their treatment recommendations solely on the prognosis of the cancer and missing the bigger picture, we can change the conversation from one about prognosis to one about patient goals, asking, *"What is an acceptable quality of life for this patient, and what is she willing to go through to get there?"* (Collins and Abrahm 2019). Ultimately, palliative care specialists strive to align with both our patients and colleagues and work to reframe a difficult situation. The communication model "Talk Palliative to Me," which I (*Molly Collins*) developed for discussing prognosis with my colleagues, helps reveal the range of perspectives and how we can work together.

Practice Points: "Talk Palliative to Me"

- What's the big picture of where things are headed for this patient?
- What's the best case, worst case, most likely case?
- How much of the best case, worst case, most likely case have you shared with the patient?
- What's my role in communicating this information moving forward, and what's yours?

CULTIVATING PROGNOSTIC AWARENESS

As patients consider the future, it is normal for them to swing between more hopeful and more realistic outlooks. This way of thinking enables many people to cope with the difficult reality of their mortality (Jackson et al. 2013; Jacobsen et al. 2018). Jackson et al. (2013, p. 894) described this process as "the cultivation of prognostic awareness," with prognostic awareness defined as "a patient's capacity to understand his or her prognosis and the likely illness trajectory." Beginning the discussion of prognosis early in the course of the disease, as we review in Chapter 1, and fostering it all along the trajectory of terminal illness greatly facilitates this awareness.

When my (*Molly Collins's*) palliative care team cared for Tiffany Boyle, we used many of the communication tools Jackson and her colleagues developed to help prepare Tiffany and her family for her death. Tiffany was only 30 years old when she was referred to our palliative care clinic for abdominal pain, nausea, and anorexia related to recently diagnosed metastatic cholangiocarcinoma with peritoneal carcinomatosis. We knew the referral carried with it another unstated and underlying request from her oncology team: to help support Tiffany, her family, and the team as we all witnessed the heartbreaking end of this too-short life. Our team's palliative care fellow, Dr. Willow, took the primary role in Tiffany's care.

Tiffany was frail, cachectic, and child-like, accompanied by an aunt whose posture always reflected the protective role she served for Tiffany. Early on, when Dr. Willow asked Tiffany what her understanding of her illness was, she and her aunt always emphasized the positive: *"I know I'll need to be on treatment forever. It will work, and I'm hopeful I'll get my strength back."* As we probed and asked her how much she wanted to know about what the future held, Tiffany's body language stiffened, and her aunt seemed to flash us dagger eyes. Tiffany was clear in her reply: "I'm not ready to talk about that right now."

We conveyed our support and that we would be there for her when she did feel ready to talk about it. This technique has been termed "talking about talking about it" (Jacobsen et al. 2018, p. 325). We explored with Tiffany how a discussion could be helpful or problematic. Jackson et al. (2013, p. 897) suggest "inquiring whether the patient can imagine a poorer health state." This could sound like, *"If time were shorter than we all hoped, what would be most important to you right now?"* If Tiffany were clinically declining, and decisions needed to be made, you can use "wish" and "worry" and name the dilemma of not addressing prognosis. You might say, *"I sense it is very difficult to talk about getting sicker, or that you may even die from your cancer, and I wish we didn't have to. I worry that if we don't talk about this, we will lose the chance to make decisions together while you're still able to. Can we think together about how we can talk about this?"*

Luckily, Tiffany's clinical situation remained stable on gemcitabine and cisplatin for the next few visits, and we focused on developing rapport and building

---

Practice Points: Strategies for Patients Who Are Reluctant to Talk about Prognosis

- Talk about talking about it.
  - *Example.* "It's really normal to worry about talking about the future. It can be scary and painful. What are some reasons you might not want to talk about this? I'd like to think with you about when and how it might be helpful to talk about this. How will we know when it is time?"
- Walk both roads with the patient.
  - *Example.* "I am also hopeful that you do as well as possible for as long as possible. And in my experience, most patients find it helpful to prepare for the possibility that things don't go as we're both hoping."
- Imagine a poorer health state with the patient.
  - *Example.* "I wonder if we should think together about what it would be like if you got sicker." Or, "If time were as short as [name a time frame slightly longer than you think the patient may have and then progressively shorten this] a few months, would you be doing anything differently?"
- When the clinical situation is urgent, align with the patient and name the dilemma of not addressing prognosis.
  - *Example.* "I sense it is difficult to talk about getting sicker, or that you may even die from your cancer, and I wish we didn't have to. I worry that if we don't talk about this, we will lose the chance to make decisions together while you're still able to. Can we think together about how we can talk about this?"

(Adapted from Jackson et al. 2013 and Jacobsen et al. 2018)

---

trust through improving her pain control and other symptoms. Though she increasingly trusted Dr. Willow, we were aware of "the elephant in the room." Dr. Willow worried that if no one discussed her prognosis or revisited a discussion about the future, Tiffany wouldn't be given the opportunity to express her emotions, acknowledge what was happening with her family, and prepare. We both envisioned Tiffany dying in the ICU attached to machines with her family saying, "We had no idea time was so short." While we prepared ourselves for this possibility, we continued to plan how we could address prognosis with Tiffany.

First, we stayed in regular touch with her oncology team, who likewise encountered resistance when they tried to talk about the future. When her disease progressed, they focused on getting Tiffany to a clinical trial at another institution, but privately shared our worries that her prognosis was tenuous. While she could possibly gain a few extra months with the trial, her prognosis was most likely a small number of months.

As our discomfort grew with ignoring that she likely had only a few months to live, Dr. Willow and I again used the "talking about talking about it" and the "hope" and "worry" strategy. We explored Tiffany's *hopes* for the trial and asked about any *worries* she had. She acknowledged her worry that the treatment wouldn't work. This allowed us to align with her hope, but also with her worry that treatment might not work as well as we all hoped. We asked Tiffany how she felt talking about that possibility, and she said she knew that at some point we would have to talk about what to do in that case, but she didn't feel ready to talk about it yet. We assured her that we would let her know if there came a point when we would need to talk about it and reiterated that we were there to support her and her family, no matter what happened.

Unfortunately, Tiffany declined quickly. Within weeks of our discussion, she was requiring support just to get to the bathroom and was admitted for nausea due to the trial drug. Dr. Willow rallied her oncologist, and together we sat down with Tiffany and her family. Her oncologist shared that the weakness and worsening symptoms were a sign that the cancer was taking over, and that further treatment would cause her more harm than good. I said that we were facing the final chapter of Tiffany's life and that though it would be difficult, we needed to discuss how to approach it. Tiffany broke down in tears, and we sat in silence as her brother held her hand. Finally she calmed and said, "I just can't do this anymore."

I recommended that we shift from fighting the cancer to gaining as much comfort and peace as possible in the time that remained and that we work to get her home, with hospice. Into the space that was created from acknowledging that this was the end, Tiffany was able to express her deep sadness, and we were able to support her in her grief. Tiffany died at home, peacefully, two weeks later.

Tiffany's story illustrates how nuanced these discussions may need to be for some patients. If you are struggling with feeling that you have a responsibility to speak the truth now, acknowledge reality, and help your patients prepare, you may harm patients who are not ready for the discussion and whose condition does not demand that you have it. To prevent this, you may find it extremely helpful to share your worries and uncertainties out loud with a trusted colleague, such as the patient's social worker or oncologist (e.g., "We aren't addressing the reality of her prognosis!") and assess whether this is the patient's problem or yours.

Steps to cultivate prognostic awareness. Jackson et al. (2013) outline the first steps to cultivate prognostic awareness: (1) understand the actual prognosis (including the range of what may be possible and likely) and likely illness trajectory; (2) assess how much prognostic information the patient has integrated; and (3) assess the patient's readiness to hear this type of information.

It is important to assess the clinical urgency when we consider moving forward with a discussion about the future. As with our patient Tiffany, "If the patient is ambivalent or resistant but doing well clinically, the clinician may decide to repeat the self-assessment in an effort to help the patient become more comfortable with the discussion" (Jackson et al. 2013, p. 898).

If the patient is ready for the discussion or clinical urgency demands it, we should proceed with discussing the prognosis and likely trajectory, tailored to what the patient is ready to hear. For example, if your patient tells you, *"I know this is all in God's hands, and no one knows for sure, but I just hope I make it to my first grandchild's birth in six months."* You might reply, *"I wish that were possible, but I worry that it may be unlikely. I would love to be wrong, but I want to help prepare you and your family for the possibility that time may be shorter than six months."*

The earlier we can start this process of cultivating prognostic awareness, the better patients seem to become at tolerating this difficult discussion, and the deeper they can go. I find this to be especially true in the outpatient setting, upstream from the end of life, when patients are often more clinically stable. The self-reflection that is required each time we ask whether it's time to have the talk may gradually build the resilience they need to think about the unthinkable. We don't do this to hammer the painful reality of mortality home. We do it because an accurate understanding allows patients to prepare and facilitates shared decision-making. Those patients who find a degree of acceptance with the reality of their situation can focus on living well in the time that remains, rather than feeling overwhelmed by their fears of the unknown that awaits them.

Practice Points: Cultivating Prognostic Awareness

- Palliative care and oncology can collaborate to formulate the patient's prognosis.
- Assure patients that your goal is to prepare them for the future, and that you will continue to provide support *no matter what happens*, whether or not they continue on antineoplastic therapy.
- Assess patients' understanding of their prognosis.
  - *Example.* "What is your understanding of the big picture with your illness, and what the future holds?"
- Assess their readiness to talk about prognosis.
- Provide prognostic information tailored to patients' readiness.
  - *Example.* "I've heard you say how important it is that you know what to expect in the future and how much time you're likely to have. I wish I had different news, but I worry that time could be as short as a small number of months."
- Respond to emotions (NURSE, Chapter 1).
- Focus on living well while tolerating the possibility of dying.
  - *Example.* "What brings you joy, meaning, and purpose? Tell me about what gives you strength despite everything you're going through?"

(Adapted from Jackson et al. 2013 and Jacobsen et al. 2018)

Even the most skilled clinicians can find this process challenging when patients remain reluctant or resistant to talking about the future. But if you persevere, most patients and families will come around. True denial—in which patients are unable psychologically to acknowledge their illness or its terminal nature—is rare.

It is much more common to see patients swing between more hopeful and more realistic outlooks (Jackson et al. 2013; Jacobsen et al. 2018). In the same breath, patients may describe planning for their funeral and attending an event in the far distant future. This is not denial or even low prognostic awareness. This is normal coping behavior and represents a process by which patients integrate reality at a pace they can handle, "walking both roads."

MAKING THE FINAL TRANSITION

The final shift from life-prolonging treatment to fully supportive care focused on quality of life is the last important challenge clinicians face as their patients approach death. If clinicians, patients, or their families are not able to cultivate prognostic awareness along the way, they are unlikely to have prepared for this moment. Some clinicians do not have the skills, training, experience, or ability to tolerate the emotional intensity of these discussions and leave them until they can no longer be avoided. Some patients and families have great difficulty tolerating much of any discussion about the what-ifs and planning for death, even with the support of a skilled palliative care team. When the cancer advances explosively or a complication arises quickly, the opportunity to have a preparative discussion is lost.

But if your patients have been able to work with you along the way to prepare for the future, it does not come as a complete surprise when you share with them that the time to transition has arrived. It is a moment to acknowledge the sadness that the cancer has worsened despite everyone's best efforts. How you and the oncology team have that conversation makes all the difference.

In one study, analysis of the reports of family members after being told that chemotherapy would be stopped and the patient transitioned to end-of-life care revealed three general patterns (Norton et al. 2019). The worst pattern was called the "Left to Die" style. Here, they recalled no discussion of end-of-life care, and the transition off therapy occurred only during or after crises. The "Beating the Odds" pattern included explicit discussions about end-of-life care options but no review of prognosis, leading to what were perceived as "chaotic" transitions to end-of-life care. We can only hope that the third option, the supportive "We pretty much knew" pattern will increase. Those families recalled clear discussions of end-of-life care and shared understanding about prognosis.

A helpful heuristic at this stage is embodied in REMAP, which stands for **re**frame, **e**xpect emotion, **m**ap out values and goals, **a**lign, **p**lan. When there are few or no antineoplastic treatments left, REMAP helps clinicians share that news with the patient and family, learn the patients' values and goals, and integrate these into a new patient-centered plan (Childers et al. 2017). The first step of REMAP is **re**frame, in which the clinician delivers a "headline": a statement that includes the information that the patient's condition has changed and that there are serious implications to that change. For example, *"I know that in the past I've always offered more treatment when your disease progressed. Unfortunately, we're in a different place now with the cancer damaging your liver and no way to reverse this. Further treatment against the cancer isn't safe and that means time is getting shorter."*

The *E* stands for "**e**xpect emotion." Seeing the emotional response is how we know the news landed, and we need to respond to the emotion before moving forward. A few moments of silence (10–20 seconds) helps patients and families process and clinicians regain their balance. Then, use one or more of the NURSE statements (see Chapter 1): **n**ame the emotion; convey **u**nderstanding and re**s**pect; provide **s**upport; and **e**xplore feelings.

Next, take a step back, even if they ask, "What are we going to do now?" and ask open-ended questions to "**m**ap out" what's most important to them. *"What are you hoping for? What are your worries?"* You can ask about situations they want to avoid and ask "what else?" to explore other goals and hopes and fears, taking into account the medical realities. Keep asking "what else?" until they have nothing else to add to your understanding.

To "**a**lign" with your patients and check that you got their values right, reflect back what you've heard. You might tell one patient, *"I'm hearing that because family is your top priority, it's important that we leave no stone unturned in looking at all possible treatment options, but you hope to be at home with your family at the end. If nothing can be reversed, you want to be at home, not in the hospital."* To another, with different goals, you might say, *"I'm hearing that extending your life no matter how poor the quality is, is your top priority. If we get to the point where treatments will no longer help extend your life—and I'm worried we may be there soon—I want to reassure you that we will work as hard as possible to ensure you do not suffer, which will probably mean we care for you in the hospital or in an inpatient hospice at the end."*

When the patient signals that you have heard him correctly, you can ask permission to move on to the "**p**lan." For example, to the first patient above, you might say, *"May I give you my recommendation? Given what you've told me, I will circle back with all your other doctors to see if they have any other ideas for treatment and get back to you later today. If they cannot offer something that would help, we should focus on supporting you at home so you can be with your family. What do you think?"*

REMAP helps keep this conversation flexible, with patients as experts in their lives and what matters most, and clinicians as the experts in what is medically possible (Childers et al. 2017)

I (*Molly Collins*) often include in this transitional discussion that the progression of the cancer was not the patient's fault, and there was nothing they could have done to prevent it, which often elicits tears or another emotional response. I learned this on my first day of palliative care fellowship from Dr. Bethany-Rose Daubman, a coeditor of this book. Although we never intend to blame our patients, we may unwittingly have done so by implying that they can control the cancer by staying active, "eating right," and doing everything asked of them. They try to *keep going* despite the challenges their deteriorating body increasingly presents to them. It is really important to acknowledge this effort and explain that what is happening is *"not your fault—you, your doctors, and your family have done everything they could, but this cancer has grown despite our best efforts."*

At our direction, and with our encouragement, families have been carefully monitoring patients throughout antineoplastic therapies, and we should be explicit about what they no longer need to do, and which interventions are no longer helpful. Close monitoring of blood tests, for example, no longer provides information needed to make the patient safer or more comfortable. Phrases such as *"It's no longer indicated"*; *"We want to stop the antibiotics and blood transfusions"*; or *"We won't be doing any more tests"* may lead the family to conclude erroneously that useful interventions are being discontinued or that *all* care is going to be stopped. Families can easily focus on the *stop* part of the message and respond, *"But we want everything done. How can you deny our father the care that he's entitled to?"*

Substituting phrases such as the following conveys a more accurate idea of caring and support and enhances the likelihood that the family will agree that fully supportive care is best for the patient: *"We want to care for your father as you would at home if you had all the help we do here. We'll do all we can to make sure he is comfortable, and we'll only do things that will make him feel better."*

"Don't you care at all?"

The focus on comfort, however, may be interpreted by other clinicians as not caring. Our palliative care team had been consulting on the care of Oma, a young woman dying from a refractory metastatic gynecologic cancer. She was much loved by her house staff and the nurses on the unit, who had known her for several months. She and her family had come from Haiti to seek help for her condition, but the tumor had continued to grow despite everyone's best efforts. It swelled her abdomen and afflicted her with abdominal pain and finally with hypercalcemia, which was also refractory to medical efforts at correction. The hydration efforts had caused painful leg edema and dyspnea.

Oma was well supported by her family and friends. Her mother had been with her throughout the months of her stay in the United States. In her last weeks of life, Oma reunited with her estranged husband. Her family was allowed to be in close attendance, and together, we were able to give her the comfort she needed, and she died peacefully under our care in the hospital.

But we did not achieve this easily, even though Oma had accepted comfort care, understanding that there was no further antineoplastic therapy to try. While the house staff and nurses shared the goals of our palliative care team, they were often puzzled by and resisted implementing our recommendations, which included discontinuing intravenous fluids that were only exacerbating her ascites and peripheral edema and stopping the monitoring of her electrolytes and calcium levels. The morning we made those suggestions, an angry intern asked me, *"Don't you care at all?"*

The answer to the mystery appeared only after her death, while we were meeting with members of the gynecologic oncology team at their request. They could not understand how we and they had observed the same patient and yet found different problems that required totally different solutions. They were saddened by Oma's death and feared that they had contributed to her suffering. They wanted to understand how to help future patients.

They asked us, *"How do you know when it's time to stop what we normally do?"* How should we think about caring for someone who is on comfort care? What criteria did we use as we made our recommendations? For example, why didn't we want them to monitor her calcium and potassium levels? Why did we oppose "fluid challenges" (i.e., rapid infusions of 500-ml bolus doses of IV fluid) when she was tachycardic, up to 150/min? *"Why,"* the nurses asked, *"do they want us to do an enema in someone only days from death?"*

It was not the details of day-to-day management that they needed to understand; they needed a new appreciation for how different the goals are when you care for dying patients. We suggested that the gynecologic oncology team treat these patients as though they were caring for them at home, perhaps with the help of a hospice team. There, the goals and priorities of the patient and family—not the disease or metabolic abnormalities—are paramount.

We suggested that instead of weighing the risks and benefits of each intervention, they ask themselves what is the *burden* versus the *benefit* of this intervention? How will it help us further the patient's and family's goals? We acknowledged that assessing the burden/benefit ratio was very different from assessing risk/benefit, with which they were more familiar. After all, only minimal risk is entailed in a venipuncture or a fluid challenge. But there is a great deal of potential burden, especially in someone whose ascites, pulmonary secretions, and edema are going to be markedly exacerbated by the fluid.

The gynecologic oncology team was troubled about these suggestions. This did not look like "care" to them: *"If we aren't drawing blood, or monitoring her vital signs, what should we do?"* They felt helpless and at sea; they felt they had no more to offer to Oma or her family.

We explained that there are many other ways to show concern. Providing excellent comfort care, for example, requires frequent observations of patients and their families and an understanding of what causes distress for dying patients. We explained that we asked them to stop the fluids to prevent her from having breathing difficulties due to excess hydration, and we asked for the enema because we surmised that obstipation due to the continuous opioid infusion and refractory hypercalcemia was causing her significant discomfort and could contribute to her risk of developing delirium. We also praised them for their frequent visits to Oma and obvious concern for her, as well as sharing how much that provided comfort to her family. By the end of this meeting, the team members said they began to understand the other ways in which they could provide care and the other goals they could try to achieve for their dying patients.

Practice Points: Moving to Fully Supportive Care

- Convey concern.
- Reassure the patient and family that you will do everything possible to keep the patient comfortable.
- Consult with the patient and family to determine the burden/benefit ratio of each test, procedure, and treatment.
- Work to tailor the diagnostic and treatment plan toward aligning with the patient's values and priorities.
- Explore the patient's and family's religious beliefs about the significance of accepting comfort care, discussed in Chapter 3.
- Reassure the patient and family that you will not abandon them.
- Be open to discussions of psychological, financial, spiritual, and existential concerns.
- Readily refer patients and their families to palliative care, to hospice, or to individual professionals who can address these concerns.

READDRESSING RESUSCITATION CHOICES

Chapter 1 includes language for discussing resuscitation, intubation, and life-sustaining treatments. But even after these discussions, many patients who have far-advanced disease choose to be resuscitated when they die, despite their oncologist's explanations that they will end their days in an ICU. Some of these patients and families, as reviewed in Chapter 3, are hoping for a miracle or have religious objections to a shift to fully supportive care.

We can sometimes gain the trust of families who are waiting for a miracle by providing meticulous patient care, respecting their views, and attempting to fulfill their needs. When we let go of the "DNR agenda," our compassion can shine through. Families who are not spending their time fighting us about code status can, with assistance from their religious leader or social worker, reflect on what is best for their loved one and reconcile their loss and their beliefs. When the end nears, they and the health care team can arrive at the same place, albeit by different roads.

Family concerns can also cause some patients to demand resuscitation, as reviewed in Chapter 2. Some patients are the center of their family constellation, the matriarch or patriarch to whom everyone has turned for advice, validation, and love. They have directed careers, patched up marriages, managed divorces, run the family business, comforted angry teenagers, and made peace between generations. When disease overwhelms such a person, and there has been insufficient time to delegate that role and its responsibilities, dying is not an option. Despite being told repeatedly by their trusted oncologist that resuscitation is futile, such patients cannot accept DNR orders. For them, communication even while intubated is preferable to death.

As reviewed in Chapter 2, through intensive work by the social worker with the family and the patient, the burden of leadership can be transferred to one or more family members. Encouraging family members to let the patient know that they will take care of each other, and that the patient's spirit will continue to guide them, can sometimes release the patient from the strongly felt obligation. When these patients remain unconvinced, you may have to resuscitate them against your better judgment.

Young adult patients are often just beginning to have their hard work pay off in successful careers or growing families. They seem to be trying to make sense of their short lives or wondering how they can possibly leave their children. Some have no religious tradition that can help them make sense of what is happening to them. For patients with existential distress, we can offer to help them tell their stories, to bring meaning to the short lives they have had (Chapter 9 reviews how we can help patients with existential distress). As you might expect, the concerns that lead parents of young children to refuse DNR status usually differ significantly from those of other patients. As we discuss below, when appropriate plans have been made for their children, many parents will see the benefit of transitioning to fully supportive care.

TALKING WITH CHILDREN ABOUT SERIOUS ILLNESS AND DEATH

Young parents, especially single parents, present a heartrending challenge. Clinicians need to explore whether we can help them with concerns about their children. Try to ensure that the children are offered support, at least from their school counselors, who should be aware of the parent's serious illness. Dr. Paula Rauch, a consultation child psychiatrist at the Massachusetts General Hospital, founded and directs the Marjorie E. Korff Parenting at a Challenging Time (PACT) Program. PACT provides guidance for parents with cancer or amyotrophic lateral sclerosis (ALS) in supporting child resilience and communicating with their children about their illness and potentially impending death. Rauch's guidelines for clinicians who work with these parents and their children include six steps. For further guidance, I strongly encourage parents and clinicians alike to visit the

PACT website (www.mghpact.org) and to read Dr. Rauch's book, written with Dr. Anna Muriel, *Raising an Emotionally Healthy Child When a Parent Is Sick* (2006).

Practice Points: Working with Parents

1. Learn about the children.
2. Maximize the child's support system.
3. Facilitate honest communication about the illness.
4. Address common questions.
5. Prepare for hospital visits.
6. Encourage parents and children to say good-bye.

(Adapted from Rauch, Muriel, and Cassem 2002)

Learn about the children. Start with something simple like asking parents to tell you about their children, including their ages and how they coped with previous personal or family challenges.

Maximize the child's support system. A mainstay of a support system for children is maintaining their normal routine. Help the parents identify who among their family and friends can assist in keeping the children's schedules as close to normal as possible, including sleeping, eating, school, friends, and out-of-school activities. If the ill parent encourages the children to form relationships with these nonparental supports, the children won't feel disloyal in doing so.

Facilitate honest communication about the illness. Parents need to spend as much time as is needed to invite questions warmly and ensure that their children have all their questions answered in a way that is appropriate for their ages. Children from 3 to 7 years old may mistakenly feel that they are the cause of their parent's illness. These children may be expressing their guilt by "anxious, inhibited behavior or outbursts of angry, oppositional behavior." Their parents need to ask the children what they think caused the cancer, so they can correct their misunderstandings. Young children do not understand that death is permanent, and they may fear that their behavior contributed to the cancer. They may need to be reassured: "You didn't do anything to cause Daddy to be sick." Older children (7 to 12) know that death is permanent, and they may need to discuss their fears and concerns about their parent leaving them. Children should be encouraged to share any stories they have heard but don't understand, and to ask any questions they want to. Parents, however, have to be careful to understand what the real question is and should feel free not to answer every question right away. Saying, "That is an important question. Let me think about it," is fine, so long as you remember to give an answer at a later time.

Address common questions. Parents often ask Dr. Rauch, "What do we call the illness?" She encourages them not to use euphemisms, but rather to name the cancer specifically. Calling it a "boo-boo" or bump may scare and confuse children who themselves have had many a boo-boo or bump. Parents also ask, "How much should we share with the children?" Dr. Rauch says, "Assume that whatever the adults are discussing will be heard by the children." They are likely to feel more frightened by being left to interpret the information alone than if they are present, informed, and can be comforted should they show distress. Although it is natural for many parents to want to protect their children from painful information, giving age-appropriate, honest explanations can prevent misunderstanding and help children cope. Another question from parents is, "Should I make my child talk about the illness?" Although it is important to let children know that a parent is available to talk if they want to, Rauch advises parents to let their children initiate the discussions. "Are you going to die?" is, Rauch says, "the question most commonly feared by parents." She advises parents to ask about "specific worries about what would happen if the parent died" (such as whom the children would live with), and to share that although the illness might be fatal, they're doing all they can to live as long as possible and as well as possible.

Prepare for hospital visits. Children should be allowed to visit the hospital if they want to, except when a parent is confused or agitated, which a young child is unlikely to understand. But they need special preparation for what they are about to see, including a discussion of their fears and expectations, and someone to take them who can leave when the child is ready to leave. After the visit, children should be asked to discuss any parts that were difficult or enjoyable or different from what they expected. For children who do not want to visit, a family member or other trusted adult can help them communicate with the ill parent by preparing letters, drawings, or other gifts, lending the parent one of the child's own best-loved toys (such as a stuffed animal), making videos, or talking on the phone.

Saying good-bye. Rauch says, "If one's children know they are loved, and why they are loved, there is usually no need to say the word 'goodbye.'" But she encourages parents and their children to say a last "I love you" in person whenever possible. If necessary, a child can say it to a parent in a coma, or after the parent has died. Children should also be given "a road map for the grief process ahead," and the surviving parent can help the children feel comfortable about going on with school and other activities after the death by encouraging them to talk about what they have been doing, just as that parent did before the death.

Using these guidelines, clinicians can often help parents make the plans needed for care of their children when they are gone. As Rauch and Muriel (2006, p. 201) write, "While this is a major loss . . . an important aspect of this is imparting your confidence that your child will go on to live a happy and productive life, while carrying the loved [one] in his or her heart." Although parents face their deaths with undiminished sadness, they are able to say what their children need to hear.

Practice Points: Age-Specific Advice

Understanding of Illness and Death	Age-Specific Advice

Infants and Toddlers (0–2)

• Can sense disruption and stress in others. • Have no understanding of death.	• Maintain routines if possible. • Start talking about feelings with toddlers.

Preschool (3–6)

• See the world from their limited point of view, which can lead to a sense of responsibility and guilt. • May separate emotions from information. • May think death is reversible.	• Anticipate feelings of guilt: "Nothing you did caused Daddy to get sick." • Keep explanations simple: "Her body is going to stop working and she will die, but we will still have memories." • Connect through play with drawing, talking to stuffed animals, etc.

School Age (7–12)

• Understand death is irreversible.	• Encourage talking about feelings. • Use simple explanations about what to expect.

Teenagers (13 and up)

• Have abstract thinking. • Can understand uncertainty. • May formulate independent ideas about what happens when we die.	• Find out how and when kids want to hear information, e.g., before or after a big event, test, or assignment. • Provide candid information about illness. • Support older children in making choices about their time and their priorities.

(Adapted from Rauch and Muriel 2006)

SUMMARY

Communication among patients, families, and clinicians is crucial as patients approach the end of life. By avoiding misunderstandings about the goals of therapy; reinstating patients' personal calendars; discussing prognosis honestly while acknowledging uncertainty; and clarifying patients' and families' priorities, clinicians can help most patients and their families make the transition to fully supportive care focused on quality of life.

PART II

Pain Control, Symptom Management, and Psychological Considerations

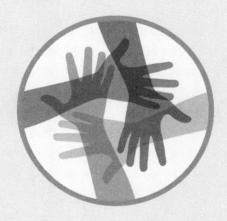

CHAPTER 6

Assessing the Patient in Pain

INTRODUCTION

Why an entire chapter devoted to assessing pain in cancer patients? Pain, after all, is something clinicians already know a lot about. It is one of the most common complaints for which patients seek their help, and clinicians routinely elicit comprehensive descriptions of the pain to aid them in diagnosis. But with all the advances in pain therapy, 39 percent of patients receiving curative therapy, 55 percent of those undergoing cancer treatment, and 66.4 percent of patients with advanced cancer reported pain, and pain was moderate to severe (≥ 5) in 38 percent (van den Beuken-van Everdingen et al. 2016). Similarly, in the largest prospective study to date of pain in outpatients with cancer, more than 3,000 outpatients with breast, lung, colorectal, or prostate cancer were enrolled, and the findings, published in 2012, were disturbing (Fisch et al. 2012). Of the more than 2,000 patients who told the investigators that they were having pain, 670 patients (34 percent) were not getting adequate pain medication. Twenty-three percent of patients with severe pain and 27 percent of those with moderate pain were getting no analgesic at all, and only 40 percent of patients with severe pain and 27 percent of patients with moderate pain were treated with a strong opioid. The odds of a minority patient having inadequately treated pain were twice those of a non-Hispanic white patient; not being on active treatment, having a good performance status, and being treated at a site where the majority of patients were minority all predicted inadequate pain management. These disparities are unsettling and suggest a lack of belief of the patient's complaints of pain, which I discuss later in this chapter.

To treat any cancer patient with pain, clinicians need to be able to assess all the causes. In cancer patients, the cancer or its treatment is likely to be the problem, although patients with chronic noncancer pain may also develop cancer and new pain. Only about 5 to 10 percent of pain in cancer patients is caused by diseases common in patients who don't have cancer. Ninety to 95 percent of cancer pain is due to the cancer, resulting either directly from tumor involvement (about 75 percent) or from treatments for the disease (about 15 to 20 percent), such as mucositis caused by chemotherapy or radiation therapy or chemotherapy-induced peripheral neuropathy.

The procedures needed to stage the cancer also cause significant distress. Pain was reported by almost 70 percent of patients undergoing bone marrow aspirate or biopsy, 14 percent undergoing lumbar puncture, and 10 percent having catheters placed (Portnow, Lim, and Grossman 2003). In 25 percent, the pain was moderate, and in another 25 percent, it was severe. NCCN guidelines (Swarm et al. 2019) include how to manage this pain, which is often accompanied by anxiety. They recommend using education about the procedure, and pharmacologic and nonpharmacologic approaches for the anxiety and the pain.

A comprehensive assessment of patients in pain must include the social, spiritual, psychological, and existential sources of distress. This chapter deals with aspects of those assessments that relate directly to the pain experience. But a more comprehensive discussion of the distress associated with these sources can be found in other chapters on these topics (Chapters 2, 3, and 9). A final component of the recommended assessment is for risk factors for opioid abuse, misuse, or diversion, which are reviewed in Chapter 7.

GUIDELINES FOR ASSESSMENT OF CANCER PAIN

Guidelines written by experts with years of experience in pain research and in consultation and treatment of cancer patients with pain emphasize the importance of a thorough pain assessment (Fallon et al. 2018; Paice et al. 2016; Swarm et al. 2019). Most mistakes in diagnosing the cause of a pain syndrome and failure to manage the problem effectively stem from neglecting one or more components of the ASCO, ESMO, and NCCN assessment guidelines. The following list is adapted from their recommendations.

Screen all patients for pain at each contact
Measure the pain and the distress it causes
    Intensity scales
    Pain assessment forms
        Interference in patient function (work, social life, sleep, sexual
            function, appetite, mood, well-being, and coping)
    Pain diaries
    Patient-reported outcomes (PROs)
        PROs and clinical decision support
Comprehensively evaluate the patient
    Telehealth
    Define temporal aspects of the pain: acute, chronic, or breakthrough
    Discover pain quality: somatic, visceral, or neuropathic
    Determine pain etiology ("make a pain diagnosis")
    Recognize cancer-related pain syndromes
Reevaluate when the pain pattern changes

The remainder of this chapter considers each of these recommendations in more detail.

Screen All Patients for Pain at Each Contact

Cancer patients who develop pain vary in their personalities and past experiences of pain, as well as in the nature of their disease, its stage, and where they are in their course of treatment. These variations cause differences in when and how they report their pain. Patients with acute cancer-related pain may report their pain promptly. They often want to know what's causing it and what can be done to fix it. Psychologically, they may tolerate this pain well, believing it is likely to resolve over a short period because in their experience, that's what happens when the pain's cause is identified and treated.

But patients with chronic cancer pain may not complain about their pain during routine office visits. They may assume that pain is an inevitable, irreversible part of having cancer, and they see no reason to waste the time with you talking about something they don't think can be changed. Or worse, they fear that increased pain must mean their disease is progressing, and so they cannot risk admitting it to themselves, let alone telling you. Instead, they ask you about the progress of their treatment, their medication side effects, or how to reverse their increasing debility. Some may fear that you will think less of them if they are unable to deal with their pain, so they do not reveal it even if you ask how they are feeling; instead, they limit themselves to telling the assistant who asks for a pain number as part of their vital signs, or the nurse in the infusion suite. While some cultures encourage reaching out when a person is in pain, and vocalizing to let others know about the pain, others teach that pain is just part of life, and it is not acceptable to complain of pain. These patients may worry that they will be considered weak if they complain (Narayan 2010).

It is left to you, then, to ask patients directly whether they are having pain, especially if they have lesions that are likely to cause discomfort. You may need to be clear with them that you don't consider it shameful to have pain, any more than it is shameful to have a cough or a broken arm. By carefully questioning them and being attentive to their responses, you can demonstrate that you consider pain to be a legitimate complaint. And by managing their complaints successfully, you can correct their misconception that pain is a necessary part of the cancer process.

Cancer patients may also be reluctant to report their pain to you because they have had prior experiences in emergency rooms or other health care settings that lead them to think that you won't believe them. They may be reluctant to admit that they need a stronger medication to relieve their pain, because in the past, especially before their cancers were diagnosed, they were treated as if they were drug addicts. We must believe the patient's complaint of pain, however, because doing so is crucial to an accurate pain assessment.

But this is not as easy as it may seem. Culture and experience play a large role in how pain is communicated, how much is tolerable, who to tell, and what kinds of pain should be reported. Hollingshead, Ashburn-Nardo, et al. (2016), in their critical literature review, describe several challenges for American Hispanic and Latinx patients. It may be more acceptable to report pain in some Hispanic and Latinx cultures, to seek comfort from the group (Flanagan 2018). But purely Spanish-speaking patients may see their lack of ability to communicate in English as a major barrier, along with immigration status and financial barriers. Compared with non-Hispanic whites, they may not think clinicians believe their complaints of pain.

Robinson-Lane and Booker (2017) reported on studies of white versus Black Americans. Black Americans may underreport their pain. For some, "claiming pain" may increase its intensity and "power in one's life." This underreporting may contribute to the findings that Black people are more likely to have their pain poorly managed. Adequate pain medication was more often prescribed to nonminority than to minority patients (Anderson, Green, and Payne 2009), Black Americans are less likely than whites to have a prescription for long-acting opioids, and Black Americans had longer wait times than white Americans. (Other ways in which culture influences pain assessment are discussed later in the chapter.)

Unconscious bias may be playing a role. Both white and Black Americans in one study reported that they thought Black Americans were less sensitive to pain and less likely to report pain than white Americans (Hollingshead, Meints, et al.

2016). White medical students and residents were found to hold false beliefs about biological differences in the experience of pain between whites and Blacks that can lead to differences in treatment recommendations (Hoffman et al. 2016).

And whether or not a patient "looks" as if he is in pain may affect whether you believe his complaint. For example, you are likely to believe complaints of pain from a patient with a broken arm, because people with *acute* pain look as if they're in pain: they appear uncomfortable and anxious and are often sweating. People with acute pain look this way because their activated sympathetic nervous system causes sweating and an increase in pulse and blood pressure. When we observe these findings, we usually believe complaints of pain.

But what about patients with *chronic* pain who do not "look" as if they are in pain? Their complaints often seem out of proportion to the amount of disease that can be documented by physical exam or x-rays. Consider the patient with metastatic breast cancer with compression fractures after radiation therapy. Her pulse and blood pressure are normal; she's not particularly anxious, and she's not sweating. Don't you find it a little harder to believe that she is in severe pain, despite full doses of nonsteroidal anti-inflammatory drugs (NSAIDs)?

If you think the objective findings don't substantiate her complaint of severe pain, you might well be reluctant to add an opioid to her regimen. But what are the objective findings for someone with chronic pain? What should you be looking for to substantiate her pain complaint? Being familiar with the presentation of patients in severe *chronic* pain makes it easier for us to decide how to treat them.

Neuropathic Pain

It was hard for Mr. Cirelli's physicians to believe he was in pain, though that was what led him to see his doctor. Mr. Cirelli was thought to have a Pancoast tumor, a lung cancer that, because of its location in the lung apex, often infiltrates the chest wall and the nerves of the brachial plexus. I met him while I was working at the Philadelphia VA in hematology and oncology. When the admitting resident called to ask me to see him, she apologized that no pathologic diagnosis had yet been made: *"His chest film shows a mass in the right lung apex, but I really haven't been able to do a thorough exam or obtain any tissue because Mr. Cirelli won't cooperate."* When I went to see him, his nurses confirmed the resident's impression, adding that Mr. Cirelli was short tempered and demanding, and that I was unlikely to get much conversation from him.

On entering his room, what I saw was a man lying quietly in bed staring at the TV mounted on the wall. In answer to my greeting, he slowly turned his head toward me, but the rest of his body stayed still. He looked exhausted, but he was not grimacing or wincing. He kept his right elbow bent with his right forearm across his chest, supported by his left hand.

In response to my questions, he said that he had been well until four months earlier, when he had noticed a mild aching pain in his right shoulder area. The discomfort had progressed, and when he developed weakness in the grip of his right hand, he saw an orthopedist, who treated him for an injured rotator cuff. When the pain worsened and a shoulder film suggested a mass in the apex of the lung, he was referred for further evaluation. He now described the pain as excruciating (the choices I gave him were mild, moderate, severe, or excruciating). It was constant, deep, and aching, and it occasionally "shot down" his arm like electricity.

He could not move his right arm without pain and could no longer sleep except for catnaps. He had lost his appetite and ability to concentrate. The pain was his central concern. He told me all this calmly but with a very depressed affect. His pulse and blood pressure were normal, and he was not sweating. I tried to examine his right shoulder area, but he could not tolerate any evaluation of his neck, right supraclavicular area, right shoulder, or right axilla, and he would not sit up for a lung examination. His right hand showed muscle atrophy typical of the C7-T1 distribution.

Mr. Cirelli's symptoms and signs were typical of someone with chronic severe neuropathic pain arising from tumor infiltration into the nerves of his right lower brachial plexus. His physicians and nurses were not familiar with the exquisite sensitivity to touch caused by this kind of nerve injury and so could not have known how agonizing any examination of the shoulder area was for him. Since he didn't resemble patients with acute pain, they mistook his distress for obstreperousness.

Patients like Mr. Cirelli who have severe chronic pain do not sweat or have tachycardia or hypertension, but they usually guard the part that hurts and often have a generalized lack of spontaneous movement. They may appear anxious or depressed, withdrawn, or angry, and may have difficulty relating to others, sleeping, concentrating, or eating.

Since I frequently cared for patients who had chronic neuropathic pain, I was able to believe Mr. Cirelli. I pointed out my findings to his physicians and nurses, then suggested that his personality might be very different if he had less severe pain. They were still skeptical but concurred that we would not be able to make a diagnosis unless we relieved his pain. At my recommendation, they agreed to a trial of high-dose dexamethasone, which is often effective for neuropathic pain, gabapentin 3 times a day (with a higher dose at bedtime to help him sleep), and a low dose of immediate-release opioid if needed every 4 hours.

Within 48 hours Mr. Cirelli was a different person. His pain was now only moderate, which was acceptable to him. He showed me how he could now move his right arm with tolerable discomfort. He readily agreed to a physical examination and to the scans and biopsy necessary to make a diagnosis. The nurses remarked on how affable and talkative he was and how helpful he had been to other patients on the floor. He was able to sleep through the night, eat, and interact with others. The relief of his chronic pain had been dramatic, and according to his family, he had become himself again.

Mr. Cirelli's neuropathic pain was a clue to his underlying pathology. Had it been recognized sooner, he would have suffered less, his lung cancer may have been discovered sooner, and his hand strength might have been preserved.

Measure the Pain and the Distress It Causes

All the guidelines stress that the patient's self-report should be the primary source of assessment. In this respect, pain is unique. Although we ask a diabetic patient about his symptoms, clinicians usually rely on blood glucose and ketone levels to adjust insulin doses. To determine the effectiveness of a pain-relief regimen, we must rely on the patient to *tell us* how his pain and function have changed after therapy. No one but the patient can accurately report his pain—not the nurses caring for him, not his family, not his friends. No matter how well trained we are or how well we know our patients, numerous studies have shown that all of us significantly underestimate the intensity of patients' pain.

Practice Points: Questions for Assessing Cultural Attitudes of Patients and Their Families

- Is touching acceptable to you?
- What word do you use for pain?
- How will we know you are in pain?
- How does your family usually react to pain?
- How do you normally treat or cope with pain?
- Which foods are comforting or healing to you?
- Do you want your family near you when you are hurting?
- How does your family react to your pain?
- Do you see a folk healer when you are sick?
- How do you explain your illness or pain?
- What does the pain mean to you?
- Does the pain mean you are getting better or worse?
- Is it OK to take medication to relieve pain? If not, why?
- Do you want immediate pain relief, or do you believe that you must wait until the pain is severe?
- What type of treatment do you want to control your pain?
- Do you read? Which languages?
- How best do you learn (reading, videos, etc.)?

(From Fink and Gates 1995, p. 34)

Of course, people differ in how they experience and report pain. If you ask five people with broken arms to rate how much pain they are having, you are likely to get five different answers. But if you give them nothing to relieve their pain and ask them to rate it again sometime later, each patient is extremely likely to give you exactly the same rating as the first time. Numerous studies have shown, in fact, that a patient's reports of pain are consistent, reproducible, and reliable. Pain ratings after treatment are just as accurate and are used to indicate the effectiveness of a specific treatment for that patient.

But culture plays a role in the meaning pain has to patients and their families and therefore when and how they report pain to clinicians and how they seek relief. If pain is part of the struggle of being human or part of your duty to God, then reporting pain or seeking its relief may be discouraged and stoicism valued. For those for whom pain is a spiritual experience, prayer and spiritual counseling may come first, before, or instead of any pharmacologic therapies (Narayan 2010; Hollingshead, Ashburn-Nardo, et al. 2016; Robinson-Lane and Booker 2017). Some patients explicitly verbally report the level of their pain, whereas others use nonverbal cues, body language, and context to signal distress. The verbal report is only part of their communication of their pain experience. As you might expect, congruence in appreciating the extent of patient distress is more likely if the clinician and patient are from the same culture. Fink and Gates (1995) offer useful questions that can help you explore the effect of culture on your patient's pain experience and expression.

Pain rating scales are of course subjective, not objective. But they are still *accurate*, and for most patients they provide a *number* that represents the intensity of a patient's pain. (I discuss later in the chapter how to assess pain for patients for whom the number does not represent the intensity of their distress.)

Equally important, physicians and nurses can ask patients whether the degree of pain relief *is satisfactory to them*. For some patients, a pain rating of 6 on a scale from 0 (no pain) to 10 (the worst pain you can imagine) is fine. These patients can tolerate the pain better than they can the side effects caused by higher doses of analgesic. For others, a level of 2 or 3 must be achieved. Mr. Cirelli, for example, told me he had "no pain" after he began taking the dexamethasone and gabapentin. When I pressed him for a number, he said it was a 2 or a 3. In my experience, he is typical of patients with well-controlled chronic pain, for whom "no pain" is a level 2 or 3.

I sometimes find it necessary to explain these concepts to nursing colleagues and house staff in the hospital so that they can help me relieve a patient's pain as quickly as possible. Since pain has become "the fifth vital sign" and is measured at least every time the other vital signs are measured, most nurses and house staff are familiar with the importance of measuring pain and do it routinely. Some even do it before and after they give a patient a medication for pain, entering both values in the electronic medical record. Those longitudinal records are helpful in guiding pain management. If, however, you find that staff is not reporting the numbers to you as you attempt to regulate the pain regimen, you might find a diabetes analogy helpful. You might say something like,

> *If you were taking care of someone with diabetes, you wouldn't call me and say, "The patient's blood glucose was bad, so I gave him some insulin and it got a little better." (That usually elicits a laugh.) Well, I won't know what to do if you tell me, "The patient's pain was bad, so I gave him an oxycodone and now it's better." If instead you said, "The patient said his pain was a 9 out of 10. I gave him 5 mg of oxycodone, and an hour later he said his pain level was a 7 and that he was not satisfied with that degree of pain relief," that would give me all the information I need: the 5 mg of oxycodone was inadequate, and I will need to order a higher dose.*

I also encourage house staff to include a quantitative pain assessment in the daily progress notes of all patients with a significant complaint of pain, just as they would include the blood glucose level in the progress notes of a patient with diabetes. Since The Joint Commission (TJC) has mandated documenting the level of pain and pain relief, hospitals have modified their TPR (temperature, pulse, and respiration) sheets to include a continuous record of patients' pain levels and whether the degree of pain relief is satisfactory to them (Figure 6.1).

The numerical scales used in the examples above and the intensity scales reviewed below have been extensively tested in research settings and found to be valid and reliable; they are easy to administer and to understand. They are designed to be used by patients, their families, their physicians, and other health professionals. If you offer various types of scales and tools, patients and their families can choose one that makes the most sense to them and then learn from someone in your office exactly how to use it.

Intensity Scales

Visual Analog Scale. A Visual Analog Scale (VAS) is a 10-cm horizontal or vertical unruled line anchored at its ends by numbers or words describing the two extremes of a symptom. In the case of pain, for example, one end is labeled "0," or "no pain," and the other end "10," or "worst possible pain." To unravel complex pain syndromes, it is useful to determine not only the intensity of various pains but the associated distress. A VAS can also be used here; the ends would be labeled "no distress" and "unbearable distress." If you feel that a patient will not be able to do these measurements easily, choose instead a scale that is already ruled in 1-cm increments, with each mark numbered. This ruled scale is not quite as accurate as the unruled one, because patients tend to choose a whole number rather than a fraction of one, but it is adequate for clinical purposes and is very reliable. If you are assessing a patient from China, Japan, or Korea, cultures whose language reads vertically, offer to present the number scale vertically, rather than horizontally (Narayan 2010). Similarly, offer to present the scale going from right to left (lowest number on the right to highest number on the left) to Hebrew, Arabic, Kurdish, Farsi (Persian), and Urdu speakers.

A disadvantage sometimes noted for these scales is that they rate only the intensity of the pain, not its quality or the degree of functional, psychological, and social disability it induces. And some people cannot understand the abstract concept that a larger or smaller number reflects increasing or decreasing pain. These patients always assign the same number even though they clearly are

TEMPERATURE

Month-Day-Year								
Post Adm/Post-Op								
Hours of Day	4 8 12	4 8 12	4 8 12	4 8 12	4 8 12	4 8 12	4 8 12	4 8 12
160 150 140 130 120 110 100 90 80 70 60 50 40 (RECTAL • ORAL ○ TYMPANIC ×) (41 40 39 38 37 36 35)								
Respiration								
Pain Intensity (10 5 0)								
Relief Acceptable (Y/N)								
Weight								

	N	D	E	N	D	E	N	D	E	N	D	E	N	D	E	N	D	E	N	D	E	N	D	E
Blood Pressure																								
INTAKE Oral																								
Tube Feeding																								
Supplements																								
Intravenous																								
Blood Products																								
TPN/PPN/Lipids																								
8 Hour Total																								
24 Hour Total																								
OUTPUT Urine																								
Emesis/NG																								
Stool																								
8 Hour Total																								
24 Hour Total																								

FIGURE 6.1. Memorial Sloan-Kettering Vital Sign Sheet Incorporating a Pain Documentation Form.
Source: From M. Bookbinder, M. Kiss, N. Coyle, et al., "Improving Pain Management Practices," in *Cancer Pain Management*, 2nd ed., edited by D. B. McGuire, C. H. Yarbo, and B. R. Ferrell (Sudbury, Mass.: Jones and Bartlett, 1995); reprinted with permission.

experiencing varying pain intensities. You can more profitably use a functional tool, such as the Wisconsin Brief Pain Inventory described below, to assess the effect of therapy for patients like these.

Nonverbal pain assessments. For patients whose cultures discourage verbal complaints of pain, nonverbal signs may reveal the degree of their distress, as they did in Mr. Cirelli's case. Patients who use prayer to cope with their pain may appear similarly withdrawn and noncommunicative. If you find someone who appears to be praying or talking with themselves, inquire if they are praying and, after apologizing for interrupting their prayers, offer your concern about their discomfort and explore what the pain has done to their function.

Pain Assessment in Advanced Dementia and Pain Assessment Checklist for Seniors with Limited Ability to Communicate. It can be challenging to assess pain in a patient who has dementia as well as cancer. Several scales have been validated in this population. A consensus recommendation from an expert panel endorsed the Pain Assessment in Advanced Dementia (PAINAD) scale (Figure 6.2) (Warden, Hurley, and Volicer 2003) and the Pain Assessment Checklist for Seniors with Limited Ability to Communicate (PACSLAC) (Herr et al. 2010). I find the PAINAD easy to use clinically. The dimensions that you are asked to observe include breathing, negative vocalization, facial expression, body language, and consolability. Patients can be scored up to 2 points in any area, and the total number of points (0 to 10) puts them in the same categories—none (0), mild (1–3), moderate (4–6), or severe (7–10)—as with the other numerical scales. Many other tools are available, some of which are validated (Herr 2011). Unfortunately, unlike for patients with dementia, there is no reliable and valid pain assessment tool for patients with delirium (Fischer et al. 2019).

Word scales. For some people, it is simpler and more intuitive to rate their pain or distress on a scale that uses words instead of numbers. Word scales (descriptive scales) have been found particularly useful for patients over 70. Instead of asking them to make a mark on a line or assign a number to quantitate the pain, ask them whether they have *no pain* or pain that is *mild, moderate, severe, very severe,* or *worst possible.* This scale is called a Simple Descriptive Pain Intensity Scale. Another word scale gives patients the choice of *none, mild, moderate, severe,* or *excruciating* to describe their pain. Patients may, however, use different words to describe the intensity of their pain, such as "hurt," "sore," or "discomfort" for mild to moderate pain; "nagging," "ache," or "miserable" for moderate; and "pain" only to describe the most severe pain (Flanagan 2018; Robinson-Lane and Booker 2017). A pain intensity scale is available for patients speaking only dialects of the Chinese languages. This scale presents the words in the vertical format, and the intensity choices range from "No Pain" to "Quite Painful/Bearable" for mild pain, "Very Painful/Indescribable" for moderate pain, "Unbearable/Excruciating" for severe pain, and "Crushing Heart and Lungs/Crucifying Pain" for excruciating pain (Liu, Chung, and Wong 2003; Flanagan 2018).

There is also a word scale for the distress caused by the pain. The patient chooses a word to indicate whether her distress level is *none, annoying, uncomfortable, dreadful, horrible,* or *agonizing.* These words have been extensively tested for their ability to discriminate among different degrees of pain intensity; to maintain the reliability of the scale, these specific words must be used.

Pain Assessment in Advanced Dementia Scale (PAINAD)

Instructions: Observe the patient for five minutes before scoring his or her behaviors. Score the behaviors according to the following chart. Definitions of each item are available in Warden et al. 2003. The patient can be observed under different conditions (e.g., at rest, during a pleasant activity, during caregiving, after the administration of pain medication).

Behavior	0	1	2	Score
Breathing independent of vocalization	• Normal	• Occasional labored breathing • Short period of hyperventilation	• Noisy labored breathing • Long period of hyperventilation • Cheyne-Stokes respirations	
Negative vocalization	• None	• Occasional moan or groan • Low-level speech with a negative or disapproving quality	• Repeated troubled calling out • Loud moaning or groaning • Crying	
Facial expression	• Smiling or inexpressive	• Sad • Frightened • Frown	• Facial grimacing	
Body language	• Relaxed	• Tense • Distressed pacing • Fidgeting	• Rigid • Fists clenched • Knees pulled up • Pulling or pushing away • Striking out	
Consolability	• No need to console	• Distracted or reassured by voice or touch	• Unable to console, distract, or reassure	

Total Score

Maximum 10

Scoring: A possible interpretation of the scores: Mild pain 1–3; Moderate pain 4–6; Severe pain 7–10

FIGURE 6.2. Pain Assessment in Advanced Dementia (PAINAD) Scale. *Source:* Adapted from V. Warden, A. C. Hurley, and L. Volicer, "Development and Psychometric Evaluation of the Pain Assessment in Advanced Dementia (PAINAD) scale," *J Am Med Dir Assoc* 4:9–15, 2003.

Just as with the number scales, physicians can use any of these word scales to get an idea of the range of pain and its associated distress patients have experienced throughout the day. Patients simply select which word best describes the most severe and which describes the mildest pain they have had that day.

Pain Assessment Forms

A minority of patients cannot use numbers or words to quantify their pain, the distress it is causing, or the efficacy of therapy. For them, I rely on comprehensive assessment forms (or tools) that include a measure not only of pain intensity but also of other functional dimensions that reflect the effects of the pain on the patient's day-to-day life. These tools are also easy to use and take no more than five to ten minutes to complete.

Wisconsin Brief Pain Inventory. One of the most widely used forms, which is extremely useful in unraveling and managing complicated pain problems, is the tool developed by the Pain Research Group at the University of Wisconsin–Madison Medical School (see the appendix for the full inventory). This Brief Pain Inventory, which can be reproduced for inclusion in the patient's chart, records the location of each pain on a diagram (Figure 6.3); the worst, least, and average pain intensity, as well as the level "right now"; the degree of relief that pain treatments have provided; and the functional consequences of the pain (i.e., the pain's interference in work, social life, sleep, sexual function, appetite, mood, well-being, and coping). It has been translated into many languages and validated in many populations (Narayan 2010).

The functional consequences, such as disturbances in physical activity, mood, walking ability, relationships with others, sleep, and enjoyment of life, can be sensitive indicators that a patient's pain is unrelieved or improved. Even patients who cannot tell you whether their pain number has changed, or cannot give you a word to describe it, report changes in their functional levels that indicate the efficacy of the treatment. Patients' families can help as well, completing the assessments at home after changes in the patient's pain-relief regimen and reporting the results to you by phone or e-mail.

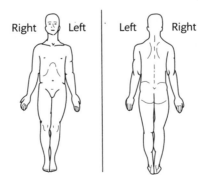

FIGURE 6.3. From the Wisconsin Brief Pain Inventory.
Source: University of Texas M. D. Anderson Cancer Center; reprinted with permission.

The functional changes noted in Mr. Cirelli's behavior, for example, heralded the relief of his pain. From a bedridden, depressed, withdrawn person with a short temper and attention span, he became voluble, helpful, interactive, and cooperative. When his pain was relieved, the disturbances disappeared.

Other useful scales include the Faces Pain Scale–Revised and the Iowa Pain Thermometer–Revised, which may be preferred by some populations (Robinson-Lane and Booker 2017).

Pain Diaries

The VAS, Wisconsin Brief Pain Inventory, Faces Pain Scale–Revised, and the Iowa Pain Thermometer–Revised provide sufficient information for designing pain-relief regimens for most patients. But there can be cases in which the regimen seems to be working only part of the time. Pain diaries, which can be as high tech as the smartphone apps I discuss later in the chapter, or as simple as pen and paper, are useful here. In the diary, patients record the time of day they took their pain medicine, the pain intensity rating before and after they took it, the type of pain medicine, and any other comments they feel are relevant (e.g., what they were doing when the pain occurred). A sample diary page is shown in Figure 6.4.

For patients who complain of being too sedated, diaries can help determine whether they're taking too much medicine or taking the correct dose but too often. And diaries are useful for patients who have *breakthrough pains*, moderate to excruciating acute pains that occur intermittently, often on a background of well-controlled chronic pain. There are three types of breakthrough pain: *end-of-dose pain*, which is pain that recurs before the next regularly scheduled dose of medication is due; *incident pain*, which is directly related to an activity (such as turning over in bed); and *spontaneous pain*, which occurs unpredictably.

Diaries are helpful in determining which kinds of breakthrough pains patients are experiencing. For many, the pattern that emerges will reveal end-of-dose pain or incident pain. You can then devise a plan to prevent the anticipated pains. For example, if the pain recurs 4 hours before the next sustained-release morphine pill is due (i.e., end-of-dose pain), you can decrease the dosing interval to 8 hours. Or if a patient's pain reliably exacerbates with movement (i.e., incident pain), a short-acting medication can be given 30 minutes to an hour before the patient gets out of bed, or an immediate-acting agent can be given 5 or 10 minutes before.

Finally, diaries are essential to solving the mysteries of those few patients who have a pain recurrence pattern that seems to make no pharmacologic sense. Miss Alexander was such a patient.

The Pain Pattern that Makes No Sense

Miss Alexander was a 32-year-old woman receiving chemotherapy for metastatic ovarian cancer. She had worked in her father's business since her high school graduation and had lived in her own apartment until the side effects of the

You can use a chart like this to rate your pain and to keep a record of how well the medicine is working. Write the information in the chart. Use the pain intensity scale to rate your pain before and after you take the medicine.

Pain Intensity Scale

0 1 2 3 4 5 6 7 8 9 10

No pain   Medium pain   Worst pain

Date	Time	Pain intensity scale rating	Medicine I took	Pain intensity scale rating 1 hour after taking the medicine	What I was doing when I felt the pain
9/1/14	2:35	6	2 ibuprofen tablets	3	Sitting at my desk and reading.

FIGURE 6.4. Pain Diary. *Source:* From the Agency for Health Care Policy and Research, Rockville, Maryland.

chemotherapy and increasing disability from her cancer forced her to move back to her parents' home.

Miss Alexander had abdominal pain that, despite my efforts at changing her medication dose and schedule, seemed never to come under satisfactory control. I asked her to keep a pain diary. In the diary she recorded that she took sustained-release morphine at 6 a.m., 2 p.m., and 10 p.m. At 7 a.m., before setting out for work, she usually took a dose of immediate-acting morphine. Using a scale of 0 to 10, she recorded her pain intensity before each dose of morphine and its intensity an hour or so later.

She had been taking the same morphine doses for about a week when she came to the office. I reviewed the diary and graphed the pain intensity (0 to 10) on the *y* axis and the time of day on the *x* axis (Figure 6.5). I noted that her pain intensity was highest on weekends and between 7 p.m. and 10 p.m. on weekdays. Her pain relief was satisfactory at all other times.

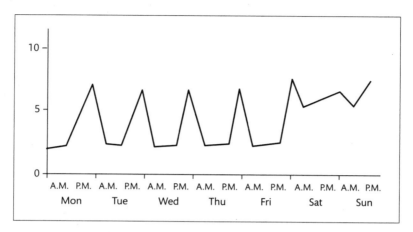

FIGURE 6.5. Miss Alexander's Pain Pattern

There is nothing I know about morphine's pharmacology that could explain why sustained-release morphine would be effective for eight hours in the day-time on weekdays and overnight, but not on weekends or weekday evenings. As I wondered what other factors might be involved, I considered that it might be difficult for Miss Alexander, a formerly independent, lively young woman, to have to return from work to her conservative family home every night and weekend. So I questioned her about this. She replied,

> When I'm at Dad's office, there's plenty to keep me occupied. I do some work, though not as much as before, and I can visit with my friends. But there's not much to do at home. And Mom keeps asking me all the time, "How are you doing? Are you having any pain? Is there anything I can get you?" or "What did the doctor say today, honey?" Oh, sometimes there's a TV program I like, or I can get caught up in a book I'm reading. The pain's not so bad, then—kind of like it is at the office. But most of the time, it's much worse.

At home, it seemed, there wasn't much to take her mind off her cancer or her loss of independence, and her pain was more intense and caused her more dis-tress. Since she had found a few things that helped, I suggested she try to continue to fill her evenings and weekends watching movies or videos, listening to music, or reading books on her iPad, and to ask her friends from the office to visit or take her with them on weekend outings. Happily, this strategy was effective, and her pain came under satisfactory control without any further changes in dose or timing of medication. The diary was the key—once I knew *when* it hurt, I could figure out *why*.

Patient-Reported Outcomes (PROs)

Pain relief was one of the first patient-reported outcomes (PROs): *What is your pain level? Is this level of relief satisfactory to you?* And it remains an important one for cancer patients and their families, both in the hospital and outside it. In the hospital or clinic setting, it is easy to ask patients to report their pain level and record its response to various treatments.

But when patients are at home, their suffering may go undetected, except by their loved ones. Patients call their oncology providers about fevers or other new infection symptoms, but they may be reluctant to call about their pain (Cooley et al. 2017). Yet, those who report PROs regularly, which are then used by their clinicians' electronic health record (EHR) to alert members of their oncology team to their uncontrolled symptoms, have experienced numerous benefits (Basch et al. 2017, 2018; Bakitas et al. 2009; Denis et al. 2019; Velikova et al. 2020; Back, Friedman, and Abrahm 2020; Basch, Leahy, and Dueck 2021). These benefits include enhancements in patient-clinician communication, clinician awareness of symptoms, symptom management, quality of life, and patient satisfaction. The patients tolerate treatment better, have fewer unplanned admission or Emergency Department visits for uncontrolled symptoms, and even show improved overall survival.

These remarkable results were achieved by several new technological strategies that enable clinicians to learn of their patient's pain and accomplish remote assessments. Patients use cell phones, tablets, or computers linked to their EHRs to report their level of pain directly to their clinicians (Basch et al. 2018). Algorithms send alerts to a triage nurse via the EHR when the pain is above a prespecified level (e.g., 7, or severe) or the trend of the symptom is worsening, and the nurse contacts the patient. The nurse assesses and makes suggestions regarding an Emergency Department or clinic visit, makes another referral, or changes the pain management regimen (Basch et al. 2018; Denis et al. 2019; Wagner et al. 2015). Algorithms in the PROMIS-T system do not even require a nurse intervention for the EHR to make appointments for the patient for needed social work, registered dietician, or health educator services (Wagner et al. 2015). The algorithms used in the eRapid system enable the EHR to provide the patient either with severity-tailored advice or a recommendation to contact the team (Basch et al. 2018; Velikova et al. 2020; Basch, Leahy and Dueck 2021; Absolom et al. 2021). The mobile app used in ePAL has led to decreased pain severity and significantly fewer pain-related hospital and Emergency Department admissions (Kamdar et al. 2018). There is an ongoing trial of PRO-TECT, involving 26 community oncology practices in 15 states, which is examining the effect of ongoing symptom monitoring with alerts to nurses for severe or worsening symptoms and review of symptoms by oncologists at office visits (Basch et al. 2020).

Some patients from underserved populations may not have access to these types of high-tech interventions. An interactive voice response (IVR) system, however, with alerts to providers if the patient reports moderate to severe symptoms, was used successfully in underserved Latinx and Black women with breast cancer; it was found to decrease patient pain and symptom severity compared with a control group who did not receive the phone calls (Anderson et al. 2015). In the future, natural language processing techniques that search the electronic record for patients who are having uncontrolled symptoms will be used to supplement PROs. They are especially important for those patients who find it difficult to quantify symptoms electronically or in person (Koleck et al. 2019). These PROs can then generate similar alerts and responses as those discussed above.

PROs and clinical decision support. PROs are an important first step in identifying patients in distress and helping them resolve that distress promptly. But the next level of care involves using clinical decision support (CDS) based on national consensus guidelines. Clinical guidelines for symptom assessment and management, like those from the NCCN, ASCO, MASCC, and other organizations, are readily available but not often used in the practice setting (Borneman et al. 2007); it can take an average of five years for a guideline to be adopted in practice (Balas and Boren 2000). Nonetheless, CDS facilitates dissemination of and adherence to these guidelines (Latoszek-Berendsen et al. 2010).

CDS provides clinicians, patients, and other health care stakeholders with pertinent knowledge and person-specific information, intelligently filtered or presented at appropriate times, to enhance health and health care (Osheroff et al. 2005). The system takes the information provided by the PROs or from natural language processing and then, using algorithms developed from accepted national consensus guidelines for symptom assessment and management, along with patient-specific data, "works behind the scenes" in the EHR to capture, analyze, and make suggestions for assessment and treatment of patients' pain and other symptoms (Cooley et al. 2013; Lobach et al. 2016).

I am part of a research group that is hoping to use CDS and the EHR to improve the ability of oncology clinicians to manage the symptoms of their patients without a palliative care referral. If CDS systems are to improve practice, they need to be part of the workflow, provide specific recommendations, be present at the time and location of decision-making, and be computer based (Bright et al. 2012; Kawamoto et al. 2005; Lobach 2013). Our group incorporated these principles in our study of CDS combined with PROs and provided thoracic oncologists with paper reports containing the severity of each symptom, along with recommendations for treating pain, anxiety, depression, dyspnea, and fatigue; an independent chart review revealed that the clinicians accepted 60 percent of our recommendations (Back, Friedman, and Abrahm 2020; Cooley et al. 2013; Lobach et al. 2016).

In the next iteration of our work on CDS, clinical guidelines will again be used to create algorithms that generate patient-specific evidence-based suggestions for symptom assessment and management, using PROs and other data available in the EHR. In this iteration, the CDS will include validation from the clinician as to the doses of medications the patient is taking, and the report generated will be visible in the EHR for the clinician's view during the patient visit; the report will provide patient-specific symptom assessment and management recommendations, along with "smart phrases" for automatic documentation and billing of whichever suggestions the clinicians adopt.

Comprehensively Evaluate the Patient

A part of any assessment of a patient in pain is a careful medical and neurological examination to identify the source and cause of the pain (whether or not that cause is reversible or even treatable), along with comorbidities that could complicate the picture, such as alcoholic or diabetic neuropathies (Minello et al. 2019). When you cannot do this assessment in person, you might be able to use telehealth facilities, often with staff on hand to perform and report to you the results of selected examinations you would do yourself if you were seeing the patient in person.

Telehealth

Telehealth or telemedicine means that the clinician is using telecommunication technology to assess, manage, and educate patients or families who are at remote locations, often their homes. It can also include consultation between professionals at remote locations, bringing the expertise of the specialist to the community, especially the rural community. For the seriously ill palliative care patient, it has obvious benefits, since patients can be evaluated in their homes, and family members and other caregivers can more easily be present (Back, Friedman, and Abrahm 2020). It is used often in the United Kingdom for patients with palliative care or hospice needs (Worster and Swartz 2017).

Technology used in telemedicine ranges from telephone calls, including video calls on phones, to videoconferencing using computers or tablets. The benefits include offering expert palliative care to patients who are in rural settings (Bonsignore et al. 2018), who have low incomes and cannot afford the time or expense of an office visit, or who are otherwise less able to come to outpatient visits because of physical disabilities. Patients report satisfaction with the more frequent access telehealth offers them, though elderly patients have more difficulty with using the technology (Worster and Swartz 2017). Telehealth could also support caregivers, but much more research is needed. Pilot studies have shown promise in various app- and web-based technologies for caregiver education, appointment scheduling, medication management, communication, decreasing negative mood, and touch-based techniques including massage (Shin et al. 2018).

As experts caution, though, implementing telehealth programs is complex, requires expert personnel and technical resources, and is tricky to get reimbursed (Calton et al. 2019). And it remains unclear whether this medium will lend itself to conversations about goals of care, hopes and worries, and wishes regarding hospital transfers and resuscitation.

Temporal Aspects of Pain: Acute, Chronic, or Breakthrough

Cancer patients usually have a mixture of chronic and breakthrough pains. To maximize pain relief while minimizing side effects, it is useful to determine both the intensity of the chronic pain and the characteristics of the breakthrough pains and to treat each with agents appropriate for them.

Long-acting agents (e.g., methadone) or sustained-release formulations of short-acting agents (e.g., transdermal fentanyl or buprenorphine, sustained-release oxycodone, morphine, oxymorphone, or hydromorphone) are used to keep the chronic pain at an acceptably low level (e.g., level 2 or 3). The peak blood level of opioids delivered in these preparations is lower than with other formulations, and they are therefore less sedating.

End-of-dose breakthrough pains, once recognized, are easy to prevent by increasing the frequency of dosing of sustained-release agents. Spontaneous pains and incident pains, which can be precipitated by movement, the Valsalva maneuver, or even flatulence, are more difficult to manage. A patient with bony metastases, for example, may have reasonable control of chronic pain without excessive sedation but develop severe pain when rising from a bed or chair. Agents with a quick onset of action (hydromorphone, morphine, oxycodone, and oxymorphone) and immediate-acting agents (the transmucosal formulations of buprenorphine or fentanyl citrate) can be added either prophylactically for activities expected to cause incident pain or episodically when spontaneous pains occur. But the higher peak opioid levels associated with these agents can cause sedation. Patients often must endure this increased sedation to achieve acceptable pain relief.

Pain Quality: Somatic, Visceral, or Neuropathic

Determining the quality of cancer pain is often helpful in identifying the site of tissue injury, because somatic, visceral, and neuropathic pains each have a characteristic presentation. Somatic and visceral pains are common in people who do not have cancer. Other than in patients with dental or disk disease, diabetic or alcoholic neuropathy, or herpes zoster, nerve injuries that cause neuropathic pain rarely occur in people who do not have cancer or AIDS.

Somatic pain. Somatic pain arises from skin and subcutaneous tissues, bone, muscle, blood vessels, and connective tissues. It is usually described as *constant, dull,* and *aching, increased by movement,* and *localized to the area of the lesion.* Patients with arthritis or bony metastases will describe their chronic pain in words similar to these. Incident pain, however, is not dull but rather a sharp, intense somatic pain caused by movement of a bone that contains a metastasis or is fractured.

Visceral pain. Visceral pain arises from organs and the lining of body cavities. The pain caused by a myocardial infarction is a typical example of visceral pain.

It is often a *poorly localized, deep, aching* discomfort, but it can feel like *cramping, squeezing, twisting,* or *tearing*. Patients with hydronephrosis caused by tumor or a distended liver filled with metastases will have this type of pain. Visceral pain can localize to more superficial structures and, if it is intense, often radiates to larger areas, usually the muscle or skin innervated by the same spinal nerves that innervate the viscus. Pain in the left shoulder and arm of a patient with myocardial ischemia is an example of this phenomenon. Abdominal pains due to bowel obstruction by tumor are also visceral, but they have the intermittent, cramping, cycling quality that characterizes a bowel obstruction from any cause.

Neuropathic pain. Neuropathic pain, the kind Mr. Cirelli suffered, arises from injury to peripheral nerves, the spinal cord, or the brain. Persistence of importins in the sensory nuclei of injured nerves in the dorsal route ganglia has recently been identified as the mechanism by which the acute pain caused by injury to peripheral nerves becomes chronic and persistent; importins may become a target for future therapy (Marvaldi et al. 2020). Neuropathic pain is the most distressing type of pain. It is usually poorly localized and often *burning* (as typically seen in diabetic neuropathy or herpes zoster) but can be described as *sharp, shooting, tingling, electrical,* or *shock-like*. With sufficient nerve damage, there may be associated *paresthesias, painful numbness, hyperesthesia,* or *sensory loss*, and, as in Mr. Cirelli, *weakness* and *muscle wasting*. *Allodynia*, pain caused by normal touch or by clothing, or *hyperalgesia*, in which a mildly painful stimulus causes severe pain, can also occur. Neuropathic pain can be limited to the site of the lesion, but it often radiates or is completely referred to distant sites.

Practice Points: Distinguishing among Somatic, Visceral, and Neuropathic Pain

- Somatic pain (e.g., arthritis, bone metastases) is constant, dull, and aching, increased by movement, and localized to the area of the lesion.
- Visceral pain (e.g., myocardial ischemia, liver metastases) is poorly localized, deep, aching, cramping, twisting, or tearing.
- Neuropathic pain (e.g., sciatica, brachial plexus metastases) is burning, sharp, shooting, tingling, electrical, or shock-like.

Pain Etiology: Recognizing Cancer-Related Pain Syndromes

Several pain syndromes are seen almost exclusively in cancer patients (Portenoy and Ahmed 2018). Mr. Young, for example, a patient with lung cancer whom I took care of when I still practiced oncology, had a referred pain syndrome peculiar to patients with cancer. About three months after completing radiation therapy to his lung lesion, he developed severe right hip pain. Findings from x-rays of his hip and pelvis were entirely normal, and the bone scan confirmed the absence of metastases in this region. But the scan did reveal a metastasis in his thoracic spine, at T12. After radiation therapy to this lesion, the referred hip pain entirely resolved.

Cancer-related pain can be acute or chronic. Acute pain related to the cancer can be due to pathologic fractures; obstruction or perforation of the bile duct, bowel, ureter, or bladder; hemorrhage within the tumor; or acute venous thrombosis. Antineoplastic agents can cause mucositis, palmar-plantar erythrodysesthesia (hand-foot syndrome) and other skin toxicities, which are discussed in Chapters 7 and 10. The acute pain syndrome causes by paclitaxel is discussed in Chapter 7. Infusion of chemotherapy into the peritoneum, bladder, hepatic artery, or peripheral veins can also cause pain. Intravenous dexamethasone, if administered too quickly, causes perineal burning and shooting pain.

Chronic cancer-related pain syndromes may be from metastases to bones and viscera, as discussed later in this chapter. But the most troublesome ones are caused by nerve damage. The cancer usually has spread to the bone or tissue adjacent to the nerve, and as it grows, it compresses the nerve or its blood supply, causing neuropathic pain and eventual nerve death. Recognizing neuropathic pain, therefore, is crucial to identifying patients with lesions of (1) cranial nerves as they exit the skull, (2) nerve plexuses (cervical, brachial, and lumbosacral), (3) peripheral nerves, and most dangerously, (4) the spinal cord (from tumors in vertebral bodies and the epidural space) (LeBlanc and Kamal 2018). Patients with primary or metastatic brain lesions have headaches if they have significant cerebral edema.

Cranial nerves. Metastases to the *jugular foramen* cause occipital and ipsilateral shoulder pain along with dysfunction of cranial nerves 9 to 12, which exit through the foramen. Disease of the *sphenoid sinus* mimics sinusitis, but patients with tumor infiltration usually have a more severe headache, and they may have diplopia due to infiltration or edema of the sixth cranial nerve. Patients with tumor infiltration of the cranial nerves have pain in the head and face in the distribution of the nerve involved, often the ninth or the trigeminal.

Nerve plexuses. Brachial or lumbosacral plexus infiltration can be particularly difficult to diagnose, but it can herald primary or recurrent tumors. In the brachial plexus, the nerves lower in the plexus (C7 to T1) are most likely to be directly invaded by tumor, as were Mr. Cirelli's. Patients with either brachial or lumbosacral plexus infiltrations present with deep, aching, often shooting pains and, later, muscle atrophy in the groups innervated. MRI (magnetic resonance imaging) may reveal tumor infiltration, and treatment can be planned.

The pain of radiation fibrosis may mimic that of recurrent cancer in the brachial plexus, but it has a different distribution. Because the clavicle protects the nerves lower in the plexus, nerves located in the upper part of the plexus (C5 and C6) are most commonly affected by radiation damage. The pain and weakness will be in the C5,6 distribution; an EMG (electromyogram) will document the abnormality.

Peripheral nerves. Peripheral nerves can be affected by various chemotherapeutic agents, causing what is called *chemotherapy-induced peripheral neuropathy* (CIPN). I discuss the agents responsible and ways to prevent and treat CIPN in Chapter 7. The post-mastectomy and post-thoracotomy pain syndromes (including pain following a port insertion) are two other important syndromes caused by injuries to peripheral nerves. Prompt recognition of these syndromes is particularly important because treatment within six months of their onset is usually effective.

The term *post-mastectomy syndrome* is something of a misnomer because it can occur in women who undergo any type of breast surgery, from lumpectomy to radical mastectomy. It is a common problem: 4 to 10 percent of women who undergo breast surgery develop this syndrome. The pain can appear immediately or as late as six months after the surgery. A patient with post-mastectomy syndrome feels a burning, constricting sensation in her posterior arm, axilla, and anterior chest wall in the area where she has lost sensation as a result of the surgery. Her chest wall may be hyperesthetic or dysesthetic. The patient finds it most comfortable to keep her arm flexed, and she may therefore develop a frozen shoulder. Post-mastectomy pain is caused by a neuroma of the intercostobrachial nerve (a branch of T1,2), which was cut during surgery. There is often an associated trigger point (a place where the pain can be reproduced by touching that part of the skin) in the axilla or anterior chest wall.

Similarly, patients who have had thoracotomies or who have ports inserted for intravenous access can develop post-thoracotomy syndrome. These patients describe an aching and burning sensation in the distribution of the incision and numbness of the skin in that area. There is exquisite point tenderness at both ends of the scar. The post-thoracotomy syndrome is caused by pulling or cutting of the intercostal nerves.

Recently, specialized glial cells in the skin have been found to form an extensive mesh-like network with unmyelinated nociceptive fibers and directly transmit signals of noxious mechanical deformation of skin, causing pain (Abdo et al. 2019). These networks may be involved with the post-mastectomy and post-thoracotomy (including post-port-insertion) pain syndromes. The glial cells and their connections may prove a target for novel therapeutics to prevent or treat these syndromes.

As you can imagine, suffering caused by either of these syndromes can be significant, especially for those whose cancer has been cured. For these patients, the pain is a reminder both of the experience and of the potential for cancer recurrence. Early diagnosis and prompt treatment can eliminate this pain.

Vertebral lesions. Patients with *odontoid* and *atlas* fractures present with severe neck pain radiating over the posterior part of the skull to the vertex, as well as neck stiffness. The symptoms may mimic meningitis and are particularly dangerous because the patient is at risk for developing paraplegia or quadriplegia from the subluxation and spinal cord or brainstem compression.

Metastases to C7. These metastases often do not cause neck pain, but patients experience pain between the scapulae. Early detection will prevent cervical cord compression, but these lesions are often missed because films are taken only of the thoracic spine, and if the findings are normal, no MRI is done. Similarly, *lesions of T12* can present as isolated hip pain, as occurred in Mr. Young. Here also, if hip and pelvis films reveal no abnormalities, a spinal MRI is indicated. For either lesion, full spinal MRI and sometimes CT will be required to plan therapy. While the C7 and T12 referred pain syndromes are important to recognize, they are fortunately rare.

Epidural disease. In cancer patients, epidural disease usually does not cause a unique pain syndrome. It presents most commonly as back pain in the area of the vertebral metastasis, with or without radiation in the distribution of the spinal nerves exiting the spinal cord at that level. Its similarity to the pain of benign disk disease is a source of dangerous diagnostic confusion.

Practice Points: Recognizing Spinal Cord Compression

- Back pain may be the only finding.
- In a patient with back pain and findings consistent with metastases on a plain film of the spine in the area of the pain, the probability of invasion of the epidural space is approximately 70 percent. A radiculopathy raises this probability to 90 percent.
- Emergency MRI is indicated in any cancer patient with back pain, even when plain films and the neurologic exam are completely normal.
- Prompt recognition and therapy are the key to preserving ambulation; only 10 percent of patients with spinal cord compression who lose their ability to ambulate will ever regain it.

If a patient without cancer complains of back pain and there are no abnormal neurologic findings, most physicians would not order a plain film of the spine, let alone an MRI. They would treat symptomatically.

But in a cancer patient, back pain may be the only clue that she has a malignant epidural process and an impending cord compression. Epidural metastatic disease must be diagnosed and treated before any neurologic abnormalities develop, because once they appear, they are often irreversible. If patients are treated while they are still ambulatory, they have about a 90 percent chance of remaining so. If they become paraparetic, the odds drop to 40 to 50 percent, and only 10 percent of patients who lose their ability to walk because cancer is compressing their spinal cord will ever walk again. Thus, evaluation of the back pain of a cancer patient must be much more aggressive than that of the patient without cancer.

Plain films are not sensitive enough. Bone scans are of little value as a screening test for patients with multiple myeloma because the results are usually normal even in the presence of extensive bony disease. And in patients with other cancers, as many as 5 percent with normal bone scans will have metastatic bony disease demonstrated on MRI.

Even with completely normal neurologic findings, and normal plain films, therefore, *a full spine MRI must be done immediately* to exclude epidural disease in a patient with back pain and cancer, whether active or dormant (Lawton et al. 2019). There is about a 70 percent chance that a cancer patient with back pain and abnormal plain films of the spine has epidural metastases. If a patient cannot have an MRI, then CT myelography, which is a more uncomfortable procedure and potentially associated with more complications, must be done.

An MRI of the complete spine is needed to guide therapy. In the 40 percent of patients whose cancer involves more than one vertebral site, a full spine MRI will reveal additional lesions above and below the area of pain, which may make the patient ineligible for surgery and will need to be included in the radiation field (Lawton et al. 2019).

Psychological, Social, Financial, and Spiritual Sources of Distress

Psychological, social, existential, financial, and spiritual sources of distress are of particular importance for patients with chronic cancer-associated pain (lasting more than three months). These patients have "meaningless" pain: the pain does not alert the patient to something that can be fixed, but rather reminds them of the cancer they had or have. Therefore, the assessment of the psychological, social, existential, financial, and spiritual responses to pain in these patients must be extensive (ASCO, ESMO, NCCN guidelines).

Asking *"How are you within yourself?"* (Byock 1997) is a wonderful way to start a conversation designed to detect the psychological, social, existential, financial, or spiritual problems that often occur in cancer patients with pain and that by themselves can cause distress even in those without pain. An evaluation in each of these areas completes the initial pain assessment. And, because patients' reactions to pain are modified by their families' reactions and abilities to cope with someone in pain, a determination must be made of how the family is functioning. For patients cared for by hospice teams, the nurse, social worker, and chaplain will routinely do these assessments and communicate the results to you.

The model developed by Betty Rolling Ferrell, MA, PhD, FAAN, FPCN, director and professor, Division of Nursing Research and Education, Department of Population Sciences at City of Hope National Medical Center, provides a framework for the assessment (Figure 6.6). This model explores the extensive effects of pain on all dimensions of the quality of a patient's life: physical, psychological, social, and spiritual (Ferrell and Rhiner 1991). We have already reviewed how to assess the physical impairments induced by pain; the spiritual impairments are reviewed in Chapter 2, and the psychological causes in Chapter 9. But I briefly review the psychological effects of cancer pain below.

Psychological effects. Psychological effects of cancer pain include both the emotional response to the pain (the affective dimension) and how the patient thinks about the pain (the cognitive dimension). Delirium, an organic mental disorder that particularly affects cancer patients, can be caused by the pain itself and is a source of great distress. Its assessment and treatment are reviewed in Chapter 9.

Affective dimension. People who have uncontrolled pain are usually unable to feel much pleasure. Happiness, even of a momentary kind, is hard for them to imagine. In addition, patients in pain are often anxious or depressed and are unable to focus their attention on anything other than the pain. Pain also exacerbates depression, which is the strongest contributing factor to suicidal ideation in cancer patients.

Anxiety and depression are, of course, not limited to cancer patients with pain—they are the most common psychological problems of all patients with cancer. Assessment and management of patients with depression and anxiety are discussed in Chapter 9.

Cognitive dimension. The cognitive dimension, which includes families' and patients' attitudes, beliefs, and knowledge about pain and its treatment, affects their interpretation of new pains and their acceptance of proposed changes in treatment regimens. For example, it may be psychologically easier for the family

Physical Well-Being and Associated Symptoms	**Psychological Well-Being**
Functional Ability	Anxiety
Strength/Fatigue	Depression
Sleep and Rest	Enjoyment/Leisure
Nausea	Pain Distress
Appetite	Happiness
Constipation	Fear
	Cognition/Attention

Social Concerns	**Spiritual Well-Being**
Caregiver Burden	Suffering
Roles and Relationships	Meaning of Pain
Affection/Sexual Function	Religiosity
Appearance	

FIGURE 6.6. Effects of Pain on Dimensions of the Quality of Life. *Source:* B. R. Ferrell and M. Rhiner, "High-Tech Comfort: Ethical Issues in Cancer Pain Management for the 1990s," *J Clin Ethics* 2:108–12, 1991.

to ignore worsening pain than to face the implications of the patient's worsening condition. In their denial of the patient's impending death, they may not adequately treat his escalating pain. Families are no better than physicians at guessing the intensity of the patient's pain, and the more different their perception is from what the patient is actually feeling, the more stress they experience (Miaskowski et al. 1997).

Practice Points: Assessing Other Dimensions of the Pain Experience

- Discover what the pain means to the patient; it will affect both their emotional response to pain and their ability to cope with it.
- Determine the patient's expectations about the extent of pain relief and work to align these expectations with what you know to be clinical reality.
- Assess the family caregiver's personal characteristics (e.g., age, sex) and how those characteristics affect caregiving efforts, especially as they relate to giving pain medications.
- Assess the family's willingness to acquire new skills, desire for information, and psychological needs.
- Take the opportunity to reassure the patient and family that every effort will be made to control the patient's pain and that the family will be supported in its caregiving efforts.

Gaining a family's cooperation begins with assessing their desire for information, willingness to acquire new skills, and psychological needs. Physicians can begin this process by addressing unasked family questions, such as:

How bad is his pain likely to get in the future?
Will we have help managing Mom's pain at home?
Who will answer our questions as they arise?

Family members can be reassured that you will continue to work with them to relieve the pain, no matter how intense it becomes, and that you will not abandon them. They will know that you'll help them cope with the stresses they are likely to experience as they care for the patient at home.

Patient-Specific Goals for Comfort and Function

In addition to the family assessment, you also need to know what patients are thinking and feeling, what are their goals and their hopes for comfort and improved function. You have to determine what the pain means to them, because this will affect their emotional response to and ability to cope with the pain. Does the patient, for example, believe his pain to be a manifestation of progressive disease? People who have this belief are more likely to be depressed or anxious or to report more pain than those who do not. Alternatively, the patient may regard his pain as a challenge. If so, he will probably cope better and be less depressed than someone who views pain as a punishment.

Effect of Therapies on Comfort and Function

You must also ascertain patients' therapeutic expectations. A patient with extensive bony metastases is unlikely to achieve complete pain relief without side effects if the only medication she takes is a sustained-release morphine preparation. She may have such an expectation, however, and question the polypharmacy that is prescribed. Once the source of confusion is elicited, the patient's expectations can be better aligned with yours.

Social and financial causes. Some patients are suffering from what Cassell, in *The Nature of Suffering and the Goals of Medicine*, describes as a loss of "personhood," as discussed in Chapter 1. Cassell has developed a "topology of person" that explores the many dimensions of how illness can affect an individual's personhood and cause suffering. Personality and character will affect the response to illness, as will "the lived past . . . a story that has taken place over time, in many places, and involving countless others" (2004, p. 43), as well as the family's lived past. The patient's cultural background, the many roles he has played (son, father, Little League coach, board chairman), and his associations and relationships are also determinants of suffering in response to illness. Grief over having to relinquish these activities and the accompanying loss of social standing can be a source of significant pain. Other sources include injuries to the body or unconscious mind, diminished possibilities of the self as a political being, loss of a secret life, dashed hopes for the perceived future, or loss of the transcendent dimension—the spirit. When disease progresses, these aspects of personhood may become damaged or lost. Knowledge that these roles may never be regained becomes an ongoing source of suffering.

Patients and their families also need an evaluation of the social and financial barriers to optimal pain relief. A basic assessment should include the family's living conditions and financial and insurance status. This information helps to determine, for example, whether financial help will be required for patients who need the more expensive pain medicines or a high-tech pain therapy, such as intravenous or epidural opioid/anesthetic infusions. It will also reveal whether financial worries are causing insomnia, which exacerbates pain.

It is crucial to determine whether the pharmacies near the patients' homes will dispense the opioids the patients need. Studies have shown that neighborhoods housing mainly non-white patients have many fewer pharmacies (Cobaugh 2017; Chisholm-Burns et al. 2017), and those that are present are much more likely not to stock or agree to order opioids, regardless of the patients' average income (Morrison et al. 2000; Green et al. 2005).

Role of the Social worker. Hospital social workers, the social workers employed by home health agencies or hospice agencies, or those in oncology practices effectively perform comprehensive assessments of patients' cultural and psychosocial needs and obtain help for families dealing with these issues. Even if families do not directly express these types of concerns, encourage them to have at least one consultation with the social worker. This consultation often allows the social worker and the patient's family to develop a relationship that can be renewed as needed throughout the course of the patient's illness.

At the time of diagnosis and during the early phases of treatment, in addition to performing the psychological and social assessment, social workers may work on insurance and other financial problems and connect the patient and family with community social service agencies. Social workers can also advise you as to which families or patients need more intensive psychological support. They may be able to provide the needed counseling and education in coping skills. If the disease later progresses, the social worker can continue to provide the patient and family members with psychological and social assessments and, for those who need it, intensive counseling or assistance in coping with impending death. We discuss these therapeutic roles of the social worker in more detail in Chapter 9.

Reevaluate When the Pain Pattern Changes

The final recommendation of the guidelines is to assess each new pain. Pain assessment is an ongoing process, directed not only at determining the efficacy of the pain-relief regimen but also at detecting new pains and identifying their causes. When the character, quality, or timing of the patient's pain changes, a new or progressive lesion is usually responsible. Disease may be advancing, a bone may have fractured, or a problem unrelated to the cancer may have developed. Frequent reassessment will detect these and enable you to institute effective therapy promptly.

SUMMARY

A comprehensive pain assessment is the foundation of effective pain therapy and is not hard to accomplish. The guidelines from ASCO, NCCN, and ESMO are straightforward, and validated measurement tools are available. The complaint of pain is often so much more than a clue to the discovery of a reversible underlying cause. Assessing for the multiple causes and modifying factors discussed in this chapter will enable you to gain a comprehensive understanding of your patients and their pain and be much more likely to be able to relieve their suffering.

CHAPTER 7

Pharmacologic Management of Cancer Pain

INTRODUCTION

Pharmacologic therapy is the mainstay of cancer pain relief. Satisfactory pain control for 90 percent of cancer patients can be achieved with oral, parenteral, transmucosal, or transdermal therapies with minimal adverse side effects. But the largest prospective study to date, an observational study of more than 3,000 outpatients with breast, lung, colorectal, or prostate cancer, found significant underprescribing of pain medications (Fisch et al. 2012). Two-thirds of these patients reported pain at their initial visit to their oncologist, and a month later, half of them (33 percent of the total) were receiving inadequate medications for their degree of pain. Patients who did not have advanced disease and who were not receiving antineoplastic therapy, and those who were treated at a center with a predominance of minority patients or who were minority patients treated at any center, were at particular risk for undertreatment. A full 43 percent of patients reporting severe pain were not receiving an opioid at their first assessment or a month later. Twenty percent were receiving no analgesic. And as reported in 2016, 39 percent of patients receiving curative therapy, 55 percent of those undergoing cancer treatment, and 66.4 percent of patients with advanced cancer reported pain, and the pain was moderate to severe (≥5) in 38 percent (van den Beuken-van Everdingen et al. 2016). So we have a lot of work to do.

To achieve good pain control for your patients, you will need to be familiar with the nonpharmacologic strategies to relieving pain discussed in Chapter 8 and proficient in using a combination of oral, parenteral, transmucosal, or trans-dermal opioid and adjuvant analgesics, along with other agents that prevent or treat opioid-induced constipation, nausea, sedation, and delirium. In the rare circumstance that the other routes are not successful or available, you can use rectal, subcutaneous (SQ), or spinal routes to achieve pain relief. Unfortunately, compounded topical creams for neuropathic, nociceptive, and mixed pains do not work (Brutcher et al. 2019). For any patient whose pain persists at unacceptable levels despite your best efforts, I suggest you collaborate with a palliative care colleague.

In this chapter I discuss the drugs you will need: non-opioid, opioid, and ad-juvant analgesic medications, as well as other treatments in addition to agents that prevent or relieve opioid-induced side effects. I review patient and family unasked questions about opioids; provide a strategy for risk mitigation for all patients for whom you need to prescribe opioids; and, for patients in whom the benefits of opioids exceed the burdens and risks, offer strategies you can use to help them accept the opioids they need. I also review anesthetic methods that can relieve pain. The special needs of older patients, of patients with active or past history of substance use disorder, of patients with hematologic malignancies (e.g., multiple myeloma and those undergoing hematopoietic stem cell transplant), and of cancer survivors are included. I discuss some common clinical situations: treat-ing patients with renal or hepatic failure; starting a patient on opioids; changing opioid doses, routes, or agents; and relieving excruciating pain rapidly. This chap-ter's tables appear at the end.

NONSTEROIDAL ANTI-INFLAMMATORY DRUGS

Nonsteroidal anti-inflammatory drugs (NSAIDs), taken by people with mild to moderate nonmalignant pain, are useful alone or combined with an opioid for cancer patients with pain from various sources. They are especially useful for patients with bone pain or tissue inflammation.

The NSAIDs include the *p*-aminophenols (e.g., acetaminophen), the salicylates (e.g., aspirin and the nonacetylated salicylates such as salsalate), the propionic acid derivatives (e.g., ibuprofen, naproxen), and the acetic acid derivatives (indomethacin, ketorolac) (see Table 7.1).

Most NSAIDs indirectly inhibit synthesis of prostaglandins by myeloid cells involved in inflammation. Prostaglandins synthesized as a consequence of injury to bones or joints help mediate the inflammatory response and the transmission of the pain signal. Recent research has identified new potential upstream targets for drugs that can limit the inflammatory response and the pain it causes, the IRE1alpha-XBP1 signaling pathway that controls prostaglandin biosynthesis (Chopra et al. 2019).

The majority of NSAIDs inhibit the synthesis or the function of both forms of cyclooxygenase (COX) enzymes required for the production of prostaglandins. COX-1 is present in the stomach, kidney, and blood vessels, whereas COX-2 is produced only in inflamed tissues. NSAIDs that inhibit COX-2 therefore minimize the inflammation associated with bone or tissue injury, whether a sports injury, arthritis, or a metastasis. NSAIDs that also inhibit COX-1, however, impair synthesis of the beneficial prostaglandins produced in the stomach and kidney and can therefore cause gastrointestinal distress and renal dysfunction.

Using NSAIDs for Cancer Pain

Although much anecdotal evidence supports their use, there is a paucity of good data demonstrating the effectiveness of NSAIDs for patients with cancer pain (Magee et al. 2019). And NSAIDs used alone usually do not provide sufficient relief for patients with cancer pain, though I have had some success with these drugs for painful bone metastases in patients receiving hormonal therapy for metastatic prostate cancer or aromatase inhibitors for breast cancer. When first prescribing an NSAID, generally start with the lowest effective dose and escalate to the maximum 24-hour dose (indicated in Table 7.1). Since both acetaminophen and aspirin have a ceiling effect (1000 mg is the ceiling dose for both agents), a patient gets no more pain relief from a 1500-mg dose of aspirin or acetaminophen than from a 1000-mg dose; he just gets increased toxicity. If the initial agent chosen is ineffective at the maximal recommended dose or the patient develops an intolerable side effect, switch to one of the NSAIDs in a different chemical class (see Table 7.1).

Selecting an NSAID

To decide which NSAID to prescribe first, I consider the cause and intensity of the pain (see Chapter 6 for assessing and determining the etiology of pain), any underlying illnesses that would contraindicate use of an NSAID, and the expected side effects. I also consider whether the patient can take oral medications or will need an intravenous or a rectal preparation.

> ### Practice Points: Selecting an NSAID for Cancer Pain
>
> - Review patients' underlying medical illnesses.
> - Give NSAIDs alone for mild pain.
> - Give oral indomethacin or intravenous ketorolac for pleuritic or pericardial pain, or pain from chest tube or feeding tube / draining gastric tube insertions. Ketorolac should generally not be used for longer than 5 days at a time. The oral form is not effective.
> - Be aware of the "ceiling" effect: the maximum pain relief obtainable from acetaminophen or aspirin is from a 1000-mg dose.
> - When pain is refractory to NSAIDs alone, add an opioid for mild to moderate pain.

Knowing the cause of the pain and its intensity can sometimes help you choose the appropriate NSAID. Oral indomethacin or intravenous ketorolac, for example, are the drugs of choice for patients with pleuritic or pericardial pain, or pain from the insertion of a chest or abdominal tube (feeding tube or draining gastric tube), and indomethacin has special efficacy for gout. They often relieve the pain of these disorders rapidly and completely. Therefore, despite the risk of gastrointestinal and renal side effects and bleeding complications from these agents, I recommend them for these patients unless they have a coagulation problem or known renal or ulcer disease. Proton pump inhibitors can be added for patients over 60, as they protect against what may be asymptomatic gastrointestinal bleeding.

Underlying illnesses also help direct the choice of NSAID. All NSAIDs should be avoided in patients with a known allergy to aspirin or with asthma, as they can produce bronchospasm in up to 20 percent of these patients. Patients at high risk for complications include those over age 60 (those over 70 are at an even higher risk) and those with a history of previous ulcer disease, NSAID-induced bleeding, or cardiovascular disease. These risks are additive. Other risk factors include concomitant use of corticosteroids or anticoagulants and use of multiple NSAIDs. To minimize gastrointestinal ulcers and bleeding frequency, high-risk patients should be started on COX-2 selective agents rather than nonselective NSAIDs (Chan et al. 2002; Laine 2003). The risk is so high for patients taking anticoagulants that they should never take an NSAID that inhibits prostaglandin synthesis.

Patients who have somatic or inflammatory pain but who also have moderately reduced platelet counts ($<100,000/mm^3$) or inherited coagulation disorders (such as hemophilia) can take the COX-2 selective agent celecoxib (Celebrex) or an NSAID that does not affect cyclooxygenase or prostaglandin synthesis, such as choline magnesium salicylate or salsalate, and not have an increased risk of bleeding (Reynolds et al. 2003). Patients taking anticoagulants such as warfarin, however, cannot take celecoxib. The interaction in the metabolism of warfarin and celecoxib causes marked increases in the INR (international normalized ratio) and an increased risk of bleeding. Two other COX-2 selective agents, valdecoxib (Bextra) and rofecoxib (Vioxx), were voluntarily withdrawn from the market because of side effects and cardiovascular safety concerns.

Patients with congestive heart failure, cirrhosis, severe liver failure from any cause, or chronic renal failure experience increased edema, worsening renal function, or hypertension if treated with either nonselective agents or COX-2 inhibitors, so both should be avoided (DeMaria and Weir 2003).

For patients with mild to moderate somatic or visceral cancer pain refractory to NSAIDs alone, they are effective when combined with an opioid. The most commonly used combination pills contain 5 mg of oxycodone along with either 325 mg of aspirin (e.g., Percodan), 400 mg of ibuprofen (e.g., Combunox), 325 mg of acetaminophen (e.g., Percocet), or 500 mg of acetaminophen (e.g., Tylox). Unfortunately, patients can take only a limited number of these pills each day because of the toxicities of the acetaminophen, ibuprofen, and aspirin. Patients who need more opioid can take higher doses of an oxycodone or other opioid preparation along with a safe dose of an NSAID. A patient with uncontrolled bone pain from metastatic breast cancer, for example, might be switched safely from 12 oxycodone/acetaminophen tablets a day, which contain 60 mg of oxycodone (5 mg × 12 pills = 60 mg), to 30 mg of sustained-release oxycodone every 12 hours along with acetaminophen 1000 mg orally every 8 hours.

Intravenous ketorolac (e.g., Toradol) is likely to be effective for someone with acute, severe somatic or inflammatory pain, such as someone who has just had a chest tube or a G-tube inserted, or one of the conditions listed above. Because ketorolac has the pain-relieving potency of an opioid, it is also used in situations in which the clinician does not want to prescribe an opioid, but the patient needs the level of pain relief an opioid can deliver. For example, ketorolac is frequently given by emergency room clinicians who wish to avoid the mental status changes that opioids can induce (see Table 7.1 for doses and frequency). A 30-mg dose of parenteral ketorolac is equivalent in pain-relieving potency to 15 mg of parenteral morphine. Ketorolac can impair renal function, however, and is therefore contraindicated for patients with renal insufficiency. And it cannot be used for chronic pain relief because it is associated with a significant incidence of acute renal failure and gastrointestinal side effects, and the oral form is not effective. A typical course of intravenous ketorolac is limited to five days of up to 4 doses per day every 6 hours standing or as needed, combined with an intravenous or oral proton pump inhibitor. If a patient responds well to the ketorolac, it may be reasonable to try oral indomethacin, since they are both acetic acid derivatives.

Intravenous or Rectal Administration

For patients who cannot take oral preparations, acetaminophen is available intravenously. Aspirin, indomethacin, and acetaminophen can be given rectally (Samala and Davis 2012) and are available by commercial suppository. Suppositories should be inserted base first, to promote retention. Though available only as a liquid, naproxen may be the best choice for rectal administration because it has the longest half-life and 80 percent bioavailability. Ten to 30 ml of the liquid suspension (125 mg/5 ml) can be given twice a day. Ibuprofen is not available in suppository form, and the liquid suspensions are available only in pediatric doses (100 mg/5 ml). A therapeutic dose of ibuprofen would necessitate giving 30 ml rectally (p.r.) every 4 to 6 hours, and this may be difficult for patients to tolerate.

Side Effects

The inhibition of prostaglandin synthesis can cause several serious abnormalities in platelet and kidney function, as well as in the lungs and the gastrointestinal tract. Because prostaglandins are necessary for normal platelet function, most NSAIDs impair platelet function and predispose the patient to bleeding. And since prostaglandins are also required to maintain renal arterial blood flow, NSAIDs may precipitate renal failure in patients, especially the elderly, with impaired flow. NSAIDs may also enhance salt and water retention and cause edema to develop in patients with congestive heart failure or cirrhosis.

Practice Points: Toxicity of NSAIDs

- Avoid NSAIDs (except acetaminophen) for patients older than 70 and for those with thrombocytopenia, coagulation defects, renal failure, cirrhosis, heart failure, or asthma.
- Use nonacetylated salicylates (e.g., choline magnesium salicylate or salsalate) for patients taking anticoagulants or with thrombocytopenia or bleeding disorders. Doses of warfarin will likely need to be lowered.
- Consider adding a proton pump inhibitor (e.g., omeprazole) to prevent gastrointestinal ulceration for patients older than 60 or for those with a history of peptic ulcer disease.
- Avoid aspirin/oxycodone, ibuprofen/oxycodone, and acetaminophen/oxycodone combinations. Rule out salicylate toxicity in a patient taking an aspirin-containing combination agent who develops otherwise unexplained mental status changes, ataxia, or tachypnea, even if there are no complaints of tinnitus.

Life-Threatening Toxicities

The side effects described above occur with therapeutic doses of NSAIDs. At toxic blood levels, however, aspirin and acetaminophen can be life threatening. Few patients would knowingly take too much aspirin, but aspirin and acetaminophen can be "hidden" in the combination products mentioned above. It's not hard to imagine that someone could have an exacerbation of her pain, double or triple the amount of Percodan or Percocet she is taking, and, in consequence, develop an overdose.

Aspirin overdose. Aspirin and the nonacetylated salicylates are metabolized by the liver; less than 5 percent is excreted by the kidneys. But the liver can metabolize only a limited amount of aspirin; if a person ingests more than that, the drug accumulates and can rapidly reach toxic levels. Patients who increase their dose of aspirin much above 6000 mg/day can easily develop salicylate toxicity, which manifests as tinnitus, ataxia, hyperventilation, delirium, and even coma. Older patients with presbycusis may be at particular risk because they cannot detect tinnitus. Despite my warnings to the contrary, a number of patients have increased their aspirin intake in this way and developed life-threatening salicylism.

The "Drunk" with an Undetectable Alcohol Level

Mr. Lafferty was taking two Percodan every 4 hours for his metastatic prostate cancer pain. His wife called to ask our advice because, she said, *"He is staggering around and talking out of his head like he used to when he was drunk all the time. But when I took him to the local emergency room, they said he couldn't be drunk; there was no alcohol in his blood."*

As it turned out, her husband had not been drinking. When she inspected his medication bottle, she found that instead of the 12 pills a day he normally took, he had taken 25 Percodan the day before. These contained 8125 mg of aspirin! I asked her to take Mr. Lafferty back to the hospital because he needed immediate medical attention.

When he again arrived in the emergency room, the triage nurse noted that he was still ataxic and confused, and I could understand why she thought he was inebriated. On further evaluation, he was also found to be hyperventilating because of the metabolic acidosis the salicylate induces. An electrolyte panel confirmed the characteristic anion gap acidosis. To minimize the deposition of salicylates in his central nervous system (CNS) and to increase salicylate clearance, the emergency medical staff gave him intravenous sodium bicarbonate. They also avoided any agents that could sedate him, because if he stopped hyperventilating, the acidosis would worsen, more aspirin would deposit in his CNS, and he would deteriorate further. Mr. Lafferty responded well to this therapy and was back to his old self within a few days.

Acetaminophen overdose. The safe chronic dose of acetaminophen is 3–4 g/day. Aspirin toxicity is not uncommon, but it would be very difficult for a patient with normal hepatic function to accidentally take enough acetaminophen to induce serious toxicity. This would require an intake of more than 20 g of acetaminophen at one sitting. Even someone taking a combination preparation of acetaminophen and oxycodone containing 500 mg of acetaminophen per pill would have to take 40 tablets over 1 to 2 hours.

In patients who have chronic liver disease, however, such as that induced by alcohol, the safe dose is 2–3 g/day. Liver toxicity can develop even with these therapeutic acetaminophen doses, and accidental overdose may occur. If you discover such an overdose soon after the patient ingests the acetaminophen, the Emergency Department is likely to treat the patient successfully with oral acetylcysteine (Mucomyst). But if the overdose is recognized late, acetylcysteine will be ineffective. Liver transplantation can be life saving for appropriate patients.

OPIOID ANALGESICS

Although NSAIDs can be useful, opioids are necessary for the vast majority of cancer patients with pain. Opioids are under development now that selectively activate mu receptors in the periphery, at the site of inflammation and pain generation (Spahn et al. 2017). In mouse models, they caused none of the usual opioid side effects of depressed respiration, sedation, or constipation, and had no addiction potential. Until these are commercially available, however, when antineoplastic and nonpharmacologic therapies, non-opioid pain relievers, and adjuvant agents are not enough, and the patient's daily activities remain unacceptably limited by uncontrolled pain, there is a role for carefully selected and titrated opioids.

Strategies for Minimizing Harm

Helping Patients and Families Weigh the Burdens and Benefits of Opioids

In the face of the epidemic of substance use disorder, the benefits of opioids for selected patients with otherwise uncontrolled symptoms may seem to be outweighed by the burdens. Shared decision-making among the patient, family, and clinician is needed for all to be confident that they are doing what's best for the patient. Patients and families share their functional goals and their concerns about adding opioids to their regimen, and clinicians share the hoped-for benefits along with the risks that adding opioids will pose and their plans for mitigating those risks.

Unasked Questions: Patients' and Caregivers' Fears about Opioids

- Risk of becoming addicted to opioids
- Fear of exhausting effective pain medication, leaving themselves with untreatable severe pain later in the course of their disease
- Preventable and treatable side effects
- Misunderstandings about religious teachings on the therapeutic use of opioids

Studies have indicated that patients, families, and clinicians share many fears and misconceptions about opioids that contribute to concerns about using them for pain, dyspnea, or cough. In my experience, patients and their families rarely initiate discussions of such concerns. Their *unasked* questions can prevent them from accepting the relief that is available.

Risks of Addiction: Risk Management

Death from prescription drug abuse has become a more common cause of death in the United States than abuse of illegal drugs. Patients' families and friends may be at risk if they use the opioids we prescribe to manage our patients' pain; the patients themselves may be at risk if they misunderstand our instructions about use of sustained-release oral or transdermal opioids or methadone.

Risks of persistent opioid use in cancer patients newly taking opioids are real.

About 20 percent of oncology patients who need opioids are at risk for developing an opioid-use disorder (Bruera and Del Fabbro 2018). Risk factors include (1) history of substance use disorder, including smoking; (2) family history of substance use disorder; (3) history of post-traumatic stress disorder (PTSD) or personal abuse, especially in childhood; and (4) depression, anxiety, or personality disorders or other psychiatric comorbidities (Dale, Edwards, and Ballantyne 2016).

A retrospective study of ~68,000 patients undergoing curative-intent cancer surgery who filled an opioid prescription from 30 days before surgery to 14 days after, found that 7–11 percent of opioid-naive patients became chronic opioid users (the equivalent of six 5-mg tablets of hydrocodone per day) up to a year after surgery. That number rose to 15–21 percent if patients then received adjuvant chemotherapy (Lee et al. 2017).

Risk mitigation is recommended for all cancer patients for whom opioids are being considered (Paice 2019). Risk mitigation includes

1. Screening for known risk factors using an accepted screening tool such as the Screener and Opioid Assessment for Patients with Pain, Short Form or Revised (SOAPP-SF and SOAPP-R), which are appropriate for patients with cancer (Koyyalagunta et al. 2013; Yasin et al. 2019), or the Opioid Risk Tool (Figure 7.1) (Scarborough and Smith 2018).

2. Careful monitoring: the frequency and content of monitoring (e.g., with urine toxicology) is based on the patient's risk score. Low-risk patients may need to be seen only every 3 months, with monthly refills, but high-risk patients should be given prescriptions for only a 1–2 week supply.

3. Having patients sign an opioid-use agreement that explains safe opioid use and storage, the purpose of the monitoring, and the consequences of opioid misuse.

4. At each visit, reviewing the patient's record on the state Prescription Drug Monitoring Program (PDMP) (anecdotally, our patients are relieved that we are monitoring them so closely).

	Enter score in box	Score (Female)	Score (Male)
1. Family History of Substance Abuse			
Alcohol	❑	1	3
Illegal Drugs	❑	2	3
Prescription Drugs	❑	4	4
2. Personal History of Substance Abuse			
Alcohol	❑	3	3
Illegal Drugs	❑	4	4
Prescription Drugs	❑	5	5
3. Age (Enter score if 16–45)	❑	1	1
4. Psychological disease			
Attention-deficit/hyperactivity disorder, obsessive compulsive disorder, bipolar disorder, schizophrenia	❑	2	2
Depression	❑	1	1

Total Score Risk Category   TOTAL _____
Low Risk 0–3, Moderate Risk 4–7, High Risk >8

FIGURE 7.1. The Opioid Risk Tool

For patients on long-term opioid therapy, some practices use the Current Opioid Misuse Measure (COMM) to help them detect opioid-use disorder–related behaviors (Butler et al. 2007; Meltzer et al. 2011). Unfortunately, though oral formulations of long-acting opioids that resist tampering (i.e., they can't be injected or inhaled) are available, there is no evidence that they have decreased opioid misuse (Bruera and Del Fabbro 2018).

Sam

Some patients do not use the opioids you prescribe at all. In the days before the opioid crisis became what it is today, when I still practiced oncology, I cared for Sam, a 44-year-old long-haul truck driver who was the father of five girls and lived with their mother, his partner of many years. His parents had trouble with alcohol and depression. He smoked and drank alcohol (to excess in the past), bowled in a league, and was a terrific dad.

Sam developed back pain, and his primary care physician (PCP) initially blamed it on the suspension of Sam's truck. When the pain persisted, plain films of his back revealed suspicious lesions, and a lung mass was found on chest x-ray. Biopsy revealed a squamous cell carcinoma of the lung, and staging showed it to be metastatic to nodes and bones, including several areas in his spine, one of which was the source of the pain.

Sam was referred to me for treatment, which initially went well. His tumor responded to systemic therapy, and his back pain resolved after radiation to the area causing pain. I treated Sam in the era when we didn't have targeted therapies or immunotherapy, and as usually happened then, his lung cancer recurred, again presenting with back pain. Sam was devastated, and he and his partner agreed to regular counseling with our social worker, along with counseling on how to talk with his children. His brother Robert was very religious, a practicing Catholic, but Sam resisted our recommendation for spiritual support.

Work was important to Sam, and to enable him to continue while he was receiving targeted XRT, I treated his pain with a bisphosphonate, NSAIDs, and immediate- and sustained-release oxycodone (Oxycontin); he declined referral for acupuncture or physical therapy. A few months later, the pain worsened, and we placed an intrathecal pump. He told me it made no difference, and I continued to increase his doses of oxycodone, including Oxycontin, to manage it. He declined trying methadone for his pain, citing people he had seen in his neighborhood who were taking methadone because they had opioid-use disorder. His urine toxicology always showed only oxycodone.

Sam's disease progressed, with brain metastases and such weight loss and debility that he could no longer work. Eventually he became bedridden and continued to complain of uncontrolled back pain. His partner enrolled him in hospice care, but he became too agitated to stay at home and was admitted to our hospital. As he lay dying, his brother Robert asked to speak to me. I thought that like many family members, he needed support, or wanted to thank me and my team for all we'd done for Sam.

Imagine my shock when, instead, Robert said he had a confession to make. He couldn't let me continue to believe that all we had done for Sam's pain had not worked. Robert told me, *"Dr. Abrahm, that pump worked perfectly. Sam had very little back pain after you put that in. But he kept asking you and his PCP for the oxys because he was selling them. He couldn't work anymore, and it was the only way he could support his kids. I couldn't let you go on thinking you hadn't helped him, and not knowing. Please forgive him and forgive me for not telling you."*

Of course, I forgave Sam. I hoped he could hear me when I told him I understood and forgave him. He died soon after that, peacefully. Sam had been smart enough to take some of the immediate-release oxycodone, so it would appear in his urine. We didn't have a PDMP to show me the prescriptions he was getting from his PCP. I wish I had used the Opioid Risk Tool, on which he would have scored as "high risk." I would have had him sign an opioid-use agreement, monitored his prescriptions more closely, and discovered the diversion before he died.

All patients and their caregivers need to understand the risks of opioids and how to mitigate them. Now, I suggest strongly that they store their drugs in a locked box to which only the patient and one designated caregiver have access. You or your staff can educate them about the opioids and their side effects, as well as how to use naloxone. The naloxone-dispensing devices (IM/SQ or intranasal) available in community pharmacies deliver doses adequate to reverse opioid overdoses (Ryan and Dunne 2018). Ask them to pick one up (or if you live in a state that requires one, give them a prescription for naloxone), teach them the signs of overdose, and urge that they make a plan for when to use the naloxone and when to call providers.

In addition to aberrancy on the PDMP, signs of substance use disorder include (1) forged prescriptions; (2) doctor shopping; (3) urine drug-testing aberrancies, which includes the absence of an expected opioid; (4) lost opioid prescriptions; (5) requesting early prescriptions; (6) unscheduled clinic visits due to pain complaints; (7) ER visits for pain; and (8) requests for opioid dose escalation without apparent change in functional status (Dale, Edwards, and Ballantyne 2016). If necessary, an addiction specialist can be added to the team while the patient still requires opioids as part of the pain management plan.

If you want to learn more about risk assessment and monitoring, several Risk Evaluation and Mitigation Strategy (REMS) courses are available online. The opioid REMS programs include basic information on the difficulty of determining which patients are at risk for opioid abuse; the rationale for using *universal precautions* when considering prescribing these agents to any patient; how to use a risk tool, such as the Opioid Risk Tool; educating patients about the safe use and proper disposal of the various forms of sustained-release oral and transdermal opioids; providing written informed consent to everyone using sustained-release opioids, including the benefits, risks, and adverse events expected; appropriate use of random urine toxicology screens and how to interpret the results; and what elements need to be documented in a pain assessment and management program. The Prescribers Clinical Support System for Opioid Therapy (PCSS-O; www.pcssnow .org) has free web-based or downloadable courses for iPhone or Android.

Opioid Risk Tool. Assessing patients' personal and family history of opioid use or substance use disorder will help you assess the risk that patients will use the opioids you prescribe for their pain for other purposes, most commonly to "chemically cope" with the anxiety that could better be addressed with more effective measures. Several validated tools are available for this purpose. Our team has chosen the Opioid Risk Tool (Figure 7.1) (Scarborough and Smith 2018) to assess the risk of opioid-use disorder. This and the SOAPP-SF and SOAPP-R are practical tools that take no more than five minutes to complete.

Patient and family education. For those patients who need opioids as part of their pain relief regimen, I find I often need to clarify misconceptions they have about what addiction to opioids is and is not (Scarborough and Smith 2018). We know that patients taking opioids for prolonged periods *will* become *physically dependent* on them: if the drug is abruptly stopped, they will experience a withdrawal syndrome. But addiction is not simply physical dependence; patients who are *addicted* want to use the drugs for their psychological effects—they *want another feeling from the medication besides pain relief (e.g., euphoria), and they cannot control their use.* They seek drugs for the escape they provide, and in their efforts "to get out of life," they continue to use drugs even when the drugs are harming them or others.

Patients with pain who need opioids but are not addicted, on the other hand, simply want "to get back into" their lives. When the pain is gone, they no longer ask for pain-relieving medication. Most patients, rather than developing drug-seeking behavior, strongly resist taking opioids because they share the clinician's concern about the risks of addiction. And if a son or daughter is or has been addicted to opioids, the patient may be reluctant to add opioids to their regimen even to control excruciating pain. These patients have expressed to me their fear that if they take the medication, they will experience the same disintegration they saw in their child.

Practice Points: Risks of Developing an Opioid-Use Disorder

- Assume that the patient or family has concerns about opioids.
- Explain your risk mitigation strategy; they will be relieved.
- Reassure the patient and family that if the source of the pain disappears, you will wean the patient safely off the opioid.
- Tell them that people with an opioid-use disorder use drugs to "get out" of their lives; patients may need opioids to get back "into" their lives, to do the things they want to do.
- Draw analogies between the need for opioids and the need for other medications, or caffeine in coffee drinkers.

Earlier in my career, I was unaware of patients' reluctance to take opioids (and their families' uneasiness about administering them). I first became aware of this when I was faced with a patient whose pain seemed unaccountably resistant to therapy.

Opioids Don't Equal "Dope"

Mr. Pugh was a 68-year-old man with refractory metastatic prostate cancer; his wife always accompanied him on his visits to my office. He was now bedridden by his pain. He was taking naproxen and acetaminophen, as well as having monthly bisphosphonate injections. I had increased his opioid dosage several times, but the pain seemed undiminished. I was mystified until the visiting nurse called me from Mr. Pugh's home to report that none of the medication bottles had even been opened. When the nurse asked why, his wife replied, *"What makes the doctor think I would give him any of that dope?!"*

Neither the patient nor his wife, of course, had ever shared with me their concerns about the opioids. I have never had a patient or a family member voluntarily disclose such fears when I first recommended opioid therapy. I suggest, therefore, that you proceed under the assumption that these concerns are present, even if not articulated. To break the ice, you might adopt an opening I have used successfully: *"People who have a substance use disorder use drugs to get out of their lives. You will be using them appropriately, to get back into yours."* For other patients, I might say, *"If you take this medicine, you know, you won't start stealing TV sets."*

That usually gets a laugh and, along with it, an admission of a worry that is not entirely a joke. What can follow is a valuable opportunity for a frank discussion of the source and nature of the fears of this particular family. They are usually surprised that you have "guessed" their state of mind, and your ability to understand them so well may help them listen more closely to what else you have to say.

Many perfectly reasonable people will have trouble understanding that taking a drug that causes physical dependence does not mean that they are "addicted" to it. Addiction carries with it dramatic negative connotations (stealing that TV set!), and it is particularly important that patients taking opioids not be locked into that word *addiction.* They should not label themselves as addicts.

It is easiest to get patients to agree to try opioids when they are likely to need them for only a short time. In such circumstances, you can reassure the patients that you'll taper them off the drugs as soon as they don't need them anymore. For example, to someone receiving radiation therapy to a bone metastasis, you might say, *"You are likely to have less and less pain as the radiation treatment works. I'll follow your progress closely and decrease the medication as you find you need it less. If you don't need the opioids anymore, I'll stop them the way I do any other medication."* It seems easier for patients to preserve their self-esteem if they consider that they are taking opioids as part of their pain relief regimen "just until the treatment has time to work." Your assurance that you will wean them gradually and safely usually removes that obstacle to their accepting your recommendation.

Clinician education: Prescribe opioids at the correct frequency. By prescribing opioids incorrectly, clinicians can cause patients with pain to exhibit what looks like drug-seeking behavior. Someone with severe pain from breast cancer metastatic to bone may exhibit such behavior, for example, if prescribed oxycodone every 6 hours as needed for pain. The pain relief provided by oxycodone lasts 3 to 4 hours at most, leaving the patient with 2 hours of unrelieved pain. Such a patient might appear to have drug-seeking behavior because she asks the nurse for medication "2 hours early," but she is simply in severe pain because of inadequate blood levels of the opioid that provided pain relief. Education of nursing and medical colleagues can prevent this misunderstanding, which causes undue suffering and, if the patient feels they are being treated as a "drug seeker," affects their self-esteem in such a way as to limit their willingness to use opioids in the future.

Fear of Exhausting Effective Pain Medication

Patients who resist taking opioids may be thinking, *"I can stand this pain now. But what if it becomes worse later? What will be left?"* Their pain may be "only" moderate now, and they fear that if they take *any* opioid, they will have "used up" the strongest medication available. Their past experiences may have contributed to such concerns. A patient of mine had cared for her husband, who was prescribed ibuprofen and a low dose of immediate-release oxycodone for pain from lung cancer that had metastasized to his hip. In addition to his systemic therapy, he had received radiation therapy, took the medications as prescribed, and resumed normal function, but several months later, the pain returned and became more severe. She recalled that she had to give him the oxycodone pills at first only when he needed them for pain when he moved, then every 6 hours, and then every 4, and by the time she called us to help her with his pain, she was convinced that he was now "resistant" to achieving pain relief from any medication. What in fact had happened was that his cancer had grown, causing more pain that needed stronger pain relief. But all she remembered was her feeling that if she hadn't given him the pain medications for the pain initially, he wouldn't have become "resistant" to them. And she therefore didn't want to accept any opioids as part of her own regimen for her severe bone pain from metastatic breast cancer.

You can explain to such patients and their families what actually caused the seeming "resistance," that their regimen can include pain-relieving medications now, and that if the pain becomes worse, 95 percent of the time there will a regimen of medication and other therapies strong enough to relieve it without unacceptable side effects.

Unfortunately, as you know, many patients may not be willing or able to articulate this concern to you. To anticipate and allay it for them, you might say something like: *"You cannot use up pain medicine; there's always plenty more where that came from. I've prescribed a low dose of the opioid as part of your regimen for now, and I can always give you more of it, or we can change to a stronger medicine later if you need one."*

Misconceptions about Side Effects

Patients may also resist taking opioids because of adverse side effects they have experienced when taking a mild opioid, for example, after a tooth extraction. I remember well the experience of a colleague of mine with codeine. When she was ending her intern year, her L5-S1 disk herniated—she had fallen on the ice that winter and, over the following months, had apparently lifted too many patients. At any rate, she was unable to stand and, as she was living alone at the time, was admitted to the hospital. After the first shot of morphine, which relieved her pain, she was given one or two additional shots of morphine.

But upon awakening the next morning in severe pain, she was offered only oral codeine. She found it so profoundly nauseating that she took it as infrequently as possible. What was worse, though, she said, was her realization, one week into her hospital course, that she hadn't had a bowel movement. She had never thought to ask for a laxative, and one had never been offered. The discomfort of the eventual evacuation, exacerbated by her herniated disk, convinced her that opioids were something she'd *never* accept again.

And she is a physician. It is easy to understand why patients with similar experiences may refuse to consider including opioids in their pain regimens, even though they may be suffering from moderate to severe pain. The anticipation of uncontrolled constipation, nausea, or a "doped up" feeling is often unpleasant enough to prompt patients to refuse. We must let patients know that we are aware of these side effects and intend to prevent as many as we can, and that we will offer treatment for those we cannot prevent. (You can find a full discussion of the prevention of constipation and the treatment of nausea and other opioid-induced side effects later in this chapter.)

Misconceptions about Religious Teachings

Finally, patients, their families, and even health care professionals may be leery about pain medicines because they have misinterpreted or are misinformed about what their religion teaches on the subjects of drugs, pain, suicide, and euthanasia. There are strictures in some religions, such as Roman Catholicism, against suicide, euthanasia, and the use of illicit drugs. Patients and their families may mistakenly think that these prohibitions apply to opioids prescribed for pain relief. They may believe that they cannot take (or give) doses of opioids that would relieve pain but might shorten life, because they would be committing suicide or assisting euthanasia.

The Church's position was stated first by Pius XII in 1957 and reiterated in the 1994 and 1997 editions of the Catechism (*Catechism of the Catholic Church* 1997, Subheading I, Euthanasia, verse 2279):

> Even if death is thought imminent, the ordinary care owed to a sick person cannot be legitimately interrupted. The use of painkillers to alleviate the sufferings of the dying, even at the risk of shortening their days, can be morally in conformity with human dignity if death is not willed as either an end or a means, but only foreseen and tolerated as inevitable. Palliative care is a special form of disinterested charity. As such, it should be encouraged.

This teaching is in contrast to the prohibition of the illicit use of drugs (*Catechism of the Catholic Church* 1997, Subheading II, Respect for the Dignity of Persons, verse 2291):

> The use *of drugs* inflicts very grave damage on human health and life. Their use, except on strictly therapeutic grounds, is a grave offense. Clandestine production of and trafficking in drugs are scandalous practices. They constitute direct co-operation in evil, since they encourage people to practices gravely contrary to the moral law.

Opioid pain medication given or taken to relieve pain is morally acceptable to the Church, even if its use results in a shortening of life. This is the so-called doctrine of double effect. If the intent of giving the medication is to relieve pain, an unintended shortening of life is acceptable. Furthermore, there is little if any credible evidence that pain medication given carefully and titrated to a patient's pain actually shortens life. The rare exception might be patients with far-advanced obstructive lung disease, in whom increasing hypercapnia might have that effect. But even in that situation, the stricture against "use of drugs" does not apply. The clinician or family member who gives medication to relieve suffering is not considered to have used drugs illicitly or to have participated in any form of euthanasia; the patient taking such medication is not considered to have committed suicide.

Physicians, nurses, nurse practitioners, physician assistants, and other health care providers may not be familiar with this teaching. One of the hospital nurses who cared for many of my patients attended an in-service class I was giving about pain, and when I discussed this subject, she burst into tears. She told me that for more than ten years, she had been giving opioid medication to terminally ill patients to relieve their suffering but had assumed each time that she was committing a mortal sin. The relief she felt was palpable. And when I have pointed out the Church's teaching on this to many Catholic patients and their families, their relief was apparent as well.

Most Orthodox Jewish opinion, as well as that of Islamic leaders, also supports this doctrine of double effect. Pain medicine can be given even at the risk of shortening life. Intent is the key in all these cases. As one of the Islamic opinions clearly stated, "Intention is beyond the verification by the law," but according to Islam, "it cannot escape the ever watchful eye of God Who according to the Qur'an 'knows the treachery of the eyes, and all that hearts conceal'" (Qur'an 40:19). Some Muslims who need pain medication, however, will resist accepting even parenteral doses during the month of Ramadan. They may not be aware that the Qur'an relieves the sick of the burden of fasting during this month.

Eliminating these powerful misconceptions can allow Catholic, Jewish, and Muslim patients to attain the relief they need, along with the spiritual reassurance that what they and their families are doing is right. Observant Buddhists pose a different challenge. Their search for awareness may induce them to refuse pain medication if it interferes with clarity of mind for their required meditation practices. Here, the suffering may affect the staff more than the patient, who accepts it as a necessary part of his spiritual life.

Practice Points: Enhancing Pain Relief if Opioids Are Needed

- Reassure patients that taking opioids now will not make opioids ineffective if they develop more severe pain.
- Reassure patients that opioid-induced side effects can be managed with additional medications or by using a different opioid.
- Explain the doctrine of double effect and correct misconceptions about religious teachings on opioids.
- Help patients identify a functional goal that can be accomplished if their pain is relieved.
- Enlist the help of family and friends to obtain a more accurate assessment of patients who do not wish to distress you by admitting they are still in pain.
- Reassure patients that increased pain does not always mean increase in disease severity.
- Use careful questioning to uncover guilt, denial, or anger that are exacerbating the suffering.

Develop a Functional Goal

For many patients, their pain, not the cancer, has robbed them of the ability to do the things they love. You can work with them to understand that if they added opioids to their pain regimen and the pain became tolerable, they could function again. The depression that can accompany severe unrelieved pain may have left them unable to set goals for themselves. Help them set functional goals by asking, *"What would you like to do that you can't now do because of the pain?"* Then, depending on the patient, suggest something like:

> *Would you like to make breakfast for your partner?*
> *Would you like to take the kids to a ball game?*
> *Would you like to go fishing?*
> *Could you go to church and sit through the service?*

Patients will often choose one of these or offer another reasonable goal. Then add, "If *you take the medicines I've prescribed, you'll be able to do that—and other things you haven't been able to do for some time."* Even patients who have felt such despair at their helplessness and inactivity that they have expressed suicidal ideas have responded to these questions by setting realistic goals, and after getting needed psychological and/or spiritual counseling, the pain (and, if needed, antidepressant) medications helped them accomplish these goals.

Unearth Hidden Agendas

Finally, some patients seem inexplicably resistant to accepting any pain therapies, including opioids. I have sometimes been successful in discovering their hidden agendas, which most commonly included unexpressed guilt, denial, and anger.

Guilt. Some patients, despite our best efforts, seem to resist all attempts to relieve their pain. I have been amazed at the range of reasons for this. One Vietnam War veteran finally admitted to me, *"I'd rather burn now than burn later."* He never told me what it was he thought he needed to atone for, but he clearly felt that the suffering he was now experiencing would save him from an eternity of punishment after he died. A week or so after our discussion, he agreed to try various agents for his pain.

I was so grateful that I had been able to convince the patient to trust me enough to reveal his feelings. If I'd initially had more insight into his distress, I could have enlisted the aid of a psychologist or chaplain to help him uncover, share, and perhaps relieve his spiritual suffering much sooner.

Alan, a patient I later consulted on with far-advanced HIV-AIDS and meningeal spread of an AIDS-related lymphoma, was just as challenging. Despite all our efforts, he continued to complain of severe pain and paresthesias in both lower extremities. In the course of discussions with our social worker, Alan revealed that he yearned to see his 8-year-old daughter, who was living with her mother, his former girlfriend. The social worker was able to locate his girlfriend and let her know that Alan was dying and that his last wish was to say good-bye to his daughter.

We never discovered what had gone on between them, but his girlfriend angrily refused. We were crestfallen and almost afraid to let him know that we had failed. But our social worker finally told him, with me in tow for support. To our surprise, Alan's face lit up with an almost beatific smile. He said, *"Well, at least I tried,"* and fell asleep. When he awoke, he was a different man. The anguish was gone and, along with it, his complaints of intractable pain. And his death was a peaceful one.

Addressing Health Care Disparities

Hispanic and Black cancer patients continue to report worse pain at the time their cancers are diagnosed, and to have their pain underestimated and undertreated more often. This undertreatment may stem from both implicit clinician bias and inability to locate a pharmacy that stocks the opioids they need (Scarborough and Smith 2018), especially for those who live in areas of so-called minority ZIP codes. Clinicians can address the disparity by inquiring whether the patient has had difficulty getting the prescription filled, working with the community pharmacy to stock the needed opioid, or changing the opioid to one the pharmacy feels it is safe to stock. State and national policy changes will be needed, however, if an effective solution is to be found.

General Guidelines for Opioid Use

Uncontrolled pain remains one of the major obstacles to cancer patients' efforts to accomplish their goals. Some of the reasons for this have already been discussed: inadequate pain assessment, clinicians' reluctance to prescribe opioids in the appropriate frequency and dose, and patients' reluctance to take them. Clinicians also may mistakenly believe that opioid medication will interfere with the ability to diagnose the cause of acute pain in the emergency setting. In fact, in a prospective, randomized trial, patients arriving at an emergency room with abdominal pain of unknown etiology were initially (i.e., for the first 60 minutes) given morphine or saline. This study found no occasions when the administration of morphine masked a physical finding or led to a decrease in diagnostic accuracy (Thomas et al. 2003).

Adhering to the following guidelines may help.

Guidelines for Opioid Use

- Use nonpharmacologic therapies, NSAIDs, and adjuvant medications to minimize opioid dose and opioid-induced side effects.

   N.B. Nonpharmacologic therapies are reviewed in Chapter 8, NSAIDs above, and adjuvants are discussed later in this chapter.

- Give an opioid dose that is adequate.

- Give opioids often enough to prevent chronic cancer-related pain from recurring.

- Use the least invasive route.

- Prevent or treat common opioid-associated side effects.

What is an "adequate dose"? An adequate opioid dose is the dose needed to provide acceptable pain relief. The goal is to work with a patient to determine what acceptable pain relief looks like for her, not to decrease pain to a particular number on the pain scale. But the higher doses often cause neurotoxicity, and it's usually better to change the patient's opioid to a different, more potent agent. For example, if a patient receiving 10 mg/hr of intravenous morphine along with appropriate NSAIDs and adjuvant medications still has pain, she would be likely to develop neurotoxicity as you increase the dose. Most patients who need these very high doses have neuropathic pain and therefore would benefit from a rotation to methadone. Later in this chapter, I review why this is so and how to do the rotation.

Scheduling of doses. Many patients with advanced cancer who have pain that rarely remits should be taking the drugs at regularly scheduled intervals around the clock rather than as needed (p.r.n.). They need a long-acting agent or sustained-release formulation of an opioid to relieve their baseline steady pain and a short-acting opioid to relieve unexpected exacerbations. Doses of a short- or immediate-acting preparation given to someone who is taking around-the-clock opioids are often referred to as *rescue* doses: they rescue the patient from breakthrough and incident pains (more about these later in the chapter). With the variety of available agents, around-the-clock pain control is often achievable.

Mild to moderate cancer pain may be intermittent, however, and for patients with this kind of pain, p.r.n. dosing may be appropriate. When they are at home, patients can give themselves pain medicine whenever they need it. But hospitalized patients can experience significant delays in receiving needed p.r.n. medication. For these patients, instead of ordering opioids p.r.n., I use a "patient-may-refuse" order. The nurse offers the medication regularly (e.g., oxycodone every 4 hours), and the patient has the option to take it or refuse it. I would not use this strategy for patients who are delirious or who are using opioids to medicate other forms of distress.

Use the least invasive route. The vast majority of cancer patients will be able to take opioids orally, transmucosally, or transdermally in a skin patch. The drugs can also be given rectally. Intravenous opioids may be needed for pain crises, or if patients become unable to take oral medications and are not candidates for transdermal opioids, as I discuss later in this chapter. Patients who are dying will seldom need intraspinal opioids, though some will need continuous subcutaneous or intravenous opioids. Avoid giving opioids intramuscularly, because it is painful and no more efficacious than giving them subcutaneously.

Selecting an Opioid Analgesic

Patient preference. For my initial choice of drug, I consider patients' preferences, which are influenced by their experiences with opioids. For example, a patient who has had his wisdom teeth extracted might have had good pain relief from short-acting combinations of oxycodone and aspirin or acetaminophen. If he now needs something more long acting, I can use that same opioid (oxycodone) in a sustained-release preparation, if his insurance will pay for this formulation. Many insurance plans require patients to try specific long-acting opioids first before others, so check with your patient's pharmacist.

If, on the other hand, the patient had a serious side effect from an opioid, I know to avoid that agent and, if possible, other agents in the same class. Unfortunately, except for transmucosal buprenorphine and fentanyl, all the immediate-acting potent opioids are structurally related to morphine. Unless the patient has a true morphine allergy, you will usually be able to switch to another opioid that is less likely to cause the troublesome side effect. If, for example, a patient has nightmares or hallucinations from morphine, you can switch her to an equianalgesic dose of hydromorphone. The rare patient with a true morphine allergy can take transmucosal buprenorphine or fentanyl (if opioid tolerant) or methadone; none of these is chemically related to morphine.

Pain intensity. Next, determine the pain's intensity. As I discuss in Chapter 6, pain intensity can be measured using various numerical, word, face, or behavioral scales. In a numerical rating scale, pain ratings of 1 to 4 are considered mild, 5 to 6 moderate, and 7 to 10 severe. The World Health Organization (WHO) has adopted an "analgesic ladder" based on these ratings (Figure 7.2) and guidelines for using it to relieve cancer pain.

In addition to these guidelines, WHO recommends a stepwise escalation that matches the potency of the opioids to the intensity of the pain. For mild pain, start with non-opioid analgesics. Moderate pain should be treated with less-potent step 2 agents or low doses of potent opioids (see Table 7.2), and severe pain with the most potent step 3 opioids (see Table 7.3). Non-opioid analgesics and adjuvant medications should be continued when indicated.

In addition, if a patient has pain that is unrelieved by the agents recommended for that step, the WHO guidelines suggest moving up to the next step. If a patient with mild to moderate pain, for example, does not get adequate pain relief from a step 2 agent, a step 3 opioid should be prescribed. The WHO ladder and guidelines have been shown to be very effective, even in dying patients. In one study in which they were used, at the time of death, only 3 percent of patients reported severe pain, and no patient died of respiratory depression due to the opioids (Mercadante 1999).

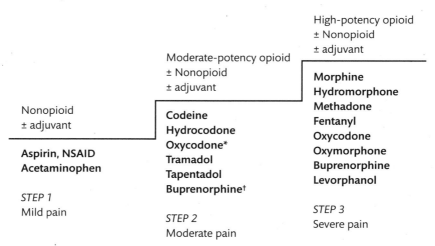

FIGURE 7.2. Analgesic Ladder. *Oxycodone (5–10 mg) in combination with aspirin, acetaminophen, or NSAID is a step 2 agent; alone, it is a step 3 agent. †At dose levels available in the United States (as of 2022), buprenorphine is a step 2 agent. *Source:* Adapted from the World Health Organization, *Cancer Pain Relief: With a Guide to Opioid Availability*, 2nd ed. (Geneva: World Health Organization, 1996).

Practice Points: Selecting an Opioid

- Consider patient preference when choosing the opioid and the opioid formulation.
- Match opioid agent with pain intensity using the WHO ladder; advance up the ladder if pain persists, even if the patient still characterizes it as "mild" or "moderate."
- Match opioid formulation to the temporal pattern of pain (i.e., continuous, intermittent, or both).
- Except for patients who have previously used codeine with good results, avoid codeine for cancer patients.
- Consider methadone for patients with severe neuropathic pain, or when drug cost is important.

Step 2 agents. In my experience, cancer pain is rarely, if ever, mild. For cancer patients with mild to moderate pain, I have found low-dose hydrocodone/acetaminophen combinations (e.g., Vicodin, Lortab) and codeine to be the *least* useful of the step 2 opioids. The dose of hydrocodone in the Vicodin or Vicodin ES preparations is not strong enough, and codeine is often nauseating and causes dysphoria. A higher-dose hydrocodone is available in a combination preparation, Vicodin HP CIII, which contains 10 mg of hydrocodone with 660 mg of acetaminophen per tablet; this combination is problematic because the dose of acetaminophen cannot be given more than every 6 hours, but hydrocodone is effective only for 4 (see Table 7.2).

Codeine. Codeine is problematic in cancer patients, for several reasons. Although the side effects of codeine may be helpful in discouraging abuse in people with nonmalignant pain, these effects are unacceptable in someone with cancer pain. Further, for codeine to provide pain relief, it must be metabolically converted to morphine by a specific hepatic enzyme. Patients who either lack that enzyme, such as many Asian patients, or are taking drugs such as cimetidine that inhibit the enzyme's function, will get little or no analgesia from codeine.

Tramadol. For certain patients, tramadol (e.g., Ultram) may be useful for cancer patients with mild to moderate pain. It is a centrally acting non-opioid analgesic that is chemically unrelated to opioids but binds to one of the opiate receptors. Approximately one-third of its analgesic effect is reversed by naloxone. The rest of the analgesia it produces may be due to its ability to decrease reuptake of norepinephrine and serotonin.

Tramadol can relieve mild to moderate somatic or neuropathic pain, including post-herpetic neuralgia (Barakat 2019); 100 mg of tramadol is more effective than 60 mg of codeine but is approximately equivalent in potency to 60 mg of codeine plus 650 mg of acetaminophen or aspirin. Side effects are similar to those caused by opioids, but in addition, tramadol may increase the risk of seizures in certain patients. Tramadol may also precipitate a serotonin syndrome in patients already taking selective serotonin reuptake inhibitors (SSRIs) (Mahlberg et al. 2004). (Serotonin syndrome is discussed in Chapter 9.)

The usual dosage of tramadol is 50 to 100 mg every 4 to 6 hours; total 24-hour dose should not exceed 400 mg. Doses should not exceed 300 mg for patients over 75, or 200 mg for patients with renal insufficiency. Tramadol may not be activated in patients with severe hepatic failure or cirrhosis, so it should be avoided in these patients. Tramadol is available in once-daily formulations, which should not exceed 300 mg per day.

Tapentadol. Tapentadol is an oral, centrally acting analgesic that both binds mu opiate receptors and inhibits the reuptake of norepinephrine (Wade and Spruill 2009). As such, it is of particular efficacy for patients with neuropathic pain, and it is effective in patients with cancer pain (Mercadante 2017). Patients receiving 50 or 100 mg of tapentadol (q4h–6) for chronic osteoarthritis pain had about the same relief as those receiving 10 to 15 mg of oxycodone but had less nausea, vomiting, or constipation (Wade and Spruill 2009). No dose adjustments are needed for mild to moderate renal or hepatic impairment. Yet, tapentadol must be used with caution along with SSRIs and selective norepinephrine reuptake inhibitors (SNRIs), tricyclic antidepressants, monoamine oxidase (MAO) inhibitors, or other agents that impair serotonin metabolism, because serotonin syndrome can result. (Serotonin syndrome is discussed in Chapter 9.)

Step 3 opioid agents. For patients with more severe pain, the potent step 3 opioids are needed (see Table 7.3). Opioids in the morphine family include, besides morphine, hydromorphone (e.g., Dilaudid), oxymorphone (e.g., Opana), oxycodone, and levorphanol (e.g., Levo-Dromoran). Any of these can be safely used for patients with normal renal and hepatic function, but all should be used with caution and at lower doses in patients with renal insufficiency. The other step 3 opioids—methadone, meperidine, buprenorphine, and fentanyl—are not structurally related to morphine. Any of these can be safely used for patients with normal renal and hepatic function but all should be used with caution and at lower doses in patients with hepatic failure.

Morphine family. Morphine is a hydrophilic opioid available orally, intravenously, and rectally in immediate-release and extended-release preparations (Table 7.3). It has an active metabolite, morphine-6-glucuronide (M-6-G), which is excreted by the kidney. If the creatinine clearance decreases by half, doses of opioids in the morphine family of agents should be reduced or their frequency of administration changed accordingly. They can be used with dose reductions in patients with moderate hepatic failure, however.

Oxycodone. Oxycodone is a useful oral opioid analgesic for patients with mild to severe cancer pain. It is listed with both the step 2 and step 3 agents because in step 2, several formulations combine a low dose (5 to 10 mg) of oxycodone with an NSAID. All provide excellent relief for this degree of pain, often induce slight euphoria, but cause only mild to moderate constipation. Many patients with moderate, intermittent pain due to bony metastases from breast, lung, or prostate cancer respond very well to these agents. For unclear reasons, women have a 25 percent higher blood level of oxycodone than men after ingesting the same dose (Kaiko et al. 1996). Oxycodone should be avoided in patients with severe hepatic impairment, and the dose reduced in patients with severe renal impairment.

Oxymorphone. Parenteral oxymorphone (e.g., Numorphan) has been used for many years for pain relief. Both immediate (e.g., Opana) and sustained-release oral forms (e.g., OpanaER) are available in the United States (Craig 2010; Sloan 2008). Oral oxymorphone is about twice as potent as oral oxycodone. The recommended starting dose of immediate-release oxymorphone for an opioid-naive patient with acute, moderate to severe pain is 10 mg every 4 to 6 hours; 5 mg of the sustained-release form can be started at every 12 hours.

Fentanyl family—fentanyl and meperidine. Of the opioids in this family, only fentanyl should be used for pain relief.

Fentanyl. Fentanyl is a lipophilic opioid with a short intravenous plasma half-life, available for oral transmucosal use (which I describe later in this chapter), intravenous administration, or in a transdermal patch, which is a fentanyl transdermal delivery system. The Duragesic patch consists of a drug reservoir lined on the bottom by a rate-limiting membrane, which itself is attached to an adherent backing (Figure 7.3). Generic patches have the drug infused throughout. The lipophilic opioid fentanyl is contained in the patch reservoir; once the patch is attached to the skin, the fentanyl diffuses from the reservoir through the rate-limiting membrane into the fat in the skin. It is then absorbed into the bloodstream from this skin reservoir. Fentanyl doses do not need to be reduced in renal failure, even in patients on dialysis.

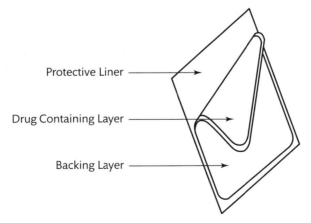

Protective Liner

Drug Containing Layer

Backing Layer

FIGURE 7.3. Duragesic Patch. After the unit is placed on the chest wall, fentanyl, contained in the drug reservoir, diffuses through the release membrane into the skin. The drug is absorbed from the skin reservoir into the bloodstream. By 14 to 24 hours after the first patch is applied, blood levels of fentanyl are sufficient to provide pain relief. New patches are usually applied every 72 hours. *Source:* From Janssen Pharmaceuticals, Inc., with permission.

Fentanyl does not cause hypotension, and because of this and its short half-life, it is often used intravenously in the intensive care unit setting.

Meperidine. You are probably wondering why meperidine (Demerol) is not included in the lists of step 2 and step 3 agents. Meperidine is not recommended for patients with cancer pain. It is inconvenient to give, and it can be dangerous.

Practice Points: Why Meperidine Is Unsuitable for Cancer Pain

- Meperidine (e.g., Demerol) relieves pain for too short a period (about 2 hours, at most).
- Meperidine has poor oral availability (75 mg IV = 300 mg p.o.).
- Meperidine's toxic metabolite, normeperidine, causes seizures; it accumulates rapidly in patients with renal insufficiency.
- Meperidine is contraindicated in patients who are also taking MAO inhibitors.

Meperidine provides pain relief for only 1 to 2 hours (see Table 7.4). And meperidine is contraindicated for patients receiving MAO inhibitors for depression or as part of a chemotherapy regimen, as it has caused hyperpyrexia, seizures, and death in these patients. Of equal concern are the potentially life-threatening side effects induced by meperidine's toxic active metabolite, normeperidine, which builds up in patients with renal insufficiency or dehydration and causes myoclonus and seizures. Naloxone exacerbates these effects and is likely to precipitate seizures in a normeperidine-toxic patient. Lorazepam is required.

Step 3 opioids that bind opiate receptors and antagonize N-methyl-d-aspartate (NMDA) receptors: methadone, levorphanol, and buprenorphine. All three opioids are uniquely positioned to decrease hyperalgesia and neuropathic pain (Davis 2012; Martyn, Mao, and Bittner 2019; McPherson et al. 2019) because they all antagonize NMDA receptors, which block the ability of opioids to relieve pain. Patients with hyperalgesia or neuropathic pain have increased levels of NMDA receptors in the dorsal horn of the spinal cord. so blocking their NMDA receptors enhances the analgesic effect of externally administered opioids.

Methadone. Methadone is not a new drug, but it is being increasingly used for cancer patients with moderate to severe, usually neuropathic, pain. It is by far the least expensive of the opioids. Methadone is structurally unrelated to the morphine family of drugs and to meperidine and fentanyl, and it can be used in the rare case of true allergy to these agents. It is also good for patients with renal insufficiency because it has no known active metabolites and does not accumulate. In elderly patients suffering from vascular insufficiency pain, which is a type of neuropathic pain, doses as low as 1 to 2 mg two to three times a day used with immediate-release opioids such as hydromorphone have been effective and cause minimal side effects (Bach et al. 2016). Methadone has been shown to be an effective adjuvant analgesic for cancer patients on chronic opioid therapy as well (McPherson et al. 2019).

In patients with Child-Pugh Class C liver disease, you should use the lowest effective doses, and only increase the dose after 10–14 days (McPherson et al. 2019). Methadone should also be used with caution in patients with structural heart disease, or with sleep apnea or other disorders of breathing. Methadone is not the best agent for patients who cannot reliably be monitored, who have cognitive impairment and don't have a caregiver who can manage the medication, who have trouble following directions or self-titrate medications, or who use opioids for reasons other than pain relief (e.g., anxiety). If you need to use methadone in a patient with current or past substance use disorder, it's important to have an addiction specialist comanage the patient (McPherson et al. 2019).

Methadone is available in oral, subcutaneous, intravenous, and rectal formulations. If you are giving methadone by the intravenous or subcutaneous route, use half the oral dose (Elsass, Marks, and Malone 2018; McPherson et al. 2019). Topical preparations of methadone (10 to 45 mg/day as a powder dissolved in PLO [pluronic lecithin organogel]) are *not* effective: the levels reached are inadequate to provide analgesia (Sylvester et al. 2011). Subcutaneous infusions are problematic because methadone causes local irritation, and the inflammation can interfere with absorption of the drug. Practices that can minimize this irritation include rotating the infusion site every few days; using intermittent boluses rather than infusions (Fürst et al. 2020); adding dexamethasone, which extends the use of the site for a continuous infusion up to 5 days; and adding bolus doses or infusions of hyaluronidase (McPherson et al. 2019).

Why is methadone particularly helpful in treating patients with neuropathic pain? Methadone contains l- and d-isomers that act as opioid receptor agonists and NMDA receptor antagonists, respectively (McPherson et al. 2019). Methadone also inhibits the reuptake of serotonin and norepinephrine (Moryl, Coyle, and Foley 2008) and blocks adenylate cyclase overactivity (Martyn, Mao, and Bittner 2019).

The difficulties with using it lie in its biphasic elimination, its metabolism by CYP 3A4 isoenzymes (one of the isoforms of the cytochrome P450 system), its effect on the QTc interval, and its controversial equianalgesic dosing range. Because of methadone's initial distribution phase, if you are using it as the only opioid, the first loading usually requires that it be given every 4 to 6 hours (McPherson et al. 2019). But methadone has a second, extended phase lasting 36 to 60 hours, which causes drug levels to accumulate. By the fifth to sixth day of treatment, methadone usually needs to be taken only twice to three times a day to maintain analgesia and only once a day to prevent withdrawal.

After the first few days of methadone therapy, therefore, the dosing interval should be decreased to two or three times a day to minimize the chance of inducing sedation or respiratory depression. Alternatively, you can give the methadone three times a day from the start and use rescue opioids for a day or two until the methadone serum levels rise. If the rescue doses are effective, this is what I do, because the patient is less likely to be oversedated or develop respiratory depression in the third or fourth day of methadone therapy. (I discuss below how to rotate patients from another opioid to methadone.) Patients should be monitored carefully for side effects in the first 5–7 days, 10–14 days for elderly patients or those with liver disease. If the pain is inadequately relieved, the methadone doses can be increased after this period (McPherson et al. 2019).

Methadone interacts with inducers and inhibitors of the cytochrome P450 system (McCance-Katz, Sullivan, and Nallani 2010). Patients must be monitored when methadone and a drug that is also metabolized by CYP1A2, CYP3A4, and CYP2D6 are given together; CYP1A2 and CYP3A4 are induced by multiple drugs and other substances (e.g., cigarette smoke), and CYP2D6 has a genetic polymorphism. Once you stabilize patients on methadone, I'd suggest that you check for methadone drug interactions on a website (e.g., "Methadone Interactions," Drugs. com, www.drugs.com/drug-interactions/methadone.html) every time you start or discontinue one of these drugs. Drug levels can increase; methadone levels can increase or decrease; and there's no way to be sure unless you check.

For example, when patients are receiving methadone, drug levels of desipramine (or other tricyclic antidepressants) and zidovudine increase. Drugs that lower the levels of methadone include antiretrovirals, phenytoin (by 50 percent), phenobarbital, carbamazepine, rifampin, somatostatin, spironolactone, and risperidone, each of which has precipitated withdrawal symptoms (McCance-Katz, Sullivan, and Nallani 2010). Drugs that raise the serum methadone levels and that are commonly used in patients who have cancer include fluconazole, voriconazole, fluoxetine, and fluvoxamine. The SSRIs may raise methadone levels in CYP2D6 rapid metabolizers (McCance-Katz, Sullivan, and Nallani 2010). The SNRIs (e.g., venlafaxine) do not. Grapefruit juice and acute alcohol use can increase methadone levels; chronic alcohol use may decrease them.

Methadone also prolongs the QTc interval. Cancer patients on therapy often have metabolic abnormalities that also prolong the QTc, such as hypocalcemia from bisphosphonate or receptor activator of nuclear factor κβ ligand (RANK-L) inhibitors, or hypokalemia and hypomagnesemia from diarrhea, vomiting, or effects of the chemotherapy on the kidney. Every effort should be made, therefore, to normalize potassium, magnesium, and corrected calcium levels before assuming the QTc is too long to allow you to use methadone.

And you may even need to measure the QTc manually because the Bazett formula that electronic systems such as GE Healthcare MUSE use to measure the QTc overestimates it (Muluneh et al. 2019). Other correction methods such as the Framingham (QT + 0.154 × 1-RR interval) may provide a shorter and more accurate correction (Muluneh et al. 2019).

Patients who at baseline have a prolonged QTc interval, or who need high doses of methadone, have developed cardiac arrhythmias (*torsades de points*; polymorphic ventricular tachycardia) and even death as a result. Most of the reports of cardiac arrhythmia were in patients on a methadone maintenance program taking more than 300 mg a day; the cancer patients who developed problems were taking more than 600 mg of methadone per day (Reddy et al. 2010).

Only the very, very rare patient will require that high a dose of oral methadone. What is the risk for most patients taking methadone? Reddy and colleagues (2010) prospectively measured the QTc intervals of cancer patients at 2, 4, and 8 weeks after they began taking methadone. Twenty-eight percent of their patients had a prolonged QTc interval at baseline, due in 75 percent to reversible conditions such as medications or, more rarely, hypokalemia or hypocalcemia; only 25 percent had structural cardiac disease. The patients with a baseline QTc interval prolongation had a much greater chance of worsening the QTc than patients without initial QTc interval prolongation, but only 1 of the 28 patients developed a QTc of greater than 500 (it was 509), and that patient's baseline QTc interval was 498 msec.

At the 8-week point, the median QTc was 373, and the median dose of methadone was 28 mg per day; the doses of methadone never exceeded 100 mg per day, and no other patients developed a QTc greater than 500 msec. These findings suggest that with the usual doses of methadone (<100 mg/day), even in patients with underlying QTc interval prolongation, significant QTc prolongation does not occur. What monitoring schedule is needed for cancer patients receiving more than 100 mg methadone per day who are not placed on other agents that prolong the QTc interval is not clear (Gourevich 2009). McPherson et al. (2019) offer recommendations for the "level of vigilance" and recommended EKG monitoring (or not) for the most common clinical scenarios.

Methadone must be used with caution, or the QTc interval monitored, however, in anyone receiving intravenous methadone or for whom drugs are needed that also prolong the QTc interval. Intravenous methadone is stabilized with a preservative (chlorobutanol) that blocks potassium channels. If your patient develops a prolonged QTc interval when switched from oral to intravenous methadone, use the preservative-free methadone if it is available at your site (McPherson et al. 2019). Common drugs used in patients with cancer that prolong the QTc interval include the quinolone antibiotics (especially levofloxacin), typical and atypical antipsychotics (such as haloperidol and olanzapine), SSRIs (but not SNRIs), metoclopramide, and certain chemotherapy agents like epidermal growth factor receptor inhibitors and tamoxifen.

Other difficulties with using methadone lie in the controversy about its equianalgesic dosing range (Moryl, Coyle, and Foley 2008; Knotkova, Fine, and Portenoy 2009; McPherson et al. 2019). All suggest that the equianalgesic dose of morphine to methadone varies as the dose of morphine increases. The latest consensus statement (McPherson et al. 2019) recommendations are 10 mg oral morphine equivalents (OMEs): 1 mg methadone for patients receiving 60–199 mg OME and who are younger than 65, and 20 mg OME:1 mg methadone for patients taking ≥200 OME and/or patients older than 65 (see Practice Point: Conversion from Other Opioids to Methadone).

Practice Point: Conversion from Other Opioids to Methadone

<60 mg OME	2.5 mg oral methadone t.i.d.
60–199 mg OME and patient <65 yo	10:1 (10 mg OME:1mg methadone)
≥200 mg OME and/or patient >65 yo	20:1 (20 mg OME:1 mg methadone)

(McPherson et al. 2019)

Why do we need relatively so much less methadone for patients on higher doses of opioids? I'm not sure, but the way I think about it, patients taking high opioid doses have a large amount of pathologic destruction of their nerves (such as cancer patients with plexopathies). The constant firing of those damaged nerves may lead their spinal cords to generate the greater number of NMDA receptors we know these patients have. And we know that NMDA receptors inhibit the ability of opioids to prevent transmission of the pain signal. When we give the patient methadone, we do two things: the d-isomer of methadone (which is 50 percent of the drug we give the patient) inactivates the inhibitory activity of the NMDA receptors (Knotkova, Fine, and Portenoy 2009), leaving the opioid receptors able once again to be inhibited by opioids, and the l-isomer binds the opioid receptors. So we need much less methadone than we would expect.

Conversion to methadone. There is no one right way to convert patients to methadone. It takes at least three days to convert my patients to methadone, because it is going to take at least three days for the dose of methadone I give the patient on Day 1 to reach a steady state (i.e., after three half-lives). There will be higher blood levels of methadone on Day 2 than Day 1, and even higher levels on Day 3. I usually need to make the change to methadone in a patient with unrelieved neuropathic pain who is taking a great deal of short-acting rescue opioid, because the sustained-release opioid or the intravenous continuous infusion is not working. The rescue doses work, but only for a short time, and the amount of drug needed may cause myoclonus or other opioid neurotoxicities.

My goal is to load the patient slowly and safely with methadone, leaving the other opioids in place just long enough for the methadone levels to finally relieve the pain. I don't want to stop the *basal* opioids (sustained-release tablets or opioid continuous infusion) too soon, because the patient would be in more pain, relying solely on rescue dosing. In most cases, patients need less and less rescue medication each day as the methadone levels rise. I am able to taper off the old basal opioid over several days, so that by day three or four, patients are taking methadone as the new "basal" medication, along with p.r.n. doses of short-acting rescue medications. If you are beginning methadone in an outpatient, check in with them daily for the first week to assess and adjust medications as needed.

Josh

Josh, a 31-year-old fireman, had a refractory, recurrent sarcoma in his pelvis. He had severe neuropathic pain that was not responding to sustained-release oxycodone. Josh did not want to come into the hospital to have his pain more quickly controlled. His partner, Steven, was a nurse, and Steven promised to keep good records of all the medications Josh took, and to call daily to let me know their effect and any side effects. If Josh didn't have such a reliable and knowledgeable home caregiver, I would have insisted he be admitted to bring his pain under better control as we rotated him to methadone.

To calculate what dose of methadone to start with, I used the morphine:methadone ratios recommended by McPherson et al (2019) as shown in the Practice Points box above. Josh was taking 200 mg of sustained-release (SR) oxycodone every 8 hours (i.e., 600 mg/day), and he had taken an additional 300 mg in oxycodone rescue doses each day for the past several days (i.e., five doses of 60 mg each). I planned to convert only the SR oxycodone to methadone.

Step 1. Calculate the equianalgesic dose of oral morphine (the oral morphine equivalents—OMEs).

600 mg of oxycodone (200 mg × 3 doses) = 900 mg of oral morphine equivalents (20 mg of oxycodone = 30 mg of oral morphine).

Step 2. Identify the correct morphine:methadone ratio.

The ratio to choose for 900 mg of oral morphine is 20 mg of OME to 1 mg of oral methadone (e.g., ≥200 mg OME, use the 20:1 ratio).

Step 3. Calculate the 24-hour methadone dose.

900/20 = 45 mg.

Step 4. Be conservative; don't exceed 30 mg/day initially no matter what the initial OME is.

Start at 10 mg of methadone p.o. t.i.d. You'll still have the rescue dosing if this dose proves too low, and you can titrate up the methadone later in the week.

DAY 1. Josh's pain level is 10/10 and not acceptable.

Recommendation: 200 mg SR oxycodone every 8 hours, along with 10 mg of oral methadone every 8 hours and whatever rescue doses of 60 mg oxycodone every 4 hours he needs (he had the oral liquid concentrate of oxycodone at 20 mg/ml).

DAY 2. Josh needed only two rescue doses, each early in the previous day, and Steven said that he had slept through the night. His pain level is 6/10 and not acceptable.

Recommendation: Decrease SR oxycodone to 100 mg every 8 hours; continue the 10 mg of methadone every 8 hours and the rescue opioid dose of 60 mg oxycodone every 4 hours as needed.

DAY 3. Josh again used only two or three rescue doses; his pain level is now 4/10 and acceptable.

Recommendation: Stop all SR oxycodone and continue only the t.i.d. methadone and immediate-release oxycodone p.r.n.

DAY 4. Josh's pain level is still 4/10 and acceptable without any excessive sedation. He needed only two doses of p.r.n. oxycodone the day before. Josh has therefore been effectively and safely converted to oral methadone, with oral oxycodone for rescue.

If your starting dose is too high. If on Day 2, Josh's pain level had been a 3 and acceptable, I would have realized that the dose of methadone was too high for him, and that if I continued it, he would be asleep and possibly even have respiratory depression by Day 3. I would therefore have decreased the SR oxycodone by 50 percent and the methadone to 10 mg p.o. twice a day.

If your starting dose is too low. If Josh had needed 300 mg rescue oxycodone on Day 1, I wouldn't have decreased his SR dose Day 2, but would have continued to monitor the as-needed usage. I don't decrease the SR opioid until there is a significant decrease in the use of p.r.n. opioid. If Josh had still had 8/10 pain on Day 3 and was taking significant rescue doses, I would have increased his oral methadone dose and continued to monitor his pain levels and use of rescue medications.

When you first do these opioid rotations to methadone, it's wise to work with someone who has experience using the drug, such as an anesthesia pain or palliative care colleague, a hospice medical director, or a clinical pharmacist who works with a palliative care or hospice team. They can check your calculations, offer cautions about drugs the patient is on that can increase or decrease methadone levels, or the QTc interval, and help you know when to increase or decrease the methadone dose and the patient's other opioids.

Levorphanol. Levorphanol is much more expensive than methadone, but it has a shorter half-life (11–16 hours). Given this half-life, dose escalations should not be made more often than every 48 hours. Levorphanol does not prolong the QTc as methadone does, and it does not require CYP 450 metabolism (Pham, Fudin, and Raffa 2015). It does have an active metabolite that is renally cleared, so it should be used with caution in patients with renal insufficiency.

Four milligrams of levorphanol are equivalent to about 30 mg of morphine (Pham, Fudin, and Raffa 2015). Recommended conversion ratios of morphine to levorphanol are 12:1 for morphine doses <100mg/day; 15:1 for 100–300 mg/day; 20:1 for 301–600 mg/day; and 25:1 for >600 mg/day (McNulty 2007). As for all opioids, once you calculate the equianalgesic dose, decrease by one-third for incomplete cross-tolerance between opioids.

Buprenorphine. Buprenorphine is a semisynthetic thebaine derivative available in oral transmucosal tablets, films, and in transdermal patches. It is a mu agonist and a kappa receptor antagonist; it does not antagonize the pain-relieving effects of other opioids, and it helps prevent hyperalgesia (Martyn, Mao, and Bittner 2019). Effective plasma levels from the transdermal patch are reached within 12 to 24 hours, and the patch is replaced every 7 days. Some patients have end-dose failure, where it does not last all 7 days; they need to change it every 5 days. Buprenorphine may be used safely in patients with renal failure or who are on dialysis, but with caution in patients with hepatic failure.

Buprenorphine has many unique aspects that make it an excellent opioid for patients with moderate to severe cancer pain (see Practice Points: Buprenorphine vs. Other Opioids) (Davis 2012; Davis, Pasternak, and Behm 2018). It is safer for patients at risk of respiratory depression because when higher doses are needed for pain relief, analgesia improves, but respiratory depression does not occur. Unlike morphine or fentanyl, buprenorphine is not immunosuppressive, and it does not cause hypogonadism. Importantly, unlike methadone, it does not prolong the QTc at doses of <20 mcg/hr. In practice, I often use buprenorphine in older patients, those on very low doses of opioids, or for patients who have had significant side effects with even small doses of short-acting opioids. I also use it in patients with carcinomatosis who struggle with intestinal hypomotility.

Practice Points: Buprenorphine vs. Other Opioids

- Less sedation, euphoria, constipation, and respiratory depression than other opioids
- Not immunosuppressive
- Less or no hypogonadism
- No QTc prolongation at doses <20 mcg/hr

(Johnson, Fudala, and Payne 2005; Davis 2012; Davis, Pasternak, and Behm 2018)

Temporal aspects of the pain. To decide which formulation of the opioid to prescribe, consider whether the pain is continuous, intermittent, or both. Most patients whose cancer is far advanced have both types of pain. To treat the continuous pain, I usually prescribe either a fentanyl transdermal patch or an oral SR preparation of an opioid with a short half-life (i.e., morphine, oxycodone, hydromorphone, or oxymorphone) as the active agent. If the total daily opioid dose needed is <80 mg OME, I can prescribe a buprenorphine transdermal patch.

Oral sustained-release preparations are formulated in a matrix that dissolves in the gut and releases opioid over 8 to 24 hours, depending on the preparation. As of 2020, only transdermal fentanyl and oral SR morphine (as in MS Contin, Kadian, and Embeda-type morphine sulfate in an extended-release capsule with a sequestered core of naltrexone) were available in generic formulations. Kadian is effective for 12 to 24 hours and is available in 20-, 50-, and 100-mg capsules. Fentanyl patches are replaced every 48 to 72 hours; SR morphine can be taken every 8 to 12 hours. Levorphanol (Levo-Dromoran), because of its half-life, is dosed every 6 to 12 hours. OxyContin and Xtampza are the SR form of oxycodone and are taken every 12 hours. Exalgo is a SR form of hydromorphone that is taken daily. OpanaER is the SR form of oxymorphone that is taken twice a day. Butrans is the buprenorphine transdermal patch, changed every 7 days, though for some patients every 5 days.

More rarely, I use methadone, an opioid with a 24-hour half-life. Because of the multiple interactions with other agents, QTc prolongation potential, and the time it takes to titrate to effective pain relief, I generally choose methadone as the initial opioid only when there is a history of allergy to morphine, the patient's pain has a large neuropathic component, I need to give a long-acting preparation through a feeding tube (it comes in a liquid formulation), or I need to use the least expensive agent.

To treat intermittent pain or brief exacerbations of continuous pain, I prescribe a shorter-acting preparation of morphine, oxycodone, hydromorphone, or oxymorphone that can begin to provide relief in about 30 minutes to an hour. For opioid-tolerant patients whose insurance will pay for the medication, I might also prescribe as a rescue dose an immediate-acting preparation of oral transmucosal fentanyl citrate, which can begin to provide relief in as little as 10 minutes and can be helpful in severe incidental pain that occurs with movement. The transmucosal fentanyl preparations have been shown to be "non-inferior" to subcutaneous morphine to manage these episodes, and patients preferred them (Zecca et al. 2017). They might even prevent hospitalizations for pain exacerbations that would otherwise require parenteral opioids. But clinicians must enroll in a risk-reduction educational program, the TIRF (transmucosal immediate-release fentanyl) REMS (Risk Evaluation and Mitigation Strategy), to prescribe transmucosal fentanyl, as I review later in the chapter.

Routes of Administration

Once you have chosen an appropriate opioid, you need to decide the route by which it should be taken. Most patients will be able to use the oral route. Those with a feeding tube in place can receive medications through the tube. For cancer patients who cannot take medications using those routes, use the transmucosal, transdermal, rectal, intravenous, or subcutaneous route. Step 2 agents (which include oxycodone in fixed combinations with NSAIDs, tramadol, and tapentadol) are available only in oral formulations. Table 7.3 indicates which formulations are available for each of the step 3 opioids listed (including pure oxycodone).

Opioids should not be given intramuscularly for either short- or long-term management of cancer pain. The injections are painful, and since absorption of the opioid is variable, they lead to unpredictable blood concentrations of the analgesic and provide suboptimal pain relief.

Oral route. More than 90 percent of patients can achieve effective therapy with oral, transmucosal, or transdermal opioids. All the step 3 agents listed in Table 7.3 are available in oral formulations, various forms of transdermal fentanyl, as well as liquids or immediate- or SR tablets, pills, or capsules of other opioids. Patients with feeding tubes can safely use crushed tablets of methadone that dissolve completely in water, liquid methadone, or liquid immediate-release morphine, oxycodone, oxymorphone, or hydromorphone. Levorphanol powder can be mixed in liquid for feeding tubes.

Oral sustained-release agents for patients with feeding tubes or difficulty swallowing tablets. Most SR preparations of morphine and oxycodone are designed to provide pain relief for 8 to 12 hours, but they may cause serious side effects if they are cut or crushed, because the full 12-hour opioid dose will be absorbed in an hour or two. There are morphine and oxycodone formulations (Kadian and Xtampza, respectively) that consist of capsules containing polymer-coated SR pellets from which the morphine or oxycodone is released. Because of this novel formulation, the Kadian or Xtampza capsules can be opened and the pellets sprinkled on food or put into a liquid such as orange juice or water; Kadian and Xtampza can be placed into a 16 French or larger gastrostomy tube in 20 ml of liquid. Do not attempt to put the beads through smaller gastrostomy tubes or a nasogastric (NG) tube. Embeda (extended-release morphine with a sequestered core of naltrexone) should not be administered through NG tubes.

Oral agents for patients without feeding tubes but with difficulty swallowing large volumes of liquids or at risk of aspiration. Concentrated (20 mg/ml) morphine (e.g., Roxanol) or oxycodone solutions (e.g., Intensol), given sublingually or buccally, are helpful for these patients. The efficacy of these agents is due largely to their being swallowed and absorbed from the gastrointestinal tract in the same way that larger volumes are absorbed. Only about one-fifth of sublingual morphine solution or about one-third of sublingual methadone solution is absorbed, even when held under the tongue for 10 minutes (Weinberg et al. 1988).

Transmucosal agents. Several immediate-acting preparations of transmucosal fentanyl are now available in the United States. To be prescribed any form of transmucosal fentanyl, your patient must be taking the equivalent of 60 mg of oral morphine a day (see TIRF REMS, www.TIRFREMSaccess.com).

Transmucosal fentanyl. The original version was available in the form of an oral sweetened lozenge containing 200 to 1600 mg of fentanyl citrate, attached to a handle. The fentanyl is easily absorbed transmucosally; it is effective in 75 percent of patients, produces rapid pain relief (in 10 to 15 minutes), and is well tolerated. There is no evidence of decreased effectiveness of this agent over time (median duration of use, 79 days; range, 1 to 423 days). The disadvantage of this formulation (brand name Actiq, but now also available in generic forms) is that the patient must "paint" the lozenge for about 3 to 5 minutes on the buccal mucosa. If the lozenge is sucked on, and the fentanyl swallowed, two-thirds of it will be wasted.

Other forms include a sublingual tablet (Abstral), a buccal tablet (Fentora), a buccal film (Onsolis), and nasal sprays (Lazenda, which is available in the United States, and Instanyl and PecFent [Lyseng-Williamson 2011], which in 2020 were not). The tablets and films are rapidly absorbed from normally moist mucosa, but the tablets dissolve poorly in patients who have undergone radiation to the head and neck and are poorly tolerated in patients with mucositis. An excellent discussion of the comparable benefits of each of these forms was published in a comprehensive review of transmucosal fentanyl (Twycross et al. 2012).

To prescribe any of the forms, clinicians must enroll in a risk-reduction educational program, found at the TIRF REMS website (www.TIRFREMSaccess.com). When the medication is prescribed, the clinician must provide the patient with information on the product (also available at the website), and both the provider and the patient need to sign a consent form that must be faxed to the pharmacy. The lowest dose of the preparation must be prescribed first, but if that dose is not effective, the dose can be titrated. Since there is no relationship between the dose of the continuous baseline opioid the patient is taking and the dose of transmucosal fentanyl that will be effective (Knotkova, Fine, and Portenoy 2009), starting at the lowest dose is clinically reasonable. Although all transmucosal fentanyl preparations provide pain relief for only about an hour, they cannot be prescribed any more often than every 4 hours.

Transmucosal buprenorphine. Sublingual buprenorphine tablets and films can provide relief for mild to moderate pain but are approved only for treatment of patients with opioid-use disorder in the United States. A buccal version (Belbuca) is approved for the treatment of pain and is typically dosed twice daily. Patients may continue to use short-acting opioids for breakthrough pain.

Topical route. Topical opioids may act through opioid receptors of all classes that are present in peripheral nerve terminals of inflamed tissue. These receptors appear in normal tissue within minutes to hours of the onset of inflammation (Stein 1995). When the epidermis is eroded, such as in pressure ulcers or cutaneous metastatic tumors, the topical opioid can bind the receptors and produce local pain relief. The gel has to be placed on open skin because it has poor bioavailability over intact skin (Paice et al. 2008). Compounding pharmacies can add morphine to the IntraSite gel that is a standard treatment for stage II or III pressure ulcers. The gels are topically applied once to several times a day and covered with a standard dressing. Data demonstrating the efficacy of topical opioids are limited, but two randomized double-blind pilot studies support the use of topical morphine in treating patients with decubitus ulcers (Paice et al. 2008; Zeppetella, Paul, and Ribeiro 2003). The opioid-containing gels can provide equivalent or better relief of pain and cause fewer side effects than the higher doses of systemic opioids. Case reports suggest they are also useful for patients with open tumor infiltrates of the skin.

Transdermal route. Both fentanyl and buprenorphine are available as transdermal patches. Fentanyl patch doses range from 12 mcg/hr to 100 mcg/hr. Total fentanyl dose does not usually exceed 400 mcg/hr, which requires multiple patches to be placed.

In the United States, we have access to only the lower-dose buprenorphine patches (Butrans), of 5, 7.5, 10, 15, and 20 mcg/hr. The total daily dose should not exceed 20 mcg/hr because at this dose, the QTc can prolong by up to 9.2 msec; and you may have to limit use of other QTc prolonging agents. These low-dose buprenorphine patches are likely to help only patients with mild to moderate pain, needing <80 mg total oral morphine equivalents per day.

In Europe, patches are available in 35, 52.5, and 70 mcg/hr options. Effective plasma levels are reached within 12 to 24 hours; in the United States the patch is replaced every 5 to 7 days, but outside the United States, every 96 hours. In one randomized placebo-controlled trial, cancer patients who were receiving 90 to 150 mg/day of oral morphine equivalents were switched to a buprenorphine patch of 70 mcg/hr with satisfactory pain relief in 75 percent (Poulain et al. 2008). A consensus panel of European pain and palliative care experts concluded that transdermal buprenorphine was a valuable treatment for patients with chronic cancer pain (Pergolizzi et al. 2009; Davis 2012).

Both fentanyl and buprenorphine can be used without dose reduction in patients with renal failure. Fentanyl is metabolized by the CYP3A4 cytochrome system in the liver, and its plasma levels can rise, and patients can develop somnolence or respiratory depression if the fentanyl is used with other drugs that are also metabolized by CYP3A4, such as ketoconazole, fluconazole, diltiazem, erythromycin, or verapamil. For the same reason, pain may return if a patient has been stabilized on a fentanyl regimen while on one of these agents and that agent is discontinued.

Because fentanyl is very rapidly metabolized by the liver, at least 12 hours are required to build up enough drug in the skin reservoir to establish an adequate blood level. By 14 to 20 hours, an effective, stable plasma concentration is reached and, in most patients, is maintained for a total of 72 hours. New patches are usually applied every 72 hours, though as many as 25 percent of patients find they need to replace the patches every 48 hours.

For many patients with stable chronic pain, transdermal fentanyl patches are useful as the sustained-release component of their pain regimen. The patches are especially helpful for those who are unable to take oral medications, who cannot tolerate other opioids, or who simply prefer a patch to taking pills even once or twice a day. In a randomized crossover study of patients who expressed a preference, significantly more preferred the fentanyl patches over oral sustained-release morphine (Payne et al. 1998).

The patch is not the best choice for managing the chronic pain of some types of patients. Transdermal fentanyl is not recommended for patients under 18 years old who weigh less than 110 pounds. And though I have not seen any studies documenting this observation, I and many of the nurses with whom I work have noticed that cachectic patients seem to get less relief using the patch. The patch must be placed on the skin over an area of fat into which the drug can diffuse. Do not place them over edematous areas, bony prominences, or tattooed skin, since the drug cannot pass through water or ink. Since many hours are required to achieve a therapeutic drug level, the transdermal system is not indicated for someone with acute severe or excruciating pain. In these patients, an opioid drip using morphine, fentanyl, or hydromorphone is more appropriate.

The patch can also be problematic for patients who have recurrent bouts of fever and infection, even simple urinary tract infections. During fevers, more drug is absorbed from the skin reservoir into the bloodstream, and the patient may develop a fentanyl overdose. In addition, if the patient becomes acidotic during sepsis, more drug will be liberated from albumin-binding sites. This "free" drug can also cause significant toxicity.

If the patient develops symptoms of overdose, removing the patch will not stop delivery of fentanyl into the bloodstream. Fentanyl continues to pass into the vasculature from the fatty skin reservoir until it is empty. Twenty-four hours after the patch is removed, the amount of fentanyl in the reservoir has decreased by only 50 percent. These patients may require a low-dose naloxone drip until the remaining drug is metabolized. To avoid precipitating a withdrawal syndrome due to the naloxone, use just enough to restore adequate respiration but allow the patient to remain asleep.

Despite these limitations, for many patients the transdermal system is a useful way to deliver a steady dose of a potent opioid. It is usually well tolerated and effective for patients who are medically stable and whose pain medication requirements do not vary markedly from day to day.

Rectal route. The rectal route of opioid delivery is especially helpful in a patient at home who is suddenly, unexpectedly unable to take oral pain medication. It is preferable to intramuscular injections and will provide effective relief. Tramadol, codeine, morphine, hydromorphone, oxycodone, and methadone can all be given rectally. These drugs are available as commercially or custom-made suppositories, as custom-made gelatin capsules that enclose the oral long-acting formulation

---

Practice Points: Clinical Implications of the Transdermal Fentanyl Delivery System

- The fentanyl is deposited into a fat reservoir in the skin, from which it is absorbed. Rescue dosing is needed for 12 to 24 hours while the reservoir is accumulating fentanyl.
- Used alone, the patch is not an effective initial treatment for patients with severe pain.
- For patients with severe pain, short-acting drugs should be used to establish the opioid dose that relieves the pain; then a fentanyl patch of appropriate strength can be placed.
- Toxicity can result from increased absorption during febrile episodes.
- In cases of overdose, 50 percent of the fentanyl is still present in the skin reservoir 24 hours after the patch has been removed.
- Patch placement is very important. Fentanyl must be placed over an area of fatty tissue such as the upper outer arm or upper buttocks; it cannot "travel" to the fat through edema fluid; tattoos also impair its absorption.
- The patch must adhere to the skin to deliver the fentanyl effectively; patches are not useful in patients with drenching sweats or in whom the patch cannot be placed flat onto the skin.

(e.g., MS Contin), or as elixirs that can be given as microenemas (i.e., in less than 30 ml of liquid) (Davis et al. 2002) through a rectal Macy catheter if this is acceptable to the patient and family.

The sustained-release morphine preparations are as effective given rectally as orally, and the same or higher opioid blood levels are achieved after 24 hours (De Conno et al. 1995). Immediate-release oxycodone is absorbed generally in about 30 to 60 minutes and provides analgesia for 8 to 12 hours, though there is a great deal of variability from patient to patient (Leow, Cramond, and Smith 1995). Hospice nurses suggest that before patients have the sustained-release tablet inserted, they have a soapsuds enema to remove any stool from the rectal vault. The tablet is then placed in the lower part of the rectum. Hospice pharmacies can often prepare customized suppositories containing the oxycodone, methadone, or morphine the patient was previously receiving.

The venous drainage from the rectum flows into a mix of portal and systemic circulation. Since morphine and oxycodone are extensively metabolized by the liver, avoiding the portal system maximizes the active blood levels you can achieve per dose but minimizes the levels of hepatically created active metabolites such as M-6-G. Unfortunately, colostomies are drained solely by the portal system; opioids placed in colostomies have less than half the bioavailability of those placed in the rectum.

Although placing sustained-release morphine or oxycodone tablets into the rectal vault is not approved by the U.S. Food and Drug Administration (FDA), morphine delivered by this route has been extensively studied and is safe and effective. Doses of rectal SR morphine as high as 900 mg/day have been used.

Intravenous or subcutaneous routes. Patients with rapidly escalating pain, and those who are not getting relief from a transdermal patch, cannot swallow, do not have feeding tubes, or have a bowel obstruction, need to have the opioid delivered by the intravenous or subcutaneous route. Opioids can be given by either route continuously (to deal with the chronic portion of the patient's pain) and as bolus doses (to treat acute breakthrough pain).

Intravenous route. Intravenous opioids have the advantage of rapid action and easy dose adjustment. They can be given continuously, as IV boluses, or as patient-controlled analgesia (PCA) boluses alone or with a continuous opioid infusion.

You may be most familiar with PCA in the postoperative patient. These patients usually do not receive a continuous dose of opioid; they simply give themselves bolus doses as needed. The pump is programmed to regulate the amount of drug given and how often a patient can dose himself; it records both how often the patient asks for a dose and how much drug he actually receives. For example, the computer may record that the patient requested a bolus dose 12 times in an hour but received it only 4 times, because the device was set to deliver a bolus dose only every 15 minutes. It also records the total 24-hour quantity of opioid delivered.

PCA is also for cancer patients. If I admit someone in pain, I often use an intravenous route with a basal opioid infusion and the PCA option or nurse-administered IV bolus doses because I can escalate doses quickly and precisely. If the patient has been taking oral opioids at home but cannot take them now, I start the basal intravenous drip at an opioid dose equivalent to what I think she has been taking at home. If the patient is in pain at home because they are taking much less opioid than I prescribed, that quickly becomes apparent, and we lower the drip rate.

Patients using a PCA can give themselves bolus doses, as needed, every 10–15 minutes, and a nurse can administer extra boluses if needed. The nurse carefully monitors the patient for pain relief and, if the patient is using a PCA, reviews the computer record for the total number of milligrams used each shift. I use this information to increase the strength of the bolus whenever needed and, every 8 to 12 hours, to adjust the continuous-infusion dose (I explain this in detail later in the chapter).

When a PCA is not used, nurses can give opioid boluses every 2–3 hours as needed, and the opioid drip rate can be increased every 8–12 hours until the patient's pain is relieved. When the required opioid dose has been determined, I transition the patient from the intravenous opioid to an oral sustained-release or a transdermal opioid at an equivalent dose along with a rescue short-acting oral opioid.

Practice Points: Advantages of Intravenous Opioids

- Prompt dose escalation in medically unstable patients with moderate pain who cannot use oral medication
- Rapid, precise, safe dose escalation for rapid relief of severe or excruciating pain
- Patient-controlled analgesia option

For patients with severe or excruciating pain, there is really no safer way to achieve adequate opioid plasma levels quickly than to do an intravenous opioid titration with IV bolus doses based on how much opioid the patient is already taking (NCCN 2020). (Later in this chapter, I provide an example of how to do this titration.) A patient might present with severe pain due to widespread bone metastases causing a combination of somatic and neuropathic pain. After careful titration, these patients are often found to need morphine infusions of 5 mg/hr or more (or 0.5 mg of hydromorphone) to relieve their pain. An infusion of 5 mg of morphine per hour would translate into 120 mg of sustained-release oral morphine every 8 hours (Table 7.4); that is, 5 mg/hr × 24 hr = 120 mg IV/day; 120 mg × 3 = 360 mg oral morphine/day. Even in an opioid-naive patient, using the intravenous boluses, adding an intravenous infusion, and adjusting doses as needed, you will be able to reach 5 mg/hr in less than 24 hours. Using oral morphine alone, reaching a dose of 120 mg every 8 hours in an opioid-naive patient is likely to take much longer.

The intravenous route is also preferable for medically unstable patients who cannot use oral medications. For the reasons mentioned above, I would not prescribe the transdermal fentanyl patch initially in these patients. If a patient with good pain control while taking oral medications needs to be NPO for surgery, I prescribe an opioid drip at a dose equivalent to his oral dose, then place him back on his oral medication as soon as possible.

Rare patients will not be able to tolerate oral medication and will have either contraindications to transdermal fentanyl patches or inadequate adipose tissue. Some of these patients will be able to use subcutaneous infusions if they are part of a hospice program, but most use continuous intravenous infusions at home, through a portable PCA pump, because of the volume of medication needed or the toxicity associated with delivering the medication subcutaneously.

If a patient has been receiving oral medications or using a transdermal patch, you simply need to convert the 24-hour oral dose to an intravenous one using the techniques detailed later in the chapter (see also Table 7.4). Many of these patients will already have an implanted vascular access device (e.g., a catheter or port) through which they can receive the infusions. If not, the patient will need a PICC line (peripherally inserted central venous catheter) to receive the continuous opioid infusion. The catheters are easily maintained for 2 to 3 months.

Subcutaneous route. Some patients who cannot take oral medications and whose pain is unrelieved by transdermal fentanyl find subcutaneous opioid infusions effective. Ambulatory patients can use one of a variety of pumps that can provide both continuous infusion (for the chronic pain) and bolus medication (for breakthrough pains). This system is often used by hospices and prevents an unnecessary trip to obtain more permanent IV access, usually a PICC.

For the subcutaneous infusions, patients have a 27-gauge "butterfly," or Silastic, needle inserted subcutaneously, usually on the anterior chest wall or in the abdomen. The site is changed every 5 to 7 days to minimize skin irritation. Many patients or their families can insert the needles themselves. Local inflammation is common but rarely is severe enough to warrant discontinuing the infusion. If it is bothersome, the patient can try changing to a different opioid to reduce the concentration or volume of the infusion or to eliminate allergic reactions to preservatives or impurities in the preparation.

Morphine and hydromorphone (e.g., Dilaudid) are the most commonly used opioids in subcutaneous infusions. They are generally nonirritating and are well absorbed. You prescribe the same doses as for a continuous intravenous infusion. Methadone is less well tolerated subcutaneously and often induces a local reaction.

While most advanced-cancer patients need only the equivalent of 100 to 300 mg/day of oral morphine, about 10 percent will need much more. But even these very high doses can be delivered subcutaneously using an equivalent hydromorphone dose. One hydromorphone preparation (hydromorphone HP) delivers 10 mg/ml of hydromorphone, and 2 to 5 ml/hr is well tolerated subcutaneously. Using this preparation, you can easily deliver 30 mg/hr of hydromorphone with only 3 ml/hr of solution. This is the equivalent of 200 mg/hr of morphine, or 4800 mg/day of parenteral morphine. If necessary, the pharmacist can prepare even more highly concentrated solutions.

Spinal opioids (epidural, subarachnoid). Spinal delivery of opioids produces pain relief because the exogenous opioids bind to receptors for the natural opiates (e.g., enkephalins) already present in the spinal cord. Nerves containing endogenous opiate receptors are present in the same area of the spinal cord that contains the synapses between afferent neurons and spinal interneurons. When either endogenous opiates or exogenous opioids bind to those receptors, they prevent the spinal interneuron from transmitting the pain signal up the spinal cord to the thalamus and cerebral cortex. Since the cortex does not receive the pain signal, the person does not experience pain.

Because epidural opioids are delivered locally into the epidural space and diffuse into the spinal fluid around the cord, they are effective at one-tenth of the doses required for the same opioid given peripherally. Subarachnoid opioids delivered directly into the spinal fluid are effective at one-hundredth of the systemic doses. Even though spinal opioids are absorbed into systemic circulation, the side effects from these much lower doses are usually milder.

Practice Points: Advantages of Spinal Opioids

- Spinal opioids can treat refractory neuropathic pain resulting from injury to peripheral nerves.
- Opioids, anesthetics, alpha-adrenergic agents (e.g., clonidine), and other drugs are infused.
- Temporary infusions can be used to
  - help patients regain sensitivity to lower systemic opioid doses.
  - determine whether the epidural route provides effective pain relief. If so, a permanent catheter may be placed.
- Patient-controlled epidural and intrathecal analgesia are available.

Spinal opioids can be used alone or with anesthetics, alpha-adrenergic agents, or baclofen (for spasticity) to improve their efficacy or to minimize the opioid-induced side effects. They can be delivered via either temporary epidural catheters or permanent epidural or subarachnoid catheters. Patient-controlled epidural analgesia (PCEA) or intrathecal analgesia, by which patients self-administer a bolus of spinal opioid, are also available.

Implantable intrathecal drug delivery systems. A randomized trial comparing implantable intrathecal drug delivery systems (IDDS) with conventional medical management delivered by an expert pain team demonstrated some surprising findings (Smith et al. 2002, 2003). This trial enrolled 202 patients who were taking at least the equivalent of 200 mg of oral morphine a day and were unable to achieve satisfactory pain relief with standard therapy, even when managed by pain experts, or who were taking less than 200 mg oral morphine equivalent per day but were suffering intolerable side effects from what otherwise was satisfactory relief of their pain. If the conventional management was ineffective, an IDDS was offered. Significantly more of the patients given an IDDS had a greater than 20 percent reduction in their pain and in side effects related to the treatment (38 percent vs. 58 percent), particularly fatigue and sedation. These differences likely resulted from the lower systemic opioid doses required to control the pain. More unexpected, however, was that patients with IDDS lived longer! The patients were more alert, less fatigued, and in less pain, and perhaps they had increased mobility; all these may have contributed to the documented increase.

Anesthesiologists who specialize in pain management typically place and manage both temporary and permanent epidural and intrathecal infusions. I offer below a general overview of the use of these routes. More detailed discussions of the devices used, the insertion techniques, and the management of the catheters are provided in the articles and books listed in the bibliography online.

Indications. Spinal opioids benefit those patients whose neuropathic pain syndrome is not responding to systemic opioids, or who require such high systemic opioid doses that, despite the use of appropriate adjunctive agents, the side effects are intolerable.

Temporary infusions or boluses of epidural opioids are most commonly used to manage postoperative or obstetric pain. Temporary catheters are placed before surgery, and opioid solutions are given as a bolus or infused (e.g., Duramorph). The infusions or boluses are repeated as needed in the next several days, and the catheter is then removed.

Temporary opioid/anesthetic or opioid/alpha-adrenergic agent (such as clonidine [e.g., Duraclon]) infusions are used in a rare cancer patient to enable him to regain sensitivity to lower doses of systemic opioids. Even in these patients, systemic opioids usually are not stopped entirely, because many patients have pain in areas outside the areas treated by the spinal infusion. For example a patient might have chest wall pain from bone metastases eroding through the skin along with severe lower extremity pain from nerve plexus involvement. The spinal catheter alleviates the lower extremity pain, but systemic opioids are needed for the chest wall pain. The systemic opioid dose is usually much lower after an epidural or intrathecal infusion is begun. Close collaboration with your anesthesia pain consultant will ensure that this is done safely without pain exacerbations or opioid-induced toxicity. The spinal opioid infusion is considered a success if the dose of systemic opioid can be lowered enough that the associated side effects become tolerable.

Other patients, such as those with chest wall pain from infiltrating cancer such as mesothelioma, or bilateral severe neuropathic pelvic pain due to recurrent colorectal, bladder, or gynecologic cancers, receive temporary catheters to determine whether opioids and anesthetics given via the epidural or intrathecal route will provide satisfactory pain relief. If the temporary infusion reduces the patient's pain by at least 50 percent, she is considered a good candidate for insertion of an intrathecal pump. Much more rarely, a permanent epidural Port-a-cath, identical to the one used for intravenous infusions, is implanted subcutaneously in the skin of the abdominal wall, and its catheter is placed into the epidural space, instead of in the vascular space. The port is attached by a needle to an external pump that delivers the medication. It is difficult, however, to identify nursing services outside the hospital setting that can manage these devices or pharmacies that can provide the solutions necessary for the infusions.

Epidural versus intrathecal catheter placement. Anesthesia pain specialists can place permanent catheters in either the epidural or the intrathecal spaces. The choice of the totally implantable intrathecal pump over the epidural for a permanent catheter depends on the experience of the clinician, the needs and life expectancy of the patient, and the expertise of the home care teams. Extensive preoperative education of the patient and the family is required before any permanent catheter is inserted.

Intrathecal catheters connected to totally implanted pumps have several advantages over epidural catheters. Intrathecal opioids act more quickly and for a

---

Neuraxial Drug Delivery Systems

- Temporary (1 to 4 weeks): percutaneous epidural or intrathecal catheter
  - Taped to patient's back (for diagnostic infusions)
  - Tunneled 1 to 2 inches from insertion site (for therapy)
- Intermediate (1 to 2 months)
  - Tunneled epidural catheter attached to implanted injection port; patient almost always must be hospitalized
- Permanent (months to years): implanted intrathecal catheter
  - Attached to totally implanted programmable pump for intrathecal infusions; patient can be at home, in a facility, or in a hospital

---

longer time. In addition, only 10 percent as much opioid is needed because it is delivered into the spinal fluid, not the epidural space. Because of the lower opioid doses required, patients experience fewer systemic opioid-induced side effects. The implanted pumps require no maintenance, and their reservoirs require infrequent (usually monthly) drug refills.

Practice Points: Comparisons of Intrathecal (IT) and Epidural Catheters

Advantages of IT Catheters

- Smaller drug volume
- Fewer systemic side effects
- Lower incidence of fibrosis if used for 3 to 6 months
- Pump refills needed only monthly vs. weekly epidural cassette replacement
- No risk of needle from cassette to port being dislodged
- No home care services required

Disadvantages of IT Catheters

- Increased incidence of meningitis
- Cost of totally implanted system

Totally implanted pumps connected to intrathecal catheters are also considered when a patient is expected to live more than 3 months, because, over time, epidural catheters are more frequently obstructed by fibrosis. They are also indicated for patients who cannot tolerate the volume of epidural infusion that they would need for pain relief.

While the intrathecal site can be beneficial, it also has disadvantages. Though intrathecal catheters allow access to the spinal fluid for sampling, infections of intrathecal catheters can more easily induce meningitis. And their insertion requires a totally implantable delivery system with a subcutaneous infusion pump, which alone can cost more than $50,000.

Drugs used in spinal infusions. Morphine or hydromorphone are the opioids most commonly used in epidural and intrathecal infusions. They are hydrophilic drugs, not very lipid soluble, and take quite a while to diffuse across the meninges and into the cord. But they also remain in the cerebrospinal fluid (CSF) and are bound to the spinal cord opioid receptors for a long time. Because they migrate to other spinal segments, the spinal catheter does not have to be placed directly over the affected segment for the infusion to be effective.

More lipid-soluble opioids such as fentanyl or sufentanil are also used in spinal infusions. They are potent spinal analgesics, but because they don't migrate in the CSF, their effectiveness depends on precise catheter placement.

Local anesthetics (e.g., bupivacaine), alpha-adrenergic agonists (e.g., clonidine), and baclofen (e.g., Lioresal) are also given by spinal infusion. Infused alone or added to opioid solutions, bupivacaine and clonidine can provide pain relief for patients who do not get relief from opioids alone, and they can minimize the side effects of the opioids by decreasing the doses needed for pain relief. Bupivacaine is the most commonly used anesthetic agent; the starting dose of intrathecal bupivacaine is 3 mg/day, and it is escalated as needed. Rarely, epidural infusions of 0.125 to 0.150 percent bupivacaine cause sensory or motor impairment. Baclofen is effective in relieving neuropathic pain and spasticity, with few associated side effects compared with oral administration. Doses used are 100 to 1,000 times less than oral doses. More rarely, somatostatin, octreotide, calcitonin, ketamine, or midazolam are infused.

Side effects of spinal opioids and anesthetics. Opioid-naive patients who receive epidural opioids for pain relief after surgery experience pruritus, nausea, vomiting, urinary retention, constipation, and more rarely, respiratory depression. The vast majority of cancer patients requiring spinal opioids, however, are not opioid-naive, and they rarely develop these side effects. If they do, small doses of naloxone (a 40-µg bolus followed by a continuous infusion starting at 5 µg/kg/hr) can reverse the side effects without eliminating analgesia. Compared with the opioid-naive patient with nonmalignant pain, cancer patients may require much higher spinal opioid doses. As these doses are absorbed into the circulation, the patient may become sedated. Very high intrathecal opioid doses can cause the patient to develop myoclonic jerking.

The side effects caused by anesthetics used intraspinally are due to the sympathetic blockade they induce as well as their systemic absorption. Depending on the location of the catheter, patients may become hypotensive initially, so they are usually given concomitant intravenous fluids when the infusion is begun. In

> ## Practice Points: Side Effects and Drug- and Catheter-Related Complications of Neuraxial Infusions
>
> - Pruritus, nausea, vomiting, and urinary retention are rare in patients already taking systemic opioids.
> - Depending on the dose infused, patients may have typical opioid-related side effects.
> - Anesthetic or clonidine may induce hypotension.
> - Placement-related complications include superficial bleeding (or, very rarely, hematomas compromising the cord or the cauda equina), abdominal or retroperitoneal organ or lung perforation, nerve root damage, seromas, postspinal headache in up to 20 percent of patients receiving subarachnoid catheters.
> - Catheters become dislodged, tear, kink, or become plugged by fibrosis or catheter-related granulomas.
> - Patients may underdose or overdose as a result of errors in refilling or programming.
> - CNS or skin infection may occur.

animal studies, bupivacaine caused both systemic and local toxicities, including seizures, cauda equina syndrome, and impaired sensation. In clinical trials, although patients might experience dose-dependent local toxicities, systemic effects were rarely seen, possibly because the bupivacaine is so highly protein bound. The neurologic side effects are not reported for bupivacaine doses of less than 25 mg/24 hr (Du Pen et al. 1992).

Catheter-induced complications. The most common complications of spinal infusions arise during catheter implantation or from the catheters themselves. Permanent catheters are inserted following administration of local anesthesia and tunneled subcutaneously to an implanted injection port or pump. During implantation, bleeding can occur superficially or, very rarely, in the epidural space, where it can cause an epidural hematoma, spinal cord compression, or a cauda equina syndrome that may require emergency neurosurgery. Other surgery-associated problems include perforation of an abdominal or retroperitoneal viscus or lung by the tunneling needle, or damage to nerve roots or the cord by the needle or the catheter itself. Patients may also develop pump pocket seromas, which usually require no specific therapy.

Catheters can dislodge, kink, or tear. Epidural catheters can also cause epidural fibrosis when in place for several months, which occasionally leads to cord compression. The fibrosis can also restrict the migration of the drug and decrease its efficacy. Catheters may even have to be repositioned.

Fibrosis is not a problem with catheters in the intrathecal space, but there can be catheter-associated granulomas. Postspinal headache due to CSF leaks occurs in up to 20 percent of patients who have intrathecal catheters inserted. If the headaches persist, epidural blood patching is necessary.

Other complications. Errors in refilling or programming the continuous-infusion pumps can lead to serious or even life-threatening complications. Anesthesia pain specialists minimize this risk by ensuring that only properly trained individuals perform these tasks and that they check their work meticulously. If an error is discovered that might cause an overdose, the patient is immediately hospitalized for observation and treated symptomatically (e.g., naloxone for respiratory depression, anticonvulsants for seizures). Underdosing due to kinks or other problems with the catheter or the infusion pumps or mixtures can result in recurrence of severe pain.

With very long-term use, patients can develop impotence (reversible with testosterone), amenorrhea, and other endocrine abnormalities. Edema of the hands and feet also occurs and is only partially responsive to elevation and diuretics.

Infection is the most serious complication. Implanted epidural catheters have an infection incidence of 8 percent, but the infection is usually limited to the skin around the injection port and the subcutaneous track of the catheter. If the injection port and catheter are removed promptly, the infection rarely progresses to an epidural abscess.

Contraindications. Certain medical and social situations preclude the use of spinal opioids. Patients with bleeding diatheses or active septicemia cannot have the catheters placed. Diabetics and immunocompromised patients have higher rates of septicemia, but these are not absolute contraindications. Epidural metastases can lead to CSF obstruction, but catheters can be placed rostral to the obstructing lesions.

As with continuous-infusion opioid therapy at home, cost and maintenance issues must be addressed. Will the patient or family be able to travel to the clinic for pump refills? Are clinicians and home care services available to refill the implanted pumps at home?

Caring for patients receiving spinal opioids. Anesthesia pain specialists along with their specially trained nurses and home care service nurses care for patients with spinal catheters and implanted pumps both as inpatients and as outpatients. They work with the patients' families and with the home care and hospice services that are helping patients and their families maintain the pumps at home.

Summary. Spinal infusions add significantly to the quality of life of those rare patients who need them. I have seen patients with severe thoracic, bilateral lower abdominal, or pelvic pain, who are unable to tolerate systemic therapy or are continuing to feel intolerable pain, experience a marked improvement in their day-to-day existence while receiving an infusion of a spinal opioid/anesthetic, with or without clonidine. I urge you not to hesitate in referring patients who might benefit from this treatment to anesthesia pain specialists.

PREVENTING AND RELIEVING SIDE EFFECTS OF OPIOIDS

For many patients, especially older ones, it is not enough that opioids relieve their pain. More than 75 percent of patients are concerned that if they take opioids, they will develop constipation, nausea, drowsiness, confusion, or manifestations of delirium such as nightmares and hallucinations. Even side effects that seem minor to us can persuade patients that these drugs are not for them, so side effects must be prevented whenever possible and treated aggressively if they occur.

Constipation

Constipation is the most common side effect of opioid therapy, occurring in almost everyone who takes opioids, even in those with colostomies. In my experience, the only exceptions are patients with total gastrectomies or those with gastric or jejunal feeding tubes, whose diet consists mainly or entirely of liquid enteral nutrition. And opioid-induced constipation absorbs significant health care resources: cancer patients with opioid-induced constipation are more than twice as likely to be hospitalized as are patients on opioids who are not constipated. The adjusted health care costs are more than $20,000 a year higher (Fine et al. 2019).

> **Searching for a Natural Solution**
>
> Mr. Samuels, a former longshoreman, was suffering from recurrent colon cancer that invaded his sacrum. As you can imagine, his pain was excruciating, and we hospitalized him to bring it under control as quickly as possible. After a few days of escalating doses of intravenous morphine, he told us that his pain control was satisfactory. We switched him to the equivalent dose of an oral sustained-release preparation, which, in his case, was 60 mg of SR morphine every 8 hours, and discharged him.
>
> When we saw him a week later, his pain was again excruciating. He told us that he didn't like the "artificial laxative" we had prescribed (lactulose syrup), and therefore he did not take any of it. When he became constipated, he quite accurately attributed his constipation to the opioids, and he stopped taking them as well. He said he preferred the pain to being constipated—that a daily bowel movement was important to him. It was only when we discussed the fact that a more "natural" laxative was available, and he purchased some senna from a health food store, that he agreed to resume his opioids.

Even patients taking step 2 opioids develop constipation. In one hospice study (Bruera et al. 1994), for example, 40 percent of those not receiving opioids, 63 percent of those on step 2 opioids, and 87 percent of those taking step 3 opioids required laxative therapy. Unfortunately, constipation is one side effect that usually does not diminish with time. The gut does not accommodate or return to its normal pattern. Guidelines strongly recommend, therefore, that you prescribe routine, not as needed, stool softeners and laxatives for any patient beginning opioid therapy (NCCN 2020; Fallon et al. 2018).

Several factors may contribute to constipation in cancer patients with pain. Inactivity, lack of a private place to defecate, poor food or fluid intake, hypercalcemia and hypokalemia, peritoneal studding with cancer, bowel obstruction, as well as damage to the spinal cord, cauda equina, or peroneal nerve plexus can induce constipation even in patients not receiving opioid pain medications. So can a number of drugs, including anticholinergics, calcium-containing antacids, calcium channel blockers, diuretics, opioid adjuvant agents such as tricyclic antidepressants and phenothiazines, octreotide, and serotonin antagonists used as antiemetics (e.g., ondansetron).

The type of opioid may also be a factor, though this is controversial. In two systemic reviews, however, transdermal fentanyl was less constipating than oral sustained-release morphine (Tassinari et al. 2008, 2009). Buprenorphine also induces less constipation than many other mu-agonist opioids (Davis 2012).

Unfortunately, the lifestyle changes and medications we normally recommend to patients with constipation who are not taking opioids are not likely to be effective for patients who need opioids. Increased water intake, increased activity, insoluble fiber therapies (e.g., Metamucil), or disodium disuccinyl docusate (e.g., Colace) are generally fine for people who are constipated and not taking opioids but won't work for patients who are taking opioids. Insoluble fiber is likely to exacerbate the problem. Even if the patient can take the amount of water needed and gets some exercise, the slowed intestinal transit time makes insoluble fiber therapy ineffective in facilitating bowel movements. And patients often feel bloated or full, further impairing what may be an already diminished appetite.

Mechanism. The difference lies in the effect of the opioids on intestinal motility (Walters and Montagnini 2010). The bowel normally empties through coordinated waves of peristaltic movements that are more frequent in the first half of the day. Inactivity itself reduces these waves and increases the colonic transit time from the normal 2 to 3 days to between 4 and 12 days.

In contrast, the bowel of a patient on opioids is in a state of muscle *fibrillation*; the intestinal muscles are unable to produce the normal coordinated peristalsis, colonic mucosal secretions are decreased, and colonic transit time and the time for water to be reabsorbed from the stool are prolonged. Although the gut has opiate receptors, it is unlikely that these effects are due entirely to the local receptors. Patients taking parenteral opioids also suffer from constipation, and switching from oral to parenteral opioids does not reverse the problem. In addition, opioids increase the tone and decrease the sensitivity of the anorectal sphincter to the presence of stool, which then does not relax appropriately. This side effect further predisposes older patients, who already have decreased sphincter sensitivity, to opioid-induced constipation.

> ## Practice Points: Treating Opioid-Related Constipation
>
> - All patients taking step 2 or 3 opioids need routine (not p.r.n.) prophylactic laxatives.
> - Discontinue insoluble fiber (e.g., Metamucil).
> - Give osmotic agents (e.g., polyethylene glycol) or agents that stimulate the myenteric plexus (e.g., senna). Reserve lactulose for lactose-tolerant patients.
> - Increase the laxative dose as the opioid dose increases.
> - Consider changing the opioid to buprenorphine.
> - In patients taking opioids without laxatives, diarrhea or urinary incontinence suggests impaction.
> - Opioid bowel syndrome may respond to motility agents (e.g., metoclopramide) or to peripheral-acting opioid antagonists (naloxegol, naldemedine, or methylnaltrexone).
> - If the syndrome does not respond to motility agents, methylphenidate and clonidine can prevent withdrawal while the opioid dose is lowered.

Therapy. Multiple bowel regimens have been published, but none has been studied in a controlled fashion. (Sources for a number of these are provided in the online bibliography.) Table 7.5 indicates the drugs most commonly used to prevent or treat constipation, along with their mechanism of action, recommended doses, and frequency of administration.

Agents that stimulate the myenteric nerve plexus, such as senna (e.g., Senokot) and bisacodyl (e.g., Dulcolax), and osmotic agents, such as magnesium hydroxide (e.g., Milk of Magnesia), magnesium citrate, lactulose/sorbitol, and polyethylene glycol (e.g., Miralax), are the most effective agents. Senna is usually given at a starting dose of two tablets twice a day and can be increased to three to four tablets two or three times a day as needed. Bisacodyl is started at two tablets at bedtime, to be repeated in the morning if necessary. It can be increased to two to three tablets two or three times a day if needed and is also effective in the form of a 10-mg suppository daily as needed. A newer agent, prucalopride, is a selective agonist of the 5HT4 receptor, which stimulates colonic motility. It has moderate effect for cancer-related, non-opioid-induced constipation (Ginex et al. 2020).

Lactulose is given at much lower doses than are needed for patients with hepatic encephalopathy. It is effective at 15 to 30 ml at bedtime but can be increased to 60 ml every 6 hours as needed. Lactulose, however, can cause excessive gas and cramping in the many patients we see who are lactose deficient (Teuri, Vapaatalo, and Korpela 1999). Other patients become lactose deficient during therapy, when chemotherapy agents denude their gastrointestinal mucosa. Should those patients become constipated because of opioids, I would use polyethylene glycol (e.g., Miralax), instead of lactulose, starting at 17 g in 4 to 8 oz of liquid once a day. All the stimulants are of course contraindicated in patients with bowel obstruction.

Newer agents add water to the gut by increasing the activity of guanylate cyclase-C enzyme (plecanatide/linaclotide) or blocking the chloride channel (lubiprostone). They are effective for patients on opioids who do not have cancer, but they have not been tested in cancer patients with opioid-induced constipation (Webster et al. 2018; Miner et al. 2017).

Naldemedine is an oral peripherally acting mu-opioid receptor antagonist that is effective for opioid-induced constipation in patients with cancer, though it can induce diarrhea. It does not cross the blood-brain barrier and so does not cause recurrence of pain or opioid withdrawal symptoms (Blair 2019). Naloxegol is also a peripheral mu-opioid antagonist. Although it is not yet approved in the United States for patients with cancer pain being treated with opioids (Jones, Prommer, and Backstedt 2016), insurance will often agree to pay for this in patients with cancer who cannot stool normally despite multiple laxatives. Naldemedine and naloxegol are both less expensive than methylnaltrexone (discussed below). When a patient requires three or more bowel agents to counteract opioid-induced constipation, I typically consider a trial of a peripheral mu-opioid antagonist if insurance will cover this.

Patients on opioids who have extensive peritoneal carcinomatosis, longstanding diabetes mellitus, or had problematic constipation in the past may remain constipated despite all these measures. Methylnaltrexone is designed for these patients. Methylnaltrexone is a peripheral opioid receptor antagonist that, unlike naloxone, does not cross the blood-brain barrier. It reverses opioid-induced constipation in about 50 percent of patients, works within 1 to 2 hours, and causes no increased pain or evidence of opioid withdrawal, although it can cause cramping as the bowels "wake up" (Table 7.5) (Becker and Blum 2009; Chamberlain et al. 2009; McNicol et al. 2008; Portenoy et al. 2008). To minimize the chance of bowel perforation, ensure that the lower bowel is emptied with suppositories and/or enemas before giving the methylnaltrexone.

General recommendations to prevent and treat opioid-induced constipation. I have found a combination of senna and an osmotic agent (sorbitol or polyethylene glycol) to be effective and well tolerated by patients on opioids. When you first prescribe tramadol or even a low dose of opioid, also prescribe a bedtime laxative, such as one or two senna tablets per day. Explain to patients that to maintain regular bowel movements, they must take the laxatives daily, even if they have had a bowel movement that day.

Patients taking step 3 opioids, such as sustained-release morphine or oxycodone or transdermal fentanyl, may need as many as six senna tablets in divided doses, along with a bedtime osmotic agent as needed (e.g., 17 g of polyethylene glycol). As mentioned above, polyethylene glycol is likely to have fewer side effects than lactulose, and it is more effective for patients with chronic constipation

---

Practice Points: Laxative Escalation

- Initial regimen:
  - Senna (e.g., Senokot) ± polyethylene glycol p.r.n. h.s. if no stool in 48h
  - or
  - Bisacodyl h.s. ± polyethylene glycol
- If ineffective:
  - Escalate doses of initial agents (e.g., two senna tablets b.i.d. or t.i.d. plus 17 to 34 g of polyethylene glycol, or 30 to 60 ml of lactulose in lactose-tolerant patients).
- If patient is obstipated:
  - Add Milk of Magnesia + mineral oil or magnesium citrate
  - or
  - Increase lactulose up to 60 ml q.i.d. or increase dose of polyethylene glycol.
- Consider adding plecanatide/linaclotide or lubiprostone (not tested in cancer patients) to increase water in the stool.
- Consider adding prucalopride to enhance colonic motility.
- Use oral naloxegol (not tested in cancer patients) or naldemedine or methyl-naltrexone SQ for patients whose opioid-induced constipation remains refractory.
- If patient is impacted, prior to using stimulants, osmotics, or methylnaltrexone:
  - Lubricate rectum, disimpact, and give enemas until clear.
  - Then institute appropriately aggressive prophylactic regimen.

(Lee-Robichaud et al. 2010). Generally, the more opioid, the more laxative a patient needs. The goal is for patients to have one soft, unforced bowel movement every one or two days.

If a patient becomes obstipated, you may need to add magnesium hydroxide (e.g., Milk of Magnesia) (30 to 60 ml) plus mineral oil (15 to 30 ml) daily or twice a day, magnesium citrate (8 oz), or enemas, as well as adding a dose of lactulose (30 to 60 ml), but these agents are less well tolerated and are not usually needed as part of a routine regimen. You can try adding plecanatide/linaclotide or lubiprostone to increase water in the gut, but they have not been tested in cancer patients. You can also increase the polyethylene glycol to two to four times a day. For paraplegic patients, 34 grams of it in 8 oz of water two to three times a day is usually effective, along with a daily suppository for local stimulation. For patients with opioid-induced constipation that is refractory to all these measures, consider adding oral naloxegol (not tested in cancer patients), naldemedine, or SQ methylnaltrexone.

Impaction. Fecal impactions can occur when patients on opioids are not prescribed a laxative or do not take one. Older patients, especially those who are confused, are particularly susceptible to this problem because their decreased rectal sphincter sensitivity allows a large mass of stool to accumulate in the rectum. These impactions may be difficult to diagnose because patients and their families may not be aware of them. Rather than complain of constipation, the patient may instead complain of symptoms caused by the pressure of the fecal mass, or urinary incontinence or diarrhea, which is actually stool passing around the impaction through a sphincter that has·become incompetent.

Since 90 percent of impactions occur in the rectum, they are easily diagnosed by digital rectal examination. They are readily treated by lubricating the rectum and doing a manual disimpaction, followed by saline rectal lavage or enemas. Glycerin suppositories or mineral oil enemas may be required to soften the impaction. After the impaction is cleared, you can institute one of the prophylactic regimens outlined above.

Opioid bowel syndrome. A very small minority of patients develop so-called opioid bowel syndrome. Unlike impaction, this syndrome is caused by a functional, not a mechanical, bowel obstruction. Patients on opioids who develop this syndrome experience nausea, vomiting, abdominal distention, and mild abdominal pain. The pain will exacerbate if higher opioid doses are used to treat it.

If there is no mechanical bowel obstruction, you will often be able to reverse the syndrome with an agent that increases bowel motility, such as metoclopramide (e.g., Reglan) orally or intravenously, or agents that reverse the opioid receptor binding, such as oral naloxegol or naldemedine, or SQ methylnaltrexone.

On occasion I have found that the syndrome would not reverse until I lowered the dose or even totally discontinued the opioid. If you must lower the opioid to less than 25 percent of the previous dose, you will need to prevent opioid withdrawal. Withdrawal symptoms after chronic opioid use are mediated in part by increased activity of noradrenergic neurons, which can be blocked by clonidine or lofexidine. Clonidine has been successfully used at 0.1 to 0.2 mg (p.o.) every 4 hours for patients who use heroin, tapered after Day 3 for a total of ten days. Cancer patients may be treated with a clonidine patch, 0.1 to 0.2 mg/24 hr. If insomnia or muscle cramps appear, chlordiazepoxide is recommended. Lofexidine, 0.2 mg titrated up to 1.2 mg twice daily, can also be used (Kosten and O'Connor 2003). A palliative care consultant or hospice medical director can help you control the patient's pain with adjuvant agents, such as ketamine, at lower doses of opioids.

Nausea

Nausea is also a common side effect of certain opioid agents. If no antiemetics are given, one-half to two-thirds of patients who take oral codeine or morphine for the first time will develop nausea or vomiting. These patients may mistakenly think that they are allergic to the opioid. If you don't warn them about this side effect, you may not be able to convince them to continue taking these agents, even if they have been effective in relieving their pain.

Practice Points: Treating Nausea in Patients Taking Opioids

- Eliminate other contributing factors (constipation, gastritis, peptic ulcer disease, gastric outlet or bowel obstruction, hypercalcemia, hyponatremia, hepatic or renal failure, CNS disease).
- Warn opioid-naive patients about transient nausea or prescribe a prophylactic antiemetic.
- Consider lowering the opioid dose for patients who develop nausea after receiving other treatments that eliminate or diminish the painful condition (e.g., radiation therapy).
- Give a different opioid agent.
- Add neuroleptics (e.g., prochlorperazine, haloperidol, olanzapine) for patients with nausea and vomiting.
- If prochlorperazine is not effective, discontinue and replace with ondansetron.
- Consider a gastric motility agent (e.g., metoclopramide) for patients with nausea, vomiting, early satiety, or bloating after eating.
- Give antivertigo agents (e.g., meclizine) if nausea is induced by movement.

To prevent nausea in opioid-naive patients, consider adding prophylactic prochlorperazine (e.g., Compazine) (10 mg p.o. t.i.d. or q.i.d.) or warning patients and their families that nausea may develop, that it is likely to last only a few days, and that you can relieve it with prochlorperazine. Some patients require as much as a week of antiemetic therapy, but most patients do not experience nausea for more than seven days despite continued opioid therapy.

If patients taking opioids develop nausea later in the course of their treatment, other etiologies must be eliminated. Other common causes of nausea in cancer patients include chemotherapy, radiation therapy, constipation, gastritis or gastric ulcer disease, gastric outlet or bowel obstruction, hypercalcemia, hyponatremia, hepatic or renal failure, or disease of the CNS. If the nausea is due to one of these problems, it will usually be relieved if you can eliminate the cause. Constipation, for example, is a common, easily reversible cause of nausea in these patients.

If none of these problems is present, late-developing nausea in a patient taking opioids may be an indication that the patient's pain is diminishing, and his opioid dose should be lowered. Consider, for example, a patient who is receiving radiation therapy for a painful bony metastasis and has been taking an opioid to relieve the pain until the radiation takes effect. Weeks later, although the pain from the metastasis has diminished significantly, the patient is still taking the same opioid dose and, as a result, develops nausea. In such a case, simply lower the dose of the opioid agent. The nausea usually disappears promptly, and the pain relief remains satisfactory.

Other patients being treated with opioids will develop nausea as they begin to take a higher dose of opioid to treat an increased intensity of pain. In these cases, if you substitute a different opioid agent, the nausea often disappears. If the patient has been receiving morphine, for example, substitute an equianalgesic dose of hydromorphone (e.g., Dilaudid) or fentanyl.

Therapy. If none of the maneuvers described above is effective, try to determine the mechanism by which the opioid is producing nausea and use the agent(s) most efficacious in reversing the problem (see Table 7.6). Treatment of chemotherapy- and radiotherapy-induced nausea is reviewed in Chapter 10.

Patients who have nausea without vomiting are likely suffering because opioids stimulate the chemoreceptor trigger zone in the medulla (the area in the brain that is responsible for chemotherapy-induced nausea), which activates the vomiting center there. These patients may benefit from neuroleptics such as haloperidol (1 to 2 mg p.o. every 8 to 12 hours or 0.5 to 1 mg parenterally every 8 to 12 hours), prochlorperazine (10 mg p.o. t.i.d. to q.i.d. or 25 mg p.r. every 12 hours), or olanzapine (Zyprexa, Zydis) (2.5 to 5 mg p.o./SL/IV daily, b.i.d. to q.i.d.), which block the transmission of the signal to the medulla's vomiting center. The 5HT3 receptor inhibitors like ondansetron (e.g. Zofran) are effective in chemotherapy- or radiotherapy-induced nausea and are often efficacious in any type of opioid-induced nausea (4 to 8 mg p.o./SL or IV b.i.d. or t.i.d.).

Delayed gastric emptying is another likely cause. Metoclopramide, with its dual sites of activity (blocking the chemoreceptor trigger zone and enhancing gastric emptying), is the agent of choice for these patients. Metoclopramide is effective even in low doses (5 to 10 mg p.o. or IV b.i.d. to q.i.d. or 1 to 3 mg/hr IV). It can also be given rectally at the oral dose, either by suppository (if available) or through rectal administration of the tablets or liquid drug.

Corticosteroids, also effective in chemotherapy-induced emesis, and mirtazapine, which has antiemetic properties, have not been studied in the treatment of opioid-induced nausea, but an empirical trial is warranted in patients who are refractory to other therapies.

Patients taking opioids who complain of nausea along with movement-induced vertigo usually benefit from agents such as scopolamine (transdermal patch or 0.3 mg t.i.d. p.o. or SQ) or meclizine (Bonine, Antivert) (25 mg t.i.d. p.o.).

Sedation

Sedation can be an important dose-limiting side effect in patients taking opioids. It can lead patients to limit the opioids they will take, even though their pain remains uncontrolled. Like nausea, sedation is most prominent when the patient first begins taking opioids and lessens within a few days, even if the dose remains the same. Studies have shown that, after the first 2 weeks of patients taking sustained-release opioids, no psychomotor impairment remains.

Practice Points: Minimizing Sedation

- Evidence about safety of driving while taking any opioids is inconclusive.
- Don't mistake "catch-up" sleep for oversedation.
- Give sustained-release agents for baseline pain control, immediate- or short-acting agents for exacerbations.
- When possible, eliminate contributing factors (e.g., medical causes or medications).
- Change the opioid dose or agent.
- Add a psychostimulant (e.g., methylphenidate).
- Consider referral to an anesthesia pain specialist.

Driving on opioids. Is it safe for patients to drive as long as they do not take immediate-release opioids sooner than 6 hours before the time they are planning to drive? The evidence is inconclusive (Pergolizzi et al. 2018). A 2012 systematic review was not able to conclude whether patients on opioids are able to drive without impairment (Mailis-Gagnon et al. 2012), and results of single studies were similarly inconclusive (Pergolizzi et al. 2018).

Evidence on cognitive impairment is also inconclusive. In one study, about one-third of cancer patients on opioids had possible or definite cognitive impairments. The largest risk factor was a very high opioid daily dose. Patients taking 400 mg or more of oral morphine equivalents daily had a 1.75 times higher chance of having cognitive impairment (as measured by the Mini Mental State Examination score <27) than those taking daily equivalent doses of 80 mg or less (Kurita et al. 2011). No opioid was more or less problematic than another. Other risk factors for patients on opioids included older age, poorer Karnofsky Performance status, less than 15 months since cancer diagnosis, and no breakthrough pain. The lack of breakthrough pain leads me to wonder whether the baseline opioid dose these patients were taking was a little too high, and whether that contributed to their cognitive problems.

In some states, patients taking opioids as prescribed may still be charged with "Driving Under the Influence" if the drugs are detected, even if they showed no evidence of impairment when stopped (Pergolizzi et al. 2018). Given that the states vary in their regulations about driving while taking any form of opioid for any length of time, it is important to caution your patients about their potential risk should they choose to drive or operate other motorized vehicles, the nature of the tests that are likely to be done, and what the legal outcomes are likely to be. Clearly document that you have counseled them not to drive (Pergolizzi et al. 2018).

In some patients, what may look like excessive sleepiness is simply a natural effect of pain relief in someone who has been sleep deprived. Patients who have just begun opioid treatment often have experienced days to weeks of severe to excruciating pain before coming to see you, and the pain has deprived them of much-needed sleep. Be careful not to mistake this natural "catch-up" sleep as oversedation. Leave the opioid dose the same for the first few days, and if the patient still complains of excessive drowsiness, with good pain relief, lower it.

Prescribe both immediate- and sustained-release formulations. A simple way to minimize sedation is to use long-acting or sustained-release opioids (i.e., methadone, transdermal fentanyl or buprenorphine, or the sustained-release opioid preparations) that have lower peak opioid levels to deliver the majority of the pain relief. Since sustained-release preparations are not flexible enough to meet the patient's changing pain needs, however, you will usually need to use both a sustained-release preparation to keep the pain at a satisfactory level most of the time and an immediate-acting agent for rescue dosing.

Contributing causes. If sedation persists beyond the first few weeks, the sedation is not acceptable, and the patient's care is not focused solely on comfort, try to determine whether a new medical problem, like hypercalcemia or hyponatremia or an unsuspected brain metastasis or a subdural hematoma, is contributing to the somnolence. Hyperglycemia, if it is causing sedation, is usually clinically apparent, as are uremia or hepatic failure, which are also likely to exacerbate the sedating effects of opioids.

In immunocompromised patients, search for CNS infections, such as viral encephalitis, toxoplasmosis, or tuberculous or cryptococcal meningitis. Carcinomatous or lymphomatous meningitis usually manifests as headaches and cranial nerve abnormalities rather than sedation.

If none of these conditions is present, review the patient's other medications, because a number of them can exacerbate opioid-induced sedation. Cimetidine, anticholinergic drugs, alcohol, and drugs that decrease glomerular filtration, such as NSAIDs and some ACE (angiotensin-converting enzyme) inhibitors, all increase drowsiness in patients taking opioids.

Sleep medications are most often implicated. Whenever possible, if insomnia is causing the daytime sedation, refer the patient for cognitive behavioral therapy for insomnia (CBT-I; Brasure et al. 2016; Sanft et al. 2021). A more extensive discussion of assessment and treatment of insomnia appears in Chapter 10.

Benzodiazepines with long half-lives, such as clonazepam (e.g., Klonopin) or diazepam (e.g., Valium), may induce daytime somnolence in patients taking opioids. If you use a benzodiazepine during the day, choose one with a shorter half-life, such as lorazepam (e.g., Ativan) (1 mg p.o.), or temazepam (e.g., Restoril) (7.5 to 30 mg p.o.).

Change the opioid dose or the agent. If sedation persists when the contributing factors are eliminated, try decreasing the dose of the sustained-release opioid by 10 to 25 percent and monitoring the patient's use of rescue medication. If the patient doesn't use more rescue doses, you can assume the pain relief is still satisfactory.

Alternatively, substitute a different opioid agent at an equianalgesic dose (I discuss how to do this later in the chapter). Just as opioids differ in how often they induce nausea, morphine, oxycodone, hydromorphone, fentanyl, and the other agents differ in how frequently they induce sedation. You may be able to achieve equivalent pain relief with less sedation simply by using a different agent.

Psychostimulants. If none of these measures is successful, consider adding a psychostimulant, such as an amphetamine. Some effective psychostimulants and their usual starting doses are listed in Table 7.7. Amphetamines have been shown to reduce drowsiness and to enhance mood. They are contraindicated for patients with arrhythmias, delirium, or psychosis; can create a substance use problem; and some patients cannot tolerate either the cardiac or the psychological side effects after starting the drugs. Even patients who can tolerate these agents may need an increased dose to maintain their antisedating and mood-enhancing effects after 3 to 4 weeks.

For selected patients, psychostimulants can be very effective, and the benefits can persist for 6 months or more. I most often prescribe methylphenidate (e.g., Ritalin). It is a CNS stimulant that increases concentrations of dopamine at the synapse by preventing its reuptake, affects norepinephrine reuptake, and binds to the serotonin transporter. Its effects peak 2 hours after it is taken, and the immediate-release form lasts up to 6 hours. The oral sustained-release formulation has its peak effect 4 to 7 hours after it is taken and lasts approximately 8 hours; a transdermal patch is also available.

There have not been any large randomized and controlled trials that demonstrate the effectiveness of methylphenidate in relieving the somnolence induced by opioids, but numerous trials of cancer patients with impaired cognition (e.g., with brain tumors) have demonstrated that this drug is effective and safe and improves cognition. Patients should begin with 2.5 to 5 mg of immediate-release methylphenidate once a day; you can add a noontime dose if necessary and escalate to higher doses (Rozans et al. 2002). Modafinil (Provigil) (100 to 400 mg/day p.o.), a nonamphetamine psychostimulant, is an agent approved for treatment of patients with narcolepsy. Patients with brain tumors or with sedation from opioids may find it increases their alertness.

If a patient needs an extra degree of mental acuity for a special event, such as a wedding, an important meeting, or an anniversary party, begin the psychostimulant a week or so before the event. Adjusting its and the opioid's dose can often provide the perfect degree of pain relief and mental alertness for the important day.

Anesthesia pain specialists. If all these techniques are ineffective and the patient remains unacceptably sedated, you might consider referring her to an anesthesia pain specialist, whose contributions I discuss elsewhere in the chapter.

Opioid Overdose

Sadly, an opioid overdose may result when a patient attempts suicide by taking more than the prescribed dose. But inadvertent overdoses are much more common than intentional ones. Patients may take the sustained-release preparation when they intended to take the immediate-release version of the same opioid. Or they may develop renal or hepatic insufficiency that is significant enough to prolong the half-life of the opioid. Patients may place new fentanyl patches without removing the old ones or can develop toxicity if they become febrile (which increases fentanyl's absorption from the skin reservoir) or septic (because acidosis increases the free fraction of fentanyl). Rarely, within hours of taking a significant dose of a sustained-release opioid, a patient may develop a bowel obstruction or other bowel catastrophe causing ileus; the opioid cannot be excreted in the usual fashion, and much more than the expected amount is absorbed, leading to an overdose. In any of these situations, family members may mistakenly ascribe the increased sedation to progressive cancer or to an expected side effect of the medication.

Diagnosis. Signs of opioid overdose in cancer patients are similar to those in patients without cancer, except that miosis in a patient who is opioid tolerant is not specifically indicative of overdose, and sedation may be more prominent than respiratory depression if the overdose is caught early. Assess for the causes listed above, particularly for any "extra" fentanyl patches.

Prevention and Management. Naloxone-dispensing devices (IM/SQ or intranasal) available in community pharmacies deliver doses adequate to reverse opioid overdoses (Ryan and Dunne 2018). Guidelines suggest that when you write opioid prescriptions, also write one for naloxone (if needed in your state), or instruct the patient or family member to pick one up at their local pharmacy (NCCN 2020). Nurses can teach them the signs of overdose and how to use the devices, and review with them their plan for when to use the naloxone and when to call 911 and you. Any patients who receive naloxone from a device need to be evaluated at a hospital.

Patients with cancer who overdose but who have been taking opioids for chronic cancer pain cannot be managed in the same way as those who have been using opioids for only a brief time, such as previously opioid-naive postoperative patients (Boyer 2012). It is important even in this situation that you *resist* the temptation to use an undiluted intravenous injection of naloxone to reverse the effects of the opioid completely. If you do administer undiluted naloxone to a patient who is opioid tolerant and who has been using chronic opioids for pain control, you may precipitate a severe withdrawal syndrome, causing the patient to wake up in excruciating pain that you will have a hard time bringing under control, even if you reinstitute opioids.

If the patient is breathing normally but cannot be aroused, simply discontinue the opioid. If significant respiratory depression has occurred, you will need to administer a dilute solution of naloxone. The low dose of naloxone usually enables the patient to reestablish normal respirations and wake up gradually without experiencing withdrawal.

Dilute naloxone can be given as either a slow intravenous "push" or a continuous infusion. For patients whose respiratory rates are between 10/min and 12/min, who are just mildly oversedated, and whose renal, hepatic, or gut function can be expected to normalize quickly, I suggest the following: dilute 1 ml containing 0.4 mg of naloxone into 9 ml of normal saline (total will be 10 ml), then infuse 1–2 ml every 2–5 minutes, giving as much of this dilute naloxone as is necessary to establish a normal respiratory rate but not enough to awaken the patient.

Patients who have developed toxic effects from a transdermal fentanyl patch, and those who have been taking sustained-release morphine or oxycodone and develop hepatic or renal failure or an ileus, are likely to require naloxone drips. These patients should be admitted to an intensive care unit (Boyer 2012). The patient with an intrathecal pump can pose a particularly difficult problem if the pump was overfilled or incorrectly programmed. Such a patient may require lavage of the CSF as well as naloxone to recover (Boyer 2012).

In addition to the naloxone drip, it is wise to institute measures that will stop the patient from aspirating and from absorbing additional amounts of the opioid. Gastrointestinal decontamination with activated charcoal can be used if the ingestion occurred no more than one hour before the patient arrived in the Emergency Department (Boyer 2012). Laxatives, oral or intravenous motility agents (e.g., metoclopramide), and enemas all help the patient eliminate the remaining sustained-release opioid from the gastrointestinal tract. Unfortunately, even after the transdermal fentanyl patch is removed, the patient will be absorbing fentanyl from the skin reservoir for 12 to 24 more hours. As the patient begins to wake up, reduce the naloxone infusion gradually to match the residual opioid level. Patients will awaken safely, without withdrawal; as pain reappears, appropriate opioid therapy can be resumed.

Opioid Neurotoxicity

Opioid neurotoxicity is an unfortunate complication of our eagerness to relieve a patient's pain quickly, especially when the patient is dying and the focus is on comfort. With rapidly escalating doses, several complications may arise (Moryl, Coyle, and Foley 2008).

Myoclonic jerking (multifocal myoclonus). Myoclonus is one of the earliest and most common manifestations. It can be seen in patients taking high doses of any opioid but is most common in patients receiving frequent, repeated therapeutic doses of morphine or high doses of oxycodone or hydromorphone. In its earliest stages, patients experience muscle jerking as they are falling asleep. With increasing opioid doses, family members or patients themselves may report muscle spasms or involuntary movements while the patient is awake. The spasms may be severe enough to exacerbate the distress from an already painful limb. Patients receiving only moderate opioid doses who develop renal insufficiency or dehydration may also develop myoclonus, possibly related to increased levels of opioids and their metabolites. If nothing is done, seizures may result.

Changing to another opioid often relieves the problem. If the patient would prefer not to change opioids, benzodiazepines, baclofen, or dantrolene can reduce the spasms. For patients with severe myoclonus or for those too close to dying for a trial of opioid rotation, lorazepam or midazolam may be particularly effective. Rarely, patients can either be resistant to a benzodiazepine or have a history of increased agitation after receiving one and refractory to baclofen and dantrolene (or unable to take medications by mouth). For these patients, I use a barbiturate infusion, usually with pentobarbital, to sedate them until the other measures reduce the myoclonus. In Chapter 11, I review how to give midazolam or pentobarbital.

Hyperalgesia. Hyperalgesia is often even more distressing than myoclonus. It is caused by "wind-up" of the central nervous system, with spreading of the pain signals throughout the spinal cord, so that pain from one arm is now caused by any limb movement. Even softly touching the skin can be painful for the patient, because the A-alpha (touch) fibers now act as C (pain) fibers and transmit a painful signal.

The treatment for hyperalgesia is to lower the opioid dose rapidly, and perhaps, if it is feasible in a dehydrated patient, to give a liter or two of intravenous fluids to flush out the opioid metabolites. Ketamine, starting at 0.02 to 0.05 mg/kg per hour by continuous intravenous infusion and titrated as needed, as rapidly as 100 percent every 4 to 6 hours (Moryl, Coyle, and Foley 2008; Loveday and Sindt 2015; Quibell et al. 2015), can provide pain relief while the opioid levels fall, but some patients may need mild sedation with a benzodiazepine. It can be difficult, but of course crucial, to explain to the patient's family why you are decreasing or stopping the opioids when the patient seems to be in such distress.

If the patient is expected to live long enough, rotate to another opioid. Start with a dose of opioid that is equivalent to the dose the patient previously tolerated without toxicity. For example, Sylvia was a 60-year-old woman who was dying at home of multiple myeloma but was not in a hospice program because she needed platelet transfusions twice a week. She had been receiving hydromorphone via a PCA with a basal infusion of 4 mg/hr. As we unraveled the story later, she had begun to moan, likely because she had developed a mild delirium, and her family had misunderstood the moans as pain and repeatedly asked the home care nurse to increase the basal rate of the hydromorphone infusion.

Over the next 48 hours, the drip rate had been increased to 16 mg/hr, and Sylvia had developed painful myoclonus and hyperalgesia. When she was admitted, she was dehydrated, so we hydrated her, then lowered the hydromorphone infusion to 4 mg/hr. We added midazolam, which quickly eliminated her myoclonus, and used low doses of liquid methadone (2 mg p.o.) to treat the increase in pain we expected her to have when the aides bathed her or changed her position in bed. We later rotated her to oral methadone, using as the base of the calculation the 96 mg a day of hydromorphone she received from her 4 mg/hr hydromorphone drip. (Earlier in the chapter, under the discussion of methadone, I describe how to do the rotation from another opioid to methadone, and more examples are found at the end of this chapter.)

Delirium

Opioid-induced delirium can be a frightening side effect for patients and their families. The first manifestation may be something as mild as nightmares, but the process can rapidly progress, and the patient can develop hallucinations and even frank psychosis. The assessment and management of delirium from all causes, including opioids, serotonin syndrome, and anticholinergic crisis, is discussed in Chapter 9.

Respiratory Depression

Respiratory depression is an unusual side effect when opioids are used to treat cancer patients in pain, as long as the opioid dose is titrated to the degree of pain, and the patient's renal and hepatic functions remain stable (Legrand et al. 2004). Opioids do marginally decrease the brain's sensitivity to carbon dioxide levels and are associated with a slight, usually clinically insignificant, degree of hypoventilation.

It is sometimes difficult to determine whether a patient's respiratory depression is due to the opioid or to something else. If an opioid is responsible, the patient will also be confused and somnolent, because opioid-induced respiratory depression is due to general depression of the central nervous system. If the patient is anxious or agitated, however, something other than opioids must be causing the respiratory depression.

Practice Points: Managing Opioid-Related Respiratory Depression

- Respiratory depression in an agitated patient is unlikely to be due to the opioid.
- Respiratory depression may indicate worsening of renal or hepatic function, hypothyroidism, persistence of drug in the bowel because of obstruction, or sepsis.
- Induce evacuation of residual opioid from the gut and remove any opioid-containing skin patches.
- If respiratory rate is dangerously low, infuse a dilute solution of naloxone until the rate returns to a safe level. Do not give enough to awaken the patient or to induce opioid withdrawal.

Occasionally, patients have underlying medical conditions that make them more susceptible to the respiratory depressive effects of opioids. Hypothyroid patients or those whose obstructive lung disease causes them to retain carbon dioxide are in this category. Hypothyroid patients with coronary artery disease and angina can be particularly problematic; they can develop respiratory arrest with even the 1 or 2 mg of IV morphine they receive for pain in the emergency room. For patients with chronic obstructive pulmonary disease, you can safely prescribe opioids if you start with very low concentrations (e.g., morphine 1–2 mg IV q3h or 2–5 mg p.o. q4h), increase the doses very slowly, and monitor the patient carefully.

Miscellaneous Side Effects

Opioid-induced *urinary retention* is also troublesome, especially for older patients or those with underlying bladder outlet obstruction. Discontinuing any agents with anticholinergic side effects is often effective, but some patients may require finasteride (e.g., Proscar) (5 mg/day p.o.) or tamsulosin (e.g. Flomax) (0.4–0.8 mg/day p.o.) to diminish the outlet obstruction, or bethanechol (e.g., Urecholine) (10 mg p.o. t.i.d., to a maximum of 50 mg p.o. t.i.d.) to relax the bladder smooth muscle that is being stimulated by the opioid.

Pruritus, which most commonly occurs in opioid-naive patients receiving epidural or intrathecal opioids, may be caused by activation of spinal opiate receptors, by opioid-induced release of histamine from mast cells, or by disinhibition of itch-specific neurons (McNicol et al. 2003). Pruritus may resolve with a change in opioid, but you may need to add ondansetron (4 mg p.o. or IV); paroxetine (Paxil) (10 to 20 mg p.o.) (Zylicz, Smits, and Prajnik 1998); nalmefene (10 to 25 mcg IV); or nalbuphine (1 to 5 mg IV) (Jannuzzi 2016). General strategies for treating pruritis can be found in Chapter 10.

Summary

Constipation, nausea, sedation, opioid neurotoxicity, delirium, respiratory depression, urinary retention, and pruritus are treatable opioid-induced side effects that can often be prevented. They can discourage patients from taking the doses of opioids they need to achieve satisfactory control of their pain. For patients with complicated pain syndromes, you may need to prescribe multiple agents to prevent or control side effects, and the patient may need to try two or three different opioids before achieving satisfactory pain control with tolerable side effects. By using these strategies you will be able to reverse or ameliorate those problems that do occur and markedly increase the comfort of your patients.

ADJUVANT ANALGESIC TREATMENTS

Adjuvant analgesics are drugs used primarily for other indications, which also produce pain relief. They are of particular value for patients with neuropathic pain, including patients with spinal cord compression (see Table 7.8) or bone pain (see Table 7.9). In the sections that follow, I describe how to use various adjuvant analgesics for the treatment of neuropathic pain, including corticosteroids, anticonvulsants, and psychotropics. I also review agents useful for bone pain, and then discuss skeletal muscle and smooth muscle relaxants.

Adjuvant analgesic agents are usually given orally or parenterally, but occasionally rectal administration is preferable. Unfortunately, though there is good information about the rectal use of opioids and NSAIDs, we have less information about administering adjuvant medications via this route.

Adjuvant Treatments for Neuropathic Pain

Patients with neuropathic pain usually benefit from adjuvant agents that can block the pain signals from the damaged nerve. When a peripheral nerve is injured, inflammatory mediators are released that cause changes in the sodium channel activity of the nerves at that site and at the dorsal root ganglion, and new calcium channels appear. These changes cause *peripheral sensitization*, which is both a lowering of the threshold for nerve firing and a spontaneous firing of the nerves. Unlike opioids, drugs that can modify the ion channels—such as corticosteroids; gabapentin, pregabalin, and the other anticonvulsants; SNRIs; tricyclic antidepressants; baclofen; NK-1 receptor antagonists; alpha-2 adrenergic agonists clonidine and dexmedetomidine; ketamine; and local anesthetics (see Table 7.8)—can provide the extra analgesia needed for satisfactory relief of the discomfort that comes from peripheral and central sensitization (Attal, Cruccu, and Baron 2010; Gilron, Baron, and Jensen 2015).

Unsuspected deficiency of functional B12 may contribute to patient symptoms and is a potentially reversible cause of neuropathic pain. Normal serum B12 levels do not exclude functional B12 deficiency in patients with advanced cancer; methylmalonic acid and homocysteine levels will be elevated in functionally deficient patients, even those with supranormal levels of serum B12 (Solomon 2016). It is not known whether B12 deficiency contributes to chemotherapy-induced peripheral neuropathy (CIPN).

Acute chemotherapy-induced pain syndrome. Paclitaxel causes a unique acute pain syndrome that occurs in 80 percent of patients receiving the drug. The syndrome is caused by damage to peripheral nerves and is more common if the drug is infused over 3 hours (25 percent incidence) than over 96 hours (2 percent incidence). Patients with this syndrome complain of joint and muscle aching and dull pains 1 to 3 days after each dose, and the symptoms usually resolve within a week

(Loprinzi et al. 2011). The intensity of the pain predicts how severe the peripheral neuropathy is likely to be. Giving dexamethasone (8 mg daily) on Days 2 and 3 after chemotherapy can attenuate this syndrome (Saito et al. 2020).

Oxaliplatin causes a different type of acute neurotoxicity that presents as a short-lived but intense paresthesia in the throat, mouth, face, and hands; jaw spasms; and cramps triggered by exposure to cold. The pain syndrome is likely due to injury to the nerve's sodium channels (Durand et al. 2012). The SNRI venlafaxine was effective in a 2012 phase III randomized placebo-controlled trial both in preventing the acute neurotoxicity induced by oxaliplatin and in decreasing the severity of subsequent chronic peripheral neuropathy (Durand et al. 2012). But a subsequent, more comprehensive study was unable to confirm either benefit of venlafaxine and recommended against another phase III study (Zimmermann et al. 2016).

Another SNRI, duloxetine (60–120 mg/day) is recommended for ameliorating oxaliplatin- or paclitaxel-induced peripheral neuropathy (Hershman et al. 2014; Majithia et al. 2016; Paice et al. 2016). The SNRIs are not without side effects; common ones include gastrointestinal intolerance (dry mouth, nausea, constipation, diarrhea) as well as somnolence, dizziness, and increased sweating. Rarely, they are hepatotoxic.

Chronic treatment-induced pain syndromes. CIPN is, unfortunately, very common. Thirty to 40 percent of people who are given microtubule inhibitors (such as vincristine and vinblastine), taxanes, proteosome inhibitors (such as bortezomib), thalidomide, and platin-containing agents (such as cisplatin, carboplatin, and oxaliplatin) develop CIPN (Grisold, Cavaletti, and Windebank 2012; Teoh et al. 2018). Almost all patients experience numbness and tingling, and about half report burning pains that are dose related and caused by often irreversible nerve damage. Sensory loss can be so severe that it includes loss of proprioception and results in ataxia and problems walking.

Symptoms lessen with time off the agents, often taking 6 months to a year to maximal recovery, but they and the associated functional impairments rarely resolve completely. Six years after treatment, 47 percent of patients are still reporting significant symptoms, including increased risk of falls (1.8 hazard ratio) (Teoh et al. 2018). The NCCN report on the management of neuropathy in cancer (Stubblefield et al. 2009) recommends screening and rehabilitation including balance training; these should be included as a part of CIPN assessment and management, though they may not be routinely offered (Stout 2017).

Prevention may be possible, but no specific agents are recommended to prevent CIPN (Loprinzi et al. 2020). The first step is to avoid using agents that can induce peripheral neuropathy in patients who have increased risk factors for CIPN. Breast cancer patients who were overweight or obese or had a low "moderate to vigorous physical activity" (MVPA) score had a greater incidence of CIPN from taxanes (Greenlee et al. 2017). In patients over 65, diabetes increased the risk

---

Practice Point: Prevention Strategies for CIPN

- Avoid using agents that produce CIPN in patients who are obese, diabetic, or inactive.
- Replace vitamin D if deficient.
- Recommend an exercise regimen.
- Use limb hypothermia during therapy.

(Glimelius et al. 2018; Greenlee et al. 2017; Hanai et al. 2018; Hershman et al. 2016; Kleckner et al. 2018; Rosenbaek et al. 2020; Sundar et al. 2017; Wang et al. 2016)

---

twofold, but patients with autoimmune disorders were half as likely to develop CIPN as those without (Hershman et al. 2016).

When agents that cause CIPN are needed, however, there are still strategies to ameliorate the problem. The severity of the CIPN induced by bortezomib and thalidomide can be decreased by normalizing vitamin D levels, because CIPN is exacerbated in myeloma patients who have inadequate levels of vitamin D (Wang et al. 2016). Vitamin D deficiency is very prevalent in this population. Sixteen percent were 25(OH)D deficient (<20 ng/ml) and 26 percent were found to be 25(OH) D insufficient (20.0–29.9 ng/ml) (Wang et al. 2016).

Limb hypothermia was effective in pilot trials in breast cancer patients on paclitaxel. In each of two trials, one of the patient's hands and feet were cooled, and the other hand and foot were not (Hanai et al. 2018; Sundar et al. 2017). Women given prophylactic cryotherapy were more likely to complete the planned dose of adjuvant paclitaxel in another trial (Rosenbaek et al. 2020). Exercise during chemotherapy reduced CIPN for patients who had received platinum, vinca alkaloids, or taxane, and was particularly effective in older patients (Kleckner et al. 2018). Calmangafodipir (an agent that protects mitochondria) used before chemotherapy in a phase II trial reduced neurotoxicity and cold allodynia from oxaliplatin (Glimelius et al. 2018).

Once the CIPN has developed, duloxetine (60–120 mg/day) is recommended for CIPN from taxanes or platinum agents (Hershman et al. 2014; Paice et al. 2016; Majithia et al. 2016). New information on the mechanism of bortezomib-induced peripheral neuropathy may lead to use of a novel medication (Emery and Wood 2018), such as an agent currently used for multiple sclerosis patients (Stockstill et al. 2018). Topical menthol (1 percent), which may bind to surface receptors, improved sleep, walking, and "catastrophizing" in patients with CIPN; neuropathy symptoms improved in 81 percent (Fallon et al. 2015). Topical lidocaine may also provide temporary relief of symptoms.

Scrambler therapy (Calmare Therapeutics Inc., Rutherford, NH), "which uses surface electrodes to capture the surface receptors of the c-fibers (which carry pain impulses) and send a 'non-pain' impulse along the usual route to the brain" (Teoh et al. 2018. p. 470), is reported in pilot trials to be more helpful for CIPN than transcutaneous electrical nerve stimulation (TENS), with 40 percent of patients on the Scrambler arm reporting a 50 percent or greater reduction from baseline in numbness, tingling, and pain during treatment days versus 20 percent of patients using TENS (Loprinzi et al. 2020). No phase III trials have been reported.

NMDA antagonists. Agents that induce CIPN induce *central sensitization*: changes in the spinal cord that occur after peripheral nerve injury. Substance P and neurokinin A released into the spinal cord by injured peripheral nerves cause changes in the activity of the calcium channels and lower the threshold for firing of spinal cord neurons. These neurons begin to respond not only to signals from the nerves that enter at their level of the cord but also to signals from nerves synapsing above and below them. In addition, more spinal cord NMDA receptors appear. These receptors inhibit the ability of opioids to relieve pain. Given all these changes, patients with central sensitization usually need treatment with agents (discussed individually later in this chapter) that affect the activity of calcium channels (such as gabapentin, pregabalin, and dantrolene) and may need agents that affect the activity of the sodium channels (such as corticosteroids or tricyclic antidepressants) or that can inhibit the activity of the NMDA receptors (such as methadone, buprenorphine, Levo-Dromoran, or ketamine).

Radiation therapy and surgery also injure peripheral nerves and can induce neuropathic pain syndromes. (These syndromes are described in Chapter 6.) Prophylactic pregabalin, discussed in full later in this chapter, may prevent post-mastectomy/post-thoracotomy neuropathic pain (Reyad et al. 2019), and may be effective for postradiation therapy pain in patients with head and neck cancer (Jiang et al. 2019; Reyad et al. 2019).

Corticosteroids. Although there is a paucity of good studies of the efficacy of systemic corticosteroids in improving the pain of cancer patients (Paulson et al. 2013; Haywood et al. 2015), corticosteroids have been reported to be effective for patients with malignant bone pain and for those with malignant neuropathic pain, such as that caused by compression of the spinal cord or nerve plexuses (e.g., brachial plexus, lumbosacral plexus) by tumor. By inhibiting synthesis of prosta-glandins and by their effect on the sodium channel that decreases firing from injured nerves, corticosteroids diminish transmission of the pain signal from the periphery to the spinal cord or from the spinal cord to the brain. By decreasing capillary permeability, they reduce edema and thereby relieve the pain of brain metastases or tumor infiltration of nerves or nerve roots. There are also clinical reports of corticosteroids relieving esophageal or gastroduodenal obstruction, but no controlled studies have been done to confirm their efficacy in these conditions.

Corticosteroids can be given epidurally, intravenously, or orally. Epidural corti-costeroids have been studied only in patients with nonmalignant pain syndromes,

---

Practice Points: Corticosteroids as Adjuvants

- Corticosteroids decrease pain due to peripheral nerve injury (e.g., acute herpes zoster or metastases to the brachial or lumbosacral plexus), spinal cord compression, and brain metastases.
- Corticosteroids decrease bone pain.
- Onset of pain relief is often rapid.
- To minimize side effects:
  - Give the minimal effective dose.
  - Consider prophylaxis for oral and esophageal candidiasis, for gastritis/ulcer disease, and for pneumocystis jirovecii if using sustained, elevated doses.
- Be alert for mood changes (euphoria or depression) and delirium.

---

but their success in some patients with radiculopathies (e.g., from disk disease) suggests that they might be beneficial as adjuncts for those with malignant epidural disease who cannot tolerate systemic corticosteroid therapy.

Corticosteroid therapy is indicated for all patients with radiologic evidence of cord compression. Corticosteroids decrease cord edema and pain and help preserve neurologic function and overall outcome after specific therapy (i.e., radiation, surgery, or surgery followed by radiation). Patients who receive high doses of corticosteroids for cord compression can experience a significant decrease of back pain within hours. There is controversy, however, about the dose that should be used because the only randomized studies were done in the 1990s and have not been repeated (Lawton et al. 2019). Patients usually receive dexamethasone (10 mg IV bolus, then 4 mg p.o. q.i.d., then tapered over 14 days after the completion of radiation therapy). Selected patients with little epidural disease and contraindications for corticosteroid therapy have been shown to tolerate radiotherapy safely without corticosteroids.

Corticosteroid therapy is also indicated as an adjuvant for all patients with radiologic evidence of cord compression while they are being evaluated for decompressive surgery. Surgery was formerly reserved for patients who had tumors that were unlikely to respond to radiation, or whose epidural disease progressed despite radiation therapy. Data from a randomized trial suggest, however, that patients who had cancers other than lymphoma, myeloma, or breast cancer, and who were treated with surgery followed by radiation therapy, either remained ambulatory longer or were more likely to become ambulatory than patients who received radiation therapy alone (Patchell et al. 2005). If you are interested in more information about assessing and treating patients with spinal cord compression, please refer to additional references in the online bibliography (Abrahm, Banffy, and Harris 2008; Lawton et al. 2019; Rades et al. 2010).

For patients with brain metastases or impending but not actual cord compression, consider tapering to 4 or 2 mg every 6 hours during the second week of radiation treatments. After the radiation is completed, taper the dose as the patient tolerates. Reinstate a higher dose if back pain, headache, or other symptoms of cord or CNS edema return.

Corticosteroids are also effective adjuvants for patients with peripheral nerve injuries, such as those with tumor infiltrating the brachial plexus (typically lung or breast cancer) or the lumbosacral plexus (typically recurrent colorectal cancer). To the opioid therapy, add 4 to 6 mg of dexamethasone orally two to four times a day. In responding patients, the pain diminishes significantly by 48 to 72 hours. To minimize the corticosteroid-induced side effects, taper the dose rapidly, watching for reemergence of unacceptable pain. In many cases, patients have been able to maintain effective pain control with alternate-day corticosteroid dosing.

Patients may not have had the opportunity to have the Shingrix vaccine, or if immunocompromised, may not have responded to it adequately. For those who get acute herpes zoster, antivirals have a more important role than corticosteroids in its treatment and that of post-herpetic neuralgia (Thakur and Phillips 2012). Corticosteroids alone have been shown to decrease the acute pain associated with herpes zoster infections, but there is no long-term benefit, and they are not recommended as standard therapy. Adding acyclovir (800 mg five times a day for 21 days) to prednisone (60 mg/day for 7 days, 30 mg/day for the next 7 days, and 15 mg/day for the last 7 days), while leading to quicker resolution of neuritis, return to uninterrupted sleep, return to usual daily activities, and cessation of analgesics, does not prevent post-herpetic neuralgia.

Antivirals should be started within 72 hours after the patient first notices the rash. Acyclovir (800 mg, five times a day), valacyclovir (1000 mg, every 8 hours), and famciclovir (500 mg, every 8 hours) have comparable efficacy and safety profiles. A meta-analysis found that acyclovir decreased post-herpetic neuralgia prevalence (15 percent vs. 35 percent in controls), and in other studies, famciclovir decreased its duration: 163 days in the placebo group versus 63 days in the treated group (Thakur and Phillips 2012).

Oral corticosteroids have also been used to increase patients' appetite and sense of well-being, but results of controlled studies of their efficacy have been conflicting. Increases in appetite in the short run (about one month) were consistently noted. In some studies, improvement in the amount of food eaten and patients' sense of well-being or quality of life was also seen, but neither weight nor survival time increased. The patients who showed the most improvement were those with neuropathic pain. For selected patients with advanced cancer, for whom appetite or sense of well-being is a significant issue, consider a course of corticosteroids (as little as dexamethasone 2 or 4 mg daily may be helpful), expecting at least a short-term benefit.

The limitation to using corticosteroids is the significant incidence of corticosteroid-induced side effects. Many of these can be prevented and others readily managed, but some of the most serious ones occur unpredictably. The corticosteroid-induced side effects and recommended treatments are described below.

Gastrointestinal disorders. Corticosteroids alone probably do not cause ulcers. Patients taking corticosteroids along with an NSAID (other than acetaminophen), however, do have a higher incidence of ulcers than those taking the NSAID alone. Therefore, consider prescribing a proton pump inhibitor (e.g., omeprazole, 20 mg/day) for patients taking both corticosteroids and NSAIDs.

Candidiasis. One of the most common corticosteroid-induced side effects, especially in patients who are debilitated or otherwise immunocompromised, is oral or esophageal candidiasis (thrush). These conditions can be distressing and may seriously decrease your patient's oral intake. It is therefore important to describe carefully to the patient and his family the signs and symptoms of oral and esophageal candidal infections (the painful, burning red tongue and the esophageal pain syndrome described below). They will then be able to call you promptly and receive appropriate therapy should an infection develop.

If you plan a prolonged corticosteroid course, you might consider starting prophylactic antifungal therapy with oral fluconazole (200 mg on Day 1, followed by 100 mg/day). For patients expected to require only a short-term course of corticosteroids, consider oral prophylaxis with topical antifungals such as clotrimazole troches (e.g., Mycelex) given three times a day. Patients will need to be monitored for esophageal candidiasis, because topical antifungals like the troches or Nystatin "swish and swallow" do not prevent it.

Esophagitis causes a distinctive pain syndrome. Even though the infection usually involves only the lower esophagus, the pain can be experienced in the mid- or even upper esophagus. You have probably experienced esophageal pain if you have swallowed a fish bone that "got stuck" or have drunk a hot liquid too quickly. As you may remember, a few seconds after you swallow, when the wave of peristalsis passes the injured area, a severe pain occurs, usually making you grimace. Patients with esophageal candidiasis will also grimace a few seconds after swallowing, when they experience the pain. You can treat esophageal candidiasis effectively with oral fluconazole (400 mg to load, then 200 mg per day for another 13 days); patients usually experience significant pain relief within 48 hours.

Mood changes. Corticosteroid-induced delirium is more common in people with a previous psychiatric history, and high-dose corticosteroids should be used with caution in such patients. For most patients, the mood changes are less marked. In some, a euphoria occurs that can be quite enjoyable. The commonly associated insomnia can be prevented by instructing the patient to take the corticosteroids before noon. Other patients develop a severe corticosteroid-induced depression, which may respond to lowering the corticosteroid dose or to discontinuing it altogether. Antidepressant drugs are not usually required.

Miscellaneous. Corticosteroid-induced *glucose intolerance* is usually easily managed with insulin. For patients with impaired mental status, the visiting nurse or hospice team can be of great assistance in regulating and administering the insulin doses. Prophylaxis for pneumocystis is needed for patients on prolonged corticosteroid therapy (i.e., 4 weeks or more of 16–25 mg of prednisolone or 4 mg or more dexamethasone equivalent per day) (Cooley et al. 2014).

Proximal muscle weakness can be quite disabling and refractory to therapy. Home physical therapy or, for those who can tolerate it, hydrotherapy can preserve some muscle function, but many patients will need assisting devices such as lift chairs to keep them independent in their daily activities. Others may require wheelchairs and support devices such as shower chairs.

Anticonvulsants. The anticonvulsants—gabapentin (e.g., Neurontin), pregabalin (Lyrica), phenytoin (e.g., Dilantin), carbamazepine (e.g., Tegretol), lamotrigine (Lamictal), topiramate (Topamax), and oxcarbazepine (Trileptal) (but not valproic acid; Gill et al. 2011)—are important adjuvant agents for patients with neuropathic pain that is *burning, sharp, cutting,* or *like an electric shock* (Table 7.8). The mechanism by which these agents relieve this pain has not yet been determined. Most of the efficacy data, other than data from studies on CIPN, come from studies on patients without cancer who have neuropathic pain.

Gabapentin is the most commonly used agent. It has demonstrated efficacy in patients with post-herpetic neuralgia and peripheral neuropathies resulting from diabetes and is empirically used for patients with neuropathic pain of any etiology, including spinal cord injury (Rekand, Merete Hagen, and Granning 2012). In 2011, a new formulation of extended-release gabapentin was FDA approved for post-herpetic neuralgia (Thomas and Farquhar-Smith 2011). To minimize sedation, especially in older patients, use low doses initially and raise the dose every 3 to 4 days (or weekly in older patients) as tolerated. Start at 100 mg orally, three times a day, or, for patients with difficulty sleeping, 100 mg in the morning and afternoon and 300 mg at bedtime. The dose for patients with renal insufficiency is 100 to 200 mg twice a day. Give patients with renal failure who are undergoing dialysis a 300-mg loading dose, and then 200 to 300 mg after each dialysis. No dose corrections are needed for hepatic failure. The minimal effective dose is usually 300 mg orally, three times a day, but if the patient reports some pain relief, the doses can be increased up to 3600 mg/day in divided doses to reduce the pain further. Sedation and peripheral edema are the usual dose-limiting side effects, but patients can also develop myoclonus. In 2020, the FDA required new warnings about an increased risk of respiratory depression in patients taking gabapentin who are also taking opioids or other CNS depressants, who have COPD, or who are elderly. Gabapentin needs to be tapered if it is no longer needed or not effective. Sudden discontinuation can cause agitation, confusion, and even seizures (Mersfelder and Nichols 2016).

Gabapentin is well absorbed at low doses, but its bioavailability falls significantly at higher doses. The 100 mg dose has 60 percent bioavailability, but the 1600 mg dose, only 27 percent. Pregabalin (Lyrica), however, is linearly absorbed at all doses, with 90 percent bioavailability and peak plasma concentration within one hour if taken on an empty stomach. Pregabalin is FDA approved for use in patients with neuropathic pain. Importantly, if a patient has suboptimal effect from gabapentin at 300 mg or more taken orally three times a day, pregabalin is likely to be effective. For pregabalin to be covered by most insurance plans, you will need to document that the patient has not responded to gabapentin.

Pregabalin has the same mechanism of action and side-effect profile as gabapentin. If you are starting someone directly on pregabalin, begin at 50 mg (p.o. t.i.d.). If the patient is already tolerant to gabapentin, the initial pregabalin dose will depend on the gabapentin dose. For example, start someone taking 300 mg (p.o. t.i.d.) of gabapentin at 50 mg (p.o. t.i.d.) of pregabalin; but start someone taking 1200 mg (p.o. t.i.d.) at 150 mg (p.o. t.i.d.; maximum dose is 200 mg p.o. t.i.d.) (Attal, Cruccu, and Baron 2010; Gilron, Baron, and Jensen 2015). In 2020, the FDA required new warnings about an increased risk of respiratory depression in patients taking pregabalin who are also taking opioids or other CNS depressants, who have COPD, or who are elderly.

Practice Points: Adjuvant Agents for Neuropathic Pain

- Pregabalin is the most useful anticonvulsant for neuropathic pain. It is well absorbed at all dose ranges and has the fewest side effects. Use gabapentin first if the patient cannot afford pregabalin. If gabapentin is ineffective, pregabalin may be effective; many insurers will cover its cost for patients not responding to gabapentin.
- Consider adding low-dose nortriptyline at bedtime to enhance pain relief with minimal additional side effects.
- Carbamazepine is best studied for tic douloureux–like pain but consider giving phenytoin to achieve therapeutic levels rapidly.

If the pregabalin does not provide sufficient relief alone, try adding (in succession) lamotrigine (150 to 500 mg/day in two divided doses), topiramate (25 to 400 mg/day in two divided doses), or oxcarbazepine (300 to 2400 mg/day in two divided doses) to improve pain control. Other active agents include divalproex (150 to 3000 mg/day in three divided doses) (Gill et al. 2011) or zonisamide (100 to 400 mg/day in two divided doses).

For patients with lancinating, electric shock–like pain that does not respond to any combination of these agents, discontinue the gabapentin or pregabalin and try phenytoin (100 to 300 mg/day) or carbamazepine (100 to 1600 mg/day, in two to four divided doses). Although carbamazepine has most often been shown to be effective, as, for example, in trigeminal neuralgia (tic douloureux), consider beginning with phenytoin. You can reach therapeutic levels of phenytoin within a day and complete a therapeutic trial in 1 or 2 weeks. If by that time the pain has not improved, discontinue the phenytoin and begin carbamazepine, increasing doses slowly (i.e., incrementally every week or two) until therapeutic levels are reached. This may take as long as a month but may help selected patients.

These other anticonvulsants cause several side effects not found in patients taking gabapentin or pregabalin, and patients on them require careful monitoring. Patients taking phenytoin may develop ataxia, nausea, vomiting, or visual problems if the dose exceeds the therapeutic range; they may also develop allergic reactions involving the skin or liver. Carbamazepine causes hypotension in ambulatory patients if the dose is escalated too rapidly, and it can (rarely) cause severe neutropenia. Lamotrigine commonly causes fatigue, dizziness, headache, rash, mental status changes, blurred vision, nausea and vomiting, and, rarely, serious allergic skin reactions and cytopenias and hepatic failure. Begin by giving 25 mg/day orally for 2 weeks, increasing to 50 mg/day orally for 2 weeks and then to 100 mg/day orally for 1 week, as tolerated. The maximum dose is 200 mg/day orally.

Topiramate commonly causes dizziness, somnolence, fatigue, mental status changes, depression, and, rarely, kidney stones, acute angle-closure glaucoma, oligohydrosis and hyperthermia, cytopenias, psychosis, and severe allergic skin reactions. Begin topiramate doses at 25 to 50 mg/day orally and increase by 25 to 50 mg/day each week. Doses above 400 mg are rarely more effective than lower doses.

Oxcarbazepine commonly causes dizziness, somnolence, confusion, diplopia, fatigue, nausea, vomiting, abdominal pain, abnormal gait, nystagmus, and, rarely, severe allergic skin reactions, cytopenias, angioedema, and hyponatremia. Oxcarbazepine doses should begin at 300 mg orally twice a day and increase by 300 mg every 3 days as tolerated, to a maximum of 2400 mg/day orally.

Levetiracetam (Keppra) is particularly difficult for patients to tolerate, as it commonly causes somnolence that does not remit with continued therapy. It also commonly causes asthenia, dizziness, ataxia, agitation, anxiety, emotional lability, behavior changes, and anemia. Begin at 500 mg orally every 12 hours, for 2 weeks, and increase by 1000 mg/day every 2 weeks to a maximum of 3000 mg/day.

SNRIs. Unlike SSRIs, which have no pain-relieving activity, the SNRIs venlafaxine (Effexor) (150–225 mg/day) and duloxetine (Cymbalta) (60–120 mg/day) are helpful for patients with neuropathic pain. Both are recommended (along with gabapentin and pregabalin) as first-line therapy for patients with diabetic neuropathy (Attal, Cruccu, and Baron 2010). Venlafaxine may be helpful for patients receiving oxaliplatin, and duloxetine helps patients receiving either oxaliplatin or paclitaxel. The SNRIs are not without side effects; common ones include gastrointestinal intolerance (dry mouth, nausea, constipation, diarrhea) as well as somnolence, dizziness, and increased sweating. Rarely, they are hepatotoxic.

Tricyclic antidepressants. TCAs are also effective as adjuvant analgesics for patients with neuropathic pain (see Table 7.8) (Guan, Tanaka, and Kawakami 2016), but their anticholinergic side effects (e.g., dry mouth, dry eyes, blurred vision, constipation, hypotension, urinary retention, and sedation) limit their usefulness. At doses far below those needed for an antidepressant effect, nortriptyline, which has the least of these side effects, is well tolerated and effective. Combining TCAs with other agents with anticholinergic activity, however (H2 blockers, e.g., cimetidine; diphenhydramine, e.g., Benadryl; or hydroxyzine, e.g., Atarax, Vistaril), can cause a *cholinergic crisis*, a life-threatening syndrome that includes high fevers and delirium. (Anticholinergic crises and other causes of delirium are discussed in Chapter 9.)

TCAs like nortriptyline add efficacy to therapy with gabapentin (and by inference, also pregabalin) (Attal, Cruccu, and Baron 2010; Gilron, Baron, and Jensen 2015). Neuropathic pain is often worse at night, so give the nortriptyline at bedtime, starting at 10 mg orally. At these doses, the TCAs are safe to give to patients with renal or hepatic insufficiency.

To avoid misunderstandings, before a patient begins taking an adjuvant antidepressant, ensure he understands that just because you're using an antidepressant to treat his pain, you don't think the pain is "all in his mind."

Baclofen. This GABA (gamma-aminobutyric acid) antagonist acts primarily at the spinal cord level and is normally used to relax spastic limbs of patients with CNS disease. It is also useful for cancer patients who have developed spasticity after spinal cord injury. Baclofen relieves trigeminal neuralgia pain and so may help those patients with cancer of the head and neck who develop a neuropathic pain syndrome similar to that of trigeminal neuralgia.

Baclofen is usually given orally, three times a day, but it can be given intrathecally if necessary. Oral doses begin at 5 mg three times daily and are escalated every three days by 5 mg at each dose to a target of 40 to 80 mg/day. This gradual dose increase minimizes the drowsiness, dizziness, hypotension, nausea, and confusion that the drug can induce. It should be used cautiously in patients with severe liver failure or end-stage kidney disease, where doses should not exceed 5 mg daily. If the patient needs to discontinue baclofen, taper it gradually to prevent the patient from developing psychiatric disorders, hallucinations, or seizures.

NK-1 receptor antagonists. NK-1 receptors are activated by substance P, which is released by efferent neurons into the spinal lamina, where it transmits the pain signal by binding NK-1 receptors there. NK-1 receptor antagonists, like aprepitant or fosaprepitant, are therefore potential adjuvant analgesics for neuropathic pain. Fosaprepitant has been effective in relieving nociceptive and neuropathic pain, in patients with sickle cell disease and severe dermatomyositis associated with ovarian cancer (Dulin et al. 2017).

Alpha-2-adrenergic agonists: clonidine and dexmedetomidine. Clonidine, usually used to treat hypertension, is also able to relieve pain and will prevent opioid withdrawal in patients who must discontinue opioids following development of opioid bowel syndrome. Used either transdermally or in intrathecal infusions, clonidine is also helpful in some patients with postoperative pain, post-herpetic neuralgia, and other types of neuropathic pain.

Dexmedetomidine. Dexmedetomidine is usually used in the ICU or in perioperative settings. It produces pain relief and sedation without inducing respiratory depression, but it can induce hypotension and bradycardia (Roberts et al. 2011). We and others have used dexmedetomidine for patients outside an ICU setting who have refractory pain, opioid-induced hyperalgesia, and/or delirium who would otherwise need palliative sedation to achieve comfort at the end of life (Mupamombe, Luczkiewicz, and Kerr 2019; Hofherr, Abrahm, and Rickerson 2020). Patients have chosen to be DNR/I and to focus on comfort measures. No monitoring is needed, but they are cared for by an expert palliative care team on a hospital unit with expert nursing staff. On these infusions they remain comfortable, alert, and interactive until their last days.

Cannabinoids. Data on the efficacy of cannabinoids for cancer patients with neuropathic pain are limited, but cannabinoids are recommended for refractory pain in patients with multiple sclerosis or HIV peripheral neuropathy (Attal, Cruccu, and Baron 2010). In two randomized controlled studies, smoked cannabis relieved the pain of HIV neuropathy (Abrams et al. 2007; Ellis et al. 2009).

**Practice Point: Potential Uses of Cannabinoids
for Neuropathic Cancer Pain**

- Reverses NMDA blockade of opioid efficacy and allows lower opioid doses for pain control.
- Reverses opioid-induced hyperalgesia.
- Decreases pain and spasticity (only studied in patients with multiple sclerosis).
- Adjuvant for neuropathic pain or refractory pain syndromes.

(Hill 2015; Nugent et al. 2017; Paice et al. 2016; Strouse 2016; Whiting et al. 2015)

Cannabinoids may be useful in (1) reversing opioid-induced hyperalgesia and NMDA blockade; (2) allowing lower opioid doses with maintenance of pain control; (3) treating chronic pain and spasticity; and (4) treating patients with chronic neuropathic pain (but cancer patients were not studied) (Hill 2015; Nugent et al. 2017; Strouse 2016; Whiting et al. 2015). The ASCO guideline for treating cancer patients with chronic pain describes cannabinoids as "worthy of consideration" as an adjuvant for neuropathic pain or chronic refractory pain syndromes (Paice et al. 2016).

Nabiximols have been shown in several placebo-controlled trials to be as effective as codeine (Johnson et al. 2010; Portenoy et al. 2012), but an oral mucosal cannabinoid extract was not effective in patients with pain from CIPN (Lynch,

Cesar-Rittenberg, and Hohmann 2014). The cannabinoid extract tetrahydrocannabinol:cannabidiol (THC:CBD) spray was an effective adjuvant in decreasing pain compared with placebo or THC spray in patients with advanced cancer and moderate to severe levels of cancer pain on chronic opioid therapy. As of 2021, it was approved only in Canada. Other trials have not shown overall efficacy of nabiximols versus placebo, except in a subgroup of younger patients living in the United States (Steele, Arneson, and Zylla 2019). There are no randomized controlled trials of CBD-alone products for pain management (Mücke et al. 2018), though patients anecdotally report that the oil is helpful for neuropathic pain.

In general, among patients using cannabinoids for chronic pain, CBD does not cause side effects, but THC causes intoxication, somnolence, and cognitive impairment (Nugent et al. 2017). Increasing the concentration of CBD may mitigate some psychoactive effects of THC alone. Cancer patients using cannabinoids have cognitive side effects, with deterioration in memory and concentration (Steele, Arneson, and Zylla 2019). In patients without cancer, additional risks identified by the National Academies of Sciences, Engineering and Medicine (2017) included increased motor vehicle crashes, smaller birth-weight children, increased development of psychosis, and exacerbation of respiratory symptoms (presumably from inhaled cannabis).

Some of the risks vary by the route the cannabis is used. People using oral cannabis more often had psychoses, intoxication, and cardiovascular symptoms (including acute coronary syndromes and myocardial infractions), while those using inhaled cannabis more often had the respiratory side effects and cannabinoid hyperemesis syndrome (Monte et al. 2019), discussed in Chapter 10.

Patients using marijuana had no increased risk of lung cancer. And it is safe to take opioids when using cannabis. In fact, there are fewer opioid overdose deaths in states that have legalized marijuana (Steele, Arneson, and Zylla 2019). As of January 2022, the FDA still considered cannabis a schedule I drug; the U.S. government considers the use of medical marijuana illegal, so it cannot be used by patients in facilities that receive federal funding, even if they bring their own products.

Ketamine. Ketamine is a pure NMDA antagonist that is typically used as an anesthetic but can be helpful in the perioperative setting for patients with sickle cell disease or cancer who are opioid tolerant, and for selected patients with neuropathic pain that is resistant to the combinations of agents discussed above. Ketamine is particularly helpful for patients with central sensitization who cannot get pain relief without sedation and who wish to be awake. Patients who are taking ketamine describe being "dissociated" from their pain. They know it's there, but it's not theirs. Unfortunately, they can also be more generally dissociated, and for some this can be frightening, as can the strange dreams and even daytime hallucinations that sometimes occur. Benzodiazepines (e.g., lorazepam, 1 mg), rather than neuroleptics, are effective in reversing these side effects (Mercadante et al. 2000).

Practice Points: Ketamine for Refractory Pain

1. Inform patients that they are likely to experience a "dreamlike" state.

2. Give a ketamine bolus of 0.1 to 0.2 mg/kg IV or 0.5 mg/kg SQ, monitoring vital signs, or start a continuous infusion of 0.02–0.05 mg/kg/hr.

3. If there is no change in the pain, double the bolus dose of ketamine at 15 minutes (for IV dosing) or 45 minutes (for SQ dosing). If using a continuous infusion, increase the infusion rate by 100 percent every 4–6 hours if needed.

4. Repeat step 3 (doubling of dose) until pain relief is achieved, and then begin a continuous IV or SQ drip to deliver the equivalent amount. For example, a patient who required a total of 12 mg of ketamine in 60 minutes should be started on a drip of 12 mg/hr. Increase the drip as needed and tolerated.

5. If a decrease in opioid dose is desirable because of opioid side effects (e.g., myoclonic jerks), decrease the opioid dose initially by 50 percent when the ketamine drip is begun, and halve again every 24 hours as tolerated.

6. Excess salivation may require additional therapy with scopolamine (Transderm Scōp), hyoscyamine (e.g., Levsin), or glycopyrrolate.

(Adapted from Moryl, Coyle, and Foley 2008)

Two randomized controlled trials, methodologically sound, found that ketamine (intrathecal [Yang, Wong, and Chang 1996] or IV [Mercadante et al. 2000]) allowed a reduction in the use of morphine and produced a significant improvement in pain control for patients with neuropathic cancer pain (Bell, Eccleston, and Kalso 2017). Ketamine is particularly useful as a bridging agent, to provide pain relief for a few days when rotating a patient to methadone or treating a patient with opioid neurotoxicity (Moryl, Coyle, and Foley 2008). Although these data, case series, and open-label studies support its use, recent reviews conclude, "Current evidence is insufficient to assess the benefits and harms of ketamine as an adjunct to opioids for the relief of cancer pain" (Bell, Eccleston, and Kalso 2017, p. 2).

Ketamine has been successfully converted to the oral route, but dosing is affected by poor oral bioavailability (Peltoniemi et al. 2016). Bioavailability is 45 percent, however, when it is given by the nasal route. Esketamine spray has been approved for depression (as discussed in Chapter 9). Nasal ketamine may also be helpful as a prophylactic (e.g., for dressing changes) or rescue pain reliever, but doses needed are not well defined (Peltoniemi et al. 2016).

Intravenous lidocaine infusion. Intravenous lidocaine is a rarely used but effective neuropathic pain adjuvant. It can also be used with bolus dosing (e.g. 100–150 mg or a maximum of 3 mg/kg/dose up to twice a day) for patients with severe pain from wound dressing changes that are not responding to pain medications or ketamine (or in whom ketamine is contraindicated) (Kintzel, Knol, and Roe 2019). The pain relief, interestingly enough, may last well beyond the infusion itself (Kintzel, Knol, and Roe 2019).

Ferrini (2000) reported on the experience of the San Diego Hospice with prolonged lidocaine infusions for hospice patients with intractable pain. The infusion was initiated in the inpatient hospice unit, titrated down to the lowest effective dose, and then continued in the patients' homes. Ferrini and Paice (2004) provide a protocol for initiating and monitoring the infusions as well.

The protocol called for starting with a 1 to 3 mg/kg intravenous loading bolus of lidocaine over 20 to 30 minutes (with careful supervision by a physician, registered nurse, or nurse practitioner), recording of vital signs every 15 minutes, and assessment of pain and side effects. If the bolus was effective, the infusion of an 8 mg/ml lidocaine solution was begun at a rate of 0.5 to 2 mg/kg/hr, with a range of 10 to 80 mg/hr. Ferrini urges caution in using lidocaine for patients with severe hepatic insufficiency or heart failure, but low doses may be tolerable and effective. You can give the lidocaine subcutaneously, but prolonged subcutaneous infusions may result in erythema and induration of the infusion site.

In Ferrini's 2000 study, lidocaine serum levels were tested in the first 24 to 72 hours and were not drawn again unless there were dose escalations or toxic side effects. Adverse effects such as lightheadedness, perioral numbness, a metallic taste in the mouth, tinnitus, and blurry vision occurred within the therapeutic range of lidocaine, which is a serum range of 2 to 6 µg/ml. When this range is exceeded, patients can develop hallucinations, dissociation, myoclonus, and hypotension (at approx. 8 µg/ml). Stop the infusion immediately if any of these occur, monitor the airway, and for the psychiatric side effects, consider adding a benzodiazepine or a fast-acting barbiturate if benzodiazepines are contraindicated. With higher blood levels of lidocaine, seizures, coma, and respiratory or cardiac arrest may occur.

Adjuvant Treatments for Bone Pain

Bone metastases cause both neuropathic and somatic pain, and there is usually an inflammatory component mediated by synthesis of prostaglandins and other cytokines. NSAIDs, corticosteroids (see Tables 7.1 and 7.8), bisphosphonates, and RANK-L inhibitors (Fournier et al. 2010; Van Poznak et al. 2011; von Moos and Skacel 2012) can therefore serve as important pharmacologic adjuvants to opioids for patients with bone pain (Table 7.9). Vertebroplasty/kyphoplasty can relieve the pain associated with vertebral compression fractures. Radiofrequency ablation also can relieve metastatic bone pain. External beam radiation is the longest-lasting palliative treatment for bone pain, and radiopharmaceuticals (e.g., radium-223 chloride [Alpharadin], samarium-153, and the older agent strontium chloride 89; Paes et al. 2011) enhance its effectiveness and are also effective used alone.

Bisphosphonates. These drugs inhibit osteoclast activity and can provide immediate relief of pain due to bony metastases or bone lesions of multiple myeloma. ASCO recommends using either pamidronate (Aredia) (60 to 90 mg IV over no less than 2 hours), or zoledronic acid (Zometa) (4 mg IV over 15 minutes) (Van Poznak et al. 2011). Both can be given to patients with hepatic failure, but denosumab (see below) is a better choice for patients with renal insufficiency. Both have been shown to decrease pain or the need for pain-relieving medications. If the pain returns, repeat doses 3 to 4 weeks apart are often effective. Both drugs have the added benefit of slowing the growth of some tumor metastases and, when given monthly, of preventing fractures from lytic bone metastases in patients with myeloma and breast cancer (von Moos et al. 2013; Stark Toller et al. 2019).

Both cause similar adverse effects. Both can cause an acute phase reaction, which includes a pain flare, fever, and aches in the joints. This acute phase reaction and renal toxicity are more frequent with zoledronic acid. Renal function should be monitored in patients who have baseline impairment or are at high risk for dehydration.

Both bisphosphonates and the RANK-L inhibitor discussed below cause hypocalcemia in vitamin D–deficient patients and an increased risk of subtrochanteric hip fracture and of osteonecrosis of the jaw (Fournier et al. 2010; Stark Toller et al. 2019). Patients with osteonecrosis from medication who were given teriparatide (recombinant human parathyroid hormone 1–34) therapy along with standard calcium and vitamin D replacement showed a greater rate of resolution of the osteonecrosis and reduced bony defects compared with patients receiving only standard calcium and vitamin D supplements (Sim et al. 2020). Teriparatide is contraindicated, however, in patients who have had previous skeletal radiation or bone malignancies, as there may be an increased risk of osteosarcoma (Ripamonti and Napoli 2020).

Vitamin D deficiency is very prevalent in the United States and in cancer patients. As many as 33 percent of the U.S. population and 20 percent of cancer patients are deficient (i.e., had 25(OH)D levels of <20 ng/ml). An additional 30 percent have levels that are inadequate for bone health (between 20 and 30 ng/ml). More than 75 percent of adults over 65 who live in the community are deficient! In addition to age, risk factors include having dark skin, osteoporosis or osteopenia, avoiding sun exposure, usually wearing a veil, living in a very polluted environment, or having Crohn's disease (DeMille et al. 2014). Patients with breast or prostate cancer who are or will receive antineoplastic procedures that will lead to hypogonadism are also at increased risk. Before starting a bisphosphonate or a RANK-L inhibitor, therefore, testing for vitamin D levels and replacement therapy should be strongly considered in these high-risk patients to avoid symptomatic and even dangerous hypocalcemia.

RANK-L inhibitors. Denosumab is a monoclonal antibody that, by inhibiting the ability of the RANK ligand (produced by osteoblasts) to bind to RANK on the surface of osteoclasts and osteoclast precursors, prevents osteoclast maturation, activation, and bone resorption. Denosumab (given as 120 mg subcutaneously every 4 weeks) therefore prevents skeletal-related complications and hypercalcemia as well as lessening bone pain in patients with breast cancer metastatic to bone. In fact, it can cause a hypocalcemia more profound than that caused by the bisphosphonates; high-risk patients (as described above) should be screened for vitamin D deficiency before receiving it.

Denosumab causes an acute phase reaction less often than zoledronic acid and does not impair renal function. When denosumab was compared with zoledronic acid in a large randomized study of patients with metastatic bone disease from breast cancer (von Moos et al. 2013), fewer patients receiving denosumab had "meaningful worsening" of their pain (defined by the authors as a greater than 2-point increase from baseline). Denosumab delayed by almost 4 months the worsening of pain from no/mild pain to moderate/severe in those whose pain did worsen, and fewer patients on denosumab had increased pain.

Vertebroplasty/kyphoplasty. Pain from benign or malignant compression fractures can be very difficult to treat, especially in older patients who develop confusion and marked worsening of constipation while using the opioid doses they need, even when they are taking NSAID adjuvants. For selected patients (those with very localized intense pain from a new or progressing fracture), vertebroplasty or kyphoplasty may be the answer. In both procedures, bone "cement" (polymethylmethacrylate + antibiotics + an opacification agent) is injected under fluoroscopic guidance into the collapsed vertebra to stabilize it; in kyphoplasty, the endplates of the vertebral body are elevated by inflatable bone tamps before the cement is injected. Both procedures can be done in the outpatient setting by an interventional radiologist, a neurosurgeon, or an orthopedic surgeon.

A 2016 systemic review by Health Quality Ontario found that cancer patients who received either kyphoplasty or vertebroplasty for cancer-related vertebral compression fractures had rapidly reduced pain, along with significant reductions in fracture-related disability and the need for opioids, compared with patients who received usual care (Health Quality Ontario 2016). Patients with malignancies are most often also treated with radiation, so it is difficult to assess the long-term contribution of the vertebroplasty, but the review and case reports indicate pain relief within 48 hours that is most likely due to the procedure (Jensen and Kallmes 2002).

The mechanism of the relief is not clear, although some authors have postulated that the injection of the cement causes destruction of nerve endings in the local tissue or necrosis of the tumor (Jensen and Kallmes 2002). Extravasation of the cement is usually asymptomatic but can rarely cause marked increase in pain that can last for days, as well as damage to the spinal cord or nerve roots from heat or pressure.

Radiofrequency ablation. Radiofrequency ablation (inducing coagulation necrosis by heating tissues to approximately 100°C) has been used to ablate focal tumors. This technique is now being used to treat painful focal tumors in bone, skin, or viscera (Gennaro et al. 2019; Goetz et al. 2004; Rosenthal and Callstrom 2012).

External beam radiation. External beam radiation is an important palliative tool for treating localized bone metastases (Shiloh and Krishnan 2018). It provides pain relief for 50 percent of patients within 2 weeks after completing radiation and for more than 75 percent of patients within 2 additional (4 total) weeks, and the relief usually lasts about 3 months. Palliative radiation given in a single large fraction is optimal for patients whose survival is expected to be 6 months or less. A single fraction produces pain relief just as fast and for just as long as the more conventional treatments involving ten fractions (Shiloh and Krishnan 2018). Longer fractionation schedules are recommended for patients with better prognoses (e.g., patients with metastatic breast cancer), because tumor recurrence requiring repeat radiation is more common after single fraction, and because the bones heal better after multiple fractions.

Stereotactic body radiation therapy (SBRT). SBRT is given to patients who need a higher dose of radiation, for example to the spinal cord, focused to avoid normal tissue. Patients who have a recurrence after external beam radiation therapy (EBRT) can therefore be retreated safely with SBRT, with local control of the tumor as high as 80–90 percent a year later (Shiloh and Krishnan 2018). Even patients whose tumors are relatively resistant to radiation, such as melanoma or renal cell cancers, respond well to SBRT, with local control rates in the 90 percent range. SBRT may also be superior to EBRT for patients with metastases to the spinal vertebrae (Sahgal et al 2020). A phase III randomized trial showed that more than twice as many patients treated with SBRT had complete reduction in pain lasting 6 months (32 percent) compared with patients receiving EBRT (16 percent) (p = .004). If other studies confirm this finding, it may be practice changing for patients with good performance status (ECOG 0–2). Something to watch for.

Radiopharmaceuticals. Systemic radiopharmaceuticals, such as the alpha emitter radium-223 chloride (Alpharadin) (Cheetham and Petrylak 2012), and the beta emitters strontium chloride 89 and samarium-153 lexidronam (Paes et al. 2011), are used for patients with diffuse bony metastases, even though studies include only patients with metastatic prostate cancer (Shiloh and Krishnan 2018).

The newest agent, radium-223 chloride (Alpharadin), utilizes an alpha particle bound to a calcium analogue that self-targets to bone metastases. It causes less marrow toxicity than the beta emitters discussed below because the range of the alpha particles is only a 2- to 10-cell diameter. Alpha particles can therefore destroy the metastasis with relative sparing of normal marrow cells. The largest randomized controlled multicenter phase III trial (vs. placebo) showed no increased adverse events in the treatment arm, along with an improvement in survival (OS 14.0 vs. 11.2 months, 2-sided p value = .0022), 30 percent decreased risk of death, and increased quality of life (Parker et al. 2013).

Practice Points: Treating Patients with Bone Pain

- For patients over 60 years old or with congestive heart failure, renal disease, asthma, or a history of gastrointestinal bleeding, the risks of NSAIDs (used as opioid adjuvants for bone pain) probably exceed the benefit.
- Bisphosphonates: Give zoledronic acid (Zometa) or pamidronate (Aredia) for pain due to bone metastases. Both can also decrease pathologic fractures in patients with metastatic breast cancer or multiple myeloma.
- RANK-L inhibitors: RANK-L inhibitors (e.g., denosumab) are equally or more effective for pain from bone metastases but can cause severe hypocalcemia in patients with deficiencies of vitamin D. Such patients will require repletion of both vitamin D and calcium.
- Use pamidronate or denosumab for patients with renal insufficiency.
- Vertebroplasty and kyphoplasty can relieve the pain associated with vertebral compression fractures caused by either osteoporosis or cancer.
- Radiofrequency ablation and external beam radiation are designed for patients with few painful bony metastases.
- For patients with refractory diffuse bone metastases causing pain, who are no longer candidates for chemotherapy, which can cause cytopenias, consider referring the patient to a nuclear medicine specialist for a systemic radio-pharmaceutical: either a beta-emitter (e.g., samarium-153 lexidronam) or an alpha emitter (e.g., Alpharadin).

The beta-particle emitters localize in osteoblastic metastases. They provide pain relief in about 60 to 80 percent of patients. Pain relief usually begins within 1 to 2 weeks and is maintained for more than 6 months in patients with breast or prostate cancer. Strontium chloride 89 can prolong the pain relief induced by EBRT, but patients who receive both are more likely to have serious thrombocytopenia (~20 percent) and leukopenia (~10 percent) than patients who receive only EBRT (Shiloh and Krishnan 2018).

Strontium-89 is chemically similar to calcium and is deposited in bone preferentially to calcium. It may therefore exacerbate hypercalcemia and should not be given to hypercalcemic patients. Strontium chloride 89 is given by slow intravenous push in the outpatient setting by a nuclear medicine physician. For 48 hours after the injection, patients should flush twice after using a toilet and should avoid using urinals and bedpans if possible. Families should be cautioned to wear disposable gloves while handling any items contaminated with the patient's urine, feces, or blood. Patients and families should also be warned that 5 to 10 percent of patients will suffer a "flare" (i.e., an increase in bone pain) 2 to 3 days after the injection, which will remit in 7 to 10 days; flares occur more often in patients with breast cancer than in those with prostate cancer. Corticosteroids or NSAIDs may relieve the pain.

Pregnancy and breastfeeding are the only two absolute contraindications to use of strontium-89, and patients should be cautioned not to get pregnant for 6 to 12 months after the injection. Patients with a GFR of less than 30 ml/min should not be treated because of the risk of prolonged myelosuppression, but those with clearances between 30 and 50 ml/min can be given a 50 percent dose reduction. Myelosuppression occurs in most patients. Strontium chloride 89 is therefore contraindicated for patients with hemoglobin less than 9 mg/dL, platelet counts of less than 100,000/mm³, or absolute leukocyte counts of less than 3500/mm³ (Paes et al. 2011).

Since samarium-153 lexidronam is also excreted intact in the urine, patients and families should exercise the same precautions as they would if the patient had received strontium, but the excretion is complete within 12 hours. The same contraindications to therapy described for strontium apply to samarium-153.

Hemibody radiation. This can relieve pain in the lower spine, pelvis, and femora in as many as 80 percent of patients with bony metastases from prostate, lung, or breast cancer, with 30 percent obtaining complete relief. The relief begins as early as 48 hours after treatment and can last as long as 6 months. Patients can develop slightly lowered blood counts and mild diarrhea (Pal et al. 2014). Antiemetics (e.g., a 5HT3 inhibitor) are needed before and for 2–3 days following treatment.

Skeletal Muscle Relaxants

Skeletal muscle relaxants include agents such as baclofen, diazepam, tizanidine, and dantrolene, which are used for spasticity, and carisoprodol (e.g., Soma), metaxolone (Skelaxin), chlorzoxazone (e.g., Parafon Forte DSC), cyclobenzaprine HCl (e.g., Flexeril), methocarbamol (e.g., Robaxin), and orphenadrine citrate (e.g., Norflex, Norgesic), which are skeletal muscle relaxants (Hardek and Pruskowski 2017). Only baclofen is FDA approved for spasticity. Used alone, they are no more effective than NSAIDs, but they do add to the efficacy of NSAIDs for patients with acute muscle injury and spasm. Carisoprodol, orphenadrine, and methocarbamol are available in preparations that include aspirin.

Skeletal muscle relaxants are not as effective for patients with chronic non-malignant pain as for those with acute pain, and they have not been studied in patients with cancer pain. Because they are metabolized by the liver and excreted by the kidneys, skeletal muscle relaxants are relatively contraindicated for patients with renal or hepatic dysfunction. In addition, they have the potential for abuse, and patients who stop them suddenly may experience a withdrawal syndrome.

Muscle relaxants cause significant side effects. Drowsiness is especially problematic and is likely to limit their use in someone receiving other sedating agents such as opioids. They can also cause dizziness, headaches, blurry vision, agitation, confusion, hallucinations, and convulsions. More rarely, patients have developed abdominal pain, nausea, vomiting, or anorexia when taking these drugs.

Cyclobenzaprine HCl is related chemically to tricyclic antidepressants, and orphenadrine citrate is related to diphenhydramine; they share the anticholinergic and antihistaminic side effects of these agents.

For cancer patients who develop an acute muscle injury or muscle spasm and who do not need opioid analgesics, a combination NSAID/skeletal muscle relaxant may be beneficial. Because of the serious side effects they can induce, do not prescribe them for prolonged periods.

A *benzodiazepine* such as diazepam (e.g., Valium), which is FDA approved for spasticity, can help cancer patients who have muscle spasms, even those induced by spinal cord injury, but it is no more effective than the other skeletal muscle relaxants or baclofen. The side effects of this long-acting agent limit its usefulness, especially for patients who require concomitant opioid therapy. Patients who have been using diazepam chronically for an anxiety or seizure disorder are likely to tolerate the combination of an opioid and the diazepam. Other patients are likely to develop intolerable somnolence.

Smooth Muscle Relaxants

Pain arising from the smooth muscle of the gastrointestinal tract is due to either stretching, as is experienced during a bowel obstruction, or intense contractions. Contractions can cause cramping, and if the contraction moves through an area of injured mucosa, such as would occur in esophagitis or in radiation injury to the rectal area, the pain can be intense. Such pain is intermittent and often difficult to control with basal opioids because a basal dose adequate to control the pain at its height causes unacceptable sedation between painful episodes. Patients receiving opioids for another cause of pain, who are opioid tolerant, however, may get significant immediate pain relief from any of the various forms of transmucosal fentanyl (oral tablet, film, or nasal spray). The onset of pain relief in about 5 minutes and the disappearance of opioid effect in about an hour make this form of opioid delivery particularly helpful for these patients.

Another approach is to relax the smooth muscle. Calcium channel blockers like nifedipine, gabapentin, or pregabalin can be helpful as can baclofen. In patients with adequate blood pressure, nitroglycerin can relieve esophageal spasm. Anticholinergic agents also relax gut smooth muscle. Dicyclomine (e.g., Bentyl) (10–20 mg p.o. up to t.i.d. p.r.n.) has minimal other anticholinergic side effects and is often effective.

Local therapies are also effective. Belladonna and opium suppositories (B&O suppositories) provide significant relief for patients with bladder or rectal spasm. Patients can use 30 or 60 mg up to four times a day. Other commonly used effective agents include oral anticholinergics, such as oxybutynin 5 to 15 mg p.o. t.i.d. or ER daily; trospium 20 mg p.o. b.i.d. (e.g., Sanctura) or one 60 mg XR capsule (e.g., Sanctura XR); and phenazopyridine, which is often used with the anticholinergic.

It is given at 100–200 mg p.o. t.i.d. p.r.n. and may stain clothing orange (De, Gomery, and Rosenberg 2017). For those with rectal spasm, it may be necessary to pretreat the rectal area with a lidocaine or hydrocortisone cream (e.g., Anusol) to enable the patient to tolerate insertion of the suppository. Refer refractory patients with rectal pain to an anesthesia pain specialist for consideration of a block of the ganglion impar (discussed later in this chapter).

ANESTHETIC METHODS OF PAIN RELIEF

Anesthetics and anesthetic pain techniques play a select but valuable role in relieving neuropathic pain for certain cancer patients. Anesthetics are available in topical and oral formulations as well as the parenteral forms that are needed to numb or ablate peripheral or spinal somatic or autonomic nerves, or to block transmissions from the spinal cord.

Blocks may be used as initial therapy for patients with post-thoracotomy syndrome, acute pain from herpes zoster (neural blockade alone), post-herpetic neuralgia, or pain from pancreatic cancer. For other neuropathic pain syndromes, parenteral anesthetic agents are indicated when the patient's pain has not been satisfactorily relieved by combinations of oral or transdermal opioids, adjuvant agents, and topical or oral anesthetics. They are delivered by anesthesia pain specialists who practice in freestanding and hospital-based pain clinics. These physicians are often leaders of multidisciplinary teams involved in research, education, and clinical care of patients with neuropathic pain. Anesthesia pain specialists can markedly improve the quality of life of the patients they treat (Careskey and Narang 2018; Narang, Weisheipl, and Ross 2016).

What follows is an overview of the techniques they use and a description of the types of patients they can help. As I am not an anesthesia pain specialist, I do not feel qualified to describe the techniques themselves in detail, but references are provided in the online bibliography.

Topical Anesthetics

Topical anesthetics are of limited general utility in cancer patients with pain, but they can be helpful in selected instances (Table 7.10). The usual preparations for cancer patients include a combination of lidocaine and prilocaine (EMLA), lidocaine alone (e.g., ELA-Max), and capsaicin (Kumar, Chawla, and Goyal 2015).

EMLA. This cream includes a mixture of two anesthetics, lidocaine 2.5 percent and prilocaine 2.5 percent. It anesthetizes the skin to a depth of about one-quarter inch (5 mm) and is used, for example, before accessing a subcutaneous port, placing a PICC, or doing a lumbar puncture, bone marrow aspiration, or biopsy. The majority of studies have taken place in children, but adults may also benefit from its use.

An hour to 90 minutes before the planned procedure, the nurse, the patient, or a family member places a mound of EMLA cream over the area to be anesthetized, using about half of a 5-g tube. Being careful to maintain a thick layer of cream, the person applying it covers the mound with a semipermeable dressing such as Opsite or Tegaderm. Immediately before the procedure, the dressing and cream are removed, and the area is prepared as usual. The skin anesthesia will remain for up to 4 hours.

Side effects of EMLA are minimal. The prilocaine in the anesthetic mixture can cause increases in methemoglobin, but when EMLA is used as recommended, methemoglobinemia has not been a problem, even in children as young as 3 months old. The only other consistent findings are changes of skin color to red or white; this rarely lasts longer than 4 hours.

Lidocaine gel, ointment, or patch. More than 25 years ago, topical lidocaine gel (5 percent) was first shown to be more effective than placebo in relieving pain in a double-blind controlled trial in patients with post-herpetic neuralgia (Rowbotham, Davies, and Fields 1995). Lidocaine ointment (5 percent and 10 percent) is also available and can be used along with capsaicin for post-herpetic neuralgia or alone for peripheral sensory neuropathy. ELA-Max, a cream containing 4 percent lidocaine, is now available over-the-counter as an alternative to EMLA cream. Because it does not contain prilocaine, there is no risk of methemoglobinemia.

Lidocaine patches (e.g., Lidoderm) are lidocaine-impregnated dressings that adhere to the skin and deliver anesthesia to the skin surface. The patch is FDA approved for use in post-herpetic neuralgia and has been reported to be effective in patients with other chronic neuropathic pain syndromes, such as diabetic neuropathy and post-mastectomy and post-thoracotomy pain.

Lidocaine patches can be placed on skin that is so hyperesthetic that even the touch of clothing is uncomfortable. Hyperesthesia can occur in patients with post-herpetic neuralgia or in those with nerve injury from surgery (e.g., post-thoracotomy, post-mastectomy, post–port placement) or from tumor invasion of either peripheral nerves or dorsal root ganglia. The patches should be applied to intact skin for up to 12 consecutive hours a day and can be cut to size or to surround an infusion port. As many as four patches can be used concurrently. Systemic concentrations of lidocaine do not reach a level at which they would affect cardiac function. Lidocaine patches should not be used where the skin is broken or over skin directly in the radiation port when the patient is receiving radiation therapy.

Capsaicin. Capsaicin cream (0.025 percent, 0.075 percent) (e.g., Zostrix, Capzacin-P) has been approved by the FDA for arthritis pain, for postsurgical neuropathic pain, and for treatment of post-herpetic neuralgia, where it can be used along with gabapentin or pregabalin (Haanpää and Treede 2012). It is also a useful addition to NSAIDs for patients with pain from bony metastases.

Capsaicin provides analgesia by depleting substance P, a peptide that is an important transmitter of nerve impulses from peripheral nerves to the spinal cord. Capsaicin is found in the seeds of hot peppers and is what causes the intense burning and numbness you've experienced if you've made the mistake of eating one!

Unfortunately, capsaicin cream is expensive, and it usually provides only partial pain relief, being effective in about half the patients with post-mastectomy and other postsurgical neuropathic pains who were surveyed, and in up to one-third of patients with post-herpetic neuralgia. Repeated applications (four times a day) for at least 4 weeks are needed. Adhesive skin patches delivering 0.025 percent capsaicin can be used but have not been tested for this indication.

Further, capsaicin's utility in relieving neuropathic pain is limited by the significant burning it causes in the skin where it is applied. Patients with post-herpetic neuralgia experience more discomfort using the cream than those with post-mastectomy pain, but it occurs in both populations and was the most common reason patients stopped using capsaicin. Some patients have found that applying a 5 percent or 10 percent lidocaine ointment prior to the capsaicin cream diminished the burning sensation; others, even with the lidocaine pretreatment, could not tolerate this agent (Watson, Evans, and Watt 1988).

Capsaicin may cause intense burning in these patients because their nerves are injured and their skin is hyperesthetic. Patients with normal skin who use capsaicin cream for arthritis or deep muscle pain notice warmth, but they tolerate it well. They rub it into the skin over the painful area once to three times a day. The area sometimes becomes warm if it is exposed to sun, but not painfully so.

Local Anesthetics Taken Orally

Mexiletine, a local anesthetic available in pill form, is an effective adjuvant for certain patients with refractory continuous or lancinating neuropathic pains (Table 7.10). It is usually reserved for patients with refractory neuropathic pain that has not responded to the agents discussed above.

Mexiletine use for patients with neuropathic cancer pain has not been studied extensively, but it is the most often used oral local anesthetic for patients with nonmalignant neuropathic pain. It is relatively safe even for patients with a cardiac arrhythmia or those receiving drugs to prevent one. The initial recommended dose is 150 mg/day orally, and it can be escalated if tolerated to doses of 300 mg orally three times a day. Dyspepsia and diarrhea may limit its tolerability.

Neural Blockade, Neuroablation, Infusion Therapy, and Cingulotomy

Neural blockade, neuroablation, and infusion therapies are the province of interventional radiologists and anesthesia pain specialists, and cingulotomy is done by neurosurgeons. Neural blockade or ablation are often employed as initial therapy for post-thoracotomy syndrome, acute pain from herpes zoster (neural blockade alone), post-herpetic neuralgia, or pain from cancers in the head and neck, chest wall, abdomen, or pelvis, and they can be helpful when the therapies mentioned elsewhere in this chapter have been ineffective.

The only patients with refractory neuropathic pain who are unlikely to benefit from neuroablative procedures are those with *deafferentation* pain. Deafferentation pain is a poorly localized, deeply aching, and distressing sensation that occurs when a peripheral nerve is "disconnected" from the spinal cord surgically or by any other process that injures a nerve. Patients with injury to the spinal cord from cancer or with tumor invading the brachial or lumbosacral plexus can develop deafferentation pain. Though such patients might experience temporary relief from a local anesthetic block, a neurolytic procedure is unlikely to be of benefit.

Neural blockade. Neural blockade is a regional anesthetic procedure that can include blocks of spinal and peripheral somatic nerves and of the sympathetic nervous system. Injections of local anesthetics such as lidocaine or bupivacaine along with a corticosteroid are used for diagnosis, prognosis, therapy, and pain prevention.

A *diagnostic* nerve block can determine which nerve is mediating the pain and whether it is a somatic or sympathetic nerve. The anesthesia pain specialist can then plan the appropriate therapeutic block or neurolytic procedure. The patient's response to this block will also allow the specialist to predict the likely outcome and the side effects of a more permanent procedure (e.g., neuroablation).

To minimize ineffective procedures, *prognostic* blocks always precede a planned neuroablative procedure; if anesthetizing the nerve does not relieve the pain, the anesthesia pain specialist does not proceed (Careskey and Narang 2018). Unfortunately, the converse is not true: a positive result from a block does not always predict a positive outcome from the neuroablative procedure.

Sometimes, *therapeutic* nerve blocks are sufficient, and a neuroablative procedure will not be needed. Interestingly, their effectiveness may outlast the known half-life of the anesthetic agent that was injected. Anesthetics, in combination with a glucocorticoid, can be injected into the spinal space or nerve roots affected by tumor, and the relief can last from days to weeks. Catheters can provide long-term delivery of local anesthetics and other adjuvant medications; they can be tunneled or be part of a Port-a-cath.

Trigger point injections can help with myofascial pains, such as those associated with post-mastectomy syndrome. A local anesthetic is usually injected into the trigger point, though dry needling or local instillation of saline or corticosteroid are also used. Before adding systemic opioids to NSAIDs for patients with myofascial pain, refer them for trigger point injections.

Subcutaneous administration of local anesthetic plus corticosteroids is often helpful for the somatically mediated acute pain of herpes zoster and for prevention of post-herpetic neuralgia. Because these injections are so often effective and have so few associated side effects, consider referring patients with these syndromes to an anesthesia pain specialist before beginning therapy with opioids or an adjuvant such as gabapentin or pregabalin.

Radiofrequency ablation. Radiofrequency ablation (inducing coagulation necrosis by heating tissues to approximately 100°C) has been used to treat patients with trigeminal neuralgia (tic douloureux) by destroying the trigeminal nerve ganglion.

Cryoanalgesia. Cryoanalgesia is performed by freezing the target nerve temporarily. The analgesia produced can last from 2 weeks to a number of months (Allano et al. 2019).

Sympathetic nerve blocks of the celiac plexus or the stellate or gasserian ganglia are usually done to determine whether the pain will respond to ablation of the ganglion in patients with pain from pancreatic cancer or cancer of the head and neck. A chemical neurolytic procedure or radiofrequency lesioning is performed if anesthetic blockade of the relevant sympathetic structure results in remission of the pain.

Sympathetic nerve blocks are also often used for patients suffering from type I complex regional pain syndrome (formerly termed *reflex sympathetic dystrophy*, or *causalgia*), which arises from injury to sympathetic nerves due to trauma, scarring, or direct invasion by a malignancy. The patient complains of burning pain in the arm or leg, and the limb becomes hyperalgesic and allodynic (i.e., even clothing touching the skin causes a burning pain). The skin may be edematous, red, or pale; may manifest decreased sweating and increased warmth; and, over time, will become atrophic. You may note such changes in the arms of patients with infiltration of the brachial plexus due to cancers of the breast or superior sulcus of the lung, or those who have received radiation to the brachial plexus. In some cases the pain syndrome will respond to a blockade alone, but in others, chemical destruction of involved ganglia or surgical rhizotomy (i.e., selective ablation of the affected ganglia) is needed.

Neurolytic procedures. Neurolytic procedures (i.e., ablation of the nerve) are indicated for patients who are expected to live only a short time, whose neuropathic pain is well localized and has not responded to other measures. Pain mediated by spinal, peripheral somatic, and sympathetic nerves can be treated by these techniques.

Neuroablation can be achieved surgically, but at present, thermal and chemical means are more commonly used. Thermal techniques include radiofrequency ablation, as discussed above, and cryoanalgesia. Chemical agents include glycerol (which is used to block the trigeminal ganglion), phenol, and ethanol. Phenol, unlike ethanol, has local anesthetic as well as lytic effects and is therefore painless when injected. Ethanol injections are so painful that they must be preceded by injections of local anesthetic, and the patient must be sedated. The usual clinical doses of phenol or ethanol are unlikely to cause side effects from systemic absorption. If phenol is injected intravascularly by accident, however, it can cause convulsions, CNS depression, and cardiovascular collapse.

Spinal neurolytic procedures. Patients suffering from recurrent gynecologic, colorectal, or bladder cancers may experience severe bilateral pelvic pain in a *saddle* distribution. Systemic opioids or a spinal opioid/anesthetic infusion usually provides these patients with satisfactory pain relief. For more than 60 percent of the very few who still have intolerable pain, subarachnoid neurolytic blockades may provide good pain relief for several months; rarely, pain relief lasts up to a year. The pain relief may be so complete that the patient abruptly discontinues all oral opioid therapy. To prevent patients from experiencing withdrawal, they are instructed before the procedure on how to taper their opioids safely.

Saddle blocks are considered when an epidural catheter cannot be used or its insertion is problematic, as can be the case for patients with frequent infections. Patients with, for example, a rectovaginal fistula or burning perineal pain from locally advanced pelvic cancers (e.g., colorectal, bladder, cervical, or endometrial cancer) may benefit from these blocks. Phenol, which is hyperbaric, is placed intrathecally and sinks to the level of S2–S4 nerves. Patients usually continue to be mobile, but the block may cause bowel and bladder incontinence. Usually, however, patients who need this block for pain relief already have diverting colostomies, ureters diverted into Indiana pouches, or renal stents to relieve obstruction caused by the tumor. Side effects (e.g., leg weakness) and pain relief depend on the concentration of phenol used. Higher concentrations of phenol can be given to patients with urinary diversions. Generally, patients have at least a 50 percent pain reduction and clearer thinking, because systemic agents can be markedly reduced. Relief usually lasts for a month, but it sometimes lasts for 2 months and, rarely, can persist for as long as 6 months.

Subdural and epidural neurolysis is used for pain in the cervical region, an area in which subarachnoid blockade is not effective. It can be helpful to patients with refractory pain due to cancer of the ear, nose, throat, or lung, or for those with bony cervical metastases.

Ablation of peripheral somatic nerves. Neuroablation of intercostal nerves can relieve post-thoracotomy syndrome, especially when performed within 6 months of its onset. This procedure can also relieve the pain of a pathologic rib fracture in someone who is not a candidate for radiation therapy. Neuroablation is also used for patients with intractable pain from metastatic lesions to tissues innervated by other peripheral nerves, such as a metastatic tumor to the forearm, which is innervated by the superficial radial, lateral cutaneous, and posterior cutaneous nerves (Turnbull et al. 2011). Because neuroablation is often so effective and has so few associated side effects compared with the doses of systemic opioids or neuropathic adjuvant agents that would be needed, consult with an anesthesia pain specialist as soon as possible.

Sympathetic nerve ablation. Some patients' neuropathic pain syndromes are caused by injury to the sympathetic nervous system. The injury can be to ganglia or to the sympathetic fibers in a nerve plexus such as the brachial or lumbosacral plexus.

Practice Points: Peripheral Neuroablative Procedures

Target	Indications
• Sacral nerves	Perineal pain
• Intercostal nerve	Post-thoracotomy syndrome
• Sympathetic ganglia:	
– Celiac plexus	Upper abdominal pain, especially radiating to back
– Inferior mesenteric (impar)	Perineal, rectal pain/spasm
– Stellate	Head and neck pain
– Gasserian	Tic douloureux–like pain
• Hypogastric plexus	Pelvic pain
• Percutaneous dorsal rhizotomy	Complex regional pain syndrome type I (causalgia) of upper extremity

Head, neck, and upper extremity. In the past, injection of the *gasserian ganglion* with alcohol was used for patients with benign or malignant causes of tic douloureux. More recently, however, for patients with pain refractory to carbamazepine or baclofen, injection of the ganglion with glycerol, thermogangliolysis, or surgical rhizotomy is used.

Sympathetic blockade of the *stellate ganglion* with local anesthetics can reduce the incidence of post-herpetic neuralgia in the upper extremity and face if used within 2 weeks of the onset of the herpes zoster. Some researchers have found that it can be effective if used within the first 2 months of appearance of the lesions.

Selected cancer patients with pain in the arms or in the head and neck or with Pancoast tumor will benefit from neuroablation of the stellate ganglion. Chemical neuroablation is rarely done, because of the damage that may be caused to nearby nervous, vascular, and brain structures by the lytic agents.

Some patients with injury to the brachial plexus have complex regional pain syndrome type I (causalgia) that does not respond to anesthetic blockade. For these patients, *percutaneous surgical dorsal rhizotomy* is considered preferable to a chemical rhizotomy because it rarely has to be repeated.

Abdominal/pelvic. Celiac plexus blocks are the most commonly used and most effective sympathetic neurolytic blocks for cancer patients. This plexus contains sympathetic ganglia that mediate pain from upper abdominal organs. Celiac plexus blocks have been found to relieve the abdominal pain of half to three-quarters of patients with pancreatic cancer. Because the blocks are so effective, some surgeons will resect the celiac ganglion or inject it with alcohol or a phenol solution at the time of definitive or palliative surgery. Anesthesia pain specialists and interventional radiologists perform the neuroablation percutaneously with fluoroscopy or CT guidance. GI specialists can do it during endoscopy.

A celiac block may also relieve pain due to cancer of the stomach, liver, small bowel, proximal colon, or abdominal metastases if it resembles the pain caused by pancreatic cancer. Celiac blocks do not have to be reserved for patients who are refractory to opioids or for whom the opioid-induced side effects are poorly tolerated. A randomized double-blind controlled trial showed that celiac plexus block done at the time of diagnosis in patients with inoperable pancreatic cancer decreased the need for systemic opioids to control pain throughout the patient's course (Wyse et al. 2011). The effects were particularly evident 3 months after randomization, and strongest in patients who did not have chemo-XRT for their cancer.

The common side effects caused by destroying the celiac plexus result from interruption of sympathetic innervation to the upper abdominal organs. They include temporary orthostatic hypotension and diarrhea due to increased gut motility. Rarely, the neurolytic solution will spread to the lumbosacral plexus or nerve roots and cause radicular pain or, very rarely, paraparesis or paraplegia.

Chemical neuroablation of the *superior hypogastric plexus* is effective in the treatment of selected patients with pelvic cancer pain, such as that caused by gynecologic or recurrent colorectal cancer. Relief can last as long as 6 months. The older procedure, chemical lumbar sympathectomy, has also been shown to be effective for pelvic pain, but the blockade is less selective.

Rectal pain/tenesmus and perineal pain respond to blockade of the *ganglion impar*, located anterior to the sacrococcygeal ligament (Mueller et al. 2020). Complications include puncture of the rectum and bladder, local infection, and abscess. Spinal anesthesia and intravascular injection may rarely occur. Evidence for pharmacologic therapy for tenesmus is too limited for a recommendation.

Percutaneous spinal cordotomy. Unilateral pain such as that caused by invasion of the chest wall by a mesothelioma or breast cancer can be responsive to percutaneous cordotomy, where lesions are made in the contralateral spinothalamic tract of the spinal cord (Fallon et al. 2018). Sustained relief is reported as high as 40–50 percent (Viswanathan et al. 2019). Patients who are not candidates for intrathecal pumps or whose pain persists despite IT pump placement may be candidates for this surgery.

Cingulotomy. Patients whose pain is intolerable despite all the other measures discussed in this chapter and in Chapter 8 are considered candidates for cingulotomy. It is reportedly effective in significantly reducing pain in 60 percent of the patients who undergo the procedure, and personality change was noted in <1 percent. The patients I've taken care of as much as a year after the procedure continue to report areas of pain, but without emotional valence. They may still require systemic or intraspinal opioids for optimal control of their discomfort, but their quality of life is much improved.

Summary. The anesthetic techniques reviewed above are often crucial to providing effective therapy for the fewer than 10 percent of patients for whom disease-directed therapy, opioids, and adjuvant agents have caused intolerable side effects or have failed to relieve their neuropathic pain. By recognizing neuropathic pain when it occurs, using the topical and oral agents judiciously, and referring appropriate patients to anesthesia pain specialists, you may enable your patients with refractory pain syndromes to experience significant relief.

RELIEVING PAIN IN OLDER PERSONS

Assessment

Staff in long-term care facilities, community nurses, and even hospice nurses underestimate intense levels of persistent pain in elderly patients and consequently undertreat them. Dementia is estimated to occur in about 5 percent of patients over 65, rising to more than 40 percent in patients over 85, and cognitively impaired patients pose a particular challenge. (Ideally, you will be able to collaborate with either the geriatrician or the geriatric psychiatrist caring for the patient.) Inadequate supplies of potent opioids, lack of trained staff to perform the assessments, and lack of pain management expertise among clinicians responsible for these patients all contribute to inadequate pain management in this setting. Even the pain of cancer patients living in nursing homes is undertreated. Most receive no opioid analgesia or only a step 2 agent for their pain.

It is often difficult to assess the degree of pain that older cancer patients experience. They have pain as frequently as younger patients and can describe its location and qualities (sharp, dull, etc.) just as accurately, but older patients less often report their pain. This may be because they ascribe any new pain to a comorbid condition such as arthritis and don't realize that it may be due to the cancer. Alternatively, they might just be more stoic, expecting to experience more pain as they age and not wanting to distress those around them.

Pain assessment in either the frail older patient or in patients who are cognitively impaired requires some modification of the techniques described in Chapter 6, where you can find a copy of the PAINAD scale, a validated tool for assessing pain in this population (Warden, Hurley, and Volicer 2003). Try to determine how well the patient performs the usual activities of daily living and gauge the success of the treatment by improvements in functional measures. If you use a pain assessment tool, choose one that the patient finds easy to use, such as a *word scale* (mild, moderate, severe, excruciating), a *pain thermometer*, or a *face scale*. Also, refer to pain behaviors, such as those listed in Table 7.11.

The key to achieving pain control in cognitively impaired patients seems to be frequent assessment. Repeated questioning is needed because, while these patients accurately report the pain they are currently experiencing, they are often unable to recall previous pain intensity. To adjust opioid doses in cognitively impaired patients, assess the intensity of their pain before they received pain medication, then repeat the assessment an hour later.

Management Considerations

Once you understand the nature of the pain an older patient is experiencing, consider two other important factors: (1) the role of family members in caring for older patients and (2) the pharmacokinetic and pharmacodynamic differences between the metabolism of pain-relieving drugs in older persons and that in younger persons.

Family members. Family members are often the key to success in managing the pain of older patients. But clinicians need to recognize how difficult this may be for caregivers, especially if they are elderly themselves. They spend a great deal of time taking care of the person in pain, often relinquishing their own jobs, hobbies, church community, or accustomed routines in the home. The caregivers are often sleepless and exhausted, feeling inadequate to the task and helpless as they watch the suffering of their loved one. They may fear causing addiction from potent opioids as much as the pain itself. Supporting and educating them is crucial to the well-being of the entire family.

Practice Points: Pain Management in Older Persons

- Assure patients and their families that you want to hear about each of the patient's pains.
- Identify a pain scale they understand and can use.
- In cognitively impaired patients, pain *now* is more accurate than remembered pain. Use the PAINAD scale.
- Involve caregivers and home nursing services in monitoring the effectiveness of the regimen and the occurrence of side effects.
- Avoid NSAIDs. If they are used, monitor carefully for side effects and exacerbations of congestive heart failure, cirrhosis, hypertension, or renal insufficiency. Consider gastrointestinal prophylaxis in patients over 65.
- Respect altered pharmacokinetics and pharmacodynamics of drugs in these patients.
  - Give lower initial doses of benzodiazepines, gabapentin, pregabalin, and opioids. Increase doses slowly.
  - Give drugs with short half-lives that are the least sedating and have the fewest anticholinergic side effects.
  - Use low doses of methadone along with short-acting opioids to provide sustained pain relief for patients with neuropathic pain (e.g., from vascular ischemia).
- Institute aggressive regimens to prevent and treat constipation.

Home nursing and home hospice services are especially invaluable to families of older persons, helping ease the caregiver's and family's physical and psychological burdens. The nurses provide expert evaluation and management of the patient's symptoms, along with patient and family education and guidelines on when to contact the prescribing physician, nurse practitioner, or physician assistant. The social workers and chaplains can address the psychosocial and spiritual needs of both the patient and the caregiver. And home health aides and volunteers can give the older caregiver a much-needed break—either by doing some of the patient care or by sitting with the patient so that the spouse can rest, take a walk, or engage in some other favored activity.

The Burden of Caregiving

The burden of the caregiver's responsibility was brought home to me by Mr. O'Hara, a 79-year-old man with metastatic bladder cancer and complete ureteral obstruction that required bilateral stents. He lived with an older sister who was dying of multiple noncancerous medical problems. Because of his own physical deterioration, Mr. O'Hara had agreed to receive home hospice services from the same visiting nurse agency that was helping his sister. They received health aide services for as much as 8 hours a day, but for the remaining 16 hours, Mr. O'Hara was the sole caregiver for his sister. And he maintained that role until her death.

After she died, he moved into a community home for older people. About a month later, the hospice coordinator got in touch with me. It seemed that Mr. O'Hara was doing so well that they wanted to discontinue the hospice services! What we had attributed to progressive cancer was actually the exhaustion and debilitation caused by caring for his dying sister. One month after her death, he had gained weight, had less pain, and seemed to need no services from the hospice staff. He did well for at least two more years, after which I lost touch.

As there was no one else to help him, and his financial resources were limited, we were unable to provide all the support Mr. O'Hara needed. But even when other people are willing to pitch in, family caregivers are often reluctant to let them. One of your major challenges, in fact, may be to convince the spouse or other person primarily caring for the patient to let others help as much as possible—to involve willing family and friends and accept community services. Primary caregivers need to accept that their own health may be endangered if they shoulder the burden alone and that, if they fall ill, there will be no one left to care for the patient at home. Accepting help may be the only solution.

Pharmacokinetic and pharmacodynamic alterations in older persons. Both the pharmacokinetics (the absorption, metabolism, and excretion of the drug) and pharmacodynamics (the effects of the drug at various serum levels) of NSAIDs, adjuvants, and opioids are different in older patients. Older persons have less muscle and more fat than younger persons, and their renal and hepatic functions are often mildly to moderately impaired, leading to less rapid hepatic and renal drug clearance. Older patients often suffer from concomitant medical illnesses, and they are more sensitive to opioid-induced sedation and confusion.

NSAIDs can be particularly problematic in the older patient. Of the choices available for mild to moderate pain, acetaminophen (<3 g per day) is the agent recommended by the American Geriatrics Society (American Geriatrics Society Panel 2009; Gloth 2011). Naproxen or low-dose ibuprofen used with a proton pump inhibitor may also be safe. The American Geriatrics Society strongly recommends that older adults take only one NSAID at a time. Topical NSAIDs, however, are endorsed as adjuvants or alone (Gloth 2011).

Other NSAIDs, including indomethacin and ketorolac especially, are likely to cause significant toxicity in older patients. These drugs are highly protein bound, and older ill patients may have low levels of serum albumin. Older patients, therefore, are likely to have higher serum levels of free NSAID than do younger patients receiving the same NSAID dose, and they develop more side effects. Older patients with congestive heart failure or cirrhosis are particularly susceptible. Those taking NSAIDs may develop dizziness, confusion, and excessive salt and water retention. Since NSAIDs may exacerbate hypertension and can induce significant hyperkalemia and renal toxicity in this population, electrolytes and renal function must be checked a week or two after NSAID treatment is started. To minimize gastrointestinal toxicity, prescribe low-dose naproxen. But for patients requiring higher doses of this agent, or whose pain is well controlled only by NSAIDs with a higher risk of inducing gastrointestinal toxicity, add a proton pump inhibitor such as omeprazole (20 mg) and periodically monitor the patient with occult blood testing.

Other adjuvants may also cause significant side effects in older patients. Do not use diazepam (e.g., Valium). The increased body fat in these patients can prolong the half-life of lipid-soluble agents, such as diazepam, and lead to excessive sedation or delirium. Local anesthetics are also associated with a higher incidence of delirium in the elderly.

Avoid using tricyclic antidepressants. They can cause orthostatic hypotension, cognitive changes, and atrial arrhythmias, which can themselves be problematic or may lead to falls. If the patient does not tolerate even dose-reduced gabapentin (e.g., Neurontin) or pregabalin (Lyrica), try desipramine (Norpramin), which has the fewest anticholinergic side effects.

The anticholinergic side effects of tricyclic antidepressants, antiemetics, and antihistamines (used to control opioid-induced pruritus) can be troublesome. They include constipation, dry mouth, blurred vision, urinary retention, and sedation. Older opioid-naive patients also should not receive prophylactic phenothiazines.

Opioids. In general, because of the alterations in metabolism noted above, older patients are more likely to have significant side effects from the usual doses of both short-acting and sustained-release opioids. Given the same dose of opioid, older patients will have significantly higher plasma concentrations than younger patients. In addition, they are more sensitive to the peak effect of the immediate-release and short-acting preparations, and they can develop excessive respiratory depression, sedation, confusion, and even paradoxical agitation. With either short-acting or sustained-release formulations, the drugs last longer, their metabolites accumulate, and toxicities increase in these older patients.

Even short-acting opioids, such as immediate-release morphine, have long-lived active metabolites that may cause problems. Immediate-release hydromorphone (e.g., Dilaudid) or oxycodone pose less of a problem with metabolites. A transmucosal fentanyl product is another option, if the patient is opioid tolerant; the intermittent pains resolve in an hour or less, which is when the fentanyl wears off. Avoid meperidine (e.g., Demerol). Older patients are particularly prone to the side effects of normeperidine, the active metabolite of meperidine, which causes dysphoria, myoclonus, and seizures.

To prevent excessive toxicity, "start low; go slow," and reassess frequently. Begin with a dose that is 25 to 50 percent less than the dose you would give to a younger adult. Rescue doses, which should be about 10 percent of the total daily dose in younger patients, initially should be no more than 5 percent in the older patient. Rescue medication, moreover, should probably be taken no more often than every 4 hours, rather than the every 2 hours recommended for younger patients.

Anecdotally, though I generally avoid long-acting and sustained-release opioids in this population, I have used 1 to 2 mg of methadone twice a day to good effect in patients over 80 who have neuropathic pain from nerve or skin lesions, like ischemic vascular ulcers. These low doses of methadone are well tolerated and remarkably effective for patients whose immediate-release opioids are not providing satisfactory pain relief or are causing excessive sedation (Bach et al. 2016). Similarly, transdermal buprenorphine (e.g., Butrans) may provide nociceptive and neuropathic pain relief with fewer side effects than many other opioids.

Use lower doses of transdermal fentanyl in well-nourished older patients, because there is a marked increase in the transdermal delivery rate of the fentanyl. This may result from the higher fat-to-water ratio in the elderly person's skin, and more fentanyl may deposit in the skin reservoir than in that of younger patients.

For short-term relief of severe, acute pain, patient-controlled analgesia can be used as successfully in older patients as in younger persons. As in younger patients, the oral or transdermal routes are preferred for treating chronic cancer pain. If parenteral opioids are needed, it's best to avoid bolus injections because of the enhanced toxicity associated with the peak effects. Continuous infusion via subcutaneous or intravenous routes is preferred. Intraspinal opioids can also be given safely. Older patients are less likely than younger patients to develop nausea or vomiting after an epidural injection.

Some special consideration must be given to opioid-induced side effects in older patients. As you might expect, older patients are more susceptible to the constipating effects of opioids. They are less active than younger patients, drink less fluid, have a more tolerant rectal sphincter, and are more often taking other medications that exacerbate constipation. It is therefore essential that older patients start a prophylactic bowel regimen along with opioid therapy.

Older patients are also prone to urinary retention due to the effects of opioids on the urinary sphincter. Urinary retention can be an important problem for patients with prostatic hypertrophy or those taking other drugs with anticholinergic side effects. Initially, these patients may require bladder catheterization to relieve discomfort, but the retention usually disappears after one to two days on opioid therapy. Rarely, patients with prostatic hypertrophy will require either a trial of finasteride (e.g., Proscar) (5 mg/day p.o.) or tamsulosin (e.g. Flomax) (0.4–0.8 mg/day p.o.) to diminish the outlet obstruction, or bethanechol (e.g., Urecholine) (10 mg p.o. t.i.d., to a maximum of 50 mg p.o. t.i.d.) or terazosin (1 mg p.o. at bedtime, increased gradually to 2 to 5 mg as tolerated and as needed) to relax the bladder smooth muscle that is being stimulated by the opioid.

RELIEVING PAIN IN PATIENTS WITH SUBSTANCE USE DISORDER

Active Substance Use Disorder

The cancer patient who has severe pain but is actively using opioids, cocaine, or alcohol aberrantly poses a difficult management problem. It is hard to trust the patient's report of pain intensity if you know his substance use disorder is active, and you may be reluctant to prescribe a high opioid dose because you don't know whether you are relieving his pain or acting as his dealer.

Consider how Dr. William Breitbart, who has extensive experience working with patients with substance use disorder who are in pain, views this issue: "I've treated about 500 patients with AIDS-related pain and a history of substance use disorder, and I've been fooled a good dozen times. But if I had allowed that experience of being manipulated and fooled to influence me, I would not have been able to help those other 488 patients" (personal communication). I share his sentiments; I would hate to miss the opportunity to help so many people for fear that a few would be "using me" in ways I don't approve of, like Sam, whom I wrote about earlier in this chapter, who was selling his Oxycontin to provide for his family. And yet I realize it is particularly hard to apply the assessment and management principles discussed thus far to this patient population. Unfortunately, there are no accepted guidelines for managing patients with cancer pain and opioid-use disorder (Goodlev et al. 2019).

To work with these patients, borrow the techniques used by the substance use disorder professionals. Whenever possible, involve a team of clinicians to manage the patient, including the patient's primary physician (or physician assistant or nurse practitioner), psychiatric clinicians, social workers, and substance use disorder professionals. You might consider also involving a palliative care or pain specialist.

> **Practice Points: Inpatient Opioid Therapy for Patients with Active Substance Use Disorder**
>
> - Control the environment.
> - Establish the therapeutic opioid dose.
> - Institute a regimen that minimizes the chance of aberrant use.

Inpatients. It is particularly important to control the environment of patients with active substance use disorder whenever they are admitted to an inpatient site. The patient should be in a private room and restricted to that room or, in some cases, to the floor. Patients should wear hospital, not street, clothing. Visitors (even family) should be restricted, and patients' possessions and packages should be searched by nursing staff. Arrange for frequent psychiatric or social work and opioid-use disorder counseling, if you can, and try to have the same nurse responsible for the patient throughout the hospital stay (i.e., "primary nursing").

During the hospitalization, substitute therapeutic opioid doses for the opioids the patient was taking "on the street." Some patients with a history of substance use disorder, who now have cancer and are unable to get the medications they need from their clinician, revert to using street drugs to self-medicate their severe pain. Your goal will be to demonstrate to them that you can relieve their pain with appropriate prescription agents and that they do not need the illegal substances for symptom control.

Finding the correct opioid dose may be particularly difficult for patients whose substance use disorder is active. You may not trust their reported pain level, and they often require very high levels of opioids (e.g., the equivalent of grams of morphine) for pain relief because of changes in their CNS created by their opioid-use disorder. Monitoring their function is more reliable; it will usually improve, as will sleep and anxiety, as the pain comes under better control. Avoid IV boluses, minimize short-acting oral opioid doses, and try to relieve the patient's pain with sustained-release or transdermal opioids.

When you have brought the acute pain under control, you need to convert the patient to a regimen that minimizes the chance of recurrent opioid-use disorder. Long-acting oral agents such as levorphanol (e.g., Levo-Dromoran) or sustained-release preparations of morphine, hydromorphone (e.g., Exalgo), transdermal fentanyl, or methadone are recommended. Avoid oral immediate-release hydromorphone (e.g., Dilaudid), combination agents (e.g., Percodan, Percocet, Tylox), immediate-release morphine, and sustained-release oxycodone for patients whose substance use disorder is active. When you write prescriptions for the long-acting opioids, give only a week's supply at a time. And warn the patient to keep the medications in a safe place, as you will not replace that supply if it is accidentally "flushed down the toilet" or "spilled down the sink."

Outpatients. After discharge, patients will need to continue to work with palliative care clinicians and psychiatric and substance use disorder counselors to maximize adherence and to prevent recurrence of aberrant use. They may be candidates for buprenorphine-naloxone (e.g., Suboxone) or methadone maintenance if their painful condition has resolved (e.g., mucositis from leukemia therapy or from bone marrow or stem cell transplant). The counselors can also provide education for the patients about the dangers of mixing the therapeutic opioids with alcohol.

Explain your expectations of how patients are to work with you, your team, the substance use disorder and psychological counselors, and the palliative care team (if you have one available to you). If you haven't had the patient sign one before, have them sign an opioid-use agreement, which will detail those expectations. These include urine drug checks (current technology can distinguish among a wide variety of opioid metabolites using both quantitative and qualitative methods), monitoring of their PDMP, and other monitoring to ensure their safety and continued appropriate use of the opioids you prescribe, as well as regular, continued visits with the counselors. Be clear that if you are to continue to provide therapy for their cancer, they must continue to work with all those clinicians.

Substance use disorder is an illness that frequently relapses, and you need to be vigilant in detecting early relapses. Behaviors exhibited by patients with substance use disorder include (1) forged prescriptions; (2) doctor shopping; (3) urine drug-testing aberrancies; (4) lost opioid prescriptions; (5) early prescription refill requests; (6) unscheduled clinic visits due to pain complaints; (7) ER visits for pain; and (8) requests for opioid dose escalation without apparent change in functional status (Dale, Edwards, and Ballantyne 2016). Several validated tools to assess substance use disorder are available (Dale, Edwards, and Ballantyne 2016; Paice 2019; Scarborough and Smith 2018). The CDC (Dowell, Haegerich, and Chou 2016) and individual states have issued guidelines for opioid use for chronic pain in patients with and without cancer, so you might discuss your state's requirements with your staff.

Rehabilitation in Remission: Mr. Salat

Patients with substance use disorder may be inspired to enter a rehabilitation program after their cancer goes into remission. Mr. Salat was such a patient. At the time I first saw him, he was 35 years old and had widely metastatic testicular cancer with lesions the size of grapefruits in his retroperitoneum and lung. He was actively using heroin, which he said helped him control the severe back pain caused by his retroperitoneal lesions. With ongoing support from his counselor and our office staff, he maintained pain relief throughout his treatment using only the opioids we prescribed.

When it was clear that his tumor was responding to treatment, I told Mr. Salat that when he was in complete remission, he was unlikely to need opioids for pain. I began to address his opioid dependence and my hope that he would be able to work with a drug counselor to avoid returning to his heroin use. He did not disappoint me: he entered a methadone maintenance program, and when I last heard from him, he was still doing well, more than 20 years later.

Patients on Methadone or Buprenorphine Maintenance

Alford and his colleagues (2006) suggest that clinicians have four main misconceptions about patients on methadone or buprenorphine maintenance: first, that their methadone or buprenorphine provides adequate pain relief; second, that if we use opioids to relieve their pain, we can cause their addiction to relapse; third, that they are at risk for sedation or respiratory depression if we treat their pain with additional opioids and continue their methadone or buprenorphine; and fourth, that they are just trying to manipulate us.

Practice Points: Opioid Therapy for Patients on Methadone Maintenance

- Don't use methadone as the pain-relieving opioid. Leave the methadone dose unchanged and titrate other opioids to achieve pain control.
- Be aware that large opioid doses may be required for patients on significant doses of methadone.
- Maintain an ongoing relationship with the patient's drug counselor.

But in fact, patients on methadone maintenance present a less difficult adherence problem because they often have well-established successful relationships with counselors. In addition to their methadone maintenance doses, however, they often require large doses of other opioids to relieve their pain (Doverty et al. 2001; Peles et al. 2005). We have several options, according to Alford and colleagues (2006), for patients on buprenorphine maintenance. These are described in detail in their paper, referenced in the online bibliography.

For patients on methadone, reassure them that you will leave the methadone dose the same and use other opioids and adjuvant agents to relieve their pain (Alford, Comptom, and Samet 2006). This allows patients to separate their opioid-use disorder from their pain issues and helps them provide you with accurate pain assessments. Even PCAs may work in selected patients whose anxiety is decreased by their ability to have some control over their pain relief.

Patients with a History of Substance Use Disorder

People who have formerly used opioids aberrantly are often reluctant to take opioids, even for excruciating pain. They and their families remember the mess drug addiction made of their lives. They are terrified that if they take opioids to relieve their pain, they will again find themselves living that nightmare.

Psychological support from a counselor familiar with substance use disorders and with opioids for pain management may be crucial to enabling patients to accept the pain medications they need for relief. Patients who formerly had a substance use disorder are sensitive to being perceived as addicts, and staff members need to receive careful instruction in how to work with these patients to help them relieve their pain. As with anyone who is at high risk of having a substance use disorder who suffers from cancer pain, monitor them carefully for signs indicating they have relapsed, such as "losing" medication, escalating doses without consulting you, obtaining medications from other clinicians, or committing prescription fraud.

Clinicians can relieve the pain of people who currently have or in the past had a substance use disorder, or who are on buprenorphine or methadone maintenance. Patients will often understand the need for the limits you set, or will at least comply with them to get their oncologic therapy. The teams you set up to support them may make it possible for them to stay with the program.

MANAGING PAIN IN CANCER SURVIVORS

More and more people are cured of cancer or are living for years as "cancer survivors" with or without active disease. It is estimated that up to 40 percent of them receive opioids to manage their pain (Salz et al. 2019). In 2016, there were more than 15 million survivors (Loren 2018), and many of them had received opioids during a portion of their successful treatment, or for residual cancer- or treatment-related pain when they came off treatment. Survivors with breast, colon, and lung cancer had mildly increased opioid use in the years following their treatment, compared with people of their age group who didn't have cancer, but this declined over time. By six years after cancer diagnosis, survivors were no longer more likely to be using opioids than others in their age group who never had cancer (Salz et al. 2019).

Other patients, though, especially those with smoking- or alcohol-related cancers, had risk factors for opioid-use disorder prior to developing their cancers. In one study of patients undergoing curative radiation therapy for cancer of the head and neck, for example, 44 percent of patients who were CAGE positive (i.e., had an alcohol use disorder) were unable to stop opioids (Bruera and Del Fabbro 2018). Even for patients without preexisting risk factors, post-traumatic stress disorder, anxiety, depression, and other life changes that cancer and cancer treatment can bring, along with moderate to severe ongoing pain, can put them at risk of opioid-use disorder.

Patients with chronic residual therapy-induced neuropathic pain or pain related to bone complications may have been prescribed opioids during cancer treatment. Many will wean off these agents, using the nonpharmacologic strategies discussed in Chapter 8, or the non-opioid therapies for bone or neuropathic pain discussed earlier in this chapter. In collaboration with patients and families, you can wean patients whom you think no longer need opioids for pain relief using guidelines from the NCCN, ASCO, and Veterans Affairs (Goodlev et al. 2019). (See "Practice Point: Opioid Taper in Survivors" below.)

Too rapid a wean can produce severe withdrawal pain, such as that experienced by Travis Rieder, the author of the heartbreaking book *In Pain*. But a 5 to 20 percent dose reduction every 4 weeks is reasonable in patients whose pain is adequately controlled and who are using nonopioid or nonpharmacologic interventions along with the opioids. Anecdotally, many of us find that patients do best when weaned off of long-acting opioids first, then the short-acting medication. If the patient was on a large dose of long-acting opioids for some time, decrease only by 2 to 10 percent every 4–8 weeks, with close follow-up. You can taper patients who are experiencing severe opioid-induced side effects more rapidly.

Practice Points: Opioid Taper in Survivors

Monitor for signs of withdrawal and treat with agents specific for the withdrawal symptom(s).

• Stable patients	Decrease by 5 to 20 percent every 4 weeks
• Refractory opioid side effects with mild pain	Decrease by 10 to 25 percent every 4 weeks
• Patients with severe opioid-related side effects, especially sedation	Decrease by 20 to 50 percent acutely, then 10 to 20 percent daily
• Patients chronically on high doses of long-acting opioids	Decrease 2 to 10 percent every 4 to 8 weeks

(Goodlev et al. 2019)

The patient may need a break in the weaning process to accommodate the withdrawal symptoms. Consider using a scale to monitor their withdrawal symptoms, such as the Clinical Opioid Withdrawal Scale (Wesson and Ling 2003). If patients develop withdrawal symptoms, treat them with agents specific for the symptom, such as antiemetics for nausea, antidiarrheals, antihistamines for anxiety, NSAIDs for myalgias, and noradrenergic agents like clonidine or tizanidine for autonomic symptoms. Avoid raising the opioid dose or adding benzodiazepines.

It is not known what percentage of survivors will not find adequate relief without opioids, but survivors who do require ongoing opioid therapy and their families will need, in addition to the involvement of their oncology, primary care, and palliative care teams, intensive multidisciplinary care from pain experts, as well as psychological help for the multiple causes of their suffering that they may be medicating with opioids. The ASCO clinical practice guideline for managing chronic pain in survivors of adult cancers (Paice et al. 2016) describes the resources these patients require. As Goodlev et al. (2019) state, "It remains difficult to balance management of survivorship pain syndromes with risk mitigation for opioid misuse, while also maintaining a low index of suspicion for disease recurrence." Worsening pain may herald such a recurrence, so the search for new disease must be extensive in patients stating their pain is no longer relieved by the current regimen (Paice et al. 2016).

MANAGING PAIN IN PATIENTS WITH SELECTED HEMATOLOGIC MALIGNANCIES

Multiple Myeloma

Myeloma patients suffer from both bone and neuropathic pain syndromes. The bone pain from lesions and fractures probably should not be treated with NSAIDs other than acetaminophen because the myeloma patient's kidneys are already subject to injury from the myeloma proteins; NSAIDs that decrease any afferent blood flow can only exacerbate that. As discussed earlier in this chapter, bisphosphonates and RANK-L inhibitors can decrease the incidence of fractures and treat bone pain.

Myeloma proteins, vertebral fractures compromising spinal nerves, and the drugs used to treat myeloma all cause neuropathic pain. The non-treatment-induced pain can be treated as discussed earlier. But the CIPN pain, especially from the effective proteasome inhibitors (e.g., bortezomib) and the immunomodulatory drugs (e.g., thalidomide, lenalidomide), can be difficult to treat. Patients may resist lowering the drug dose, however, and choose instead to tolerate the side effects of marked tingling in hands and feet, pain, and numbness. In addition to fatigue and constipation, in fact, pain and tingling in hands and feet were the most prevalent symptoms in at least 50 percent of patients with myeloma (Samala et al. 2019).

Hematopoietic Stem Cell Recipients

Patients undergoing hematopoietic stem cell transplants suffer from multiple sources of pain. Many are similar to the pain experienced by other cancer patients, such as procedural pain from bone marrow aspirates or biopsies, pain from CIPN and post-herpetic neuralgia, or mucositis (discussed in Chapter 10). Pains unique to transplant recipients include those caused by G-CSF and by skin and abdominal graft-versus-host disease (GVHD).

Procedural pain. Procedural pain can be minimized by using local anesthetic or anesthetic creams such as EMLA or ELA-Max on the skin prior to the procedure. But the anesthesia only extends about a quarter inch down. The distress from the marrow aspirate or biopsy will not be affected. Some clinicians routinely use intravenous conscious sedation with each marrow aspirate or biopsy. Even if the opioid in the conscious sedation is not enough to eliminate the acute pain, benzodiazepine (usually midazolam) eliminates the *memory* of the discomfort, which can be helpful if repeated marrows are needed. Hypnosis (discussed in Chapter 8) can also help decrease the incidence, severity, and memory of procedural pain.

The hematopoietic growth factor G-CSF is given to increase the yield of a stem cell harvest. The increased myeloid cells in the marrow cause a deep, aching pain in the sternum, back, hips, and legs that is usually responsive to NSAIDs, such as naproxen twice a day if the platelet count and renal function allow (Ma et al. 2018).

GVHD. GVHD can cause painful maculopapular skin rashes that start on the palms and soles, but eventually can affect the face and trunk. These patients are treated with topical creams as well as corticosteroids for at least 6 weeks; cyclosporine for 3 to 6 months may be needed as well (Ma et al. 2018). The diarrhea of GVHD can be associated with severe cramping pain that is also treated with corticosteroids and other immunosuppressive agents. Symptomatically, opioids and anticholinergics may be helpful, such as dicyclomine (Bentyl) or glycopyrrolate (Ma et. al. 2018).

COMMON CLINICAL SITUATIONS

Patients with Renal or Hepatic Impairment

Using pharmacologic agents safely in patients with end-stage renal or hepatic failure requires vigilance. The most common agents that should be used with caution in patients with significant renal (Sande, Laird, and Fallon 2017; Wilcock et al. 2017) or hepatic failure (Wilcock et al. 2019) are listed in Tables 7.12 and 7.13, respectively.

Starting Patients on Opioids

As discussed early in this chapter, many patients and their families, at least initially, resist accepting a prescription for opioids. To overcome their objections, I recommend conducting at least a ten-minute discussion in which you accomplish the following:

- Assume that patients and families are harboring common fears and misconceptions about opioids and explore these with them.

- Explain the difference between tolerance and addiction. I have found the following phrases to be useful. They describe patients' fears but also their hope to accomplish their goals: *"People with an opioid-use disorder use drugs to 'get out' of their lives; but patients with cancer may need opioids to get back 'into' their lives, to do the things they want to do."*

- Reassure them that taking medication now does not jeopardize achieving pain relief if the pain worsens.

- Explain the likely side effects (e.g., constipation, sedation, nausea) and how you can prevent or treat these:

  - They may feel somewhat sleepy for the first two or three days, but the drowsiness will pass, and the pain relief will remain.

  - Constipation will persist as long as they continue to take opioids, and it requires ongoing therapy. Advise them to replace any insoluble fiber laxatives with the laxatives you prescribe, to take them whether or not they have had a bowel movement that day, and to take more laxatives if they need them.

  - Nausea is not a sign of opioid allergy. It resolves over four to seven days and can be treated during that time if it is troublesome.

Initiating a treatment regimen for mild (level 1 to 4) to moderate (5 to 6) pain. For *mild* neuropathic pain, begin gabapentin 100 mg orally twice a day or pregabalin 25 mg orally twice a day and titrate up as needed; or if there are no contraindications, consider tramadol 12.5 to 25 mg orally or tapentadol 25 mg every 4 to 6 hours and titrate up as needed and tolerated. For patients with *mild* somatic or visceral pain, such as from bony metastases, begin with an NSAID such as acetaminophen or ibuprofen every 6 to 8 hours. If the pain relief remains unsatisfactory to the patient, either add low doses of tramadol or tapentadol as above, or a step 3 agent (i.e., morphine 7.5 mg, hydromorphone 2 mg, or oxycodone 5 mg) every 4 hours.

For outpatients with moderate pain (level 5 or 6 on a 0 to 10 scale), treat as follows:

- Begin with either (a) 15 mg of morphine, 4 mg of hydromorphone, 10 mg of oxycodone, 5 mg of oxymorphone, 50 mg of tramadol, or 50 to 100 mg of tapentadol orally every 4 hours as needed. For patients with somatic or visceral pain, add an NSAID such as acetaminophen or ibuprofen every 6 to 8 hours. Add polyethylene glycol daily and one or two senna tablets twice a day (or choose another laxative from Table 7.5). If the pain is neuropathic, do not use an NSAID as an adjuvant to the opioid. Instead add gabapentin 100 mg orally three times a day and titrate to a therapeutic level, at least 300 mg orally three times a day, over several weeks.

- Identify a pain scale and/or a functional goal that would indicate adequate pain relief that the patient and family feel comfortable using. Ask the patient to record, at least twice a day, her pain level before and about one hour after she takes the drug, along with any side effects.

- The day after each opioid dose change, check with the patient to determine whether the pain relief is now satisfactory.

- If the pain relief is satisfactory but the patient has developed side effects, treat them as described earlier in this chapter.

- If the pain is persistent throughout the day, relieved for only 1 or 2 hours with the immediate-release opioid, and recurs before the next dose, start an equivalent amount of a sustained-release (SR) morphine, hydromorphone, hydrocodone, oxycodone, oxymorphone, or fentanyl preparation, adding an immediate-release (IR) form for pain between regularly scheduled doses (rescue doses). The rescue dose should be 10 percent of the total daily opioid dose (5 percent initially in older patients). It is sometimes necessary to round up or round down the calculated opioid dose to accommodate the dosages available in SR or IR preparations. I give examples of how to do these calculations later in the chapter. If appropriate, continue the gabapentin for neuropathic pain, the NSAID, or add an amount of NSAID equivalent to the amount in the combination tablet that the patient formerly took.

Treating Pain that Recurs before the Next Dose

Converting from a combination product to acetaminophen or NSAID + a sustained-release form of the same opioid (oxycodone)

Initial combination agent: oxycodone 5 mg + acetaminophen 325 mg, 12 tablets per 24 hours (60 mg of oxycodone and 3900 mg of acetaminophen) (2 tablets every 4 hours)

- Total oxycodone dose: 5 mg/tablet × 12 tablets = 60 mg
- Equivalent SR oxycodone: 30 mg every 12 hours
- Add opioid rescue dose (10 percent of 24-hour dose): 10 percent of 60 mg ≈ 5 mg of IR oxycodone
- Add back acetaminophen ≤3000 mg per 24 hours or NSAID if needed

---

Initial opioid regimen for opioid-naive outpatients with severe (level 7 to 10) pain. The step 3 opioids are indicated for initial therapy of patients with severe pain. They include hydromorphone (e.g., Dilaudid) for older patients or for patients with renal or hepatic failure, as well as morphine, oxycodone, and oxymorphone. Begin with the starting doses listed in Table 7.3. Some patients need to be admitted to bring their pain under control. Later in the chapter, I review how to treat a patient in a pain crisis.

Do not use a fentanyl patch for initial therapy for a patient in severe pain; it takes 12 to 20 hours to achieve a therapeutic level of fentanyl after the patient applies a fentanyl patch. Because of the concerns described earlier in this chapter, do not use methadone as the initial agent, unless you are experienced in its use.

Treating Pain that Is Unrelieved by a Step 2 Agent

Converting from a combination agent to a sustained-release preparation containing the same opioid (oxycodone) at a higher dose

- Initial combination agent: oxycodone 5 mg + acetaminophen 325 mg, 12 tablets per 24 hours (60 mg of oxycodone and 3900 mg of acetaminophen) (2 tablets every 4 hours)
- Increase the oxycodone by 50 percent: 60 mg + (60 mg × 50 percent = 30 mg) = 90 mg of oxycodone ≈ 40 mg of SR oxycodone every 12 hours.
- Adjust rescue dose of oxycodone: 10 percent of 80 mg ≈ 10 mg; rescue dose: 10 mg of IR oxycodone every 2 hours p.r.n.
- Add back acetaminophen ≤3000 mg per 24 hours or NSAID if needed.

Whichever opioid you choose, prevention of constipation is crucial. Prescribe, for example, two senna twice daily with a daily osmotic agent (e.g., 17 g of polyethylene glycol [Miralax]) at bedtime; exclude the osmotic agent if it causes diarrhea. Instruct all patients to take the laxatives even if they have had a bowel movement that day. The stool softener docusate (e.g., Colace) does not add to the effectiveness of senna and does not need to be given with it (Pasay et al. 2017).

For patients with moderate to severe neuropathic pain, gabapentin (or pregabalin if the insurance will cover that agent) and a corticosteroid will be most effective. Start with gabapentin taken three times a day, the highest dose at bedtime when neuropathic pain is at its worst and the sedating effect of the gabapentin will be welcome (e.g., 100, 100, 300 mg p.o.). If the pain is severe, add corticosteroids, a higher dose at first, tapering as the gabapentin doses gradually increase. For example, start 8 mg oral dexamethasone taken before noon, followed by 4 mg at 8 a.m. and 2 p.m. daily for 4 days, 2 mg at 8 a.m. and 2 p.m. daily for 4 days, and 2 mg a day for 4 days. If the gabapentin is well tolerated, increase the dose over several weeks until pain relief is improved or the patient has a dose-limiting side effect. If the gabapentin is ineffective at 300 mg taken orally three times a day, the insurance will usually allow the switch to pregabalin; start at 50 mg pregabalin twice daily by mouth and titrate up to 150 mg twice daily if needed. If the neuropathic pain persists, consider increasing the pregabalin to t.i.d. or adding another of the anticonvulsants listed in Table 7.8.

Changing Opioid Dose, Opioid Agent, or Route of Delivery

Adjusting the dose. The initial dose of opioid is, unfortunately, no better than an educated guess. Doses often need to be adjusted upward or downward both during the first few weeks of therapy and later in the patient's course of treatment, as the disease process advances. Explain this to patients and ask which is preferable to them: rapidly relieving the pain or avoiding side effects such as sedation. If patients and their families want immediate pain relief regardless of the side effects, I am comfortable with using a higher initial dose. If they express a great deal of concern about the potential side effects, I am more conservative with the initial dose, but I supply rescue medication, carefully monitor the patient, and raise the basal dose until the relief of the constant portion of the pain is satisfactory. Ideally, patients with constant, not intermittent, pain need to use rescue doses of IR opioids only once or twice a day; the bulk of the pain relief should be provided by the oral SR or transdermal opioid or methadone. Patients without constant pain, whose pain is intermittent incident pain, will benefit most from taking IR opioids when they have pain. Adding SR opioids may cause excessive sedation in these patients.

Initial Oral Opioid for Opioid-Naive Patients with Severe Pain

- Morphine sulfate 7.5 mg p.o. or 5 mg oxycodone p.o. q2h p.r.n. for patients under 65 years old with normal renal and hepatic function
- Hydromorphone 4 to 6 mg p.o. every 4 hours for patients 65 or older or patients with renal or hepatic failure
- Transition to a SR after starting with an IR opioid: IR morphine or oxycodone every 2 hours p.r.n. for 24 hours; then give total daily dose in SR form if the patient is not sedated and continues to require p.r.n. doses

Example.

  7.5 mg IR morphine (½ of a 15-mg tablet) × 12 doses = 90 mg of morphine

  SR dose: 30 mg q8h SR morphine with 10 mg IR morphine rescue (e.g., 0.5 ml of a 20 mg/ml morphine solution)

Example.

  5 mg IR oxycodone × 12 doses = 60 mg oxycodone

  SR dose: 30 mg q12h SR oxycodone with 5 mg IR oxycodone rescue

- Starting with an SR opioid

Example.

  Morphine SR 15 mg q12h or oxycodone SR 10 mg q12h with 5 mg IR oxycodone rescue

Initial Transdermal Fentanyl Transition for Patients with Severe Pain

- Start with morphine sulfate 7.5 mg p.o. or 5 mg oxycodone p.o. q2h p.r.n. for patients under 65 years old with normal renal and hepatic function
- Once patients have been on the equivalent of at least 60mg/day morphine, they may be transitioned to a fentanyl patch

Example.

7.5 mg IR morphine (½ of a 15-mg tablet) × 8 doses = 60 mg of p.o. morphine

Initial dose of transdermal fentanyl: 25 µg/hr patch, which is approximately equivalent to 50 mg of morphine every 24 hours

Add rescue doses* of 7.5 mg of IR morphine or 5 mg oxycodone every 2 hours p.o., or 0.5 ml of a 20 mg/ml morphine or oxycodone solution sublingual every 2 hours (i.e., 5 mg of IR morphine or 5 mg of IR oxycodone sublingual)

*Patients should expect to use rescue doses until fentanyl blood levels are adequate (i.e., for at least the first 12 to 24 hours after receiving the patch).

Using Rescue Doses to Increase Sustained-Release Opioid Dose for Patients with Constant Pain

Example.

A patient with chronic abdominal pain from pancreatic cancer taking 60 mg of SR morphine every 12 hours took six rescue doses, 10 mg each, of IR morphine (0.5 ml of a 20 mg/ml morphine solution) for pain that recurred when the rescue dose "wore off."

Total morphine dose taken in 24 hours: 120 mg + 60 mg = 180 mg

New SR morphine dose: 60 mg every 8 hours; rescue dose: 15 mg IR morphine

To safely escalate the opioid dose in a patient with constant pain after the patient has been taking an SR preparation for 24 to 48 hours,

- Ask the patient to record all rescue doses he takes.
- If the total amount of drug he takes as a rescue dose is more than 25 percent of the total SR dose, increase the SR dose by the amount in the rescue doses.

Changing opioid agents. Patients commonly need to change opioid agents because of intolerable side effects. Much has been written about the challenges of making these changes, given that the equianalgesic tables we use are far from perfect (Knotkova, Fine, and Portenoy 2009; Fine, Portenoy, and Ad Hoc Expert Panel 2009). Using an equianalgesic table such as the one provided in this chapter (Table 7.4; or at https://pinkbook.dfci.org) will give you somewhere to start; you should be able change agents safely while maintaining adequate control of the patient's pain.

Just as I do when I ask the patient to start on opioids, I always let patients know that this is an inexact science, and that they're likely to be either more sedated or in more pain than they'd like to be for the first few days as we work to get the dose of the new agent adjusted. Knowing which of these they can tolerate (sleepiness or uncontrolled pain) helps me know where to start in the range of "acceptable" doses of the new opioid.

In Table 7.4, the columns indicate the equianalgesic oral and parenteral opioid doses for the listed drugs. For example, 30 mg of oral IR morphine equals 20 mg of oral IR oxycodone or 7.5 mg of oral hydromorphone (e.g., Dilaudid); 10 mg of parenteral morphine equals 1.5 mg of parenteral hydromorphone; and 10 mg of parenteral morphine equals 7.5 mg of oral hydromorphone or 20 mg of oxycodone.

For patients using a fentanyl patch for pain relief, and who have adequate fat reservoir but wish to change to an oral or parenteral formulation of a different opioid, I make the conversion assuming the patient is receiving a full fentanyl dose from the patch. I know it took 12 hours for a therapeutic blood level to be achieved, and that there is ongoing release of fentanyl from the fat reservoir, so I take that into account. I use only immediate-release rescue opioids as needed for the first 6 hours after the patch is removed. At 6 hours, you can begin an infusion of parenteral opioids or begin oral SR opioids at a dose that is 50 percent of the dose you will use at 12 hours. After 12 hours, you can begin the full, calculated dose of the SR opioid or IV opioid infusion.

An adequate fat reservoir cannot form, however, in patients who are very thin or have arm edema or extensive arm tattoos. Patches may not adhere because of skin oils or sweat. If you wish to change their treatment to an oral or intravenous opioid, the safest way to do this is to assume that the patients are not absorbing *any* of the fentanyl and make your calculation of how much of the new opioid is needed using *only* the amount of rescue opioid they have taken in the past 24 to 48 hours. To be safe, I use the same method described above to transition to the other opioid: using only rescue for the first 6 hours after they remove the patch, using half the calculated new opioid SR or IV infusion dose for the next 6, and only starting the full calculated opioid oral or infusion dose at 12 hours after the patch was removed.

For example, consider a very thin patient who cannot take oral medications, is not getting adequate relief from a 200-µg/hr fentanyl patch placed on the arm, but the 24 mg of as-needed IV rescue hydromorphone she was given in the previous 24 hours has provided intermittent pain relief. I assume that without the patch, she'll need at least 1 mg/hr hydromorphone (24 mg/24 h). I'd order the patch to be

Converting from Sustained-Release Morphine to Sustained-Release Oxycodone or Extended-Release Hydromorphone

Example.

 Current SR morphine dose: 60 mg p.o. every 12 hours (total dose: 120 mg/24 hr)

 Equivalent SR oxycodone dose: 40 mg every 12 hours (total dose: 80 mg/24 hr)

 2/3 (dose reduction for incomplete cross-tolerance) × 80 mg = 55 mg

 New SR oxycodone dose: 30 mg every 12 hours; rescue dose: 5 mg IR oxycodone

Example.

 Current SR morphine dose: 60 mg p.o. every 12 hours (total dose: 120 mg/24 hr)

 Equivalent p.o. hydromorphone (e.g., Dilaudid) dose: (120 mg/30) × 7.5 = 30 mg

 2/3 (dose reduction for incomplete cross-tolerance) × 30 mg = 20 mg

 New ER hydromorphone dose*: 24 mg extended release (two 12-mg tablets) p.o. every 24 hours (or 4 mg IR every 4 hours); rescue dose: 2 mg IR hydromorphone

*ER hydromorphone (i.e., Exalgo) comes in 8, 12, 16, and 32 mg tablets. (N.B. I prefer not to give two strengths of an ER opioid if possible, to minimize the chance of incorrect dosing.)

removed and continue that patient's effective rescue dose, which was 2 to 3 mg of IV hydromorphone every 2 hours as needed for the first 6 hours after the patch was removed. At 6 hours, I would order a hydromorphone drip at 0.5 mg/hr and continue the rescue doses. Twelve hours after the patch was removed, I would increase the drip to 1 mg/hr.

Some patients may develop an allergy to the adhesive in the patch. If these patients were taking fentanyl because they poorly tolerated other opioids, the fentanyl can be given as an SQ or IV infusion at the same rate as the patch.

The data that appear at the bottom of Table 7.4 apply only to equivalencies between fentanyl (delivered by transdermal fentanyl patch in micrograms per hour) and the total amount of parenteral or oral morphine taken in 24 hours. For example, the equivalent morphine dose for a patient with a 50 µg/hr fentanyl patch is 33 mg of intravenous morphine in 24 hours, or 100 mg of oral morphine in 24 hours. Similarly, the equivalent fentanyl dose for a patient on an intravenous morphine drip of 4 mg/hr (i.e., 96 mg IV in 24 hours) is 150 µg/hr. A decrease in opioid dose for incomplete cross-tolerance (see below) does not need to be taken.

Except when converting from fentanyl to morphine or vice versa (Table 7.4), it is not sufficient simply to calculate the equianalgesic dose of the new opioid. Patients who take an opioid for several weeks become tolerant to many of the side effects that opioid induces, but they may not be as tolerant to the side effects caused by the new opioid. If their pain is well controlled and they take a full equianalgesic dose of the new opioid, they may develop significant sedation or respiratory depression. To take into account this "incomplete cross-tolerance" between opioids, in patients with well-controlled pain, prescribe about *two-thirds* of the calculated equianalgesic dose of the new opioid. If the pain is not adequately relieved, however, give the full equianalgesic dose of the new agent. In all cases, 10 percent of the 24-hour dose of the new opioid becomes the new rescue dose.

It is much more difficult to convert patients safely to methadone, especially from high doses of other opioids. As I discussed earlier in this chapter, the equianalgesic ratios change as the nonmethadone opioid dose increases. Values range from a ratio of 10:1 at morphine equivalents of 60–199 mg daily, to 20:1 at morphine equivalents of greater than 200 mg daily. First, determine the oral morphine equivalent of the average total amount of opioid the patient has taken daily for the previous two days (a discussion of how to do this appears later in this chapter). If the total oral morphine equivalent was 300 mg on the first day and 400 mg on the second, the average total daily amount would be 350 mg; use that amount to determine the methadone dose according to the ratios in the box below.

Morphine Equivalent Methadone Doses

Oral Morphine Equivalent (mg/24h)	Morphine: Methadone Ratio
<60	2 to 7.5 mg/d
60–199 and patient <65	10:1
≥200 mg or patient ≥65	20:1

(McPherson et al. 2019)

For the patient taking an average of 350 mg of morphine a day, the ratio would be 20:1 (350/20 = 17.5 mg total daily dose, given in divided doses, usually three times a day, or 5 mg p.o. t.i.d.). I describe in detail earlier in the chapter how to convert a patient from oxycodone to methadone. If you have questions about this conversion procedure, consult a palliative care clinician (including a clinical pharmacist) or anesthesia pain specialist.

Changing the route of delivery. Changing from transdermal fentanyl to the intravenous route and vice versa is relatively straightforward, since the doses are equivalent. But the patient will be absorbing fentanyl from the fat reservoir for some time after the patch is removed, which will contribute to the pain relief and the side effects. My practice, which others have also reported (Kornick et al. 2001), is that 6 hours after the patch is removed, begin the continuous infusion at half the fentanyl patch dose. For example, if the patient is on a 50 mcg/hr patch,

---

Changing from Oxycodone to Methadone in a Patient with Severe Pain Uncontrolled by the Oxycodone

Example.

A patient takes 100 mg of sustained-release oxycodone every 8 hours (300 mg every 24 hours) for the past 48 hours along with 30 mg p.o. immediate-release oxycodone every 3 hours p.r.n. (total 6 doses per day over the past 48 hours).

Transition only the SR oxycodone to methadone, continuing the rescue IR oxycodone.

300 mg oral oxycodone = 450 mg oral morphine

Morphine to methadone ratio: 20:1

Equianalgesic methadone dose: 450 mg/20 = 22.5 mg of methadone

New opioid: 7.5 mg p.o. methadone q8h, beginning Day 1

N.B. The methadone will take 3–5 days to achieve the full pain-relieving effect of the initial dose. Continue the SR oxycodone until the rescue dosing markedly decreases, usually by Day 3 (suggested procedure referred to as "RULE" below).

Day 1: Give 100 mg of sustained-release oxycodone q8h and 7.5 mg of methadone q8h; continue 30mg IR oxycodone as needed q4h
  — Patient takes three 30 mg doses over 24 hours

Day 2: RULE: If the patient has used ≤3 doses of p.r.n. IR oxycodone, halve the SR oxycodone.
  — Give 50 mg of sustained-release oxycodone q8h and 7.5 mg of methadone q8h; continue 30 mg IR oxycodone as needed q4h.
  — Patient takes two 30-mg doses over 24 hours.

Day 3: RULE: If the patient has used ≤3 doses of p.r.n. IR oxycodone, stop the SR oxycodone
  — Discontinue SR oxycodone and continue 7.5 mg of methadone p.o. q8h; continue 30 mg IR oxycodone as needed q4h.

---

remove the patch at noon, and begin a fentanyl infusion at 25 mcg/hr at 6 p.m. At midnight, increase the rate to 50 mcg/hr. Provide as-needed bolus dosing in case of breakthrough pain.

When changing back to the transdermal patch, it will take some time for enough fentanyl to be deposited in the fat reservoir under the patch for blood levels to develop that provide pain relief. Therefore, I recommend decreasing the drip dose by 50 percent at 6 hours after placing the patch and stopping the infusion 12 hours after the patch was placed. For example, if the patient is on a 50 mcg/hr infusion, place the patch at noon and decrease the fentanyl infusion to 25 mcg/hr at 6 p.m. At midnight, discontinue the infusion. Provide as-needed bolus dosing in case of breakthrough pain.

Some Common Oral-to-Parenteral Opioid Conversions

Morphine: ratio of oral dose to parenteral dose = 3:1

Example.
   Oral dose: 100 mg q12h; 24-hour total dose = 200 mg p.o.
   Equivalent IV/SQ dose: 200 mg p.o./3 = ~66 mg/24 hr IV (i.e., ~3 mg/hr).

Hydromorphone: ratio of oral dose to parenteral dose = 5:1

Example.
   Oral dose: 12 mg every 4 hours; 24-hour total dose = 72 mg p.o.
   Equivalent IV/SQ dose: 72 mg p.o./5 ≈ 14 mg/24 hr IV or SQ (i.e., 2.3 mg IV every 4 hours or 0.6 mg/hr). Round to nearest dose that can be administered: 2–2.5 mg IV every 4 hours.

Changing from the oral to the parenteral route of opioid agents except fentanyl requires a change in opioid dose. A large proportion of an oral opioid dose is metabolized in its first pass through the liver; these metabolites cannot cross the blood-brain barrier to provide pain relief.

Trainees need to be reminded that it's important to specify the route by which the opioid should be given. I was once called by the nurses because a house officer had written an order for "6 mg of hydromorphone IV or p.o. q4h." The patient had been taking the oral hydromorphone dose but was going to be NPO for surgery. Luckily, the nurse did not give the 6 mg intravenous bolus; if she had, the patient would have received the equivalent of 30 mg of oral hydromorphone.

Converting from multiple oral agents to a single parenteral agent. While converting from an oral to a parenteral route of the same opioid is fairly straightforward, other conversions can be more challenging. Not infrequently, when patients are admitted to the hospital, they are taking several different oral opioids, and these must be converted to a single parenteral medication. To start an infusion using morphine, I calculate the patient's total daily oral opioid dose in oral morphine equivalents, reduce the doses of other opioids by one-third to adjust for incomplete cross-tolerance, and add all the morphine equivalents together to get the total oral morphine equivalent for 24 hours. I divide that total by 3 to get the total intravenous morphine equivalent over 24 hours. Finally, I divide that amount by 24, which becomes the continuous-infusion rate for the intravenous morphine.

Here are two sample calculations of patients whose pain control is satisfactory, but who need to be switched from oral to parenteral opioids. The first is a patient with myeloma who broke her femur and needed to have a pin placed before she received radiation (see "Converting from IR Oxycodone plus SR Morphine to an Equivalent Parenteral Morphine Dose"). She would be NPO in the

---

**Converting from IR Oxycodone Plus SR Morphine
to an Equivalent Parenteral Morphine Dose**

- Calculate oral morphine equivalents taken in the past 24 hours and decrease doses of other opioids by one-third to adjust for incomplete cross-tolerance.

Current Medications	Oral Morphine Equivalents
IR oxycodone 60 mg	60 mg (i.e., 2/3 × 90 mg, reducing for incomplete cross-tolerance)
SR morphine 120 mg	120 mg
Total	180 mg oral morphine equivalents

- Calculate the IV morphine drip rate.

Oral Morphine Equivalents	Parenteral Dose	IV Drip Rate
180 mg	60 mg (180 mg/3)	2.5 mg/hr (60 mg/24 hr)

---

perioperative period and would be expected to have postoperative pain in addition to her chronic pain from her myeloma. She had been taking 60 mg of SR morphine every 12 hours, with two 5-mg oxycodone every 4 hours as needed for breakthrough pains. Since the fracture, she had in fact taken 12 oxycodone tablets a day in addition to the morphine.

The second is a patient who was taking 180 mg of SR oxycodone a day and hydromorphone for rescue (see "Converting from IR Hydromorphone plus SR Oxycodone to an Equivalent Parenteral Morphine Dose"). He took 24 mg of oral hydromorphone on the day before admission. Intravenous hydromorphone could be used, but for this example, assume that you wish to prescribe morphine.

Some patients are admitted with persistent pain despite taking oral opioids. Because their opioid doses should be increased by 50–100 percent, I do not decrease the equianalgesic dose for incomplete cross-tolerance. I give them the exact equivalent in morphine, which, in effect, is a 33 percent increase in dose. For example, you might want to start an intravenous morphine drip for a patient whose average pain intensity is 8 despite taking two 5-mg oxycodone every 4 hours (i.e., 10 mg oxycodone × 6 doses = 60 mg IR oxycodone) and 60 mg of SR oxycodone every 12 hours.

If you are converting a patient from oral to parenteral opioids who has not received intravenous opioids before, it is important to explain to him why you are using this route. I learned this from a young patient with testicular cancer who was admitted with severe retroperitoneal pain caused by metastases.

Converting from Oral SR Oxycodone plus IR Hydromorphone to an Equivalent Parenteral Morphine Dose

- Calculate oral morphine equivalents taken in the past 24 hours and decrease doses of other opioids by one-third to adjust for incomplete cross-tolerance.

Current Medications	Oral Morphine Equivalents
SR oxycodone 180 mg	180 mg (i.e., 2/3 × 270 mg, reducing for incomplete cross-tolerance)
Hydromorphone 24 mg oral	64 mg ([(24 mg / 7.5) × 30] × 2/3, reducing for incomplete cross-tolerance)
Total	244 mg oral morphine equivalents

- Calculate the IV morphine drip rate.

Oral Morphine	Parenteral Dose	IV Drip Rate
244 mg	81 mg (244 mg / 3)	3.4 mg/hr (81 mg / 24 hr) Round to nearest dose that can be administered: 3.5 mg/hr

Dire Implications of a Morphine Drip

Joe was an 18-year-old student whose family physician had discovered a testicular mass several months before. Joe had insisted that he wanted to finish the school year before having any diagnostic procedures. He made it through graduation but soon after was admitted for pain control from extensive painful retroperitoneal adenopathy.

To relieve his pain I suggested a morphine drip with morphine boluses as needed. When I next went to see Joe, he was in tears. I asked what was the matter, and he replied, "I knew from Dr. Porter that I was sick, but he never told me I was about to die!" I was taken aback and told him that, on the contrary, he had every chance of being cured by the chemotherapy. When I asked what had made him think he was terminally ill, he said, "Well, the nurses told me you started a morphine drip. And the only time I ever heard of that being used was on my Aunt Jane; they started one on her just a few days before she died."

Since this experience, I have been careful to explain to a patient why I am choosing intravenous opioids, saying something like,

> I know you are having severe pain, and I want to lower the level of the pain as fast as I can. To do this, I need to give you opioid medications, like morphine, and I need to give them as an infusion. This doesn't mean you're about to die; it's just that this is the fastest way I can bring your pain under control. As soon as I know what dose of opioids you need, I'll switch you to oral medications.

I have frightened many fewer patients since I adopted this technique.

Converting from Oral IR and SR Oxycodone to a Parenteral Morphine Infusion for a Patient in Persistent Pain

- Calculate oral morphine equivalents taken in the past 24 hours. Given uncontrolled pain, you do not need to reduce dose for incomplete cross-tolerance.

Current Medications	Oral Morphine Equivalents
IR oxycodone 60 mg	90 mg
SR oxycodone 120 mg	180 mg
Total	270 mg oral morphine equivalents

- Calculate the IV morphine drip rate.

Oral Morphine	Parenteral Dose	IV Drip Rate
270 mg	90 mg (270 mg / 3)	3.75 mg/hr (90 mg / 24 hr) Round to nearest dose that can be administered: 3.5 to 4 mg/hr

---

Changing from pills to a transdermal fentanyl patch and vice versa. The technique for changing patients from oral medications to a transdermal fentanyl patch includes not only determining the equianalgesic dose (Table 7.4) but also providing pain relief during the time it takes for the patch to begin providing adequate analgesia. This is easy to do if the patient is taking an SR morphine, hydromorphone, or oxycodone preparation. Exalgo relieves pain for 24 hours, Kadian relieves pain for 12 to 24 hours, and the other SR preparations relieve pain for about 8–12 hours, which is almost the same amount of time it takes for the patch to begin providing adequate pain relief. Therefore, instruct the patient to take the last dose of the SR opioid pills (or 50 percent of the Exalgo dose) at the time she applies the first patch and to use the rescue doses if needed. If her pain is constant, not episodic, and 72 hours after the patch is placed, the patient's pain control is not satisfactory or her rescue doses exceed 25 percent of the total daily opioid dose, increase the dose of the fentanyl patch by an amount equivalent to the amount of rescue medication taken. Further dose titrations may be needed over the ensuing weeks.

To convert from a fentanyl patch to oral medications, as I review above when discussing how to make other transitions from fentanyl patches, you must take into consideration the significant amount of fentanyl that remains in the skin reservoir after the patient has removed the patch. Therefore, ask the patient to remove the patch and to take rescue medication if pain recurs. At 12 hours after they've removed the patch, since the serum level of the fentanyl is still significant, the patient should take half the equianalgesic dose of the oral SR opioid agent. Twenty-four hours after the patch is removed, the serum fentanyl level will no longer be therapeutic, and the patient may take the full equianalgesic dose of oral SR opioid.

Converting from Oral Opioids to Transdermal Fentanyl

Example.

A patient taking SR morphine 150 mg p.o. every 12 hours would like to switch to transdermal fentanyl.

Refer to Table 7.4 for the fentanyl dose that should be prescribed for each oral morphine dose. A further one-third decrease is not required.

Current Medications	*Transdermal Fentanyl Equivalents*
SR morphine 300 mg	150 µg/hr
Rescue dose: 30 mg IR morphine	

Give the last dose of 150 mg of SR morphine at the time the patch is placed.

Increasing the Dose of Transdermal Fentanyl

Example.

A patient who had been maintaining excellent pain relief using a 75 µg/hr fentanyl patch (equivalent to 150 mg of morphine) had for the past three days required six 15-mg doses daily (total 90 mg) of IR morphine (i.e., about 33 percent of the total daily opioid dose) for increased constant pain.

Refer to Table 7.4 for the fentanyl dose equivalent to the oral morphine dose.

Current Medications	*Transdermal Fentanyl Equivalents*
Fentanyl 75 µg/hr	75 µg/hr
IR morphine 90 mg	45 µg/hr
New patch strength	125 µg/hr (closest dose to patches available)

Calculate new rescue dose.

Fentanyl Dose	*Oral Morphine Equivalents*
125 µg/hr	250 mg
Rescue dose	10 percent of 250 mg ≈ 30 mg IR morphine

Converting from a Transdermal Fentanyl Patch to Oral Opioid

Example.

A patient using a 100-µg/hr transdermal fentanyl patch is to be switched to the equivalent SR morphine dose.

Referring to Table 7.4, select the equianalgesic dose.

Current Fentanyl Dose	*Morphine Equivalent*
100 µg/hr	200 mg morphine/24 hr

Rescue dose: 20 mg IR morphine (e.g., 1 ml of a 20 mg/ml elixir)

- Patient removes the patch and takes IR morphine every 3 hours p.r.n. for the next 12 hours.
- Twelve to 18 hours after the patch was removed, the patient begins 50 mg of SR morphine every 12 hours, with p.r.n. IR morphine q3h. At 24 hours, he starts 100 mg b.i.d. SR morphine.

Rapidly Relieving Excruciating Pain

Rarely, you will see a patient in the ED or an inpatient who has a pain "emergency": the pain has been severe, debilitating for at least 6 hours without relief from the medications the patient has tried, and has escalated over the past several days. The patient is in agony, and you want to relieve the pain as soon as possible. You can do this most expeditiously by "stacking" morphine or hydromorphone intravenous bolus doses. To do this safely, however, the patient must be monitored very closely. While the bolus doses are being given, the patient should be under continuous observation, with continuous pulse oximetry, and recordings at least every 15 minutes of vital signs, verbal pain scores, mental status changes (e.g., using the Richmond Agitation Sedation Scale [RASS]), and other adverse events, until the pain level has fallen to less than 5. This process usually takes several hours.

Rapid dose escalation is usually needed to overcome severe pain in both opioid-naive patients and those who are already taking opioids. In both situations, prescribe a bowel regimen and ensure close monitoring for opioid-induced nausea, sedation, and respiratory depression. For patients with severe neuropathic pain, consider adding corticosteroids (e.g., dexamethasone). With careful patient observation, opioid doses can be increased substantially without excessive toxicity. Suggestions for dosing of IV boluses and recommended monitoring parameters for both types of patients are given in the boxes describing the treatment of severe pain.

Treating Severe Pain in an Opioid-Naive Patient

- Begin a bowel regimen; consider adding corticosteroids for neuropathic pain.
- Monitor the patient for nausea, sedation (RASS), respiratory depression due to opioids.
- PCA option:
  - Begin with loading dose, basal rate, and bolus dosing.

    Hydromorphone for patients with renal failure:

    > 0.2 to 0.5 mg loading dose + 0.01 mg/kg basal rate + 0.2 mg boluses every 10 minutes p.r.n.; nursing bolus up to 2 times per hour, 0.5 mg

    > *Sample calculation.* For a 70-kg man, hydromorphone basal rate = 0.7 mg/hr. For patients over 65 or patients with CO_2 retention, begin at 0.3 mg/hr.

    Morphine for other patients:

    > 2 to 5 mg loading dose + 0.05 mg/kg basal rate + 2 mg boluses every 10 minutes p.r.n.; nursing bolus up to 2 times per hour, 4 mg

    > *Sample calculation.* For a 70-kg man, morphine basal rate = 3.5 mg/hr.

    > For patients over 65 or patients with CO_2 retention, begin at 0.3 mg/hr.

  - Ensure continuous pulse oximetry.
  - Check vital signs including level of sedation (RASS) every 15 minutes.
  - Reevaluate pain hourly.
  - Double PCA bolus doses every 2 hours and adjust nursing bolus dose to be twice the PCA dose until pain level falls below 5 or becomes tolerable.
  - Increase the basal opioid infusion rate every 12 hours as needed, adjusting rate by the p.r.n. opioids received.

    Example.

    > A patient receiving 3 mg/hr IV morphine received 3 mg IV morphine q3h over the past 12 hours (total 12 mg).

    > New IV morphine basal rate: 3 mg/hr + 12 mg/12 hr = 4 mg/hr

- IV bolus option
  - Start continuous pulse oximetry.
  - Give 2 to 5 mg of IV morphine; evaluate vital signs and pain relief 10 minutes later.
  - If pain level is severe and unchanged, double the bolus dose; check vital signs and RASS; reevaluate pain 10 minutes later. If still unchanged, repeat.
  - When pain level decreases but is still ≥5, repeat the same bolus dose; check vital signs and RASS; reevaluate pain level 10 minutes later. If still ≥5, repeat.
  - When pain level <5, give the effective bolus dose q3h as needed for next 8–12 hours.
  - When pain control is adequate, begin continuous infusion or oral or transdermal opioid based on the opioid used in the past 8–12 hours.

(continued)

Example.

Morphine to reduce pain level to <5: 35 mg over 2 hours (5 mg + 10 mg + 20 mg)

Three additional 20-mg boluses required in the next 6 hours. Total morphine taken in 8 hours: 95 mg IV. Because the half-life of morphine is 4 hours, 50 percent of the 95 mg will have been metabolized.

Options: morphine drip at 6 mg/hr (47.5 / 8) or oral or transdermal opioid equivalent to 6 mg/hr parenteral morphine with 10 mg IV morphine q2h p.r.n. rescue

---

Treating Severe Pain in a Patient Already Taking Opioids

- Continue the bowel regimen.
- Start continuous pulse oximetry; monitor the patient for nausea, sedation (RASS), or respiratory depression caused by the increased opioid dose.
- IV bolus option:
  - Continue the previous continuous IV, oral SR, or transdermal opioid; use 10 percent of the previous 24-hour opioid dose as the IV bolus dose every 15 to 30 minutes, depending on the monitoring available.
  - Ensure continuous pulse oximetry and check vital signs and RASS every 15 minutes.
  - Reevaluate the pain level 15 minutes after each dose is given.
  - Double the bolus dose if the pain is severe and unchanged; when pain level decreases but is still ≥5, or (i.e., moderately severe), give the same bolus dose.
  - When the pain has been brought under control, adjust the oral/transdermal dose by the amount of rescue opioid required.

  Example.

  Sustained-release oral morphine: 100 mg every 12 hours

  Current rescue dose: 15 mg IR morphine every 2 hours p.o. = 5 mg every 1 hour IV

  IV rescue doses (mg) over the first 4 hours: 5 + 10 + 10 = 25 mg IV morphine

  Total IV rescue doses over 12 hours: 50 mg IV morphine = 150 mg oral morphine. Add 50 percent of that to the basal opioid dose.

  New oral morphine dose (mg): 200 + 75 = 275 mg sustained-release oral morphine per day or 140 mg SR every 12 hours.

  New rescue dose: 30 mg IR morphine p.o. q2-3h p.r.n.

(continued)

- PCA option:
  - Start IV morphine PCA with basal rate at twice the current rescue dose. Basal rate: 1 mg/hr IV morphine, with boluses of 0.5 mg morphine IV every 10 minutes p.r.n.
  - Start continuous pulse oximetry and check vital signs and RASS every 15 minutes, pain hourly.
  - Double bolus doses every hour until pain level falls below 5 or becomes tolerable. Continue the effective bolus dose.
  - Increase the basal rate every 12 hours p.r.n., adjusting for bolus doses taken and half-life of morphine.

  Example.

    A patient receiving 1 mg/hr IV morphine required 12 boluses of IV morphine in the past 12 hours (0.5 mg + 1 mg + [2.0 mg × 10]).

    Total IV rescue doses over 12 hours: 21.5 mg/12h = 1.8 mg/h; add 50 percent of that to the basal opioid dose.

    New basal rate: 1 mg/hr + 0.9 mg/hr = 1.9 mg/hr

When satisfactory pain relief is finally achieved, the patient usually falls asleep. This is not a signal to decrease the opioid infusion rate. The patient is not overdosed; he is simply exhausted by loss of sleep due to the excruciating pain. If the patient is difficult to arouse, hold the infusion for an hour and then restart it at 50 percent of the previous dose. When the patient awakens, continue careful evaluations of pain intensity and side effects. Once the pain has been controlled for a day or two, the patient is likely to require less opioid per hour to maintain the same level of pain relief.

Opioid-tolerant patients who develop excruciating somatic pain are likely to respond to infusions of hydromorphone, with bolus doses both to establish an initial level and to provide rescue for incompletely relieved pain. If you use morphine, the amounts needed are more likely to cause neurotoxicity (e.g., myoclonus) than the doses needed of the much more potent hydromorphone. Calculate an equianalgesic starting dose from the opioids the patient has been taking that have not relieved her pain, and do not decrease for incomplete cross-tolerance, because you know the patient needs a 50 to 100 percent increase in opioids because of her severe pain.

Susannah, for example, was a 35-year-old woman with metastatic breast cancer and increasing bone pain who had been taking 100 mg of sustained-release morphine every 8 hours for several months when her disease progressed and her pain level "got out of control." When she was admitted for evaluation of the cause of the increased pain, she told us she had taken six 30-mg rescue doses in the past few days without relief. Her total oral morphine per day was, therefore, 300 mg + 180 mg = 480 mg. Knowing that 30 mg of oral morphine is equivalent to

1.5 mg of IV hydromorphone, to calculate her drip rate, I divided 480 mg by 30 = 16 and multiplied that by 1.5 = 24 mg of IV hydromorphone per 24 hours, or 1 mg/ hour. I discontinued her oral morphine, started with a loading bolus of 2 mg of hydromorphone, a hydromorphone drip of 1mg/hr, and added boluses of 1 to 2 mg of hydromorphone every 2 hours as needed to enable her to tolerate the workup.

Patients with neuropathic pain will be harder to control. Josh, discussed earlier in this chapter, was rotated to methadone at home to good effect. But patients with severe pain crises or whom you cannot monitor carefully at home will need admission. If you are rotating opioids because of neurotoxicity, consider adding a ketamine infusion to control the pain with fewer opioid boluses (Moryl, Coyle, and Foley 2008). When ketamine is not an option, consider dexmedetomidine (Precedex). Anesthesia pain and palliative care specialists can be consulted to help you manage these complex patients.

SUMMARY

As clinicians, we strive to help even our sickest patients accomplish the goals they have set for themselves. To succeed, we must relieve uncontrolled pain. The pharmacologic agents and other treatment modalities discussed in this chapter, along with the nonpharmacologic techniques reviewed in Chapter 8, enable us to control the pain of 95 percent or more of our patients with cancer without excessive sedation, minimizing the associated side effects. When our patients have accomplished their final tasks, they will—despite the urgings of the poet Dylan Thomas to the contrary—"go gentle into that good night."

Tables

TABLE 7.1 Nonsteroidal Anti-inflammatory Drugs (NSAIDs)

Chemical Class	Generic Name	Interval	Initial Dose (mg)*	Max. 24-hr Dose (mg)
p-aminophenol salicylates	Acetaminophen†	q4-6h	650	4000
	Aspirin†,‡	q4-6h	650	4000
	Salsalate	q8-12h	750–1000	3000
	Diflunisal	q12h	500	1500
Propionic acid derivatives	Ibuprofen	q4-6h	400	2400
	Fenoprofen	q4-6h	200	2400
	Ketoprofen†	q6-8h	25	225
	Naproxen†,‡	q6-8h	250	1000
	Oxaprozin	q12-24h	600	1200
Acetic acid derivatives	Indomethacin†,‡	q8-12h	25	150
	Tolmetin	q8h	400	1800
	Diclofenac†	q8h	50	150
	Sulindac	q12h	150	400
	Ketorolac	q6h	15–30 mg IV q6h (p.o. 10 mg q6h)	120 mg per day (p.o. 40 mg)
COX-2 "selective"§	Etodolac	q8-12h	200–400	1200
	Nabumetone	q12-24h	1000/24 hr	1500
	Celecoxib	q12-24h	100–200	400
	Valdecoxib	q12-24h	10	40

*In the elderly and in patients with renal insufficiency, start at one-half to two-thirds of these doses.

†Bioavailable p.r. via custom-made suppository or microenema (Davis et al. 2002).

‡Available in suppository form.

§Rofecoxib (Vioxx), withdrawn in September 2004. Valdecoxib was withdrawn in 2005.

TABLE 7.2 Commonly Used Step 2 Opioids: Preparations Available

Name	Initial Dose (mg), Oral*	Dose Interval (hr)	Dose Adjustments Needed	Preparations Available†
Hydrocodone	10	3–4	None	IR, comb
Codeine	60	3–4	Severe hepatic or renal failure	IR, comb, IM, SQ, p.r.
Oxycodone‡	5–10	3–4	Severe hepatic or renal failure	Comb, p.r.
Tapentadol	50	6	Moderate hepatic failure; severe renal failure	IR, ER
Tramadol	50	6	Cirrhosis or renal failure	IR, p.r. comb

Source: H. Knotkova, P. G. Fine, and R. K. Portenoy, "Opioid Rotation: The Science and the Limitations of the Equianalgesic Dose Table," *J Pain Symptom Manage* 38:426–39, 2009.

*For patients weighing over 110 pounds who have moderate to severe pain.

†Preparations: IR = oral, immediate-release; comb = oral combination preparation with an NSAID (acetaminophen, aspirin, ibuprofen, etc.); IM = parenteral—suitable for intramuscular use; SQ = subcutaneous; p.r. = per rectum via commercial or custom-made suppository or microenema (Davis et al. 2002).

‡See also Table 7.3 for oxycodone not in a combination preparation; that is, IR, sustained-release (SR), liquid (liq), or liquid concentrate (liq conc) oxycodone.

TABLE 7.3 Commonly Used Step 3 Opioids: Preparations Available

Name	Initial Dose (mg)*		Dose Interval (hr)	Dose Adjustments Needed	Preparations Available†
	Oral	*IM/IV*			
Morphine	15–30	10	3–4	Renal failure	IV/SQ, IR, p.r., liq, liq conc
Morphine, SR	15–30	n/a	8–12	Renal/hepatic failure	SR, p.r.
Morphine, SR	30	n/a	24	Renal/hepatic failure	SR
Hydromorphone	4–8	1.5	4	Hepatic failure	IV/SQ, IR, p.r.
Hydromorphone, SR‡	12	n/a	24	Hepatic failure	SR
Oxycodone	10	n/a	3–4	Renal failure	IR, liq, liq conc, p.r.
Oxycodone, SR	10	n/a	12	Renal/hepatic failure	SR
Oxymorphone	10	IV	4–6	Renal/hepatic failure	IR, liq, p.r.
Oxymorphone, SR	5	n/a	12	Renal/hepatic failure	SR
Fentanyl‡	n/a	25 µg/hr	72	Hepatic failure	Transdermal
Buprenorphine	n/a	5 µg/hr	5–7d	Hepatic failure	Transdermal
Fentanyl	200 µg	n/a	2	Hepatic failure	Transmucosal
Buprenorphine	75 µg	n/a	daily	Hepatic failure	Transmucosal
Methadone	5	2.5	6–8	Hepatic failure	IV/SQ, IR, liq, p.r.
Levorphanol	2	1	4–6	Renal failure	IV/SQ
Demerol§	N/R	N/R	N/R	Renal failure	IV, IR

Source: H. Knotkova, P. G. Fine, R. K. Portenoy, "Opioid Rotation: The Science and the Limitations of the Equianalgesic Dose Table," *J Pain Symptom Manage* 38:426–39, 2009.

*For patients weighing over 110 pounds who have moderate to severe pain.

†Preparations: p.r. = per rectum via commercial or custom-made suppository or microenema (Davis e tal. 2002); IV = parenteral—suitable for intravenous use; SQ = subcutaneous; IR = oral, immediate release; SR = oral, sustained release; liq = liquid; liq conc = concentrated liquid solution; N/R = not recommended.

‡Only use as an initial dose if the patient is already taking the equivalent of oral morphine.

§Not recommended for use other than for a limited time (see text).

TABLE 7.4 Commonly Used Opioids: Equianalgesic Doses

Drug	Oral/Rectal Dose (mg)	Parenteral Dose (mg)
Morphine	20–30	7–10
Hydromorphone	7.5	1.5
Oxycodone	15–20	7.5–10
Methadone*	20	10
Levorphanol	4	2
Oxymorphone	15	1
Meperidine†	300	75
Transdermal buprenorphine	5–10 mcg/hr	n/a
Transdermal fentanyl	12.5 mcg/hr	12.5 mcg/hr
Transmucosal fentanyl	800 mcg	n/a

Conversion from fentanyl transdermal patch to parenteral or oral morphine

Fentanyl (mcg/hr)	Morphine (mg/24 hr)	
	p.o.	*IM/IV*
25	50	17
50	100	33
75	150	50
100	200	67
125	250	83
150	300	100

Source: H. Knotkova, P. G. Fine, R. K. Portenoy, "Opioid Rotation: The Science and the Limitations of the Equianalgesic Dose Table," *J Pain Symptom Manage* 38:426–39, 2009.

*For dosing of methadone, see discussion in text and Practice Points box.

†Not recommended for cancer patients (see text).

TABLE 7.5 Laxatives to Prevent and Treat Opioid-Induced Constipation

Drug	Mechanism	Initial Dosage
General		
Senna	Myenteric plexus stimulant	1 p.o. b.i.d.
Senokot-S	Senna + stool hydrating agent	1 p.o. b.i.d.
Bisacodyl (Dulcolax)	Myenteric plexus stimulant	1 p.o. h.s.
Milk of Magnesia (MOM)	Osmotic	30 ml p.o. q.d.
Lactulose	Osmotic	15–30 ml p.o. h.s.
Polyethylene glycol	Osmotic	17 g in 4 oz water p.o. q.d.
MOM + mineral oil	Osmotic	30–60 ml MOM + 15–30 ml mineral oil q.d. or b.i.d.
Plecanatide*	Adds water to gut	3 mg p.o. q.d.
Linaclotide*	Adds water to gut	72–145 mcg p.o. q.d.
Lubiprostone*	Adds water to gut	24 mcg p.o. b.i.d.
Prucalopride	Stimulates colonic motility	2 mg p.o. q.d.
Opioid Bowel Syndrome		
Metoclopramide (Reglan)	Vagal stimulant	5–10 mg p.o./IV q.i.d. to 20 mg p.o./IV q.i.d.; or 1–3 mg/hr IV
Clonidine	Prevents withdrawal	0.1–0.3 mg transdermal patch
Methylnaltrexone	Peripheral opioid antagonist	Weight-based subcutaneous injection
Naloxegol	Peripheral opioid antagonist	25 mcg p.o. q.d. (decrease to 12.5 if Cr Cl <60 mL/min)
Naldemedine	Peripheral opioid antagonist	0.2 mg p.o. q.d.

*Effective in patients on opioids who do not have cancer; not tested in cancer patients.

TABLE 7.6 Antiemetics

Etiology of Nausea	Drug	Dose
Initiation of opioid therapy	Prochlorperazine (Compazine)	10 mg p.o./IV t.i.d. to q.i.d. or 25 mg p.r. b.i.d.
Stimulation of chemoreceptor trigger zone	Haloperidol (Haldol)	1–2 mg p.o. b.i.d. to q.i.d., 0.5–1 mg IV b.i.d. to q.i.d.
	Prochlorperazine (Compazine)	10 mg p.o./IV t.i.d. to q.i.d. or 25 mg p.r. b.i.d.
	Olanzapine (Zyprexa, Zydis)	2.5–5 mg p.o./SL/IV q.d. to t.i.d.
	Ondansetron (Zofran)	4–8 mg p.o./IV b.i.d. to t.i.d.
Delayed gastric emptying	Metoclopramide (Reglan)	10–20 mg p.o./IV b.i.d. to q.i.d. or 1–3 mg/hr IV
Vertigo	Scopolamine (Transderm Scōp)	1 patch q72h
	Meclizine (Bonine, Antivert)	25 mg t.i.d. p.o.
Unclear	Ondansetron (Zofran)	4–8 mg p.o./IV b.i.d. to t.i.d.
	Olanzapine (Zyprexa, Zydis)	2.5–5 mg p.o./SL/IV daily, b.i.d. to q.i.d.
	Lorazepam (Ativan)	0.5–1 mg p.o./SL/IV q4h

Note: For nausea, initial steps should be (1) treat cause, if identified; (2) consider changing to a different opioid agent (see text); and (3) use adjuvants to decrease opioid dose (see Table 7.5, opioid bowel syndrome). IV = intravenous; p.o. = oral; SL = sublingual dissolving tablets/wafers.

TABLE 7.7 Psychostimulants

Drug	Dose
Methylphenidate (Ritalin)	2.5–5 mg p.o. every morning; may repeat at noon if needed
Dextroamphetamine (Dexedrine)	2.5–5 mg p.o. every morning; may repeat at noon if needed
Modafinil (Provigil)	200 mg p.o. every morning; can increase to 400 mg/day

Note: For sedation, initial steps should be (1) treat cause, if identified; (2) use SR and IR preparations effectively; (3) discontinue other sedating agents (see text); and (4) use adjuvants to decrease opioid dose (see Table 7.5, opioid bowel syndrome).

TABLE 7.8 Adjuvants for Neuropathic Pain

Class/Drug	Dose	Comments
Corticosteroids		
Dexamethasone	10 mg bolus; 4 mg p.o./IV q.i.d.; taper as tolerated	Spinal cord compression
	4 mg p.o./IV b.i.d.	Other neuropathic pain initial dose
Anticonvulsants		
Gabapentin (Neurontin)	900–3600 mg/day p.o.	Initial dose: 100 mg b.i.d. to t.i.d.; increase by 100 mg q3-7d
Pregabalin (Lyrica)	150–600 mg/day p.o.	Initial dose: 50–75 mg b.i.d. to t.i.d.; increase by 100–150 mg q3-7d
Phenytoin (Dilantin)	1000 mg load; 200–300 mg/day	Cannot be given IM
Carbamazepine (Tegretol)	200 mg p.o. h.s., increase q3d	Suspension available for rectal administration. Do not exceed 1200 mg/24 hr
Lamotrigine (Lamictal)	100–200 mg/day p.o.	Initial dose 25 mg/day p.o.; increase by 25 mg/day q2 weeks
Topiramate (Topamax)	200–400 mg/day p.o.	Initial dose 25–50 mg/day p.o.; increase 25–50 mg/day q. week
Oxcarbazepine (Trileptal)	2400 mg/day p.o.	Initial dose 300 mg p.o. b.i.d.; increase by 300 mg q3d
SNRI		
Duloxetine (Cymbalta)	120 mg/day p.o.	Initial dose 30 mg p.o. daily; Increase by 30 mg q 1-2 weeks
Venlafaxine (Effexor)	225 mg/day p.o.	Initial dose 37.5–75 mg p.o. daily Increase q2 weeks as needed
Tricyclic antidepressants	Begin at 10–25 mg p.o. h.s.; increase to therapeutic dose (50–150 mg in divided doses)	Side effects: anticholinergic, sedation, cardiac arrhythmias, orthostatic hypotension
Amitriptyline (Elavil)		Amitriptyline: most sedating
Nortriptyline (Pamelor)		Nortriptyline: least orthostatic hypotension; minimal sedation
Desipramine (Norpramin)		Desipramine: least sedating, minimal cardiotoxicity; may need 150–300 mg for therapeutic effect
Clomipramine (Anafranil)		
Baclofen	40–80 mg/day p.o.	5 mg p.o. t.i.d.; titrate as needed
NK-1 receptor antagonists		
Fosaprepitant	150 mg IV q.d.	Case report (Dulin et al. 2017)

TABLE 7.8 (*cont.*)

Class/Drug	Dose	Comments
Alpha-2 adrenergic agonists		
Clonidine	3 mg patch daily	1 mg patch; increase as needed
Dexmedetomidine (Precedex)	0.1–1.5 mcg/kg/hr (optional bolus 0.4–1 mcg/kg over 10–30 minutes MD administered	Case reports (Hofherr, Abrahm, and Rickerson 2020)
NMDA antagonist		
Ketamine	0.1–0.2 mg/kg IV or 0.5 mg/kg SQ initial; then 0.02–0.05 mg/kg/h infusion	Double dose q15min until pain is relieved; then begin drip at equivalent amount per hour; scopolamine may be needed for increased salivation
Local anesthetic		
Lidocaine	1–3 mg/kg IV over 20–30 min, followed by infusion of 0.5–2 mg/kg/hr (i.e., 10–80 mg/hr)	Close monitoring of vital signs and patient symptoms required

TABLE 7.9 Adjuvants for Bone Pain

Drug	Dose	Comments
Bisphosphonates		Caution in renal insufficiency
Zoledronic acid (Zometa)	4 mg IV over 15 min q4 weeks	
Pamidronate (Aredia)	60–90 mg IV over 2 hr, q3-4 weeks	
RANK-L inhibitor		
Denosumab	120 mg SQ q4 weeks	Often effective for weeks to a few months; can cause symptomatic hypocalcemia
Radiopharmaceuticals		
Radium-223 chloride (Alpharadin)		Induces least cytopenias of the radiopharmaceuticals
Samarium sm153 lexidronam		Induces significant cytopenias
strontium chloride 89		Induces significant cytopenias; contraindicated in hypercalcemic patients

Note: For NSAIDs and corticosteroids, see text and Tables 7.1 and 7.8.

TABLE 7.10 Topical and Oral Anesthetics

Drug	Preparation	Comments
ELA-Max	Cream (lidocaine 4%)	For procedure-related pain
EMLA	Cream (lidocaine 2.5% + prilocaine 2.5%)	For procedure-related pain; may help in post-herpetic neuralgia
Lidocaine	Ointment (5%, 10%), gel (5%), patch (5%)	Post-herpetic neuralgia; peripheral sensory neuropathy
Capsaicin	Cream (0.025%, 0.075%)	Bone pain; post-herpetic neuralgia; avoid heat to areas where cream is used
Mexiletine (Mexitil)	Pill	Initial dose: 150 mg q.d.; do not exceed 300 mg t.i.d.

TABLE 7.11 Pain Behaviors in Elderly Patients Who Are Cognitively Impaired

Facial expressions
Slight frown; sad, frightened face
Grimacing, wrinkled forehead, closed or tightened eyes
Any distorted expression
Rapid blinking

Verbalizations, vocalizations
Sighing, moaning, groaning
Grunting, chanting, calling out
Noisy breathing
Asking for help
Verbally abusive

Body movements
Rigid, tense body posture, guarding
Fidgeting
Increased pacing, rocking
Restricted movement
Gait or mobility changes

Changes in interpersonal reactions
Aggressive, combative, resisting care
Decreased social interactions
Socially inappropriate, disruptive
Withdrawn

Changes in activity patterns or routines
Refusing food, appetite changes
Increase in rest periods
Sleep, rest pattern changes
Sudden cessation of common routines
Increased wandering

Mental status changes
Crying or tears
Increased confusion
Irritability or distress

Source: Table 3 in AGS Panel on Persistent Pain in Older Persons, "The Management of Persistent Pain in Older Persons," *Journal of the American Geriatrics Society* 50:S205–S224, 2002. Blackwell Publishers; reprinted with permission.

Note: Some patients demonstrate little or no specific behavior associated with severe pain.

TABLE 7.12 Agents to Be Used with Caution / Avoided in Renal Failure

Use with Caution

Antidepressants	Amitriptyline, citalopram, nortriptyline
Antiemetics	Domperidone, haloperidol, levomepromazine, metoclopramide, promethazine hydrochloride
Antiepileptics	Clonazepam, gabapentin, levetiracetam, oxcarbazepine, pregabalin
Antipsychotics	Haloperidol, quetiapine
Benzodiazepines	Clonazepam
Other	Loperamide, paracetamol, tizanidine

Avoid Using

Antidepressants	Duloxetine, mirtazapine, venlafaxine
Antiepileptics	Phenobarbital, phenytoin
Antipsychotics	Risperidone
Benzodiazepines	Diazepam
Opioids	Codeine, hydromorphone, morphine, oxycodone, oxymorphone
Other	Baclofen, pamidronate, zoledronic acid

Source: Wilcock et al. 2017.

Note: Renal failure defined as Cr Cl < 10 ml/min/1.73m^2.

TABLE 7.13 Agents to Be Used with Caution / Avoided in Hepatic Failure

Use with Caution

Pain Medication	Acetaminophen
Opioids	Buprenorphine, fentanyl, diamorphine, morphine
Antidepressants	Amitriptyline, citalopram, mirtazapine
Antiemetics	Metoclopramide, ondansetron
Antiepileptics	Oxcarbazepine
Benzodiazepines	Lorazepam
Antipsychotics	Olanzapine, quetiapine, risperidone
Other	Baclofen, dexamethasone, glycopyrrolate, lansoprazole, octreotide, omeprazole, scopolamine, spironolactone

Avoid Using

Pain medication	NSAIDs
Opioids	Codeine, hydromorphone, oxycodone, tramadol
Antidepressants	Duloxetine, sertraline, venlafaxine
Antiemetics	Haloperidol, prochlorperazine
Antiepileptics	Carbamazepine, phenobarbital, phenytoin, valproate
Antipsychotics	Haloperidol
Benzodiazepines	Clonazepam, diazepam, temazepam
Other	Loperamide, tizanidine

Source: Wilcock et al. 2019. Text includes detailed discussion of nuances in use of agents in various types of severe hepatic impairment.

CHAPTER 8

Nonpharmacologic Strategies in Palliative Care

Although integrative oncology and complementary and alternative medicine (CAM) techniques do not replace drug therapies, many of them are valuable adjuncts. Whenever possible, they should be incorporated into plans to relieve patient distress. These techniques, though generally low tech, involve skilled practitioners: acupuncturists; yoga, Reiki, qi gong, and tai chi teachers; physiatrists skilled in rehabilitation and exercise therapies; therapists trained in massage or in physical, occupational, or speech and language therapy; and social workers, psychiatrists, and psychologists with expertise in cognitive therapies such as mindfulness and hypnosis, as well as music and art therapists. Other useful therapies include psychological counseling for anxiety and depression (discussed in Chapter 9), and spiritual counseling (discussed in Chapter 2). Because many of the techniques can be performed by properly trained laypersons, the practitioner often serves as both therapist and teacher, instructing patients or family members in how they can perform techniques by themselves.

CAM is used by up to 80 percent of cancer patients (Latte-Naor and Mao 2019), but you may be unaware of your patient's use of CAM because only 14 percent of patients using them tell their providers (Latte-Naor and Mao, 2019). The reasons include the patients' worries that the oncologist will disapprove, their feelings that CAM use isn't relevant to their care, or simply that their oncologist didn't ask (Davis et al. 2012).

Patients who do tell their oncologists are more satisfied with their physicians (Frenkel and Cohen 2014). Clinicians who select appropriate integrative CAM therapies as adjuncts, therefore, can open an important line of communication with patients who are either using or considering using these treatments. At a minimum, your patients will be much more likely to tell you which of these CAM agents or practices they have adopted.

The National Center for Complementary and Alternative Medicine has defined five domains of CAM therapies: (1) alternative medical systems, (2) manipulative and body-based methods, (3) mind-body interventions, (4) biologically based therapies, and (5) energy therapies. Alternative medical systems include philosophies and practices that are completely independent of the usual, *allopathic* medical approach. Homeopathic, naturopathic, Ayurvedic, and Native American medicine are examples of *alternative medical systems. Manipulative and body-based* methods include chiropractic, osteopathy, massage and vibration, position and exercise, qi gong, tai chi, and transcutaneous electrical nerve stimulation (TENS). Among the *mind-body* interventions are education, cognitive and behavioral interventions, hypnosis, mindfulness and mindfulness-based relaxation therapy, and art and music therapy. *Biologically based* treatments include special diets, such as the macrobiotic, Atkins or Ornish diets; herbal treatments; megadose vitamin therapy; or use of particular substances not proved effective by conventional medical studies, such as laetrile. *Energy therapies* focus on energy fields within the body (biofield therapies) or outside the body (electromagnetic fields). Therapeutic Touch, Reiki, and healing touch are examples of these therapies. The American Society of Clinical Oncology (ASCO) 2016 practice guideline, "Management of Chronic Pain in Survivors of Adult Cancers," included only (1) physical medicine and rehabilitation, (2) integrative therapies (including acupuncture, massage, and music therapy), (3) interventional therapies, (4) psychological approaches, and (5) neurostimulatory therapies, but ASCO did not find evidence to support recommending one approach over another (Paice et al. 2016).

In this chapter, I review a selected group of integrative and CAM techniques that have the most evidence supporting their effectiveness in relieving pain and other sources of distress in cancer patients: alternative medical systems (acupuncture, acupressure, and yoga), manipulative and body-based methods, speech and language therapy, and mind-body interventions. Readers interested in a more comprehensive discussion of the domains not reviewed here can refer to the work of Dr. Barrie Cassileth (2011).

ALTERNATIVE MEDICAL SYSTEMS

Alternative medical systems embrace a theory of strengthening what promotes health of the mind, body, and spirit; diminishing what causes illness; and addressing how health and balance can be regained, which differs from that of standard medical practice. The oldest of these, traditional Chinese medicine (TCM) has been used for centuries. A comprehensive discussion of TCM is beyond the scope of this book, though I review studies of one its components, acupuncture. If you are interested in a recent review describing the evidence for the efficacy of TCM in treating cancer symptoms, please consult Smith and Bauer-Wu (2012).

Acupuncture, Acupressure, and Auriculotherapy

Acupuncture is part of classic Chinese medicine in which, as described by Helms (1999, 2020),*

> The language . . . reflects nature and agrarian village metaphors and describes a philosophy of man functioning harmoniously within an orderly universe. The models of health, disease, and treatment are presented in terms of patients' harmony or disharmony within this larger order, and involve their responses to external extremes of wind, heat, damp, dryness, and cold, as well as to internal extremes of anger, excitement, worry, sadness, and fear. Illnesses likewise are described and defined poetically, by divisions of the yin and yang polar opposites (interior or exterior, cold or hot, deficient or excessive), by descriptors attached to elemental qualities (wood, fire, earth, metal, and water), and by the functional influences traditionally associated with each of the internal organs.
>
> Acupuncture anatomy is a multilayered, interconnecting network of channels that establishes an interface between an individual's internal and external environments, permitting energy to move through the muscles and the various organs.

---

*From Joseph M. Helms, "An Overview of Medical Acupuncture," accessed May 24, 2020, http://www.medicalacupuncture.org, modified from Helms 1999; used with permission from Dr. Helms.

In acupuncture, needles are inserted beneath the skin and manipulated to provide symptom relief. Practitioners use their knowledge of acupuncture meridian points, extra-meridian odd points, and new points to choose the appropriate areas of the skin to stimulate, either mechanically or electrically. Acupuncture alters the pain experiences of healthy volunteers tested in a variety of pain-inducing experiments (e.g., tooth pain). In general, from 14 to 40 minutes after stimulation, pain relief becomes apparent and often lasts for up to several days.

It is thought that pain relief through acupuncture requires peripheral nerve stimulation, because anesthetizing the skin into which the acupuncture needle is inserted abolishes the effect. The spinal cord is also involved in a segmental, bilateral fashion, as was demonstrated by experiments with patients who were hemiplegic or paraplegic.

The delay in the onset of pain relief after stimulation suggests that inhibitory signals descending from the central nervous system are mediating the pain relief. The patient's hypnotic susceptibility may also be a factor—those who are not at all susceptible to hypnosis do not get pain relief from acupuncture. Release of endogenous endorphins, metenkephalin, dynorphins, serotonin, and oxytocin may contribute as well (Filshie, White, and Cummings 2016).

It is difficult to comment on the efficacy of *real* versus *sham* acupuncture (in which the needles do not pierce the skin) because of the nature of the currently available studies. The existence of extra-meridian and new points makes choosing placebo sites difficult. In addition, there is no consensus on the ideal design for the sham intervention (Zhang et al. 2014). If a component of symptom relief may arise from a patient's susceptibility to hypnosis or the placebo effect, then this could account for improvements that may be seen in both sham and real arms of studies. This does not mean that acupuncture is ineffective, just that its efficacy has not yet been definitively demonstrated, and we may not fully understand the mechanisms by which it works.

Oncology acupuncture is now a specialty within acupuncture (Lu and Rosenthal 2018). The studies on acupuncture for cancer pain have had structural flaws, and the results are mixed. A *Cochrane Review* in 2015 (Paley et al. 2015) found the data insufficient for recommending it for cancer-related pain. Two other systematic reviews (Choi et al. 2012; Garcia et al. 2013) felt it could be recommended especially as an adjunct to analgesics. And the NCI conference on acupuncture recommended it for cancer pain (Zia et al. 2017). Acupuncture may have some efficacy in the chemotherapy-induced peripheral neuropathy (CIPN) caused by bortezomib (Han et al. 2017) or other agents (Bao et al. 2020; Wardley et al. 2020), in breast cancer survivors (Lu et al. 2020) with CIPN, in head and neck cancer survivors (Pfister et al. 2010), and in acute postoperative cancer patients (Lu and Rosenthal 2018).

Acupuncture is helpful for patients with several other symptoms. It is useful for patients with dyspnea from chronic obstructive pulmonary disease (von Trott,

Oei, and Ramsenthaler 2020), reduces treatment-related hot flashes (Smith and Bauer-Wu 2012; Zia et al. 2017), alleviates the dry mouth patients experience after being treated with radiation therapy for cancer of the head and neck (O'Sullivan and Higginson 2010), improves nausea and vomiting (Zia et al. 2017), and helps relieve cancer-related fatigue (Molassiotis et al. 2012; Zia et al. 2017). According to the American Academy of Medical Acupuncture, the World Health Organization lists acupuncture as effective for spasm of the esophagus and cardia, hiccups, constipation, and paralytic ileus.

Acupressure involves stimulating the same acupuncture points, but pressure is used instead of needles. Acupressure may have a role in pain relief (e.g., headache, backache) and in reducing nausea associated with pregnancy, motion sickness, or surgery, but the data are conflicting. Acupressure has been found helpful for acute chemotherapy-related nausea but not for delayed nausea or emesis (Smith and Bauer-Wu 2012; Lyman et al. 2018).

In one high-quality randomized controlled trial (RCT), *auriculotherapy* (electrical stimulation of the outer ear) was effective for cancer patients with a variety of chronic neuropathic pain syndromes (Alimi et al. 2003; Paley et al. 2015; Levy, Casler, and FitzGerald 2018).

Yoga

Yoga is a 5,000-year-old practice that was designed as "a comprehensive system of health and well-being for the mind, body and soul. The word is believed to derive from the Sanskrit root 'juy' meaning to bind, yoke, union, and/or to concentrate one's attention" (Lewis 2020, p. 719). Yoga therapy is a distinct profession, with certification through the International Association of Yoga Therapists (www.iayt.org). As part of a yoga therapy program, yoga therapists can provide clinical services to patients, as well as teach staff and family (Robinson, Walter, and Godsey 2019). Yoga therapy interventions can be done for patients in a chair or in bed. Therapies may include awareness practice, breath practice, movement of the head and neck, seated cat-cow, yoga nidra, and guided imagery (Robinson, Walter, and Godsey 2019).

Of the eight major branches of yoga, hatha yoga is the most often used in the medical context. The practice of hatha yoga has been shown to have significant effects in increasing strength and flexibility, normalizing heart rate and blood pressure as well as depth and pace of breathing, and increasing metabolic rate. It has been shown to improve the pain of patients with osteoarthritis and carpal tunnel syndrome. Breathing using yoga techniques substantially reduces the chemoreflex response to hypoxia so that patients with congestive heart failure can improve their exercise tolerance (Raub 2002). Rigorous trials have shown that yoga during cancer treatment can help patients enhance sleep, decrease fatigue, and experience less depression, distress, and anxiety (Danhauer et al. 2017; Lewis 2020).

The practice of hatha yoga is designed for newcomers and focuses on basic physical postures. A session usually includes an initial shavasana (relaxation), asanas (physical postures), pranayama (breathing exercises), chanting (working with sound), shavasana again, and meditation. Patients who are bedridden can practice yoga using specially modified asanas. In fact, the effects on anxiety, strength, flexibility, and breathing can help bedridden patients become sufficiently reconditioned to graduate to more vigorous physical therapy. Patients who are anxious about their medical procedures or the limitations, losses, and other changes induced by their disease or its treatment can benefit greatly from yoga training and practice. They can be taught how to regain control of situations that seem out of their control and to increase their self-esteem and endurance. The growth of virtual platforms like YouTube makes yoga instruction more accessible, including the wide availability of "classes" tailored to a variety of needs, illnesses, and physical limitations.

Yoga practice for practitioners and families has similar benefits, but a full discussion is beyond the scope of this chapter. Yoga instruction may be helpful in your efforts to "be present" to your patients' suffering, which is one of the hardest things anyone ever has to do. An experienced yoga practitioner can teach you and your team many ways to use your breath to steady yourselves before, during, or after difficult clinical encounters. You can also do certain yoga postures at your desk, or while waiting for an elevator, to help decrease stress and increase energy.

MANIPULATIVE AND BODY-BASED METHODS

Manipulative and body-based methods for relief of pain and other causes of distress include various cutaneous interventions, massage and vibration, transcutaneous nerve stimulation, and positioning and exercise (Cheville, Smith, and Basford 2018). All these therapies can be given in the patient's home by family members or by therapists. They, along with qi gong and tai chi, can add significantly to any pharmacology-based regimen.

Cutaneous Interventions

Cutaneous interventions are of particular value when the pain is localized, when muscle tension or guarding is apparent, or when the patient is waiting for a diagnostic procedure, for treatment, or for a pain medicine to take effect. Cold and warmth are routinely used in benign orthopedic and arthritic conditions. They are also very effective for cancer pain, especially that caused by bony metastases or nerve involvement.

Cold has been noted to be particularly helpful for patients suffering from skeletal muscle spasm induced by nerve injury. It interrupts the cycle of nerve ischemia caused by muscle spasms and decreases itching and hyperesthesia. Cold also seems to help patients with inflamed joints, possibly by creating numbness, and may also decrease the release of chemical mediators of pain.

Cold wraps, gel packs, ice bags, and menthol are common ways of delivering cold. Cold massage can be done by filling a small paper cup with water, freezing it, and then massaging the painful area with the ice that forms in the cup. The mechanism of pain relief induced by the ice massage is thought to be *hyperstimulation analgesia* or *counter-irritation*. According to this *gateway* theory of pain, a different stimulus can paradoxically relieve pain by bombarding the spinal relay system with inconsequential messages that block the transmission of the more severe pain signal. You may have experienced the effect of counter-irritation after getting an insect bite or stubbing your toe, if you rub your toe or, rather than scratch a bite, slap or scratch the skin an inch or so away from the bite. In most cases, the itch or pain disappears.

Patients usually tolerate cold well, but rarely, they may develop a hypersensitivity syndrome that clinically resembles cold urticaria. Cold should not be used for analgesia in patients with peripheral vascular disease or for the rare patient with cryoglobulinemia or cold agglutinin disease.

Dry or moist heat can be delivered using a heating pad, a tub full of water, a hot water bottle, plastic wrap, a handmade bag filled with rice, or a commercial hot wrap, which maximizes patient mobility. To avoid burning the skin, sessions should not last more than twenty minutes. Dry heat can also be created by topical capsaicin creams (0.025% to 0.075%) or 0.025% capsaicin adhesive patches, as described in Chapter 7. Patients should be cautioned against using a menthol product with heat because this, too, may cause the skin to burn.

Heat is contraindicated in areas where the patient is anesthetic and in areas with inadequate vascular supply, such as an extremity in a patient with atherosclerotic or diabetic vascular insufficiency (Cheville, Smith, and Basford 2018). Tissue necrosis can result from the increased metabolic demands in the heated area. Heat is also contraindicated for patients with bleeding disorders, which can be exacerbated by the increase in blood flow.

Cold and heat can be used to prevent the incident type of breakthrough pain. Some patients find alternating the two treatments to be soothing, while others find it most helpful to combine them with any of the imaging and relaxation techniques or the other cutaneous techniques summarized below.

Massage and Vibration

Massage slows heart and respiratory rates, lowers blood pressure, and even lessens pain and anxiety. It can also deliver a nonverbal message of affection and support.

Massage is specifically helpful for patients with muscle spasm resulting from tension or nerve injury. It is also generally useful for anxious patients, those who

---

Manipulative and Body-Based Methods

- Cutaneous interventions
- Massage and vibration
- Transcutaneous electrical nerve stimulation (TENS)
- Positioning and exercise
- Qi gong and tai chi

---

are limited in their ability to communicate, or those who can benefit from the closeness such touch can offer. Some patients, however, find it too personal or see it as an invitation to more intimacy than the person giving the massage intends.

Massage can include stroking, compression, percussion, or vibration and can be done with the hands, with ice, with vibration, with aromatherapy (Wilkinson et al. 2007), or with added heat (see below). Massage should not be offered to patients with coagulation abnormalities or thrombophlebitis, whom it might harm. Nurses, physical therapists, and massage therapists can all do massage and teach caregivers of bed-bound patients the basic techniques.

Vibration, either from the hands or from an electrically powered device, is also useful for pain relief. It facilitates muscle relaxation and, possibly by counter-irritation (i.e., stimulating large-diameter fibers), may also decrease sensation in the painful area. It is indicated for the same patients who can benefit from massage, but it can also help patients with neuropathic or phantom limb pain or substitute for the TENS machine (see below). A variety of devices are available, offering multiple settings and additional heat. The patient should work with the therapist to determine the optimal setting and duration of treatment.

In the absence of specific contraindications, massage can be recommended for nausea related to autologous bone marrow transplantation, anxiety, cancer-related fatigue, pain, and lymphedema (Wilkinson, Barnes, and Storey 2008; NCCN 2020a, 2020b). Aromatherapy with massage reduced anxiety and depression for the first two weeks after the intervention, in a randomized controlled trial (Wilkinson et al. 2007). Except for cancer pain, where meta-analysis supports the efficacy of massage therapy (Lee et al. 2015), evidence for efficacy of massage in each of the other areas comes from one or more small RCTs.

Transcutaneous Electrical Nerve Stimulation

Transcutaneous electrical nerve stimulation (TENS) has documented utility in several nonmalignant pain syndromes, but its effectiveness has not been demonstrated in patients with cancer pain (Hurlow et al. 2012; Cheville, Smith, and Basford 2018). TENS machines are portable battery-operated stimulators that activate the large-diameter fibers of peripheral nerves, thereby diminishing transmission of the pain signal.

The machines are attached to small electrodes that are placed on the skin over the nerve that is thought to be sending the pain signal, and a special current is then applied. When low-intensity, low-frequency current is applied, the patient's original pain is replaced by a feeling of numbness or pins and needles. If higher-intensity, low-frequency (acupuncture-like) current is applied, muscle contraction may occur.

TENS machines are especially helpful for patients with *dermatomal* pain, such as that of post-herpetic neuralgia, fractured ribs, diabetic neuropathy, or radiculopathy due to disk disease or spinal cord compression. There have also been reports of its utility in post-mastectomy pain and phantom limb pain. It may take as long as a week of use for the maximal pain relief to be achieved, and the relief provided by the TENS machine usually lasts no more than two or three months.

TENS units cannot be used for patients who have demand pacemakers, and electrodes cannot be placed over the eye, near the carotid sinus, or over metal implants (doing so may cause short circuits). TENS should be used with caution in patients who are emotionally disturbed or intellectually disabled, patients with dementia, or for those with lymphedema, which has been reported to worsen with the use of TENS. In routine use, the most common complication, occurring in 10 percent of patients, is allergic dermatitis from the tape used to secure the electrodes. If the conducting gel is used improperly, electrical skin burns can also occur.

Properly trained and experienced physiatrists and physical therapists are key to the successful use of TENS machines. They choose the appropriate stimulator and electrodes, place the electrodes on the skin, and pick the correct electrical wave form and intensity. They also educate the patient and the family about the procedures required, as well as the potential usefulness and limitations of the machines.

Because of the difficulty of treating patients with neuropathic pain, despite the relative paucity of studies using this machine, a novel therapy that is related mechanistically to TENS therapy is also worth discussing. It involves the use of the *Scrambler* device, which delivers weak electrical impulses, which are thought to stimulate the C fibers that may be involved in transmitting neuropathic pain. In a phase II randomized controlled two-part crossover trial of patients with chemotherapy-induced peripheral neuropathy, Scrambler therapy reduced pain significantly compared with TENS machines (Childs et al. 2021). Further studies of this technology are under way.

Positioning and Exercise / Physical and Occupational Therapy

NCCN and American Cancer Guidelines recommend at least 150 minutes of moderate-intensity exercise every week for patients with cancer, especially those receiving active therapies, to minimize fatigue and maximize self-esteem and quality of life (Latte-Naor and Mao 2019; NCCN 2020b).

For patients with bone metastases, thrombocytopenia, and other medical conditions that limit safe exercise, physiatrists and occupational therapists can create individualized exercise plans. These therapists are also familiar with the proper equipment for patients with limited mobility (beds, wheelchairs, shower- and bath-assisting devices, toilets, braces, orthotics), and they can teach positioning, range-of-motion exercises, energy-conservation techniques, and safe methods for transferring patients from beds to chairs. For patients with only one limb, the therapist can demonstrate how to dress, undress, and use assisting devices.

Positioning. Cancer patients with pain may lose the spontaneous pain-relieving movements that healthy people use to minimize tissue ischemia. To relieve their pain and minimize complications such as frozen joints, decubitus ulcers, or contractures, nurses, aides, therapists, or family members need to help patients change their position. The goal is to achieve a *loose-packed* position that minimizes stress on joints. Recommended joint flexion angles are 45 degrees at the elbow and 30 degrees at the hip, and the hip should also be abducted 20 degrees. This does not need to be exact, however; patients can be helped into any position that is comfortable for them.

Custom-made cushions or pillows for beds or chairs, as well as cradles to keep bedclothes off the legs, can be helpful (Cheville, Smith, and Basford 2018). Electric beds with specially designed mattresses that distribute the patient's weight uniformly are also important. For selected patients, the physical or occupational therapist may also recommend splints, orthotics, or support devices.

Dyspnea and discomfort in the chest due to excessive secretions can be ameliorated by a combination of chest physical therapy, teaching better coughing techniques, correctly positioning the patient, and teaching ways to relax the head, neck, shoulder girdle, and thorax.

Therapeutic exercise. Exercise plans carefully constructed by trained physical therapists can maximize patient mobility, minimize pain, and help patients function independently for as long as possible. Exercise is especially important for patients with limited joint motion due to pain, paraparesis, or paraplegia to prevent even more loss of function.

Therapeutic exercise is key for patients with muscle-related pain. It is effective for post-treatment shoulder pain in breast cancer patients and arthralgias from aromatase inhibitors, as well as for decreasing pain during chemotherapy (Cheville, Smith, and Basford 2018). The exercise can be done with or without assistance from a physical therapist, aide, or trained family member. Range-of-motion exercises can be done *for* the patient by one of these caregivers. In cancer survivors, exercise can improve not only physical function and body composition, but also psychological well-being and quality of life.

Contractures, deformities, and pressure sores are painful conditions that can often be prevented by exercise regimens. Canes, walkers, manual or electric wheelchairs, chairs in which the seat lifts the patient to a standing position, and other assistance devices should be used as needed to maintain as much mobility as possible.

Lymphedema in breast cancer patients was minimized by identifying and then screening patients periodically using the prospective surveillance model (PSM) (McLaughlin et al. 2020). Once a patient develops early lymphedema, as evidenced by as little as a 5 percent increase in arm volume or by bioimpedance analysis, compression garments should be prescribed by a lymphedema therapist, who will manage the patient. Severe lymphedema often responds to an aggressive daily regimen of massage, compression bandages, and exercise, after which the now smaller limb can be fitted with an elastic compression stocking or glove. Surgical interventions include lymphovenous bypass for early lymphedema and vascularized lymph node transplant or debulking procedures for patients with more advanced lymphedema (McLaughlin et al. 2020).

Qi Gong / Tai Chi

As Zeng, Xie, and Cheng state in their 2019 systematic review and meta-analysis,

> Qigong, often used to enhance vital energy or life force, balances a patient's spiritual, emotional, mental, and physical health, and aims to reduce fatigue, anxiety, and depressive symptoms. Qigong practices are used to increase the qi, circulate it, use it to cleanse and heal the body, store it, or emit qi to help heal others. Tai Chi is also a form of ancient and traditional Chinese medicine that integrates movement (physical postures), meditation (focused attention), and controlled breathing to achieve a state of mental calm and relaxation. Tai Chi aims to improve the health of cancer patients through increased mind-body awareness, and especially when incorporating Qigong practices can add a stronger meditative aspect to enhance physical and emotional balance. (p. 1)

In cancer survivors, both qi gong and tai chi have been shown to improve fatigue, insomnia, depression, and quality of life (Maindet et al. 2019). Patients whose cancer centers offer complementary and integrative therapy programs can learn these techniques from practitioners in those programs. Home instruction and information on where to find training is also available from the Tai Chi Foundation (https://taichifoundation.org) through their DVDs. Many videos are also available on the web. In the United States, there is no standard training or licensing for qi gong or tai chi instructors.

SPEECH AND LANGUAGE THERAPY

Speech-language pathologists can help patients regain the ability to communicate and enable some patients with swallowing difficulties to eat again (Chahda, Mathisen, and Carey 2017). They are key members of the teams caring for patients with head and neck cancer (Hansen et al. 2018) and those with cancer-induced vocal cord paralysis. Speech, language, and swallowing problems affect about a quarter of the patients enrolled in hospice programs (Jackson, Robbins, and Frankel 1996). It is important to refer patients early whenever problems can be expected. Patients with brain metastases, for example, who may develop cognitive decline, or patients who may lose their ability to speak postoperatively or following prolonged intubation for respiratory compromise can benefit from a therapist's training them in other communication techniques (e.g., using a communication board) well before they are actually impaired.

After initial assessment, the therapist monitors changes, provides exercises to enhance audibility and clarity of speech, and teaches ways to compensate for loss of speech. The therapist can also provide clarification and education to family members, helping them cope with the changes, anticipate what is ahead, and learn how to maximize their ability to connect with the patient. Such techniques can be key to including the patient in discussions about hopes, worries, and goals of care, including resuscitation options.

Speech-language pathologists are also called in to assess and provide therapeutic suggestions for patients with difficulty swallowing due to oral and pharyngeal dysfunction. They can assess aspiration risk and suggest safer postures or positions for eating or how the food consistency can be modified to diminish the chance of aspiration. Referrals are indicated as soon as the patient or family notices frequent choking or coughing after eating, or difficulty handling normal oral secretions.

MIND-BODY INTERVENTIONS

Pain and psychological distress are, ultimately, cognitive experiences. The neospinothalamic and paleospinothalamic pathways carry pain stimuli from the periphery to the thalamus, and from there the pain signal is transmitted to numerous cortical projections. When the cortex has been severely damaged (e.g., by prolonged hypoxia), there are reflex reactions to noxious stimuli but no experience of pain.

The cortex is also intimately involved in modifying the transmission of those ascending pain signals. It has extensive input into descending neural pathways that carry inhibitory messages via the dorsolateral funiculus to the dorsal horn entry zones in the spinal cord, where they inhibit transmission of an ascending pain stimulus. Thus, if we can change the way a patient views his disease or his pain, we may be able to lessen his suffering without eliminating the noxious stimulus (Loscalzo 1996). A meta-analysis of studies that investigated psychosocial interventions to decrease pain in cancer patients (e.g., educational interventions and training patients in new ways to think about their pain) confirmed their efficacy (Gorin et al. 2012). Mind-body therapies, especially meditation, hypnosis, suggestion, and cognitive behavioral therapy (CBT) were found to produce moderate improvements in pain in patients on opioid therapy (Garland et al. 2020).

Pain-CBT, one of the mind-body therapies, has been effective for patients with nonmalignant pain, but the data are mixed for cancer patients (Goodlev et al. 2019; Syrjala et al. 2014). CBT for insomnia is the first-line therapy for patients with insomnia, and cognitive techniques can also modify nausea and dyspnea. CALM (Managing Cancer and Living Meaningfully) is an intervention that reduces depressive symptoms in cancer patients, as do supportive-expressive therapy and psychotherapy (Syrjala et al. 2014; Rodin et al. 2018).

Mind-Body Interventions

- Education and reassurance
- Diversion of attention; virtual reality
- Relaxation and breathing
- Guided imagery
- Mindfulness meditation and mindfulness-based stress reduction
- Hypnosis
- Biofeedback/neurofeedback
- Music therapy
- Art therapy
- Counseling

Something as simple as a room with a view, in fact, has been shown to diminish postoperative suffering and decrease the number of days spent in the hospital (Ulrich 1984). Ulrich (1984) compared the experiences of cholecystectomy patients housed in rooms with two different types of views: a view of a brick wall or of a stand of trees. The rooms were otherwise identical. Those with the wall view did much worse than those with the tree view. They went home one day later, and nurses recorded four times as many negative comments about these patients (e.g., "upset and crying," "needs much encouragement"). In addition, during the second to fifth postoperative days, those with the wall view asked for significantly more analgesic doses, and the type of analgesic they took was most often an opioid. Those with the tree view most often took aspirin or acetaminophen.

What patients were looking at significantly affected their recovery. A tree view led to less pain and an earlier discharge. To produce the mental equivalent of a tree view for your cancer patients, consider referring your patients for any of the mind-body interventions described below. With these adjunctive techniques, you can sometimes eliminate several sources of distress not amenable to other therapies.

Education and Reassurance

A diagnosis of cancer carries the risk of transforming a *person* into a *patient*. Clinicians who are patients are at least at home in the hospital setting and are aware of the procedures they will have to undergo during their cancer staging and treatment. Though they still experience anxiety about their prognosis and the effects of the treatment, they are at least in familiar surroundings.

People who are not clinicians or other health care workers enter an alien environment when they become patients, and they have no idea what to expect. They do not know what tests will be ordered, or why, or what those tests will entail. Education and reassurance can be very helpful in ameliorating their anxiety.

Practice Points: Preparing Patients for Procedures

- Explain which tests are planned and why they are important.
- Describe what the procedure will be like, including elements from as many senses as possible (sight, smell, sound, feeling, taste).
- If surgery is planned, rehearse the major events the patient will experience while awake.
- Anticipate and correct common misunderstandings about test results.

When, for example, you send patients for their first CT scan, MRI, or echocardiogram, ask someone on your staff to explain the procedure to them. It is important to include as many senses as possible in the description: what the room will look and smell like, what temperature it will be, what noises the machines will make, who will be there, and what will happen during the procedure.

To describe a CT scan, the staff member might say something like,

> *You'll be in a hospital gown on a gurney, waiting outside in a cold hall, and then you'll be wheeled into an even colder room. You'll lie on a table under the CT scanner, and you'll have a small needle connected to plastic tubing in a vein in your arm. When they put the dye in the tubing, it will go into your bloodstream, and you're likely to feel very warm and maybe even flushed. Don't worry, that's normal and will pass. There will be plenty*

of people there to help you, so let them know if you have any questions.
You'll be awake the whole time.

As the patient listens to this thorough description, he has a chance to rehearse the procedure in his mind and raise any questions that occur to him. Later, as he actually goes through the procedure, he will become calmer and calmer as the predictions come true. Confident in his knowledge of what is coming next, he can relax.

Similarly, rehearsing a planned surgery is helpful. In one study, two groups of patients who were to have the same surgery were given either just the usual pre-anesthesia evaluation or a rehearsal of what was planned for the next day, including how much pain they should expect and how they could deal with it (Egbert et al. 1964). The patients in the group that received the rehearsal needed less anesthesia and less pain medicine after the operation, and they went home almost three days earlier than the patients in the other group.

In addition to rehearsing planned procedures, it is often useful to anticipate the possible findings and explain these to patients. If you don't, they are sure to come to their own, often incorrect, conclusions. Take, for example, a woman with newly diagnosed breast cancer who has to undergo staging tests.

The Importance of Dispelling Misconceptions

Except for extensive osteoarthritis, my aunt Ruth had been healthy all her life and rarely saw a physician outside the family setting (her brother, niece, and nephew were all doctors). When she was 75, she noticed a small breast lump, and it proved to be cancerous. When I called, she told me she was scheduled for bone and CT scans to help plan her therapy. She was understandably apprehensive, but I was able to reassure her that this was all routine and that, at her age, it was likely that the cancer was still localized.

Luckily, as we were talking, I remembered her osteoarthritis, and I imagined what that would look like on a bone scan. So I said to her,

Now, Auntie Ruth, I need to explain about your bone scan. The scan can't tell the difference between cancer and arthritis in a bone. It will be abnormal wherever you have a bone that is arthritic, and because you have so much arthritis, the scan is likely to light up like a Christmas tree. They will want to take an x-ray of everywhere that lights up. When that happens, remember what I told you and don't worry—it's not the cancer; it's your arthritis.

When I next called to see how she was doing, she said,

You know, it went just as you said it would. After the scan, they came in and told me I would have to have several x-rays. I was very upset because I was sure the cancer had spread everywhere. Then I remembered what you told me—that everywhere I have arthritis would be abnormal on the scan. So I calmed down right away and felt much better.

As it turned out, all the abnormalities were due to her arthritis; her other test results were also negative, and she never recurred after her local therapy. I was able to prevent her distress by anticipating both the results of the bone scan and her reaction to them and then educate and reassure her. She, in turn, was able to use what she had learned to deal with her initial fears.

Education can also lessen the intensity of pain, especially when a patient is misinterpreting its source. A patient of mine with lung cancer and liver metastases developed acute jaundice. He was usually rather stoic but now seemed extremely distressed, even between bouts of colicky pain. He told me that he was convinced that his jaundice meant that his disease had progressed and that he was dying. Not only was he relieved when I told him that the jaundice and colicky pain was due to an inflamed gallbladder, but his pain intensity dropped by a third and his distress by over a half, and he regained his usual coping skills.

Dr. Henry Beecher, an army surgeon in World War II, found that the degree of pain his patients reported and the amount of analgesia required to alleviate their pain correlated more with *the setting and significance* of the wound than with the extent of the injury. As an army surgeon, Dr. Beecher treated extensively wounded soldiers who had survived the assault on Anzio. He found that they requested minimal or no analgesia for their wounds (Beecher 1946). Later, in his civilian practice, he found that with injuries comparable to those sustained by the soldiers, his civilian patients required much more analgesia. For these civilians, the injuries meant disruption of their usual lives and routines, loss of income, and impaired functioning. For the soldiers, however, the injury had guaranteed a ticket home. The meaning of the pain had altered the intensity of the pain experience and changed the analgesic requirements (Beecher 1956).

Whenever possible, educate patients, even if they don't directly ask, to diminish their fear and thereby decrease the intensity of the distressing stimulus.

Diversion of Attention

Diversion of attention is particularly useful in decreasing the pain and distress of cancer patients undergoing diagnostic procedures. If, for example, a patient is scheduled to have a breast biopsy under local anesthesia, you might suggest that she take along her phone with headphones and listen to music or a book or lecture during the procedure. The surgeon and anesthetist usually don't mind, and the patient will be spared having to listen to the operating room chatter.

Patients should also be encouraged to find activities at home or in their community that engage their attention and therefore distract them from their pain. Music (either listening to or playing an instrument), television, the internet, movies, card playing, visitors, crafts, or interesting scenery can all be useful distractions.

Virtual Reality

Virtual reality headsets provide diversion of attention "on steroids." A systematic review of immersive virtual reality in burn patients found that it decreased the pain, anxiety, and stress of dressing changes, physical rehabilitation, and physiotherapy (Scapin et al. 2018), and it was also effective as a method of distraction in procedural pain (Indovina et al. 2018). It is likely, therefore, to be of help for patients with cancer who may have painful dressing changes and who undergo numerous painful procedures, especially patients with hematologic malignancies.

Studies are limited, but a meta-analysis of those few available reported its efficacy in reducing fatigue in patients with cancer, with a trend toward improvement in anxiety, depression, and pain (Zeng et al. 2019). Virtual reality is also helpful for patients receiving chemotherapy (Schneider and Hood 2007), hospice residents (Johnson et al. 2020), and terminal cancer patients (Niki et al. 2019). Other than motion sickness, no adverse effects have been reported.

Relaxation and Breathing

Sometimes, however, the pain is too insistent for diversion of attention to be effective, and a technique directed specifically at lowering the pain intensity is required. Relaxation and breathing techniques are designed to do just that. They can free muscles from tension so that they hurt less. Stress decreases, and patients become more relaxed; they experience less pain and are better able to cope with any residual pain.

For patients with low levels of pain or stress, relaxation alone may be effective. For those with more intense pain, who usually require pharmacologic therapy, relaxation therapies can be effective adjuvants. The best studied of these techniques are breathing modification and progressive muscle relaxation.

You are probably most familiar with the use of breathing techniques to control the pain of childbirth (e.g., the Lamaze method), but they are also effective for patients experiencing other types of pain (see the sample relaxation exercise below). Progressive muscle relaxation can be used by most patients, but because of the need to tense certain muscles before they are relaxed, it should be avoided in the minority whose lesions make the muscle-tensing maneuvers too painful.

Relaxation alone (i.e., without systematic tensing followed by relaxation) is often a component of a hypnotic trance induction (see below) but can also be helpful in itself. The trained therapist or a trained family member helps the patient learn a sequence of muscle relaxation exercises, or a sequence of muscle tensing that is followed by muscle relaxing. There are various regimens, each prescribing a different number of sessions each day. Each session can last from five to twenty minutes and can be repeated up to three times a day.

When the sequence is complete, usually the muscle tension has diminished markedly, and the patient is much more comfortable. The patient's blood pressure, pulse, and respiratory rate decrease; peripheral vasodilatation and concentration increase. During the exercise, the patients are very still, remaining in the same position unless given permission to move "if needed" by the therapist; they are silent and seem oblivious to external surroundings (this is also what a person in a hypnotic trance looks like).

In short, they look relaxed, and their vital signs confirm that they are. And in this relaxed state, patients are more susceptible to suggestions made by the therapist about how to control their symptoms and how to feel better about themselves. The patients themselves report that, indeed, they feel much better in several ways: they feel more in control, sleep better, are less nauseated, eat and drink more, and experience less pain and less anxiety. Comparable patients receiving the same psychological supportive therapy but not taught these techniques do not experience these benefits.

Sample relaxation exercise. For each patient interested in learning progressive relaxation, I improvise a custom-made script. Each script includes breathing modification, progressive relaxation, imagery, and suggestions that build self-esteem. If I have taught the patient to use images to decrease pain (see "Hypnosis," below), I incorporate these into the script as well.

To create the most evocative imagery, I try to determine whether the patient has an aural, visual, or kinesthetic imagination. I also take a thorough travel history, noting which sites she liked and which she would rather avoid, and I record any allergies, fears, and phobias. I would not want to ask someone who cannot swim to imagine she is sailing or suggest to someone who is allergic to ragweed that she's walking in a field. That would hardly be conducive to relaxation!

Before I begin the relaxation exercise, I make sure the patient is comfortably positioned, in a quiet room with subdued lighting, if possible. Then I begin talking. Here is a sample script for a patient named Susan Harrison. In the script, CAPITAL letters indicate emphasis, not a louder voice, and the number of dots in each ellipsis indicates how long I pause before saying the next word. For example, . . . is a short pause, ... a longer one. I begin by directing her breathing, and then I time my words to her inhalations and exhalations:

> *Susan . . . I'd like you to close your eyes . . . that's right . . . Now take a deep breath in . . . . and out . . . . in . . . . and out . . . . .* [I am breathing at the same rate, to model the behavior for her, taking longer with the exhalations.] *And with each breath in . . . that's right . . . and out . . . . .* [talking more slowly now] *you can begin to feel more . . . . . and more . . . . . comfortable . . . If at any time you need to move . . . to make yourself EVEN . . . MORE . . . COMFORTABLE . . . you can do that . . . . . The only voice . . . you need to pay attention to . . . is mine . . . . . No other sounds . . . need disturb us . . . . . And with each breath in . . . and out . . . . . you're able to LET GO . . . of more . . . and more* [said on the inhale] . . . . . .

tension [said on the exhale] *... more ... and more ... of anything ... that might be on your mind ... letting it* [said on the inhale] *... all out* [said on the exhale, in a lower-pitched voice].

Now I begin the progressive muscle relaxation, using imagery.

Maybe ... you'll find yourself ... on a beach in the midmorning ..... or by a stream .... or a small lake ..... You are walking along ... at a comfortable pace ... or lying on a soft patch of ground ..... The sun ... is gently warming ... the back of your neck ..... your shoulders ..... all the way down ... your arms ..... to the tips of your fingers ..... feeling warm ... and COMFORTABLE ..... and the warmth ... is now spreading ... from the back of your neck ... ALL THE WAY DOWN [said in a lower voice] *your back ..... to the bottom of your spine ... down the back of your legs ... and the front ... to the tips of your toes ..... the muscles of your neck ... shoulders ... arms ... back ... and legs .... unwinding ..... like a braid unwinds in the water ..... more and more comfortable ..... more and more loose ... like a rag doll ..... free ..... and loose ..... and .... FINE ..... Notice the feel of the soft ... warm ... breeze against your skin ..... the smell of the air ..... the light ... as it comes through the trees ... or glints off the water ... the feel of the ground under you ..... and the wonderfully safe .... comfortable ... free ... feeling of this place ..... YOU'RE DOING VERY, VERY WELL.*

If I'm doing hypnosis work to diminish her pain, I begin that here; at the end of the work, I bring her back from this special place, gently.

And each time ... you sit ... or lie down comfortably at home ..... in a quiet ... dark ... private ... space ..... and practice ... closing your eyes ... breathing in ... and out ..... and then feeling the sun gently warm your muscles ... ALL THE WAY DOWN ..... unwinding them ... like a braid unwinds ... in the water ..... it will be easier ... and easier ... for you to get back here ... to your special place ... to this wonderful ... peaceful ... very relaxed ..... feeling ... This is something you can do for yourself ... YOU ARE VERY GOOD AT IT ... and it is very good for you ..... It is important that you take this time out of time for yourself ... whenever you need it ... And you can bring that feeling back with you ... as you gently return ... feeling very pleased ... with how VERY well ... you have done today ... and you will do again ... gently ... safely ... comfortably ... BACK [with the pitch and volume of my voice rising to the end of the sentence, as the signal for her to come back].

My patients and I both feel relaxed and refreshed after these sessions. Given the time it takes to describe the technique, take the history, and conduct the first relaxation experience, I usually reserve 30 minutes for this initial session. Subsequent sessions usually take only 15 minutes.

Relaxation exercises are easy for patients to practice at home. Each session can take as little as 5 to 10 minutes or can last 30 minutes or more—whatever the patient prefers. Many people ask me to record the session to play at home to help them practice the exercise. I ask them to be sure to let me know, after they use the recording, how I can improve it for them. They might, for example, have specific suggestions for a different special place they'd like me to describe during the session. A note on referring patients to specialists in relaxation techniques is included at the end of the discussion of hypnosis.

Guided Imagery

Guided imagery (GI) is a cognitive technique: "GI involves the generation or recall of different mental images, such as perception of objects or events, and can engage mechanisms used in cognition, memory, and emotional and motor control. The images are typically visualized within a state of relaxation, possibly with a specific outcome in mind (e.g., pain relief)" (Posadzki et al. 2012, p. 96). Both a 2011 systematic review of randomized trials of its effects on musculoskeletal pain (Posadzki and Ernst 2011) and a 2012 systematic review of randomized clinical trials of its effect in patients with non-musculoskeletal pain found few trials (<20), and most of these were poorly conducted. A majority of acceptable trials found guided imagery to be effective, while the minority found guided imagery to be no more effective than progressive relaxation, standard care, or no treatment. Given the paucity of trials and their nature, however, no definitive conclusions can be drawn about the use of guided imagery to alleviate pain.

Mindfulness Meditation and Mindfulness-Based Stress Reduction

The three general types of meditation are concentrative, contemplative, and mindfulness. Transcendental meditation and meditation in which the practitioner focuses on a word, mantra, or image are concentrative. Prayer is a type of contemplative meditation. Classic examples of mindfulness meditation are the Vipassana and Soto Zen traditions.

The patient practicing mindfulness meditation pays attention to everything that is going on "right here, right now," even if this includes painful or frightening physical sensations or emotions. The patient is encouraged to *observe* these feelings and thoughts as they arise during the meditation and to separate the sensations themselves from the emotions they are feeling *about* the sensations.

Such observation can often help the patient later reframe the *meanings* of the sensations so that they are less frightening or less able to provoke anxiety.

During a mindfulness meditation, if memories of past events and emotions, or visions of future events, arise, they can be noticed, and the patient then refocuses on the present. Through the concentration on present sensations and emotions, patients with cancer can learn to be still, to allow time to pass, to "watch" the pain or anxiety from afar, to be curious about it but separate from it. Medications take time to effect change; with mindfulness, patients can achieve emotional distance from a troubling turn of events, work towards acceptance, regain control of themselves, and make decisions more easily.

Dr. Jon Kabat-Zinn, who integrated mindfulness into his stress-reduction practice, has demonstrated in seven RCTs significant health benefits for persons who maintain a routine practice of mindfulness-based stress reduction. Medical and premedical students can also reduce their stress with routine mindfulness practice (Shapiro, Schwartz, and Bonner 1998).

In one exemplar mindfulness meditation program, participants learned four types of meditation: (1) body scan meditation, (2) sitting meditation, (3) walking meditation, and (4) loving-kindness meditation, along with hatha yoga postures (Carlson 2010). Patients were given CDs, downloaded recordings, or an app and were asked to practice these meditations in 45-minute sessions, 6 days a week. They also practiced different informal meditations each week, which involve being mindful during normal daily activities.

Patients who practice mindfulness meditation generally have less pain, anxiety, depression, and fatigue (Carlson et al. 2001). In a pilot study at the Dana-Farber Cancer Institute and Brigham and Women's Hospital, patients undergoing stem cell or bone marrow transplantation who practiced mindfulness meditation showed an immediate decrease in heart rate and pain, lowered anxiety, and increased feelings of control (Bauer-Wu et al. 2008). Mindfulness was shown to help obese patients with musculoskeletal pain, increase their self-compassion, decrease their tendency to *catastrophize* the pain sensation, and find ways to cope and function with the same degree of pain they previously could not manage (Wren et al. 2012); similar findings might be expected in cancer patients.

More recent data are almost exclusively from studies of patients with breast cancer undergoing active therapies or who are survivors. In a randomized study in breast cancer patients who did not have pain, patients who were trained in mindfulness-based stress reduction showed improved mood, anxiety, depression, anger, fatigue, and confusion; better emotional, physical, and social well-being, as well as well-being related to their roles; and fewer menopausal symptoms at the last time tested (three months after the training) compared with women who received only standard therapy (Hoffman et al. 2012). A 2017 meta-analysis confirmed that mindfulness-based stress reduction is safe and effective in decreasing anxiety and depression 6–12 months after the training (Haller et al. 2017). Mindfulness-based stress reduction has mixed effects for insomnia (Teoh et al. 2018) but has improved post-treatment pain in survivors and symptoms generally (Compen et al. 2018). Research in this area and in the benefits of mindfulness meditation is growing, and results of new studies may help define the role of mindfulness meditation for patients with cancer and their families.

An evidence-based review on the use of mindfulness meditation in oncology patients was written by a former colleague of mine, Mary Jane Ott, MN, MA, RNCS, a trained family therapist, Reiki master, and teacher of yoga and mindfulness-based stress reduction (Ott, Norris, and Bauer-Wu 2006). Mary Jane used to begin our palliative care team meetings with a meditation, often starting by bringing our attention to the fact that "we have arrived." She helped us focus on the present so that we could attend to the tasks before us, and as she ended, we would often hear her urge us to be "right here, right now." For each of us, those 2 to 5 minutes brought our scattered minds to the room in which we were gathered, and when we were done, we were refreshed and focused in a way that greatly enhanced the work we needed to do.

For those who want training in mindfulness, many courses are offered in person, through apps, and online, and Dr. Jon Kabat-Zinn has written many useful texts, some of which are available as DVDs. I have used a workbook with an accompanying CD as a guide through the introductory course (Stahl and Goldstein 2010). Internet-based mindfulness-based cognitive therapy has been found to be just as effective as face-to-face mindfulness training in improving mental health–related quality of life, mindfulness skills, and positive mental health, and in reducing fear of cancer recurrence and rumination compared with usual therapy (Compen et al. 2018).

Hypnosis

Relaxation therapy is helpful in itself, but it is also used by practitioners of hypnosis as an induction into the trance state. Hypnosis is an ancient and powerful technique that has numerous medical, dental, obstetric, dermatologic, and psychiatric uses. It is particularly effective in relief of pain and other symptoms in cancer patients, and can even decrease bleeding (as Rasputin knew well).

Aesculapius and his followers used hypnosis-like techniques, as did Franz Anton Mesmer. John Elliotson and James Esdaile, British surgeons familiar with Mesmer's work, also believed that the power of the mind could be used to fight pain. Esdaile (1850) performed thousands of operations in India with hypnosis as the only analgesia, with convincing results, though when he returned to England, he was ridiculed. James Braid, a Scottish contemporary of Esdaile, mislabeled the phenomenon *hypnosis*, meaning a sleeplike state, only to discover later that patients under hypnosis are not asleep.

In the second half of the nineteenth century, the French physicians Ambroise-Auguste Liébeault and Hippolyte-Marie Bernheim promoted hypnosis and introduced the concepts of suggestion and suggestibility. They considered hypnosis to be a function of normal behavior. Sigmund Freud studied with Bernheim, who was a noted neurologist, but when Freud found that he did not need trance for the work he was doing with his patients, he abandoned it.

As long ago as the 1950s, hypnosis was accredited as a safe, effective procedure in both the United States and England. During the last two decades, experienced practitioners have noted an increase in its use for habit control and for relief of pain of malignant and nonmalignant origin as well as other causes of distress.

Hypnosis is a set of techniques through which patients can be taught to regain control over situations in which which they have lost much control. They can minimize their suffering while waiting for pain or antiemetic medications to take effect and can minimize the amount of medication they need, along with the associated side effects. Appetite may be enhanced, and insomnia reduced. Patients often experience newly gained independence and power, which can help even bedridden patients achieve appreciation of their own capabilities and gain a heightened sense of self-control and self-respect.

If you are interested in being trained in hypnotic techniques, I recommend that you attend one of the monthly four-day training sessions held by the American Society of Clinical Hypnosis (www.asch.net). The society holds classes for beginning, intermediate, and advanced practitioners, and you will be able to use hypnosis as soon as you finish the initial training, though I encourage you to get additional training at the more advanced levels.

Definitions. Several terms have special meaning in a discussion of hypnosis. These include *trance, induction, self-hypnosis, heterohypnosis, suggestion, distraction, dissociation,* and *negative* and *positive hallucinations.* A hypnotic *trance* is a state of altered awareness in which communication between the patient and the hypnotist is facilitated. *Induction* is the method used to help attain the hypnotic state. The hypnotist does not induce a trance but assists the patient to experience one. If the trance is induced by the patient, it is called *self-hypnosis.* Trance induced by the hypnotist is called *heterohypnosis.* Frequently, a trancelike state is spontaneously induced by events of everyday life. An athlete who is "playing through the pain" can do so because he is in a trance; trance can also occur at the theater, as when a play is so engrossing that you discover, only when the lights go on, that the seats that were empty on both sides of you are now occupied.

A *suggestion* is an idea that is presented to a patient in a trance and is therefore accepted with a minimum of analysis, criticism, and resistance. *Distraction* is a diversion of attention. *Dissociation* means that the patient perceives that one part of the body or personality has been split from another, or that the body is in one location, but in some form, the person is elsewhere. A *negative hallucination* eliminates the perception of something that is objectively present. For example, if one

---

Practice Points: Using Hypnosis in Managing the Symptoms of Cancer Patients

- Hypnosis itself is not therapy, but therapy can take place while the patient is in a trance.
- Almost everyone can experience a useful trance.
- The more motivated patients are, the more they will benefit from work in a trance.
- Hypnosis helps patients suffering from insomnia, anxiety, feelings of helplessness, or feelings of loss of control.
- Patients modify the experience of distressing symptoms through imagery and metaphor.
- Patients with chronic, "meaningless" pain learn how to "put the pain away for now" and to experience only "today's" pain, not yesterday's or tomorrow's.

---

is in a trance, a loudly flapping window shade will not be heard if the suggestion is made not to hear it. *Positive hallucinations* induce the perception of something that is not objectively present. They can be auditory, visual, or tactile. It is not hard, for example, to induce an injured child to watch a favorite program on an imaginary television while his wound is being treated. Any or all of these modes may be helpful in blocking pain perception.

Misconceptions. Despite its medical utility, hypnosis is subject to numerous misconceptions. The prevalence of "hypnotists" in casino shows or on cruise ships turning people into chickens may account for some of these. Used for medical or dental purposes, however, hypnosis is not an entertainment but a therapeutic technique. Patients in trance are *not* asleep. Their eyes may be open, and they may be sitting comfortably or walking while in a trance. No one can be made to enter a trance unwillingly, and what occurs during the trance is entirely up to the subject. Nothing can be done that violates the individual's moral or ethical beliefs. People leave the trance state whenever they want to do so—the hypnotist cannot keep them there against their will.

Hypnosis itself is not therapy, but therapy can take place while the patient is in a trance. The hypnotist teaches the patient how to experience a state of trance and may give helpful suggestions while the person is in a trance. The hypnotic state itself facilitates the giving and receiving of suggestions relative to specific goals.

Hypnotic susceptibility. Almost everyone can experience a useful trance. Only 5 to 10 percent of the population cannot experience trance to any degree. About 10 percent of people are so adept that they can use suggestions made during a trance as their only anesthetic when they undergo surgery. Differences in degrees of suggestibility, which can be assessed, may affect what can be accomplished by hypnosis. For pain relief, however, results of controlled studies differ; some have found a correlation between degree of hypnotizability and pain relief achieved, and others have found no such correlation.

Clinically, the ability to benefit from a trance depends on the degree of the patient's motivation. The patient has to want to use trance to solve a problem, such as pain. In general, creative individuals with a good work history, many friends, good family relationships, and leisure activities, who are not severely depressed, tend to make the best subjects. Even depressed people can benefit, however, if they are well motivated.

Utility in cancer patients. Hypnosis has many uses for cancer patients. It can help treat nausea, vomiting, anorexia, sleeplessness, anxiety, and feelings of helplessness and loss of control. The *rehearsal technique* recommended above to decrease the anxiety of patients about to undergo various tests is particularly vivid for a patient in a trance and has special efficacy in helping patients deal with anticipated pain or discomfort prior to surgery, radiation, or chemotherapy.

In carefully controlled studies, hypnosis has also proved to be of significant benefit in relieving acute nonmalignant pain (e.g., dental), acute iatrogenic pain, and cancer pain. In these studies, patients who used hypnosis had significantly less pain than those who did not. More controversial, it seems, is whether hypnosis is more beneficial than other cognitive techniques that reduce pain. Most studies have shown equivalency, though in some areas, hypnosis was superior.

While in a hypnotic trance, patients can use images or metaphors to change the intensity of their pain or other symptoms. For example, you can ask the patient to visualize a car speedometer with a 0-to-100 scale. Ask her to move the indicator to the number that reflects the intensity of her distress. Next, suggest that she imagine the indicator moving to a higher number and ask if the symptom has also increased in intensity. It usually has. Then suggest that she move the indicator to a position lower than it was initially, and as she does, she will usually experience a lower intensity of the symptom. With appropriate suggestions, the diminished symptom intensity will persist when she comes out of the trance.

It is important to determine which images are likely to be most compelling for a given patient. The speedometer image will be useful for people who are mechanically inclined or who just like to drive. But it may not be helpful for someone with different interests. For those who are musical, you can use the image of the volume control on a radio. For visual people, you can suggest they use a rheostat to change the symptom intensity just as they do the intensity of light in a room. Visual people also find they can change the "color" of their symptom, from a hot, painful color such as red to a cooler, more comfortable one such as blue.

If a patient has chronic pain that is not serving as a danger signal, you can help him find an old trunk in the attic in which he can "put the pain" and "check on it" whenever he feels the need. He will still react to new pains or to changes in the existing pain, which he can report to you for evaluation. Children like to go to the deck of a spaceship and search for the colored wire and matching light switch that correspond to their pain. When they find them, they turn the switch—and the pain that came with it—to "off." You can create any number of metaphors and images once you know the patient's personality and his likes and dislikes.

You can also alter time subjectively, as you know if you've ever been to a boring lecture or an exciting sports event. Using hypnosis, you can prolong patients' pain-free periods and shorten the painful ones. And you can use patients' memories of other episodes of anesthesia, such as spinal anesthesia, to teach them to bring back that numbness to relieve their pain. They can also be taught to develop anesthesia in a glovelike distribution and to use that "anesthetized" hand to spread a feeling of numbness to painful body parts.

Distraction. Montaigne once wrote, "We feel one cut from the surgeon's scalpel more than ten blows of the sword in the heat of battle." Our peacetime warriors, the weekend football and basketball players, experience the same phenomenon— it is not until after the distraction of the game is gone that the bruises or even broken bones become apparent. Distraction, then, is a powerful modifier of the pain experience.

Without even realizing it, most of us use distraction when we need to do something that may make a patient uncomfortable. Performing a pelvic or rectal exam, for example, we engage our patient's attention by talking about something interesting. I have seen hematologists extract sternal bone marrow samples with no other anesthesia than the fascinating story they were telling—they were out the door before the patient even realized a needle had been stuck in his chest, marrow extracted, and a Band-Aid placed on the wound.

Distraction is much more powerful, however, when the patient is in a hypnotic trance. Trance is especially likely to be effective in the emergency room, when it is spontaneously induced by both the injury and the setting. You might have a patient with a serious limb laceration, for example. Using your voice and nonverbal cues, such as a hand on the shoulder, to help induce or simply deepen the trance, you can suggest that the patient imagine that the injured limb is covered with newly fallen snow, which is lightweight and cool. You can then suggest that the coolness and comfort are spreading throughout the injured limb. This image is likely to lessen the bleeding as well. While the wound is being closed, you can ask the patient to concentrate on guessing how many stitches it will take. Engrossed in that discussion, and in trance, she will often be distracted from the associated pain. This technique is especially effective with children.

Dissociation. Bedridden patients can often use dissociation during trance to escape from their pain. They can "go" to their favorite vacation spot and retrieve enjoyable experiences while in a trance, through self-hypnosis or heterohypnosis. The hypnosis practitioner doesn't even have to be there to help them; she can make them a recording on their phone or tablet filled with suggestions that enhance the patient's ability to dissociate.

Patients can also be taught during trance to dissociate a painful part of their body; they will then experience that body part as "not there" or "not theirs." The former is a negative hallucination; the latter is dissociation. A patient might, for example, dissociate the body part in anticipation of a painful procedure. Putting in an IV, for example, can be less painful if you make the suggestion that the arm is not really part of the body and that what happens to it doesn't need to affect how the patient feels.

You can further enhance patients' comfort during this procedure by helping them induce anesthesia in the arm. When they are in a trance, you might suggest that they use the cool sensation created by the alcohol swab to help them recall any previous feelings of numbness they've had, and then to extend the feeling of coolness in the arm to that numb feeling; when the needle enters the skin, they will feel it, but it won't hurt. When the procedure is completed, you must suggest that the sensation will return to normal; otherwise, the arm might stay numb for some time and not respond normally to a painful stimulus.

You can listen to sample hypnotic sessions for cancer patients with dyspnea, dysphagia, or pain at the Johns Hopkins University Press website (see the enhancements section at the back of the book for a link to the audio file).

Making a referral for relaxation therapy or hypnosis. While you can do a great deal with the techniques outlined above, some patients will benefit from more intensive work with someone fully trained in the use of hypnosis and relaxation techniques to relieve their symptoms. You may find, however, that patients resist such referrals. They may misinterpret your suggestion as implying that you don't really believe they are in distress, such as from pain. Or they may just be afraid of the techniques themselves. Preface the referral by saying something along the following lines:

> *The pain syndrome you are experiencing is a very complex one, but there are many effective treatments for it. Remember when you were first diagnosed with cancer, and I felt that you would benefit from both surgery and radiation treatments? That probably seemed reasonable to you. Well, I think we also need to use a number of different treatments to relieve your pain.*
>
> *In addition to taking the medications I will prescribe, I want you to learn some other techniques to lessen your pain. Two of these are hypnosis and relaxation therapy. People with the kind of pain you have can benefit a lot from these techniques. And since you won't need as much pain medicine, you'll have fewer side effects from it. Unfortunately, I am not really an expert in teaching relaxation techniques, but* [the psychologist, psychiatrist, social worker, nurse] *is and would be happy to teach them to you.* [The practitioner] *would also be happy to teach these skills to anyone in your family who is interested. Your work with* [her] *will be confidential, just as it is with me.*

> *You, your family,* [the practitioner], *and I will continue to work to-*
> *gether to try to decrease your pain, and I'd very much like to hear which*
> *treatments you are using and how they are working.*

Implicit in such an introduction is your belief that the patient is really in pain. You have also communicated your faith in the colleague you've recommended and in the techniques that person will suggest.

Biofeedback/Neurofeedback

Biofeedback, in its narrowest sense, is an electronic teaching aid that helps patients monitor certain physiological functions, such as muscle tension or skin temperature, and modify them. It has been found efficacious for patients with various nonmalignant conditions, including spasmodic torticollis, spasticity, or paresis resulting from cerebrovascular accidents and urinary or fecal incontinence, as well as for the elderly. It is also effective in mild hypertension and in some patients with migraine or tension headaches, but it is no more effective than other methods of relaxation for these conditions

Neurofeedback involves processing a person's EEG and feeding that information back to the patient in an auditory or a visual form to enable them to modify their own brain disorder. It has been used for patients with stroke, epilepsy, ADHD, migraine, insomnia, autism spectrum disorder, major depressive and anxiety disorders, substance use disorder, and psychoses (Hetkamp et al. 2019). There are no controlled studies, however, of the efficacy of either biofeedback or neurofeedback for patients with cancer pain, fatigue, depression, or insomnia (Hetkamp et al. 2019).

Music Therapy

Introduced into palliative care in the United States and in Canada in the 1970s by Lucanne Magill, Susan Munro, and Balfour Mount, music therapy involves the use of music by professionals who use music to form therapeutic relationships with patients who have physical, psychological, social, or spiritual distress (Magill 2001, 2010; O'Callaghan 2010). Music therapy can be done with individuals or groups in the outpatient, home, or hospital setting.

Music therapists are specially trained individuals who involve patients in reflective or active music making, as well as song writing. Reflective music exercises involve selecting pieces designed for relaxation or making personal playlists for the patient and then listening to this meaningful recorded music.

Music therapy is particularly useful in assisting patients with life review. It takes them back into memorable times of their life through the music that was associated with those times. Patients can also work with therapists to create music-related legacies. They can put music that has been meaningful to them into a playlist, rewrite the lyrics of familiar songs, or create new songs that reflect what they need to say. Observational studies indicate that patients, families, and staff have positive responses to this therapy, as long as they can choose the music or musical style. Not only were they able to remember good times, but also in many cases they felt "transported" to new, pleasant experiences (O'Callaghan 2010). A review of research issues in music therapy for adult cancer patients found many challenges in performing the research but also evidence of improvement in pain and other physical symptoms, psychological distress, and mood (Hanser 2006).

A *Cochrane Review* of music therapy for patients with cancer noted that while the quality of evidence was low overall, music therapy induced reductions in anxiety and improvements in depression, pain, and quality of life but had little effect on fatigue or physical functioning (Bradt et al. 2016). A later systematic review that included 40 studies, 31 of which included a control group (Gramaglia et al. 2019), also remarked on the poor quality of the studies but confirmed these findings. In most of the studies, patients were listening to rather than creating music, so-called receptive music therapy techniques. Overall, patients experienced decreases in pain, anxiety, and depression in 64 percent, 75 percent, and 69 percent of the studies, respectively, and improved quality of life in 54 percent of them. Women with breast cancer appeared to receive the most benefit. Reduction in anxiety was more pronounced when the therapy was delivered by a trained music therapist. Music interventions are also effective in decreasing the pain of adult ICU patients (Richard-Lalonde et al. 2020).

Even in the absence of formally trained music therapists, research supports a music medicine "intervention" (i.e., listening to music) to relieve patients' pain, anxiety, nausea, or vomiting (Olofsson and Fossum 2009; Yangöz and Özer 2019). Suzanne Hanser and her colleague Susan Mandel produced a useful handbook with accompanying CD that patients and families can use to manage their pain and stress (Hanser and Mandel 2010).

Practitioners of music thanatology use music to alleviate the distress of dying patients (Horrigan 2001). Therese Schroeder-Sheker is a harpist, singer, composer, clinician, and educator who founded the field of music thanatology thirty years ago, creating both the Chalice of Repose Project and the School of Music Thanatology at St. Patrick's Hospital and Health Sciences Center in Missoula, Montana. Training in music thanatology requires five semesters plus a one-year internship.

Schroeder-Sheker recommends a polyphonic instrument to "deliver prescriptive music": a piano, organ, lute, guitar, or harp, or a keyboard that simulates these instruments. She considers the harp to be "particularly effective" in this work. Instrumentalists position themselves on either side of the patient's bed; Schroeder-Sheker always uses two harpists for the vigils she conducts. Vigils can last for an hour or more.

Before and after each session, music thanatologists assess the patient's pulse rate and strength, pattern of breathing, temperature, and any indications in the face or movements of the body that suggest distress. The music is synchronized to the dying patient's heartbeat and respirations and can produce a profoundly calming, peaceful result. Breathing becomes deeper and easier, grimacing and muscle tremors resolve, and a deep sleep begins in patients who were unable to sleep before the session.

Art Therapy

Art therapy enables patients and families to use symbolic representations to express and explore their thoughts, hopes, and fears. Patients under active treatment, or bereaved family members (including children and adolescents), can participate. They create an art piece and then, with the help of the art therapist, reflect on its implications. Often the *process* is more important than the quality of the artwork. The making of the piece may enable the patient to express feelings that otherwise would be suppressed. Anger or frustration that cannot be directed at the physician or at God can manifest, for example, as pounding on clay; these emotions can be noted and then discussed with the art therapist. Hope, gratitude, and love can also be expressed in artistic creations when words do not come easily or do not suffice.

Art therapists are trained at a postgraduate level and certified. They can work in the outpatient setting or in homes, hospices, or hospitals. Art therapy is particularly helpful when patients or their families are having difficulty communicating verbally about their struggle with the illness and what it has meant for their lives, either because of language or cultural differences or because of unease with talking about such important issues. Physical, social, psychological, and spiritual struggles; concerns about body image; and lack of self-esteem are all areas that can be explored by art therapists. Studies supporting the benefits of art therapy suggest it can contribute to patients' sense of well-being (Reynolds, Nabors, and Quinlan 2000), global quality of life, and depression (Bozcuk et al. 2017), but more research is needed.

SUMMARY

The integrative oncology and CAM strategies for managing pain and other sources of suffering in cancer patients add an important dimension to the treatment plan. Acupuncture can be a significant adjunct to symptom management. Yoga practice brings together mind, body, and spirit, strengthening, refreshing, and energizing them all. Patients, their families, and the treatment team can benefit from yoga practice. Many of the manipulative and body-based methods for providing relief to patients can be performed by friends and family and can be a significant source of satisfaction for these caregivers. Working with a speech and language therapist, patients can enhance their ability to both communicate and eat. These approaches, along with art and music therapy, enhance the lives of patients with cancer. The practice of relaxation, of mindfulness meditation, or of hypnosis can offer a sense of control and hope, meaningfulness, and self-worth throughout the course of illness. The meditative techniques similarly can enhance the lives of their families and of the clinicians who care for them.

CHAPTER 9

Psychological Considerations

with Hermioni L. Amonoo, MD, MPP

INTRODUCTION

In 2003, the National Comprehensive Cancer Network (NCCN) first recognized the magnitude of the problem of psychological distress and issued guidelines for the evaluation and treatment of cancer-related distress. Panel members for the most recent version of the NCCN Distress Management Guidelines (NCCN 2021) included representatives from all the disciplines involved in the delivery of supportive psychosocial services and counseling in NCCN institutions, including medical and surgical oncology, nursing, social work, chaplaincy, psychiatry, psychology, and supportive care, along with a patient advocate.

The guidelines offer proposed standards of care, screening tools (including a distress "thermometer" and checklist of practical, family, emotional, spiritual/religious, and physical problems), assessment and treatment algorithms for patients suffering from dementia or psychological distress (delirium, mood disorder, adjustment disorder, anxiety disorder, substance use disorder, personality disorder), and indications for referral to psychiatric, social work, and pastoral services.

The 2021 guideline documented a surprisingly high cancer-related distress prevalence of 20 to 61 percent. Why so high? Patients may not want to share their distress with their clinicians, worrying that it may harm their relationship and affect the treatments they are offered. And clinicians are unlikely to have been trained in or have access to distress assessment tools. Even if they recognize the distress, they may not know which patients need treatment, which nonpharmacologic and pharmacologic treatments they can use safely, and when they need to refer the patient to a psychiatrist.

Some distress is part of normal coping with the illness and does not require treatment from the medical team. So, before we delve into different distress symptoms, we review psychological support and counseling, which can also be instrumental in helping patients manage the normal distress that accompanies managing a serious illness. In the remainder of the chapter, we discuss different distress symptoms, including adjustment reactions, existential distress, anxiety, depressive symptoms, personality traits, and delirium.

PSYCHOLOGICAL SUPPORT AND COUNSELING

The news of a cancer diagnosis is often accompanied by myriad emotional reactions, both positive and negative. Some of the common negative emotions include fear, guilt, shame, anxiety, dysphoria, and anger. Some of the common positive emotions include hope, optimism, gratitude, and determination. Your first encounter offers an excellent opportunity to explore your patient's emotions and can guide your choice of psychological supports. As you directly explore their psychological reactions to their cancer, patients may, for the first time, begin to process how they are feeling about having cancer and actually articulate this to a health care provider—exploration provides an opportunity to help patients start to make meaning of their emotional reactions to their cancer diagnosis and for treatment planning. Despite the limited time of your visit, you can start to build rapport and offer support.

How? Expand the scope of your history of the disease by asking questions that reveal not just how the cancer was found but also the emotional effects of the experience. The questions suggested by the *Serious Illness Communication Guide* (i.e., patients' hopes and worries) and by Faulkner and Maguire (1994), British experts in communicating with patients with cancer, are useful places to start.

Consider Joe Palermo, a 65-year-old man who has experienced symptoms of benign prostatic hypertrophy (BPH) for several years. Prostate specific antigen (PSA) levels were borderline during that time and were not elevated subsequently. On routine digital rectal exam, however, Joe's internist found a nodule that on biopsy proved to be cancer. Further studies indicated that the cancer had not spread beyond the prostate. Joe's internist referred him to Dr. Kew, the radiation oncologist, because Joe was interested in receiving radiation therapy rather than surgery.

> **Practice Points: Assessment of New Patient**
> - Medical history
> - Experiences seeking advice
> - Effects of treatment
> - Current state of the patient's disease and its effects
> - Current psychological state
> - Current mood state
> - Overall level of functioning
> - Other important life events
> - Nature of social support
>
> *(From Faulkner and Maguire 1994)*

In the course of a normal medical history, Dr. Kew would ask Joe how long he had had the symptoms of BPH, how troublesome they were, and when the nodule was discovered, and then would review the biopsy and staging studies with him. She would then explain the risks and benefits of the proposed radiation treatment.

This typical history, however, provides Dr. Kew with only the sketchiest view of Joe as a person who must cope with this new cancer diagnosis and plan of treatment. She knows nothing of Joe's emotional experiences in the context of his new cancer diagnosis: how is he feeling about the diagnosis and the staging procedures? What are his fears and hopes, such as about having sex or remaining continent? Does he need more intensive psychosocial support during the planned therapy?

To get to know the patient better, Faulkner and Maguire (1994) suggest the following to help explore these other areas.

Seeking advice. After the medical history, Dr. Kew should review with Joe his experiences seeking advice from physicians about his cancer. She might ask Joe whether he feels there were any delays in getting to the diagnosis (e.g., did he regret not having earlier studies done to evaluate his borderline PSA? Were they offered? Did he refuse them? How does he feel about refusing them?). Dr. Kew can also explore how Joe felt when his internist found the nodule, how he felt about the staging procedures, and what his concerns and hopes are now, as he anticipates the radiation treatment. What led him to the radiation therapist rather than back to the urologist who did the biopsy? Has anyone he knows ever gone through treatment for prostate cancer? What happened to them, and how does Joe feel about that?

Faulkner and Maguire suggest that, after the treatment begins, follow-up visits can be used to question more than just the physical side effects of the treatment. For example, Dr. Kew would normally question Joe about diarrhea, dysuria, skin changes, rectal pain, and fatigue, as well as do a complete review of systems. But in addition, consider how much more Dr. Kew will know if she also asks questions about other areas (Faulkner and Maguire 1994, pp. 36–42).

Effect of treatment. Typical questions to explore the effect of Joe's treatment would be (p. 36): *"How has the treatment been affecting you? What has the effect been on your day-to-day life? Has it had any effect on your ability to continue working, and to maintain your normal social life, hobbies and interests?"* Faulkner and Maguire also recommend asking questions that explore Joe's relationship with his partner (including their sexual relationship), his mood, and his ability to concentrate. Checking in on how the patient thinks things are going can help Dr. Kew dispel Joe's misconceptions and clarify the goals of the treatment.

Dr. Kew asks Joe and his wife, Bonnie, about how he is coping. Bonnie tells her that after three weeks of daily therapy, the reality of his cancer diagnosis has just begun to sink in, and she thinks he has been having a great deal of difficulty dealing with the feelings that have begun to emerge. Joe reports that he has developed insomnia and a poor appetite; he admits to feelings of hopelessness and helplessness, and he no longer looks forward to things he used to enjoy, like playing poker with his friends.

Current psychological state. What is wrong? Joe may have just begun to face the psychological hurdles presented to patients newly diagnosed with cancer (pp. 1–6):

1. Uncertainty about the future: Will I be cured? How do I plan if I don't know how much time I will have?

2. The search for meaning: How do I make sense of what I have done during my life? Did I leave a mark? Will I be remembered?

3. Loss of control: Is there anything I can do to increase my chance of cure? What if there isn't?

4. The need for openness: Who should I tell? What will they think?

5. The need for emotional support: I don't want to be a burden. Do I have enough support from my friends or my family?

6. The need for medical support: Can I count on my oncologist? My primary care physician? What if there's nothing more they can offer?

The distress associated with these questions can persist and transform to symptoms that meet criteria for full-blown psychiatric disorders. In fact, as we discuss later in this chapter, if they persist for more than six to eight weeks after the cancer diagnosis, they would represent an adjustment disorder with anxiety or a depressed mood or even a major depression. By including in her assessment the questions that can reveal psychological distress, Dr. Kew will be able to refer Joe for the psychological help he needs.

> ### Practice Points: Psychological Hurdles of the Newly Diagnosed Cancer Patient
>
> - Uncertainty about the future
> - The search for meaning
> - Loss of control
> - The need for openness
> - The need for emotional support
> - The need for medical support
>
> *(Adapted from Faulkner and Maguire 1994)*

Overall level of functioning; other important life events. Receiving radiation therapy for prostate cancer is, of course, likely to cause multiple physical discomforts that might seriously interfere with Joe's ability to lead a normal life. Joe began to need to defecate so frequently that he began to limit his trips away from home to places within two minutes of a restroom. A few weeks later, Bonnie says, he just stopped trying to leave home, giving up his poker group because he didn't want to explain to his friends why he wanted them to move the game permanently to his house. Bonnie is afraid that even if Joe is cured, the price he has paid will have been much too high. *"What use is living if it's going to be like this?"*

Dr. Kew discovered Joe and Bonnie's misunderstanding about the permanence of the treatment-related changes because she explored how Joe's work was going and whether he had been keeping up with social activities. She now can offer treatment for his symptoms and help them make plans for when the side effects are likely to abate. Joe is less likely to develop a serious depression if he believes that he will soon return to his normal life.

Faulkner and Maguire caution, however, that the changes people report in their moods may be unrelated to their treatments. The real cause may be an unrelated problem, such as losing a job, or the serious illness or death of a close friend or relative. By pursuing the etiology of what you perceive as a significant personality or mood change in your patients, you are likely to uncover the true cause of the distress.

Counseling

Psychological therapy. Social workers, psychologists, and psychiatrists are equipped with an array of cognitive and behavioral techniques that can help the patient and family lessen their distress. These clinicians can offer support and education and can help patients develop coping skills. They can help patients explore, make meaning, and lessen the effects of psychological distress (e.g., depression, anxiety, adjustment reactions).

Psychotherapy can be offered to the patient (either individually or in a group) or to caregivers, the family, or significant friends. Groups can be particularly helpful for cancer patients because of the well-established and studied benefits of social support from such groups. Those who have passed through one or another stage can share their successes with others now facing the same problems. By becoming teachers, patients and their families can increase their own sense of self-worth.

Patients and caregivers can benefit from counseling and psychotherapy to develop positive emotional experiences as well as build the skills to manage changes in lifestyle, function, and relationships that usually accompany cancer treatment and recovery. One does not need to show signs and symptoms of psychiatric disorders before these benefits of psychotherapy can be experienced. In addition to more traditional psychotherapy, guided imagery, hypnosis, meditation, relaxation, and other integrative techniques could also be beneficial in helping patients cope with their cancer treatment and recovery. We discuss these techniques in depth in Chapter 8.

Practice Points: The Role of Psychiatrists and Counselors in the Care of Cancer Patients

- Therapists provide psychological and emotional support and education about cancer and its treatment(s); they teach coping skills.
- Therapists facilitate communication of the patient's and family's concerns to and among health care providers.
- Therapists evaluate and address the psychological needs of the family.
- Therapists recognize and treat adjustment disorders, anxiety, depression, and delirium.

Support. Using a crisis intervention model, therapists can support cancer patients by providing emotional support and by being there for them throughout the disease process. Patients with cancer need continuity but instead usually see several specialists during the process of diagnosis and treatment—the general internist, radiologist, and medical, surgical, or radiation oncologist. The therapist can provide the needed continuity and, when necessary, can be the spokesperson for the family and patient if they are unable to explain their needs to their cancer treatment team.

Education. The therapist can also provide information about the disease and help the patient gain useful self-knowledge. Therapists who work with cancer patients are usually well-informed about the disease and its treatment, and patients may find it easier to ask them the questions they are reluctant to "bother" their oncologist with. Therapists can also help dispel misconceptions, such as those about taking pain medications, discussed in Chapter 7. They can clarify therapeutic goals and reinforce the legitimacy of reporting treatment-related side effects if they arise.

But therapists also anticipate the emotional and psychological stresses that patients are likely to face and can help them prepare by rediscovering coping strategies that have served them well in the past. Cancer is rarely the first major crisis a person has faced. The first may have been something as simple as passing an important examination or as complex as being in a front-line unit in combat. Therapists can help patients recall a crisis that they managed successfully and then, along with the patient, analyze the strategies that worked and decide how to apply the same techniques to the current crisis: being a cancer patient.

Skill development. The task of helping patients develop new skills also puts therapists in the role of teachers, as they instruct patients in relaxation and other cognitive coping techniques. The therapist can also teach patients another skill that is crucial to obtaining the best care during their illness: how to explain their needs to health care professionals.

Patients are unaccustomed to being assertive with physicians or nurses; but they may need to assert themselves if they are to retain their rights as people, even as they are being forced to take on the role of patient.

In hospital settings, common courtesy is often forgotten even when no medical emergency has supervened. There is no reason, for example, that a person must stop eating breakfast because it is convenient for a house officer or a phlebotomist to draw a blood sample at that moment. If the timing is important, the patient is owed both an explanation and an apology for the inconvenience.

There is also no need for a patient to suffer because she is afraid to tell the physician that the pain regimen isn't working. Therapists can help patients feel comfortable relinquishing this Good Patient role. Not only will the patient then be able to retain her sense of control and self-esteem even in the hospital setting, but she is much more likely to share all her concerns with us and frankly inform us if our symptom-oriented therapies are not working.

Treatment of related psychiatric disorders: anxiety and depression. Psychotherapy for anxiety and depression is effective; it can be combined with psychopharmacological agents and, in selected patients, can substitute for them. And counseling can help unravel complicated relationships that are causing distress to patients and their families. It is often difficult for patients and their families to realize that they would benefit from psychiatric or psychological help (Breitbart et al. 2015). They might misinterpret your offer of a referral as indicating that you think they are "crazy."

When I (*Janet Abrahm*) was still practicing oncology, I often needed to spend a little time explaining why I thought patients and families needed the referral and how, specifically, I expected the therapist to help them. The Abernathy family benefited significantly from the counseling they received.

The Benefits of Psychological Counseling

John and Mary Abernathy were the parents of Patricia, a 26-year-old woman with extensive, refractory sarcoma. Patricia required large doses of opioids along with adjuvants for her pain, but she felt that the pain was well controlled, and she enjoyed going to movies and sports events with friends as her energy level allowed. Over several months, despite satisfactory pain control, the hospice nurses noted a gradual change in Patricia, which I confirmed on a visit to her parents' home, where she lived.

Patricia looked very sad, was eating less, and told me that even when she felt up to it, she had no desire to see friends or go out with them as before. Her mother brought in a tray with her lunch, and after she left, Patricia dissolved in tears. She said she was feeling terribly guilty for being such a burden to her family, that she could not contribute a thing to the running of the household, and that she was just of no use to anyone. She did not want to end her life herself, but she didn't think it was really worth living anymore. She asked that I not tell her parents how she felt because that would just distress them further.

After I left her room, Patricia's parents also shared their concerns with me. They had noticed the change in their daughter but had ascribed it to "all the dope" I had prescribed for her pain. They didn't want to let Patricia know how upset they were about her changed condition, but they wanted something done to alleviate her distress.

Before leaving that day, I spoke with Patricia and her parents together about the differences in their perceptions and the communication difficulties they were having. I told everyone that I thought Patricia was depressed, that depression commonly affected patients whose cancer was as far advanced as Patricia's, but that I had every hope that the depression would respond to treatment. I suggested that in addition to individual therapy for Patricia, family therapy might help them understand each other's concerns and improve their ability to share them, and they agreed to try it.

The therapist later informed me that Patricia improved considerably, as did communication within her family. The therapist continued to provide support and counseling until Patricia's death, and she helped Patricia's parents cope with their bereavement.

If you're able to convince your patients and their families to accept this type of help, you will have opened the door to a complementary therapeutic experience for them. In their relationship with the therapist, they can ventilate and explore their feelings about the cancer without expressing any "unacceptable" doubts to you, to your staff, or to other family members.

With careful preparation, many patients will at least explore the possibility and accept the referral without feeling either betrayed or rejected by you. While you are focusing on the medical care, the social worker or other therapist can identify psychological or social problems that otherwise might never come to your attention and yet would be sources of distress for your patients and their families. And as part of a hospice team, therapists are often available 24 hours a day and can be helpful in emergencies.

Coping

Coping strategies entail the behaviors, actions, and thoughts patients use to manage stress. Cancer patients employ various coping mechanisms to manage their cancer and treatment. Our patients need coping mechanisms for various stressors, including managing the side effects from treatment, needing to make urgent decisions, and on many occasions managing uncertainties about life (Nipp et al. 2016).

Some coping mechanisms are more helpful than others. Helpful coping mechanisms include planning, acceptance, positive framing, and humor. Denial and self-blame are not so helpful. Research has shown that coping strategies such as acceptance positively correlate with patient's quality of life and mood, while strategies such as self-blame negatively correlate with these outcomes (Nipp et al. 2016).

A good understanding of patients' coping strategies can help clinicians provide better support for them. Coping can be difficult to assess, especially since many patients lack insight into their own coping strategies. One strategy a psychiatrist or psychologist might use to help patients describe their coping strategies is to administer a validated instrument such as the Brief COPE questionnaire, a 28-item self-report measure (Carver 1997). Oncology and palliative care clinicians can obtain collateral information, if possible, from family members and other clinicians who have known the patient for a long time, which can provide insights about how the patient has managed different stressors over time.

A patient's psychological resources, burden of ongoing active medical problems, and ability to discuss coping strategies all will affect whether the patient can use positive coping. Palliative care and oncology clinicians can foster helpful coping strategies by doing the following: (1) take an inventory of patients' strengths and help them find ways of channeling some of those strengths to their recovery; (2) assess the nature of patients' social support and explore with them how to make the support system more robust; (3) allow patients to share life stories, especially sentinel events that they consider successful, as a way to highlight their coping strengths; (4) validate patients' experiences and emotions about treatment, recovery, and uncertainties; and (5) consider consulting a mental health clinician in selected patients to ensure that patients do not have a comorbid psychiatric illness that is fueling unhelpful coping strategies.

> ### Practice Points: Fostering Positive Coping
>
> - Take an inventory of the patients' strengths and help them find ways of channeling some to their recovery.
> - Assess the nature of patients' social support and explore making the support system more robust.
> - Allow the patient to share life stories, especially sentinel events that the patient considers successful.
> - Validate patients' experiences and emotions about treatment, recovery, and uncertainties.
> - Consider whether there are underlying psychiatric illnesses that warrant a psychiatry referral.

ADJUSTMENT DISORDER

The normal adjustment to cancer and treatment varies among individuals. A person's coping style, defense mechanisms, and external resources such as social support can provide clues as to how a person will adjust to the stress of cancer and the distress of the cancer treatment cycle.

Evidence suggests that the maladaptive coping mechanisms discussed earlier in this chapter can cause emotional distress, especially for patients needing to manage a cancer diagnosis or undergo a prolonged course of treatment. Difficulty coping can also result in an *adjustment disorder*.

Adjustment disorders are characterized by more intense emotional or behavioral reactions to stressful or unexpected events than would normally be expected; and these reactions are so intense that they have a negative effect on the patient's overall function. Signs and symptoms of an adjustment disorder include anxiety, depressed mood, and insomnia, and the patient can manifest or experience them at any time during treatment or recovery.

Some patients will react immediately, and others will display a delayed reaction to any distress that they are having. That's what happened to Selina Basset, a patient I cared for when I (*Janet Abrahm*) still practiced oncology. When she heard the bad news, her response didn't occur while she was still with me in the office; it happened later, when she was at home. Her distress was difficult to diagnose, because her delayed response manifested as signs and symptoms that are also found with known metabolic or other complications of cancer.

Selina was then a 61-year-old corporate lawyer who visited her internist for unexplained weight loss and a cough she could not shake. Chest x-ray showed a mass near the right lung hilum, and she was referred to an interventional pulmonologist, who recommended a biopsy. Mrs. Basset requested a consultation with a medical oncologist before agreeing to the procedure, and I was able to see her later that same day.

After examining her, I reiterated her physicians' concern that the mass was likely to be cancerous and that it needed to be biopsied. She seemed to accept what I considered to be quite distressing news in a matter-of-fact way. She said she would agree to the procedure, and she called later to inform me that she was having routine blood work done and staging scans, and that they were scheduled for the following Thursday. She had important work pending that she did not want to postpone.

The following Tuesday, however, I received a call from her husband, concerned because his wife was acting strangely: *"Selina asks the same questions over and over and seems not to pay attention to the answers, and she isn't sleeping much. What do you think is the matter?"*

I first wondered whether she could be hypercalcemic or have brain metastases but dismissed hypercalcemia as unlikely. After all, as recently as four days before, other than the weight loss, she'd had no abnormal physical or laboratory findings. Also, her husband did not report any other symptoms or signs that would support brain metastases.

It was more likely that Mrs. Basset was experiencing an acute anxiety reaction or an adjustment reaction that was causing her agitation. If the hilar mass proved to be cancer, she would be suddenly transformed from an independent, healthy, successful career woman into a patient with a possibly *fatal* condition. Although she had not discussed this fear with me, her internist, or her husband, it may well have precipitated her psychological distress, which would explain the behavior her husband described.

Patients like Mrs. Basset may respond to an anxiolytic agent such as lorazepam (e.g., Ativan) in the short term, but if they have not coped well with bad news in the past or do not have other sources of psychological support, they often benefit from working with a psychotherapist or a psychiatrist.

Therapists have various important roles to play in helping patients and their families deal with the disease and its treatment. Therapists can also help a patient understand the cancer, its treatment, and the expected range of emotional and psychological responses. And they are often more aware than are patients, their families, or their friends of how effectively the oncology and palliative care teams can manage symptoms such as pain or nausea. They can convince patients that it is safe (and important) to reveal their symptoms to their clinicians so that they can relieve them.

Mrs. Basset benefited from the lorazepam and welcomed the referral to a psychologist. She was found to have stage IV small cell lung cancer. She told me that the therapist had been an important source of support and information as she struggled to decide whether, since her cancer was not curable, she should even undergo what was likely to be very toxic therapy. Mrs. Basset said she felt freer to share with him certain concerns, rather than "bother" me, her husband, or her friends with such things. *"My idea of appropriate talk during a mah jong game,"* she said, *"doesn't extend to discussing how my sex life would change on chemotherapy."*

EXISTENTIAL DISTRESS

The distress that accompanies a cancer diagnosis and treatment can transform into existential distress for some patients. The four key components of existential distress are meaninglessness, existential isolation/loneliness, lack of freedom or control, and fear of death. When existential distress is not addressed, it can exacerbate physical symptoms and overall distress resulting in preoccupation with stopping treatment or giving up completely on care.

Patients experiencing existential distress usually have a lot of questions, such as, Who am I? Do I have any reason to live? What will happen when I die? What is my reason for hope? As we discuss in Chapter 1, according to Dr. Eric Cassell, patients suffer when there is a threat to the intactness of their personhood and when they lack purpose. Patients suffer most when they do not have enough personal resources to cope with existential threats, and a cancer diagnosis is a good example of such a threat.

Symptoms of existential distress include depression and anxiety; the key is to distinguish existential distress from other psychological disorders. Judy Smith is a good example of a patient in existential distress who was misdiagnosed as having anxiety. Judy was a 35-year-old woman with metastatic breast cancer who was admitted to the hospital for nausea and vomiting. Over the course of her hospitalization, she was noted to be very anxious, and she frequently used her call button to ask for nursing staff. Palliative care was consulted to help with her symptom management.

During the palliative care clinician's visits with Judy, she frequently talked about her loss of self and her law career, which she had spent so much time working toward. She was afraid that metastasis to her brain would cause her to lose her mind. She worried for her 5-year-old daughter and what her daughter's life would be like after she died. She also expressed concern for how her family would cope without her.

Judy agreed that these thoughts about the future and her sense of self were driving her fear of being alone, her need to be with someone at all times; that was why she kept asking for a nurse to be in her room when her family was not around. She did not want any anxiolytics because she did not want to compromise her mental state or get drowsy.

So how can we bring comfort to a patient like Judy?

First, we need to recognize that she is having an existential crisis and identify it as such to other clinicians. Connecting with a patient as a human being, taking a narrative history (i.e., exploring why this patient's illness is stressful to her sense of self), and helping her enlist sources of resilience actively can be helpful ways of addressing existential distress. These therapeutic principles are grounded in existentialist traditions pioneered by Victor Frankl and Yalom's *meaning-centered* existential approach, Chochinov's dignity promoting therapy, acceptance and commitment therapy, and hope modules. If you are interested in learning more about any of these, please consult the references at the end of this chapter. Involving psychiatry to provide these therapies in the outpatient or inpatient setting can be helpful; they will determine whether the patient has not only existential distress, but also a psychiatric disorder. Working in collaboration with the spiritual care team can also be helpful for some patients in managing existential distress, as discussed more fully by Reverend Katie Rimer in Chapter 3.

In Judy's case, we affirmed that her concerns about loss of self were reasonable. After all, before her illness, she had functioned as a high-powered attorney; now she found herself in the role of a patient with metastatic brain disease. We encouraged her to share her strengths (e.g., assertiveness, resourcefulness, caring for her family and people around her), and we reflected back to her how she has continued to use these strengths in her current role. We used that reflection to remind her that many aspects of her authentic self were not completely lost to metastatic brain cancer and terminal illness.

Regarding her concerns about her daughter and family, we reminded Judy to let us know which milestones and aspects of her family's future she wanted to be present for. We suggested she could write or create audio or video recordings of special messages she would like her family to have after she was gone. Because she was naturally someone who loves to give and contribute to her family, she responded positively to those suggestions and felt empowered to create these messages for them.

Judy's newly focused energy and strength on what she could still do for her family reduced her sense of loneliness and idleness in the hospital. She found less need for nursing staff in her room because she had other ways of controlling her distress.

ANXIETY

Anxiety is prevalent in the cancer population. All patients need time to recover from the initial shock of a cancer diagnosis, but by six weeks, all but 15 to 30 percent will have recovered their psychological equilibrium and not have developed either an anxiety disorder (10 to 20 percent) or a major depression (5 to 10 percent). Even patients who have recovered may find that their overall distress symptoms increase during stressful conversations with the oncology team, such as discussions of prognosis and the treatments planned, or after treatment is completed. It is useful, therefore, to do routine, often monthly, surveillance screening for anxiety and depression. Patients at high risk for anxiety include younger patients, women, patients with a history of substance use disorder, and patients from lower socioeconomic strata (Stark et al. 2002).

Anxiety often peaks during the initial cancer therapy, but it can persist for as much as a year, even when the patient has had a curative procedure. Anxiety lessens during adjuvant chemotherapy but peaks again at the cessation of the therapy, falling gradually as the remission lengthens. If the cancer recurs, as the disease advances, the incidence of anxiety increases, and the incidence of major depression rises to between 23 and 58 percent. Anxiety disorders can negatively affect various health outcomes in the cancer population, including decreased quality of life (Stark et al. 2002), but even patients with advanced disease can often be treated effectively.

The differential diagnosis for anxiety is broad, including psychiatric disorders such as panic disorders, general anxiety disorders, phobias (Stark et al. 2002), substance use disorders, or delirium. It is also always important to rule out potential medical causes of anxiety, including thyroid, neurologic, pulmonary, and cardiac disease.

Patients' anxiety manifests in various ways. Some of the signs of anxiety are cognitive (e.g., difficulty concentrating, feeling on edge) while others are physical (e.g., sleep problems, fatigue, loss of appetite, headache, muscle tension). Some patients may experience uncontrolled worry, a sense of impending doom, motor tension, restlessness, autonomic hyperactivity (e.g., palpitations, sweating, dry mouth, tightness in the chest), nausea, vomiting, diarrhea, feeling on edge, difficulty concentrating or relaxing, insomnia, or irritability. Anxious people often feel out of control and helpless. Some patients may experience anxiety only before each chemotherapy treatment or before hearing results of follow-up scans. Others are chronically anxious. Their anxiety may exacerbate, but they are never anxiety-free.

Assessment of the anxious patient includes exploring what the patient thinks might be contributing to the anxiety, what makes it better, what makes it worse. Ask whether he uses alcohol or other drugs to ameliorate it. Don't stop the questioning until you feel fairly confident that you know what this patient is afraid of, or you know that you've gone as far as he'll allow in the questioning. Your inquiry may reveal, for example, painful memories of the suffering of a close family member or friend who had cancer many years ago, fears of disfigurement, needle phobias, or claustrophobia, all of which may respond to directed interventions.

Several validated instruments, such as the Generalized Anxiety Disorder screener (GAD-7), can also provide useful insights. For some patients who are not talkative or expressive of their emotions, validated instruments can start the conversation and help you identify an approach to treatment.

Finding one cause for a patient's anxiety should not stop you from listening for additional psychological or spiritual problems that also cause anxiety. Mrs. Hanrahan was such a patient.

Curiosity, Not Certainty

Mrs. Hanrahan was a 59-year-old woman with extensive metastatic lung cancer that had been increasingly resistant to therapy. She had worked for years as a superintendent of schools in a moderate-sized town and was married, with four children. We were asked to see her for shortness of breath and for the recent onset of episodes of rapid heartbeat that had occurred in the night during her summer vacation in Maine. She had practiced relaxation and yoga in the past but was unable to get her symptoms under control using these methods.

On initial questioning, we found that her dyspnea at rest was improved by increased oxygen but was still problematic with exercise. She was waking up at night with a sensation that her heart was pounding, and when that occurred, she increased the oxygen, to some effect. She also had these episodes during the daytime; they responded to lorazepam.

As we listened, we were thinking about how we could treat the dyspnea with more oxygen and the related anxiety with a different benzodiazepine, along with focused instruction to help her improve her use of yoga and relaxation techniques. But we suddenly realized that we really didn't know what had caused the anxiety. We had just assumed it was related to the pulmonary process. So we pursued the questioning a bit further.

Mrs. Hanrahan told us that during her vacation, she had decided to retire from her position and not return to school in the fall. She also said tearfully that several of her children were having a great deal of difficulty coping with her increasing debility.

As she talked and cried, with her husband comforting her, we realized how close we had come to missing the most important part of the story. She was suffering from so many new losses as well as existential distress—her position at work, her independence, her roles as mother and wife. Freed from the administrative burden of her job, she could focus considerable attention on her declining health and her powerlessness to help her family. Clearly these were important contributors to her anxiety, and we would need solutions other than oxygen, anxiolytics, and yoga if we were to have any chance to make it better.

As Mrs. Hanrahan explored with us these potential causes of her anxiety, we were able to help her identify the meaningful work that remained for her to do with her loved ones, her students, and her colleagues. She realized she now had new goals, purposes, and functions, and was able to reframe her roles, redefine her personhood, and begin to heal.

We knew that enrolling in a hospice program would be helpful for both her and her family (see Chapter 11), and she and her husband agreed. They understood that they would still see her oncologist, and if new, promising therapies appeared, he would let her know, and she could disenroll in the hospice program. She went home having made an appointment with her yoga instructor and with a liaison from her local hospice.

Evaluation of a *chronically* anxious patient usually requires referral to a psychiatrist. She will take a thorough psychiatric history, seeking evidence of generalized anxiety, depression, social phobia, panic disorders, obsessive-compulsive disorder, post-traumatic stress disorder, or other sources of trauma accumulated throughout the patient's life, especially those with life-limiting illnesses (Ganzel 2018). They will also look for contributing medical causes, including cardiovascular, endocrine, metabolic, neurologic, and respiratory conditions.

**Practice Points: Common Medical Conditions
Contributing to Anxiety**

- Cardiovascular: angina or infarction, arrhythmias, congestive heart failure, hypovolemia, pericardial tamponade
- Endocrine: hypercalcemia or hypocalcemia, hypothyroidism or hyperthyroidism
- Metabolic: hyperkalemia, hypoglycemia, hypoxia, hyponatremia, fever
- Neurologic: akathisia, encephalopathy, partial complex seizure disorder
- Respiratory: asthma, chronic obstructive pulmonary disease (COPD), pneumothorax, pulmonary edema, pulmonary embolism
- Medications: glucocorticoids, antiemetics that cause akathisia (e.g., Compazine, Reglan), bronchodilators and beta-adrenergic agonists, stimulants (methylphenidate), antidepressants (e.g., fluoxetine, which also causes akathisia), caffeine, "rebound" from ultra-short-acting benzodiazepines (e.g., Xanax)
- Withdrawal syndromes: alcohol, benzodiazepines, opioids, cannabis

(Adapted from Noyes and Hoehn-Saric 1998, 555)

Patients with anxiety respond to both nonpharmacologic and pharmacologic therapies. Relaxation, hypnosis, and behavioral training benefit patients with anxiety, and these are discussed in detail in Chapter 8. Although cognitive-behavioral therapy (CBT) has been found to be the most effective way to address anxiety and should be pursued with cancer patients who have the mental capacity and the time to engage in treatment, pharmacological therapies can work more quickly and are also able to address other physical symptoms that result from the cancer.

Pharmacologic therapies for anxiety (other than that associated with delirium) include benzodiazepines, antidepressants such as selective serotonin reuptake inhibitors (SSRIs), antihistamines (e.g., hydroxyzine), buspirone, and atypical antipsychotics (e.g., quetiapine [Seroquel] or olanzapine [Zyprexa]). Of the pharmacological agents, antidepressants offer the best longstanding and most efficacious way of managing anxiety. Since antidepressants may take 2 to 4 weeks to work, they should be seriously considered and initiated early in the treatment trajectory, especially for patients who have had longstanding and untreated anxiety.

Patients taking tamoxifen should avoid SSRIs known to inhibit CYP2D6, including fluoxetine, duloxetine, bupropion, and especially paroxetine (Juurlink 2016). Mirtazapine, venlafaxine/desvenlafaxine, or citalopram/escitalopram are better choices. A patient on irinotecan was reported to develop rhabdomyolysis on an SSRI (Richards et al. 2003).

Benzodiazepines offer a quicker option for treating patients with mild anxiety (Table 9.1). Lorazepam (Ativan) (0.5 mg to 1 mg p.o. or sublingual t.i.d., p.r.n.) is recommended for intermittent anxiety. Clonazepam (Klonopin) (0.25 to 0.5 mg p.o. b.i.d., with 0.5 to 1 mg at bedtime) can also be used for patients with chronic anxiety that is mild to moderate.

TABLE 9.1 Pharmacologic Treatment of Anxiety and Depression

Class/Drug	Dose	Comments
Anxiety		
Benzodiazepines		Consider initiating as PRNs and determine standing doses based on patient need and use
Lorazepam (Ativan)	0.5–2 mg q1–4h max 10 mg/24 hr	Tablets, sublingual tabs, and liquid available; tablets can be used p.r.
Clonazepam (Klonopin)	0.5–1 mg p.o.	Can be given h.s., or up to t.i.d.; tablets have been used p.r. Do not exceed 4 mg/24 hr.
Alprazolam (Xanax)	0.25–2 mg p.o. t.i.d.	Severe rebound effect; not recommended for chronic use
Diazepam (Valium)	5–10 mg p.r. h.s.	Useful for patients unable to take oral medication
Oxazepam (Serax)	15–30 mg p.o. h.s.	For insomnia from anxiety
Temazepam (Restoril)	7.5–30 mg p.o. h.s.	For insomnia from anxiety
Zolpidem (Ambien)	5–10 mg p.o. h.s.	For insomnia from anxiety
Akathisia		Discontinue metoclopramide, haloperidol, or other typical or atypical antipsychotic agents
Propranolol	40 mg p.o. t.i.d.	Metoprolol IV can also be used
Mirtazapine	7.5–15 mg p.o. daily	
Zolmitriptan	7.5 mg p.o. daily	
Depression		
Selective serotonin reuptake inhibitors (SSRIs)		
Citalopram (Celexa)	20–60 mg p.o. daily	May cause minimal sexual dysfunction Prolongs QTc at high doses
Escitalopram (Lexapro)	10–20 mg p.o. daily	May cause minimal sexual dysfunction Prolongs QTc at high doses
Sertraline (Zoloft)	50–200 mg p.o. daily	Likely to have drug-drug interactions

(continued)

TABLE 9.1 *(cont.)*

Class/Drug	Dose	Comments
Paroxetine (Paxil)	20–60 mg p.o. daily	Sedating; can be difficult to discontinue; very likely to have drug interactions
Fluoxetine (Prozac)	20–80 mg p.o. daily	Stimulating; causes anorexia; very likely to have drug interactions
Fluvoxamine (Luvox)	25–200 mg p.o. daily	Very likely to have drug interactions
Serotonin and norepinephrine reuptake inhibitors (SNRIs)		
Venlafaxine (Effexor)	75–225 mg p.o. daily	Used alone or added to SSRI; must be tapered off
Venlafaxine extended release (Effexor XR or Venlafaxine ER)	37.5–100 mg p.o. daily or b.i.d.	Used alone or added to SSRI; must be tapered off
Duloxetine	10–20 mg p.o. daily or b.i.d.; maximum 20–60 q.d. or b.i.d.	
Psychostimulants		May be used cautiously with another class of antidepressant (e.g., SSRI)
Methylphenidate (Ritalin)	5–60 mg p.o.	Divided doses (8 a.m., noon)
Dextroamphetamine (Dexedrine)	5–60 mg p.o.	Divided doses (8 a.m., noon)
Others		
Clorazepate (Tranxene)	15–60 mg/day p.o.	For anxiety from alcohol withdrawal
Mirtazapine (Remeron)	15–45 mg p.o. h.s.	At low doses also enhances appetite and decreases nausea
Bupropion (Wellbutrin)	100 mg p.o. daily; 450 mg p.o. in 4 divided doses	Activating; can be added to SSRI or SNRIs
Bupropion extended release (Wellbutrin XL)	150–300 mg p.o. daily	
Trazodone (Desyrel)	50–400 mg p.o. h.s.	Sedating; may prolong QTc
Tricyclic antidepressants		
Amitriptyline, doxepin, clomipramine, desipramine, nortriptyline	10–25 mg/day p.o. h.s.	Increase to therapeutic dose (50–150 mg in divided doses); very likely to have drug interactions; may prolong QTc.

In some patients, however, anxiety may unpredictably worsen in response to lorazepam. Benzodiazepines in general can also worsen delirium, to which many cancer patients are susceptible. Alprazolam (Xanax) (0.25 to 2.0 mg p.o. t.i.d. to q.i.d.) is rapidly effective but has a rebound effect that causes a return of the anxiety in a short period and should mostly be avoided unless a patient has been taking this medication for a long time prior to cancer diagnosis and treatment.

Oxazepam (Serax) (15 to 30 mg p.o. at bedtime), temazepam (Restoril) (7.5 to 30 mg p.o. at bedtime), or zolpidem (Ambien) (5 to 10 mg p.o. at bedtime) can be used to treat anxiety occurring at bedtime. Clorazepate (Tranxene) (15 to 60 mg/day p.o.) is used for anxiety and acute alcohol withdrawal.

It is also important to keep in mind that patients can become dependent on benzodiazepines, especially if their prognosis is longer than weeks to months. Dependency on benzodiazepines is common after long-term use, and the risks and benefits should be discussed openly with patients prior to initiating these medications. It is often helpful to assess patients' use and symptom relief from benzodiazepines to determine an appropriate timeline to taper off the medication.

The combination of benzodiazepines and opioid medications in patients who have cancer pain can also increase the risk for dependency and death and should be constantly reassessed. When patients require long-term use of benzodiazepines, and there is a history of or concern for substance use disorder, collaboration with an addiction psychiatrist or mental health clinician can be helpful in exploring the breadth of resources (both pharmacological and behavioral interventions) that are needed for the effective assessment and management of the patient.

If the anxiety is due to drug-induced akathisia, discontinue the agent (e.g., metoclopramide, haloperidol) and start a beta-blocker: oral propranolol (40 mg orally t.i.d.) or intravenous metoprolol at an equivalent dose (Avital et al. 2009). Zolmitriptan (7.5 mg p.o. daily), in a double-blind comparative study (Avital et al. 2009), and mirtazapine (15 mg p.o. daily), in a double-blind placebo- and propranolol-controlled trial (Poyurovsky et al. 2006), have also shown efficacy comparable to propranolol in reversing the akathisia, but patients in the Poyurovsky study were given the lower dose (only 40 to 80 mg) of propranolol daily.

Post-traumatic Stress Reactions or Disorder

Recently, serious illnesses such as cancer, and cancer treatment, have been identified as precipitators of post-traumatic stress reactions or disorder (PTSD). Cancer patients suffering from PTSD "relive" the cancer treatment and experience nightmares, flashbacks, or continuous thoughts about it. Untreated PTSD can lead to increased depressive symptoms and can lower the patient's quality of life. The prevalence of PTSD in cancer populations is high, and cancer patients are three times more likely to develop it than the general population (Chan et al. 2018). It is not uncommon for patients to be anxious only when they attend medical appointments, and the phenomenon of hypertension occurring only in that setting has been well described.

PTSD and childhood sexual abuse. Although PTSD symptoms in cancer patients are not age dependent, patients who have a prior history of abuse, especially of *childhood sexual abuse*, are more susceptible to post-traumatic stress reactions (Wygant, Hui, and Bruera 2011). The 2006 WHO definition of childhood sexual abuse is "the involvement of a child in sexual activity that he or she does not fully comprehend, is unable to give informed consent to, or for which the child is not developmentally prepared, or else that violates the laws or social taboos of society. Children can be sexually abused by both adults and other children who are, by virtue of their age or stage of development, in a position of responsibility, trust or power over the victim" (WHO and ISPCAN 2006, p. 10). The actual prevalence of childhood sexual abuse is unknown, but estimates are as high as one in three women and one in six men in the United States (Wygant, Hui, and Bruera 2011).

When a patient who has been abused has a diagnosis of cancer, even the physical examination can seem intensely intrusive, as can the testing involved, and the patient may have memories of the abuse or feel they are reexperiencing it. A history of childhood sexual abuse should be suspected in patients presenting with far-advanced cancers that are visible (such as breast cancers eroding the skin) as well as those who have a large number of unexplained symptoms; a substance use disorder or alcoholism history; difficulty managing anger, anxiety, panic attacks, or claustrophobia; difficulty trusting others; or problems getting along with numerous health care teams. A suggested screening question is: "Have you ever been touched in a manner that made you feel uncomfortable?" (Wygant, Hui, and Bruera 2011).

It is easy to see how someone with these concerns would be anxious at the time of physical examinations, or repeatedly miss appointments for staging examinations despite seeming to want to please the physician. A social worker or psychologist should, whenever possible, be part of the team caring for patients with suspected or confirmed childhood sexual abuse. Counseling, teaching self-comforting skills, and reinforcing that the patient is currently safe can help decrease anxiety.

DEPRESSIVE SYMPTOMS

Depressive symptoms are prevalent in the cancer population and are associated with several negative health outcomes. It can be difficult to discern which patients with advanced disease are depressed. Many of the usual somatic signs (e.g., anorexia, sleep disturbances, fatigue, or weight loss) are not helpful, because they may be due to the underlying illness. Depressed patients, however, will also feel sad, cry, be unable to get pleasure from any activity, or feel globally worthless, guilty, hopeless, or helpless.

The cancer type can affect the prevalence of depressive symptoms. They are found in 33 to 50 percent of patients with pancreatic cancer, 22 to 57 percent of patients with oropharyngeal cancer, 11 to 44 percent of those with lung cancer, and 1.5 to 46 percent of those with breast cancer (Massie 2004). Well-established validated instruments, such as the Patient Health Questionnaires (PHQ-2 and PHQ-9), can help you diagnose depression in your patients.

But you don't have to use a questionnaire. Terminally ill patients who responded "Yes" to the screening question "Are you depressed?" were likely to be confirmed as depressed in a more comprehensive evaluation. Useful follow-up

> **Practice Points: Signs of Depression in Cancer Patients**
>
> - Appearing depressed or describing a feeling of depression
> - Crying
> - Anhedonia, inability to get pleasure from any activity
> - Feelings of worthlessness, guilt, hopelessness, or helplessness
>
> *Note:* Anorexia, sleep disturbances, weight loss, and fatigue occur in many patients with cancer; these signs do not identify those who are depressed.

questions include: How do you see your future? What do you imagine is ahead for you with this illness? What aspects of your life do you feel most proud of? Most troubled by? Are you getting less enjoyment from your favorite things?

Depressive symptoms can also be manifestations of any number of medical, social, spiritual, or psychiatric disorders. Common metabolic and medication-related causes of depression in cancer patients include thyroid disease, hyponatremia, hypercalcemia, CNS tumor, high-dose interferon therapy, opioids, beta-blockers, and corticosteroids. Stress from financial or family concerns or from simple sleep deprivation are also often contributory. Like anxiety, the differential diagnosis for depressive symptoms is broad and can include a major depressive disorder, adjustment disorder with depressed mood, persistent depressive disorder (dysthymia), demoralization, bipolar disorder, or delirium. Collaborate with a psychiatrist to clarify the diagnosis when patients are not responding to trials of antidepressants.

As you consider psychopharmacology and psychotherapy treatments for depression, first optimize pain control, because uncontrolled pain is a major risk factor for depression and for suicide. Several pharmacological agents are often effective in alleviating depression, but antidepressants are the most efficacious long-term treatment. The first choice of antidepressant agent should be either one of the selective serotonin reuptake inhibitors (SSRIs), such as sertraline, citalopram, or escitalopram, or one of the serotonin and norepinephrine reuptake inhibitors (SNRIs), such as venlafaxine/desvenlafaxine and duloxetine.

Either an SSRI or an SNRI can be the first choice when immediate onset is not needed; either may take 4 to 6 weeks to show effect. Initial doses are usually small to minimize side effects, which are mostly gastrointestinal (because of the high number of serotonin receptors in the gastrointestinal tract). The starting dose (see below) is given for 3 to 7 days. The dose is then increased every week or every other week until the patient notices a benefit, or the maximum dose is reached. If the patient is very depressed, a stimulant (like methylphenidate) and an SSRI or an SNRI may be started simultaneously, and the stimulant can be titrated off

4 weeks later. Of note, however, stimulants should be used with caution. They can increase the risk of psychosis, especially in cancer patients who have a high risk for delirium due to other medications or ongoing medical problems.

Patients taking tamoxifen should avoid SSRIs known to inhibit CYP2D6, including fluoxetine, duloxetine, bupropion, and especially paroxetine (Juurlink 2016). Mirtazapine, venlafaxine/desvenlafaxine, or citalopram/escitalopram are better choices. Patients on irinotecan have been reported to develop rhabdomyolysis on an SSRI (Richards et al. 2003).

The SSRIs and SNRIs can be directly substituted for one another without cross-tapering (Howard et al. 2012), but they should not be stopped suddenly; they should be tapered if they are to be discontinued. If a patient develops a bowel obstruction or mucositis or for some other reason is unable to take oral medications, and you have not had the opportunity to taper the antidepressant, your patient may complain of *discontinuation syndrome*, characterized by insomnia with vivid dreams, nausea, ataxia, paresthesias, and anxiety or agitation. You may need to use a lorazepam taper to treat the anxiety that is likely to occur within days if the patient is on paroxetine (Howard et al. 2012), or up to a week later if the patient was taking one of the other agents.

Suggested Initial and Maximal Doses for SSRIs

- Citalopram (Celexa): 10 mg/day orally for the first week. If no response, increase by 10 mg weekly to the maximum dose of 60 mg/day. Doses greater than 40 mg of citalopram have been associated with a prolonged QTc, so if the higher doses are needed, check an EKG and minimize other drugs that prolong the QTc (e.g., levofloxacin, metoclopramide, methadone).

- Escitalopram (Lexapro): 5 mg/day orally for the first week, then increase to the maximum dose of 20 mg/day. High doses of escitalopram have been associated with a prolonged QTc, so if the higher doses are needed, check an EKG and minimize other drugs that prolong the QTc (e.g., levofloxacin, metoclopramide, methadone).

- Fluoxetine (Prozac): 5 to 10 mg/day orally for the first week; increase by 10 mg every 2 weeks to the maximum dose of 80 mg/day, as it has a long half-life.

- Fluvoxamine (Luvox): 25 mg at bedtime for the first week; increase to the maximum dose of 200 mg/day as needed.

- Sertraline (Zoloft): 12.5 to 25 mg/day in the morning for the first week, then increase to 50 mg for an additional week. It is important to note that the minimum therapeutic dose of sertraline is 50 mg. Increase as needed by 25 mg to the maximum dose of 200 mg/day. Sertraline can be especially helpful for patients with predominant anxiety symptoms—anxiety usually responds to higher doses of antidepressants, and sertraline provides room for higher doses without the concerns for cardiac side effects seen with citalopram and escitalopram.

- Paroxetine (Paxil): 10 mg orally at bedtime; increase to a maximum of 40 mg/day as needed.

Suggested Initial and Maximal Doses for SNRIs

- Duloxetine (Cymbalta): 10 to 20 mg orally in the morning or twice a day; increase as needed to a maximum dose of 20 to 60 mg once or twice daily.
- Venlafaxine (Effexor): 18.75 to 37.5 mg orally twice a day for the first week; increase by 75 mg per week to a maximum dose of 150 mg twice a day. Missing any dose of venlafaxine can cause symptoms similar to those experienced with opioid withdrawal, so the patient must be weaned off the drug carefully.
- Venlafaxine extended release (Effexor XR or venlafaxine ER): 37.5 mg orally every morning or twice a day for the first week; increase by 75 mg per week to a maximum dose of 100 mg twice a day.

The exact mechanism by which mirtazapine (Remeron) treats depression is unknown. It binds central alpha-2, 5-HT2, and 5-HT3 receptors; increases norepinephrine release; and enhances the activity of a serotonin receptor via pre- and post-synaptic receptor antagonism. In addition to norepinephrine and serotonin receptors, it also binds histaminergic, muscarinic, and dopamine receptors, hence its sedating (e.g., useful for insomnia) and appetite-enhancing properties.

Start mirtazapine at 7.5 to 15 mg orally or sublingually at bedtime and increase it to a maximum of 60 mg per day by mouth. Mirtazapine (15 mg) can be directly substituted for an SSRI (e.g., fluoxetine 20 mg, citalopram 20 mg) (Howard et al. 2012). It is important to note that the antidepressant property of mirtazapine is usually predominant at higher doses: 30 mg to 45 mg. At these doses, however, the sedating and appetite-enhancing properties are somewhat diminished; only at lower doses does the drug block histamine receptors rather than serotonin receptors. Although patients can have dry mouth and constipation, mirtazapine has fewer side effects and drug-drug interactions than other classes of antidepressants and can be safe for long-term use in cancer patients and those nearing the end of life.

Bupropion is an aminoketone used both for smoking cessation (as Zyban) and for patients with depression (as Wellbutrin) (100 mg p.o. b.i.d. to a maximum of 450 mg given in four divided doses, or bupropion XL 100 mg daily, increasing to a maximum of 200 mg p.o. b.i.d.). It is *activating* and particularly helpful for patients with retarded psychomotor function, in whom anxiety is not a major problem. QTc prolongation was seen in a case of massive overdose, but not otherwise (Goodnick and Jerry 2002).

Trazodone (Desyrel) is also sedating. Initial doses are 50 mg orally at bedtime, to a maximum of 400 mg a day. Trazodone may prolong the QTc.

Tricyclic antidepressants (e.g., amitriptyline, nortriptyline, desipramine, doxepin, imipramine) are less useful for cancer patients with advanced disease because of their side-effect profile. But if the patient also has neuropathic pain, you can try to enhance tolerance of the drugs by starting at very low doses (10 mg at bedtime) and increasing by 10 to 20 mg weekly. If there is no effect, check blood levels to ensure that the therapeutic range has been reached. Checking EKGs to detect conduction disturbances, including prolonged QTc, may be necessary when giving higher doses.

The most rapidly acting antidepressants are the psychostimulants dextroamphetamine and methylphenidate (2.5 to 5 mg at 8 a.m. and noon, maximum 60 mg), which often act within a few days. These stimulants can also result in psychosis, however, or produce delirium in patients who are at a high risk due to active medical problems or other medications, like corticosteroids.

There is also increasing evidence for the antidepressant effect of ketamine, an NMDA receptor antagonist, especially for cancer patients, even those with advanced disease (Goldman, Frankenthaler, and Klepacz 2019). The mechanism of action for ketamine's rapid antidepressant effects is unknown. The comprehensive literature review by Goldman and colleagues reported that for patients with depression, starting them on IV ketamine and then switching to oral or intranasal may be most effective. More research is needed to establish the efficacy of ketamine in cancer patients.

Increasing evidence also suggests a role for psychedelics such as psilocybin in decreasing depression and anxiety in patients with life-threatening cancer. In a 2016 double-blind RCT by Griffiths et al. at the Johns Hopkins University, high doses (22 or 30 mg/70 kg) of psilocybin resulted in large decreases in clinician- and patient-rated measures of depressed mood, anxiety, and death anxiety, coupled with increases in quality of life, meaning, and optimism, and these changes were sustained after six months. More research needs to be done to determine the full breadth and efficacy of these agents on psychological distress in this population.

Choice of agent. Both side effects and drug-drug interactions influence the choice of antidepressant. Major side effects of the SSRIs and SNRIs include hyponatremia, sexual dysfunction or loss of libido, somnolence, and gastrointestinal complaints (e.g., nausea, diarrhea, vomiting, and foul-smelling flatus). Citalopram, escitalopram, venlafaxine, duloxetine, and mirtazapine are the least likely to have drug-drug interactions; sertraline is likely, but fluoxetine, fluvoxamine, paroxetine, and all the tricyclic antidepressants are *very likely* to interact with other drugs cancer patients are taking.

Rarely, patients can develop serotonin syndrome when other agents are added, like fluconazole, that inhibit the metabolism of the SSRIs (i.e., inhibitors of CYP2C19 and 3A4), which causes a marked increase in SSRI blood levels (Levin et al. 2008). We discuss serotonin syndrome in detail later in the chapter when we review delirium.

Consulting psychiatry. If the patient does not respond to first-line agents, has a history of psychosis, or has had a trial of multiple agents, consult a psychiatrist. You should also make a referral to a psychiatrist if you are unsure of the diagnosis; the patient is psychotic, confused, or delirious; the patient previously had a major psychiatric disorder; there are dysfunctional family dynamics; or the patient is suicidal or is requesting assisted suicide.

The psychiatrist will not necessarily advise hospitalization for patients at the end of life; the psychiatrist will, however, help the hospice or home care agency and the family take appropriate precautions. Patients with pancreatic cancer are 11 times more likely to commit suicide than the people in the general population and are at particular risk in the early postoperative period (Turaga et al. 2011). Factors that make other cancer patients more likely to attempt suicide include advanced illness and poor prognosis, uncontrolled pain, depression and hope-lessness, delirium and disinhibition, loss of control and helplessness, preexisting psychopathology, prior history of attempted suicide, family history of suicide, and exhaustion and fatigue.

PERSONALITY DISORDERS

Oncologists frequently find themselves trying to care for patients who don't clearly have an anxiety disorder or depression, who are not delirious, but who stress the team to the maximum. Patients like Duane, who one minute is praising you to the skies, and the next, is outraged and threatening you when you won't refill an opioid prescription to replace one that was accidently left in his motel room on vacation. Or Susanna, who, despite long discussions in the office, calls repeatedly to ask for help making the most trivial decisions. Or Arthur, who misses appoint-ments, doesn't follow instructions regarding medications, and repeatedly calls all members of your staff seeking support and problem solving but rarely follows through. How can you understand what is causing their behavior, and who can help you and your staff manage these patients? How can you treat these people safely with chemotherapy or opioids?

I (*Janet Abrahm*) was relieved to learn from Drs. Meyer and Block, in their review "Personality Disorders in the Oncology Setting" (2011), that patients like these, "difficult" patients, have clearly described personality disorders and that there are well-defined ways to approach managing their otherwise confusing and exasperating behavior. Meyer and Block clarify what makes taking care of patients like these a "difficult encounter."

In their extremely useful paper, they describe how these patients present, their behaviors with the oncology team, our possible reactions to them, how we can respond to them, what medications might be helpful, and even what we can say in response to the challenges they present us with. Having read it, I now understand better how to create effective boundaries that will make the patients feel safer, and how to moderate the chaos they bring to clinic staff or the inpatient care team.

Types of personality disorders. Meyer and Block list seven personality disorders that are particularly problematic in medical settings: paranoid, antisocial, narcissistic, borderline, histrionic, dependent, and obsessive-compulsive.

Duane is antisocial. He initially seems charming, but he is really manipulative, and you may find that he has fired other providers or has found himself on the wrong side of the law. Meyer and Block suggest that our reaction to him may be "sympathy, followed by anger and fear," and the best strategy for dealing with him is to acknowledge your feelings and set limits on his behavior to protect yourself and the staff. If you need to treat his anxiety, don't use benzodiazepines, which he may easily divert; use an SSRI.

Susanna is "dependent," and your reaction to her is likely to be fatigue, then guilt for not taking her calls, and finally aversion. Again, acknowledge your feelings, set limits, then reassure her that you're committed to her care, but let her know the recurrent calls to staff for nonemergencies are making it harder for them to take care of her. Her anxiety may respond to SSRIs or low-dose benzodiazepines.

Arthur is narcissistic, and although he behaves well when everything is going OK, when it isn't, he can become angry and expect special treatment from you, demanding you be there for him whenever he needs you. You may in turn become angry at him and wish to attack back. Meyer and Block suggest that instead we work to partner with him, letting him know that this is the way to ensure he receives the best care, and align with his ability to achieve whatever goals he sets. If patients like Arthur are depressed, or have mood lability, then SSRIs for the depression, or mood stabilizers or antipsychotics, are recommended.

The most disruptive disorder in the clinical setting is likely to be the "borderline" patient. This is someone everyone in the office knows about and has tried to help at one time or another. She may have fired several previous doctors and nurses. When she is admitted, the nursing staff may be up in arms, and social work, patient relations, even security may be involved. These patients are impulsive, emotionally labile, and afraid that we will abandon them. Their impulsivity may manifest as substance use disorder, being sexually promiscuous, or missing appointments and medication doses. They feel especially uneasy during transitions, such as discharge from the hospital, or completion of adjuvant chemotherapy, and are likely to present then with new symptoms or problems.

These "borderline" patients need a team that is empathetic but has low expectations, one in which all the caregivers meet as frequently as necessary, even daily, to ensure they are on the same page. Team members or office staff must be alert to the possibility that the patient may try to turn staff against each other because of how the patient perceives she has been treated. Psychiatrists should be part of these teams whenever possible. Limits must be set and clearly stated and restated, along with ongoing reassurance that the oncology team is committed to care for the patient. The patient must be told, even though the reaction may be anger or outrage, that chemotherapy and opioids require regularity of visits and collaboration with the plan of care. If the patient is depressed or anxious, SSRIs can be helpful, along with atypical antipsychotics for anger or impulsive behavior. Patients given opioids must be monitored very closely, and benzodiazepines should be avoided because of their abuse potential.

I hope that after reading this section, you are saying to yourself, "Oh, that was what was going on with Mr. X!" or "That really describes Mrs. Y!" Once you learn to recognize these patients early in your relationship with them, you will find it useful to discuss with your staff the patient's sense of what is going on, what the patient likely needs for support, who on the team are able to give that support, and what the boundaries should be. You can make a plan for each office visit or admission delineating who will be the point person caring for this patient, who will support that person in that role, and when to pre-meet and debrief about patient encounters. It sounds like a lot of work, and it is, but without it, the staff is likely to be continually disrupted as long as the patient is in the practice or on the inpatient unit. With appropriate teamwork and boundary setting, these patients may be able to receive the care they need from the team safely and consistently.

Dr. Groves, a well-respected Harvard psychiatrist, also provides insights on working with the "hateful patient," whom he describes as presenting in one of four stereotypes: dependent clingers, entitled demanders, manipulative help-rejecters, and self-destructive deniers (Groves 1978). Although he wrote his paper in 1978, many clinicians still find that Grove's characterizations of these stereotypical patients ring true in their practices. He provides suggestions similar to Block and Meyer about how clinicians can work effectively with these patients so that their behaviors do not undermine the quality of care they receive.

DELIRIUM

Delirium is the most common organic brain syndrome affecting cancer patients. It is characterized by a fluctuating course of a clouded state of consciousness, decreased attention, distractibility, and sensory misperceptions (e.g., hallucinations). The signs of delirium include incoherent speech, disturbed sleep-wake cycle, and increased or decreased activity. Delirious patients may also have anxiety, fear, irritability, depression, euphoria, or apathy.

The primary driver of delirium is usually medical. Life-threatening causes include Wernicke's encephalopathy from B vitamin deficiency, withdrawal reactions from medications or substances, hypoxia or hypoperfusion of the central nervous system, hypoglycemia, hypercalcemia, renal or hepatic failure, intracerebral metastases or hemorrhage, infection, meningitis/encephalitis, or poisoning. Patients with Parkinson's disease who develop Lewy body dementia can mimic those with delirium, as they have hallucinations and psychoses. While rarely caused by pain, delirium can be caused by the medicines used to treat it, and delirium can present as uncontrolled pain. The dying process itself also can cause delirium.

Miss Monroe was a patient of mine (*Janet Abrahm*) when I was practicing hematology and oncology; she experienced delirium from a number of causes.

The Problem of Delirium

Miss Monroe was a 62-year-old elementary school teacher who developed multiple myeloma. She was sent to me from her general internist, who had made the diagnosis during his evaluation of her complaints of back pain and anemia. MRI revealed that her pain was due to an epidural spinal cord compression, and she was just finishing radiation therapy for this when she had her first episode of delirium.

Miss Monroe was accompanied on her visit by her niece, Samantha, who lived with her while going to college. Samantha had noted that her aunt was not always herself these days. Miss Monroe had previously been a steady, matter-of-fact kind of person, friendly, generous, and caring. Her students loved her, and her colleagues respected her. Lately, however, her behavior had become erratic. Although much of the time she seemed her old self, at other times she appeared euphoric, at others depressed and tearful, and at still others angry for no apparent reason. She forgot things she never would have forgotten before and seemed increasingly distant. Samantha missed the nightly talks they used to have about school and the strategy sessions for getting through the next day or week.

What Samantha had noticed were the early signs of delirium. Miss Monroe's memory was impaired; she wasn't thinking clearly; she had poor judgment; and her mental status varied from normal to abnormal throughout the course of the day. Because her calcium, sodium, and blood glucose levels were normal, we believed her delirium was caused by the high-dose corticosteroids she had begun taking when her spinal cord compression was diagnosed. Steroid-induced delirium is by no means rare: in one study, as many as one-quarter of the cancer patients treated with high-dose prednisone or dexamethasone developed delirium (Weissman 1988).

Because her radiation therapy treatments were completed, her corticosteroids were tapered rapidly—and her mental status quickly returned to normal. But later in the course of her illness, she had progressive bony disease that was refractory to therapy and began taking sustained-release morphine preparations for the pain. When the dose was escalated to improve pain control, Miss Monroe herself noticed a problem.

"I think I must be going crazy," she told me at one clinic visit. *"A few months ago, I was having nightmares, but that sort of made sense to me. After all, I'm under*

a lot of strain here; my cancer seems to be getting worse and not better, and a few bad dreams were not something I even considered mentioning to you. But lately, I'm seeing things that Samantha doesn't see and talking with people I know can't be real because they died years ago! What is happening to me?"

Once again, Miss Monroe was suffering from delirium, manifested this time by hallucinations. The morphine was responsible. Her earlier nightmares had been caused by the morphine, and raising her dose had made the problem even worse. Her symptoms disappeared when she was switched to a different opioid.

Her final bout with delirium occurred as she was dying at home. She had declined hospice services, and Samantha was doing the bulk of the caregiving. Samantha called me in tears at 3 a.m. to report a sudden major change in her aunt. Earlier that day Miss Monroe had been resting comfortably. Now, when Samantha had tried to give her some pain medication, she had refused and accused Samantha of trying to poison her. Samantha wasn't even sure that her aunt recognized her. Miss Monroe was restless, throwing off the bedcovers or "picking" at them, and was shouting at her, swearing, and refusing to be touched. Samantha said that she was about to call the police but thought maybe I had some idea of what was going on.

I told her that the symptoms and signs indicated that her aunt had another, more severe form of delirium: Miss Monroe was confused and disoriented; her speech was not always coherent; she got worse at night; and she had no insight into her problem. I reassured Samantha that none of this was her fault, that more than three-quarters of dying patients experience delirium. I advised her on which medication to administer. Luckily, Miss Monroe responded promptly. Three days later, she died peacefully at home.

During her illness, Miss Monroe displayed many of the symptoms of a hyperactive delirium, which occurs in about a third of delirious patients: agitation, hallucinations, disordered thinking and perception, delusions, labile mood, and what is termed *psychomotor behavior*—picking at bedcovers, for example. Another third of delirious patients, however, experience a quiet delirium that can go undetected unless sought. Such patients are not agitated—they may be resting quietly in bed, but when asked, they may have paranoid ideation, or may confirm that they do not feel safe. That was how her delirium manifested when she wouldn't let Samantha give her medications. The final third show evidence of both hyper- and hypoactive delirium. All types of delirium can be distressing, and hyperactive and mixed delirium often require pharmacotherapy. Almost three-quarters of delirious cancer patients who recovered remembered their experience and found it profoundly distressing (Hui et al. 2010).

The causes of Miss Monroe's delirium included corticosteroids, opioids, and the terminal illness itself. She did not receive lorazepam (Ativan), which, paradoxically, can cause an agitated delirium. She was also not receiving anticholinergic agents, which, when combined with drugs with anticholinergic side effects, can cause a *cholinergic crisis*, a life-threatening syndrome that includes high fevers and delirium. H2 blockers (e.g., cimetidine), tricyclic antidepressants, and anticholinergic agents (e.g., diphenhydramine [Benadryl] or hydroxyzine [Atarax, Vistaril]) all have significant anticholinergic side effects and can contribute to a cholinergic crisis, as I discuss below.

Practice Points: Assessing Delirium

- Delirium is characterized by:
  - an acute fluctuating change in mental status.
  - a disturbance of consciousness with reduced ability to focus, sustain, or shift attention.
  - a disturbance that develops within a short time and fluctuates throughout the day.
- Symptoms include insomnia and daytime somnolence, nightmares, irritability, distractibility, hypersensitivity to light and sound, anxiety, difficulty in concentrating or marshaling thoughts, hallucinations, delusions, emotional lability, attention deficits, and memory disturbances.
- Patients may appear hypoactive, depressed, euphoric, or extremely agitated.
- Precipitating factors include metabolic derangements (hypercalcemia, hypo- or hyperglycemia, hypo- or hypernatremia, hypoxia, renal or hepatic failure), drugs (especially opioids, corticosteroids, and anticholinergic agents), nutritional deficiency (especially of B vitamins), infection, structural brain lesions, and encephalitis.

Drug-Induced Delirium

Drugs are a major cause of delirium. We have already discussed delirium induced by opioids, benzodiazepines, and psychostimulants. Both cholinergic crisis and serotonin syndrome can manifest as delirium. Both can be induced by a combination of drugs commonly used to support cancer patients, both are difficult to recognize, and both are life threatening if not caught early and treated aggressively.

Practice Points: Managing Patients with Drug-Induced Delirium

- Change the opioid or lower the dose.
- Evaluate appropriate patients for contributing medical conditions (e.g., brain lesions, electrolyte imbalance, hypoxia, infection, nutritional deficiency, renal or hepatic dysfunction).

- Discontinue contributing medications (e.g., acyclovir, amphotericin B, anticholinergics or agents with anticholinergic side effects, antiemetics, psychostimulants, short-acting benzodiazepines, corticosteroids, cefepime).
- Review the recent antineoplastic drug regimen for contributing agents (e.g., asparaginase, fludarabine, bleomycin, carmustine, cisplatin, cytosine arabinoside, etoposide, 5-fluorouracil, hexylmethylmelamine, ifosfamide, cyclophosphamide, interferon, interleukin-2, methotrexate [high-dose], procarbazine, vinblastine, vincristine, CAR T-cell therapy, immunotherapy).

Cholinergic Crisis

Mr. Martinez was a patient with metastatic pancreatic cancer whom I (*Janet Abrahm*) saw in palliative care clinic. His family complained to his oncologist, Dr. Greenleaf, that his pain medication was "making him act funny." They wanted it stopped. Over the past week, they said, he had become intermittently confused and agitated. His vision was blurry, he was weaker, and he occasionally appeared to be hallucinating. Dr. Greenleaf suspected another cause, because Mr. Martinez's opioid regimen had not been changed in many weeks; his pain was still well controlled by a 100 µg/hr Duragesic (transdermal fentanyl) patch, along with twice daily Dilaudid (hydromorphone) for rescue.

Dr. Greenleaf evaluated Mr. Martinez and thought he might be becoming delirious. She explained that Mr. Martinez needed opioids of some type to control his pain and admitted him to the hospital to evaluate him for other causes. She asked me to recommend several agents that she could safely prescribe and contacted Dr. Blair, a psychiatrist.

Dr. Greenleaf said that Mr. Martinez, like many patients with pancreatic cancer, was depressed, and that for four months before this incident, he had been taking amitriptyline. His response to the amitriptyline had been excellent. Two weeks before the events Mr. Martinez's family reported, Dr. Greenleaf had added cimetidine and hydroxyzine (Atarax) for new gastritis and severe pruritus due to increasing biliary obstruction. His family added that a week ago, Mr. Martinez had doubled his hydroxyzine dose when his pruritus worsened. On admission, he was found to be febrile, with very dry mucous membranes, and delirious.

Given this new information, I thought it was less likely that the opioids were causing Mr. Martinez's delirium than that the combination of amitriptyline, cimetidine, and an increased dose of hydroxyzine had precipitated a *cholinergic crisis* manifesting as a hyperactive delirium.

Dr. Blair agreed. Dr. Greenleaf discontinued cimetidine and hydroxyzine, added omeprazole for gastritis and cholestyramine for the bile acid–induced pruritus, and substituted a different opioid, intravenous morphine, for pain management. Because Mr. Martinez had not developed the crisis when taking amitriptyline and opioids alone, and because amitriptyline had been of significant benefit, we thought it could safely be continued. Dr. Blair suggested haloperidol (Haldol) to control Mr. Martinez's agitation and disordered mentation. Ten days later Mr. Martinez's mental status had greatly improved, and he no longer required haloperidol. I advised Dr. Greenleaf to use oral sustained-release morphine and immediate-release oral morphine for rescue, instead of restarting the fentanyl patch.

Practice Points: Cholinergic Crisis

- Increased salivation
- Increased tearing and blurry vision
- Muscular weakness, paralysis, fasciculation
- Diarrhea
- Hyperactive delirium

We explained to Mr. Martinez and his family why the delirium had developed and why it was safe for him to continue taking opioids and amitriptyline. On this regimen, he was able to maintain excellent symptom control without recurrence of a cholinergic crisis until his death two months later.

Serotonin Syndrome

Angela Forsythe was a 64-year-old woman with recurrent glioblastoma multiforme, who was being treated with dexamethasone and a fentanyl patch of 25 mcg/hr to control her headaches. She was also taking citalopram for depression and had been doing well.

Angela came in for a routine visit during which her oncologist, Dr. Wang, reviewed the results of her MRI, which showed stable disease, and he introduced the idea of home hospice care. Angela complained of oral pain and difficulty swallowing. Dr. Wang diagnosed oral and esophageal thrush and began a course of fluconazole. A week later, Angela's daughter called our palliative care program nurse because of a change in her mother's condition. Her arm and leg muscles seemed to be jumping for no reason, and she was much more confused and didn't respond to questions. We urged Angela's daughter to bring her mother to the hospital.

In the Emergency Department, Angela was confused and had severe cognitive deficits, especially with memory; a flat affect; and periods of "absence," when she wouldn't respond to questions. She had mild myoclonus and hyperreflexia, tachycardia, and tachypnea. Her repeat MRI showed no change from the previous week, and there were no new metabolic abnormalities. Her only new medication was the fluconazole.

After Angela was admitted to the hospital, serotonin syndrome was confirmed as the likely etiology of her symptoms. Her family revealed that Angela had begun to develop the change in her behavior about three days after the fluconazole was started, and an EEG done after admission showed nonconvulsive seizure activity, responsive to lorazepam. The citalopram was discontinued, lorazepam was used for anxiety and myoclonus, and her mental status returned to its prior state within a few days.

Serotonin syndrome can be caused by an overdose of an SSRI (selective serotonin reuptake inhibitor). But more typically in patients who have cancer, it is caused by adding an agent that inhibits the metabolism of the SSRI, causing an increase in SSRI blood levels. SSRIs are metabolized in the liver by CYP2C19 and 3A4, so inhibitors of these cytochromes, like fluconazole, can easily cause the syndrome. The typical findings of serotonin syndrome are found in the Practice Points box below (Levin et al. 2008, p. 374).

Practice Points: Serotonin Syndrome

- Neuromuscular hyperactivity: tremor, clonus, myoclonus, hyper-reflexia, and, in the advanced stage, pyramidal rigidity
- Autonomic hyperactivity: diaphoresis, fever, tachycardia, tachypnea, and mydriasis
- Altered mental status: agitation and confusion in advanced stages

---

Angela had many, but not all, of these findings. Her dexamethasone prevented the diaphoresis and fever, and the fentanyl prevented mydriasis. Had she been receiving lorazepam for anxiety, she would not have had myoclonus, either. She was fortunate that her clinicians had a high degree of suspicion and were able to confirm her diagnosis and treat her promptly, so that she recovered to her baseline.

Practice Points: Drug Combinations Reported to Cause Serotonin Syndrome

Paroxetine + fentanyl	Citalopram + fluconazole
Citalopram + oxycodone	Escitalopram + fentanyl
Citalopram + tramadol	Duloxetine + linezolid
Citalopram + trazadone/linezolid	Methadone + linezolid

(Kotlinska-Lemieszek, Klepstad, and Faksvåg 2019; Levin et al. 2008; Mahlberg et al. 2004; Mastroianni and Ravaglia 2017)

Therapy for delirium. Whenever possible, consult a psychiatrist for patients with delirium, and when the patient's condition permits, initiate treatment for the underlying cause. It is fortunate that the initial episode of delirium reverses in 50 percent of patients, even when the cause remains unknown (see Table 9.2). Subsequent episodes reverse only 25 percent of the time (Lawlor et al. 2000). Dr. Eduardo Bruera, a noted hospice physician, educator, and researcher, was able to identify an etiology for the delirium in only half of his terminally ill patients. But he and others have identified some simple but effective measures to help these patients (Kang, Shin, and Bruera 2013):

- Ask a nurse, friend, or family member to sit with the patient to decrease her anxiety and help with orientation.
- Move the patient to a well-known favorite room.
- Leave a night light on.
- Put a clock and a calendar within sight, along with favorite familiar objects.

If these techniques do not work, pharmacologic therapy often does. Antipsychotic medications are commonly used as first-line pharmacological agents for managing the neuropsychiatric symptoms (e.g., agitation, hallucinations, paranoia) of patients with agitated delirium, although recent evidence on their efficacy is mixed, especially considering the potential significant side effects, such as extrapyramidal symptoms and akathisia. In one excellent RCT, patients with delirium who received antipsychotics did worse than patients in the control group who received ideal supportive care (Agar et al. 2017). Most of these patients had hypoactive delirium, so it is not clear whether the benefits of antipsychotics exceed the risk in those patients. And the ideal supportive care the patients in that control group received is difficult to replicate in our current United States health care system.

Haloperidol (1 to 2 mg p.o. at bedtime or b.i.d. to t.i.d. and every 4 hours p.r.n.), a butyrophenone, will diminish the patient's agitation, clear her sensorium, and improve her ability to think clearly. If it needs to be given parenterally, start with or 0.5 to 1 mg IV two to four times daily, because the parenteral dose is approximately twice as strong as the oral dose. Do not exceed doses of 20 mg in 24 hours to avoid inducing the often-fatal neuroleptic malignant syndrome (NMS), which presents with rigidity, high fever, encephalopathy, and widely fluctuating pulse and blood pressure (Caroff et al. 2011). It is important to note that haloperidol works best by "stacking" doses; if 1 mg does not work, repeating the 1 mg dose will not be effective. You have to titrate to 2 mg, then 4 mg, and so forth. In patients suffering hallucinations from Lewy body dementia, however, the agent of choice is pimavanserin (e.g., Nuplazid), an atypical antipsychotic that binds serotonin 5HT2A receptors. The dose is 34 mg/day except in patients also receiving strong Cyp3A4 inhibitors, who should receive only 10 mg per day.

TABLE 9.2 Treatment of Delirium

Drug	Dose	Comments
Typical and atypical antipsychotics		
Haloperidol (Haldol)	1–4 mg p.o. or 0.5–2 mg IV SQ h.s. or b.i.d. to t.i.d.	Can add the same dose q4h p.r.n. Do not exceed 20 mg in 24 hr.
		Maintain the patient on the effective dose (divided into a b.i.d. dose) for 3–4 days, then taper over 1 week, as tolerated.
Olanzapine (Zyprexa, Zydis)	2.5–5 mg p.o./SL/IV h.s. to b.i.d.	Can add 2.5 mg q4h p.r.n. Do not exceed 30mg total dose in a 24 hr.
Aripiprazole (Abilify)	5 mg p.o. daily	Do not exceed 30 mg; does not prolong and may shorten QTc.
Chlorpromazine (Thorazine)	25–100 mg p.o., IV or p.r., b.i.d. to q.i.d.	May cause significant hypotension.

Note: In delirious patients, attempt first to identify the underlying cause and begin to correct it as you give the agents listed. Make the patient's surroundings as familiar as possible. Ask a family member or friend to sit with the patient.

SL = sublingual dissolving tablets/wafers

Caution: Any benzodiazepine may exacerbate delirium, especially in older adults (>70).

It is always best to consult psychiatry to manage these medications. When the patient's delirium comes under control, continue the haloperidol at the same dose and frequency that was effective, and then taper it over several weeks, as tolerated. The patient's mental status may not return to normal for several days, but her agitation and fear usually resolve within one or two days.

If the haloperidol is not effective, discontinue the haloperidol and start olanzapine (Zyprexa, Zydis) 2.5 to 5 mg sublingually or orally, or IV twice daily plus 2.5 mg every 4 hours sublingually, orally, or IV as needed, not to exceed 30 mg in 24 hours. If patients develop akathisia from these agents, discontinue them and start a beta-blocker, as discussed earlier in this chapter, at the end of the discussion of anxiety.

All patients on antipsychotics (except those receiving only comfort-focused care) should have their QTc routinely checked because a prolonged QTc raises the risk of developing dangerous arrhythmias such as *torsades de pointes*. The atypical antipsychotic aripiprazole (Abilify) does not prolong, and may shorten, the QTc. Start at 5 mg by mouth daily and increase as needed to a maximum of 30 mg a day. Strong CYP3A4 inhibitors like fluconazole may greatly increase serum concentrations of aripiprazole, and it is important to reduce aripiprazole doses by half in patients who receive both agents. The advantage of aripiprazole over haloperidol is the lower incidence of extrapyramidal symptoms (Kasper et al. 2003), especially at doses of haloperidol needed by patients with hyperactive delirium (Boettger et al. 2011), and the lack of prolongation and perhaps even reduction of the QTc interval (Goodnick and Jerry 2002).

All three agents (i.e., haloperidol, olanzapine, and aripiprazole) are effective for patients with delirium. If the delirium was induced by corticosteroids, opioids, or metabolic abnormalities (e.g., hypercalcemia), treat the delirium while you are trying to reverse the underlying cause; the patient is likely to respond even though the precipitating cause is still present.

For some patients experiencing a particularly agitated delirium who may not be able to tolerate an antipsychotic, mood stabilizers such as valproic acid can be helpful (Sher et al. 2015). The evidence for specific dosing for delirium is limited, but anecdotally, 125–250 mg IV three times a day is a good place to start. Patients' liver function tests should be monitored routinely because valproic acid is metabolized by the liver.

For patients who are refractory to these agents, when sedation is acceptable, chlorpromazine (e.g., Thorazine) (25 to 100 mg p.o., IV, or p.r. b.i.d. to q.i.d.) is usually effective. Chlorpromazine induces orthostatic hypotension, is more sedating, and has a higher incidence of anticholinergic and cardiovascular side effects than haloperidol or olanzapine. Chlorpromazine is particularly helpful for patients with terminal delirium who are not getting out of bed, and in whom the sedation is usually an acceptable price to pay for control of the delirium. The treatment of patients with terminal delirium is reviewed in Chapter 12.

Practice Points: Managing Patients with Agitated Delirium

- Obtain a psychiatric consultation when available; aggressively treat any underlying medical conditions.
- Begin therapy directed at reversing the underlying etiologies whenever possible.
- Surround the patient with the familiar (people, objects, and sounds).
- Frequently reorient the patient to place, day, date, and time.
- Give haloperidol, 0.5 to 1 mg IV or 1 to 2 mg p.o. and repeat q6h with 1 to 2 mg q2h p.r.n. until either the agitation resolves or 20 mg has been given within 24 hours.
- For refractory patients who can take oral medication, give olanzapine, 2.5 to 5 mg (p.o., s.l., b.i.d.), and 2.5 mg q4h p.r.n. and not to exceed 30 mg within 24 hours. Olanzapine can also be given IV at the same dose and frequency.
- For patients with QTc prolongation, consider aripiprazole (Abilify), 5 mg p.o. daily; may increase as needed to a maximum of 30 mg.
- If they cannot not tolerate antipsychotics, try valproic acid 125–250 mg I.V. t.i.d. p.r.n. to manage agitation.

SUMMARY

In this chapter, we have reviewed psychological support and counseling, discussing how it can be instrumental in helping patients manage the normal distress that accompanies a serious illness. We then reviewed how palliative care and oncology clinicians can assess and address distress symptoms typical of patients with cancer, including adjustment reactions, existential distress, anxiety, depressive symptoms, personality traits, and delirium. We also indicated when it is important to bring in psychologists and psychiatrists to care for particularly distressed patients, especially those refractory to the initial therapies suggested.

CHAPTER 10

Managing Other Distressing Problems

Patients with cancer suffer from any number of disorders that cause distress without causing pain. This chapter focuses on the most common and most distressing of nonpain problems and their treatment.

ORAL PROBLEMS

Many simple measures can help patients maintain oral comfort. These include removing poorly fitting dentures; replacing vitamins and minerals that, if deficient, can result in mucositis (e.g., vitamins B, C; zinc); presenting food at moderate temperatures; avoiding dry, acidic, or highly spiced foods; and minimizing alcohol and tobacco use.

Oral comfort can also be maximized by continuing routine prophylactic oral care, even for patients who are very debilitated (Table 10.1). Regular mouth care can be carried out by the patient or the family; it can help stimulate the patient's appetite and diminish discomfort from various causes. Patients should be encouraged to continue brushing daily using a soft-bristle brush, flossing, and rinsing with an antibacterial mouthwash (that does not contain alcohol) or a solution of bicarbonate in water (e.g., 1 tsp. in a cup of water). More detailed oral care protocols are described in sources listed in the bibliography online.

Despite these preventive regimens, about half of cancer patients will develop oral discomfort, the most common causes of which are candida infections; treatment-induced mucositis; or xerostomia resulting from mouth breathing, previous radiation therapy, or medications for pain or other symptoms. Simple methods of treatment are often effective.

> **Practice Points: Maintaining Oral Comfort**
>
> - Remove poorly fitting dentures.
> - Correct vitamin and mineral deficiencies.
> - Present foods at moderate temperatures.
> - Avoid dry, acidic, or highly spiced foods.
> - Minimize alcohol and tobacco use.
> - Continue routine prophylactic oral care, including brushing, flossing, and rinsing with an alcohol-free antibacterial mouthwash.
> - Monitor for oral candidiasis and treat early.

Candida

Etiology. As many as 90 percent of cancer patients have contracted an oral candida infection by the time they die. About 50 percent are colonized before chemotherapy, but more than 70 percent are colonized after chemotherapy or radiation therapy, and almost 40 percent of patients receiving radiation therapy to the head and neck or on chemotherapy have clinical oral fungal infections. Oral and esophageal infection with candida can also arise in patients who have recently been on a course of antibiotics, which alter the normal protective oral flora. Other patients are predisposed to developing yeast infections due to immunosuppression resulting from therapeutic steroid doses or malnutrition (albumin of <3 g/dL).

Manifestations in immunosuppressed patients. Oral thrush presents most often as a burning tongue and pain when eating. Examination of the oral cavity may reveal only a beefy red tongue (in those who have recently been taking antibiotics) or white plaques (which are easily wiped off, but with bleeding) along the sides of the tongue or cheeks, on the gums, or on the roof of the mouth. Patients who leave their dentures in place between meals are particularly prone to develop both angular cheilitis and candidal infections on the roof or floor of the mouth; these appear as red edematous areas.

Candidal esophagitis can contribute to anorexia by causing dysphagia. The lower esophageal sphincter area is most commonly involved, but the pain or the sensation of food "sticking" can be present in the throat or chest as well as in the upper abdomen. Topical antifungal medications that are effective for oral thrush unfortunately do not prevent esophageal candida infections.

Therapy. Topical agents (e.g., clotrimazole troches or nystatin suspensions) are recommended and usually tried first, but for various reasons, they are often not effective in this population (Bays and Thompson 2019). The troches do not dissolve when patients have concurrent xerostomia, for example. Moreover, swishing a suspension of nystatin, which tastes terrible, four or five times a day, or taking troches that dissolve in the mouth every 5 or 6 hours is inconvenient for a patient with advanced cancer.

Fluconazole, on the other hand (200 mg loading dose followed by 100 mg p.o./day for prophylaxis or for 7 days for established oral infection), provides effective prophylaxis and therapy for oral thrush (Bays and Thompson 2019). For esophagitis, the doses need to be increased and the course prolonged (400 mg loading dose followed by 200 mg p.o./day × 14 days). Itraconazole (100 to 200 mg tablets or oral suspension daily) and amphotericin B 100 mg/ml oral solution (1 ml t.i.d. to q.i.d.—swish and spit out) are also effective.

Herpes Simplex Virus

Oral HSV infections commonly cause morbidity in patients with hematologic malignancies as well as in as many as 50 percent of patients with head and neck cancer treated with chemo- or radiation therapy (Elad et al. 2010). Patients about to undergo bone marrow or stem cell transplant or leukemia therapy routinely receive antiviral prophylaxis with acyclovir or valacyclovir to prevent reactivation, and both are equally effective in preventing HSV reactivation (Elad et al. 2010).

Treatment-Induced Mucositis

Treatment-induced mucositis is one of the most common and most distressing side effects from chemotherapy and radiotherapy and from bone marrow and stem cell transplants.

Prevention. Oral cryotherapy was well tolerated and decreased the oral thermal hyperalgesia that oxaliplatin can induce (Bauman et al. 2019). Multiagent combination oral care protocols (usually including an intensive regimen of oral cleansing with frequent saline and antiseptic rinses daily) without chlorhexidine help prevent oral mucositis during chemotherapy, radiation therapy for head and neck cancer, and hematopoietic stem cell transplantation (HCST) (Hong et al. 2019). Photobiomodulation using low-level laser therapy can prevent oral mucositis in patients undergoing HSCT and can also prevent the associated pain in patients receiving radiation therapy with or without chemotherapy for head and neck cancer (Paglioni et al. 2019; Zadik et al. 2019). Concern has been raised, however, about the long-term effects of the therapy, including potential decreases in survival (Sonis 2020). Photobiomodulation is not effective for the management of mucositis, however.

Keratinocyte growth factor-1 (KGF-1) infusions are recommended for mucositis prevention for patients undergoing autologous HSCT being conditioned with high-dose chemotherapy and total body irradiation (TBI) (Logan et al. 2020). Oral cryotherapy has been an effective protectant for patients undergoing autologous

HSCT with high-dose melphalan-conditioning protocols or with solid tumors receiving bolus 5-fluorouracil (Correa et al. 2020).

Treatment. Many agents have been tried, but data are mixed on the results. Multiagent combination oral care protocols (usually including an intensive regimen of oral cleansing with frequent saline and antiseptic rinses daily) are helpful also for treatment (Hong et al. 2019). Topical morphine (0.2%) has been found to be effective for mucositis pain of patients with head and neck cancers treated with combination radiation and chemotherapy (Saunders et al. 2020). So-called magic mouthwash, consisting of diphenhydramine, lidocaine, and antacid, or a doxepin-containing mouthwash, provided more short-term pain relief than placebo mouthwash, 85.5 percent ($p = .02$ vs. placebo) and 79.5 percent versus 68.4 percent respectively (Sio et al. 2019), supporting the claim that "magic mouthwash may have meaningful benefits" (Elad and Yarom 2019).

Xerostomia

Etiology. Dry mouth is a common complaint, occurring in 56 to 77 percent of patients with far-advanced solid tumors (Fleming, Craigs, and Bennett 2020; Frowen, Hughes, and Skeat 2020). Some have received radiation that diminished their saliva production, and others are taking medication that is causing xerostomia as a side effect. Therapy is often effective in these patients and in patients for whom a clear underlying cause is not apparent.

I find it useful to review the patient's medications to see which could be contributing, and then discontinue these and, if necessary, substitute other agents that are less likely to induce this side effect. In addition to the antihistamines and anticholinergics, certain anticonvulsants, antipsychotics, hypnotics, beta-blockers, opioids, and diuretics can contribute to xerostomia. The more of these agents patients are receiving, the more likely they are to develop xerostomia.

Cancer therapy also induces xerostomia (Jensen et al. 2010a, 2010b; Mercadante et al. 2021). Patients who receive conventional, 3D-conformal, or intensity-modulated radiation therapy (IMRT) that includes the parotid, submandibular, and minor salivary glands all develop some degree of permanent xerostomia. Patients who are candidates for IMRT that spares the parotid, however, less often develop salivary dysfunction, and the xerostomia is less severe (Jensen et al. 2010b). The 2021 guidelines (Mercadante et al. 2021) recommend using IMRT to prevent these complications. Acupuncture and systemic bethanechol during radiation therapy can reduce the risk of subsequent xerostomia. Antioxidants, including vitamin E, should not be used during head and neck radiotherapy, and evidence remains insufficient to recommend for or against the prophylactic use of oral pilocarpine, amifostine, or low-level laser therapy, among other potential therapies, during radiotherapy (Mercadante et al. 2021). Many of these patients gradually recover full salivary secretion over one or two years. Xerostomia caused

> **Practice Points: Therapy for Xerostomia**
>
> - Minimize the number of medications that produce xerostomia.
> - Try sugar-free sour lemon drops or other sugar-free hard candy.
> - Encourage continued good routine oral hygiene, adding a fluoride-containing toothpaste for selected patients.
> - Try pilocarpine (Salagen), bethanechol, or cevimeline (Evoxac) to ameliorate radiation-induced xerostomia.
> - Acupuncture can improve salivary flow.

by conditioning total body irradiation and chemotherapy for HSCT or other forms of chemotherapy or immunotherapy is also usually transient (Jensen et al. 2010b).

Therapy. Topical mucosal lubricants or saliva substitutes, as well as sugar-free sour lemon drops or other sugar-free acidic hard candies, are useful for patients with mild xerostomia (Jensen et al. 2010a). Acupuncture, transcutaneous electrostimulation, acupuncture-like transcutaneous electrostimulation of the salivary gland, or oral pilocarpine or cevimeline may also be useful (Mercadante et al. 2021). To prevent mouth pain and protect the teeth, I ask patients to avoid foods that contain sugar and encourage them to continue routine oral hygiene, supplemented, in some patients, with fluoride rinses.

For those without cardiac contraindications, the muscarinic agent pilocarpine (Salagen) (5 to 10 mg p.o. t.i.d.) an hour before meals has been shown in randomized controlled clinical trials to be effective in inducing saliva production in patients who have undergone radiation to the oral cavity or neck (Jensen et al. 2010a). The cholinergic agonists cevimeline (Evoxac) (30 mg p.o. t.i.d.) and bethanechol, both of which work through muscarinic receptors, are also effective (Jensen et al. 2010a).

Acupuncture (but not sham acupuncture) increases salivary flow and reduces xerostomia-induced problems, and with follow-up therapy, the effects have been reported to last as long as three years (Blom and Lundeberg 2000). Mucosal lubricants and saliva substitutes can be used by patients who do not respond to any of these therapies.

GASTROINTESTINAL PROBLEMS

Ascites

Ascites is most common in patients with ovarian or breast cancer but also occurs in those with any cancer that involves the peritoneum; other genitourinary, gastrointestinal, or lung cancers; and in those with malnutrition and liver failure.

Ascites that is refractory to the usual diuretic measures (Aldactone [spironolactone] ± oral furosemide) can be difficult to manage. Adding oral hydrochlorothiazide or discontinuing oral furosemide and substituting intravenous furosemide infusions (100 mg over 24 hours) or Bumex (bumetanide) (0.5 to 2 mg/day p.o. or 0.5 to 1 mg IV—do not exceed 10 mg/day) may be effective. For other patients, not until their disease advances and their oral fluid intake diminishes does the ascites stabilize or decrease.

TIPS and peritoneovenous shunts. If patients have only a few months to live, repeated paracentesis may be the most appropriate therapy. Patients who need frequent paracentesis often have a Port-a-cath or PleurX catheter placed in the abdominal wall to facilitate the repeated taps.

But for those patients with a reasonable life expectancy for whom ascites is a major problem, consider a referral for a transjugular intrahepatic portosystemic shunt (TIPS) or percutaneous insertion of a peritoneovenous shunt (i.e., a Denver shunt). TIPS is indicated for patients with ascites from portal or hepatic vein obstruction (not peritoneal carcinomatosis). In a prospective randomized trial of patients who had nonmalignant ascites, patients given TIPS had longer assisted shunt patency (31 months versus 13 months $p < .01$), longer efficacy (85 percent versus 40 percent at 3 years), and longer survival (28.7 versus 16.1 months), but ascites was controlled more quickly with the peritoneovenous shunts (73 percent vs. 46 percent at one month) (Rosemurgy et al. 2004). For patients with malignant ascites, Denver shunts can be placed percutaneously (Yarmohammadi and Getrajdam 2017); they are particularly useful for patients with metastatic breast or ovarian cancer, who live a relatively long time.

Constipation

Constipation is a frequent and distressing problem for patients with cancer. While it occurs in about 15 percent of the general population, it is reported in 32 to 87 percent of patients with advanced cancer (Davies et al. 2020). Constipation can exacerbate anxiety, depression, delirium, anorexia, and nausea and vomiting, and even precipitate hospital admissions.

Prevention. For patients with cancer, as for those without, adequate exercise, oral hydration, and fiber intake are the basics for maintaining regular bowel movements. But exercising and maintaining this intake can be an added burden for patients with cancer. And their usual strategies, for example, taking insoluble fibers such as psyllium, are actually counterproductive if they are unable to take in enough water or are on opioid therapy. Cancer patients often take a number of medications that can exacerbate constipation by dehydrating the patient, slowing gut peristalsis, or increasing the tolerance of their anal sphincters, leading to less frequent defecation. I discuss opioid-induced constipation in Chapter 7. But other medications, especially anticholinergics and octreotide, can also contribute.

Practice Points: Constipation

- Ensure adequate privacy.
- Discontinue contributing medications, when possible, including insoluble fiber.
- Use conventional laxatives (e.g., senna, polyethylene glycol, lactulose; if normal renal function, milk of magnesia, magnesium citrate).
- If refractory, consider adding linaclotide, plecanatide, lubiprostone, or prucalopride.
- If opioid related, consider adding methylnaltrexone, naldemedine, or naloxegol.
- If no stool in response, consider suppositories and enemas.

(Davies et al. 2020; Ginex et al. 2020)

Therapy. Both the European Society for Medical Oncology (ESMO) and the Multinational Association of Supportive Care in Cancer (MASCC) have issued guidelines for treatment of constipation in patients with cancer (Davies et al. 2020). The principle recommendations are listed in Practice Points below. Detailed drug doses for all the agents mentioned can be found in Chapter 7. In addition, in a randomized, parallel, sham-controlled trial, electroacupuncture was found to be more effective than sham acupuncture in significantly increasing weekly complete spontaneous bowel movements for patients with severe chronic *functional* constipation (Liu et al. 2016). Patients with cancer were not excluded but no information was given on whether participants had cancer.

Diarrhea

Etiology. Diarrhea is less common than constipation or nausea and vomiting, but it is found in 4 to 10 percent of terminally ill cancer patients. Common cancer-related etiologies include newly acquired lactose intolerance (e.g., after chemotherapy); chemotherapy-induced gastrointestinal toxicity, especially prominent with 5-fluoruracil and irinotecan; drug effects (metoclopramide or excessive laxatives) or side effects (caffeine, theophylline, antibiotics); intermittent bowel obstruction; fecal impaction; sphincter incompetence (e.g., due to rectal cancer or spinal cord lesions); chronic radiation enteritis; infection; graft-versus-host disease; or products of neuroendocrine tumors. Small cell lung cancers, for example, can produce vasoactive intestinal peptide (VIP), calcitonin, or gastrin. These and other substances from rarer tumors, such as gastrinomas, pheochromocytomas, medullary carcinoma of the thyroid, and especially malignant carcinoid, can cause voluminous diarrhea.

Prevention and therapy. In patients with pelvic malignancies treated by chemotherapy plus radiation therapy or radiation therapy alone, probiotics including

Lactobacillus spp were effective in preventing treatment-induced diarrhea (Bowen et al. 2019).

Specific treatment for the conditions noted above is often effective. Treatment for the diarrhea related to graft-versus-host disease (GVHD) includes resting the gut by making the patient NPO, using antimotility agents, judiciously using opioids for abdominal cramping, and giving small doses of octreotide IV (e.g., octreotide 500 mcg every 8 hours for seven days; Ippoliti et al. 1997), taking care not to induce an ileus.

Evidence defining the optimal antidiarrheal therapy or nutritional support for these patients is not yet available (Kornblau et al. 2000; van der Meij et al. 2012). In a phase II study, an amino acid mixture *enterade* rather than a glucose-based rehydrating solution was effective in reducing diarrhea following bone marrow transplant, and it is under study in patients with neuroendocrine tumors. A retrospective chart review indicated it was also effective in chemotherapy- or immunotherapy-induced diarrhea (Chauhan et al. 2020).

The diarrhea caused by the serotonin and substance P secreted by carcinoids is often controllable with octreotide (150 to 300 µg SQ b.i.d. to t.i.d. or continuous IV or SQ infusion). The use of simple subcutaneous pumps, or instruction of family members in the technique of subcutaneous injections, enables patients to be treated at home. Carcinoid-induced diarrhea may also respond to cyproheptadine. If the diarrhea is refractory to these agents, the addition of telotristat ethyl (Xermelo) has been effective (Kasi 2018).

When specific treatment is unavailable or is ineffective, patients can still be treated symptomatically. Rehydrate them orally using a solution of salted, sugared water such as Gatorade, or intravenously if necessary, and instruct the patient to avoid fats and milk products until the diarrhea resolves. For the diarrhea itself, use loperamide (Imodium), 4 mg by mouth initially, then 2 mg after each loose stool, to a maximum of 16 mg/24 hours, or diphenoxylate/atropine (Lomotil), orally to a maximum of 20 mg/24 hours. If this is ineffective, try tincture of opium, 15 to 20 drops orally every 4 hours.

Dysphagia, Nausea, and Vomiting

Dysphagia, nausea, and vomiting are often amenable to therapy in patients with cancer, even when the cause is irreversible.

Dysphagia

Etiology. Dysphagia can be induced by esophageal candidiasis, as mentioned above; by cancers, especially of the head and neck or of the esophagus; or by the chemotherapy and radiotherapy used to treat them. In one study, about half of patients with solid tumors on therapy reported some symptom of dysphagia, most often for solids (Frowen, Hughes, and Skeat 2020). Almost 90 percent of patients with cancer of the head and neck complained of dysphagia, and more than 60 percent of those with lung, bone and soft tissue, upper gastrointestinal, or colorectal cancer also reported some degree of dysphagia.

Treatment. Patients with dysphagia may benefit from referral to speech and language pathology therapists, which we discuss in Chapter 8. Patients with unresectable esophageal cancer can achieve significant reduction of their dysphagia from short courses of chemo/radiotherapy (Kawamoto et al. 2018). For sicker patients, single-dose brachytherapy was found to be as good as esophageal stenting (see below) in relieving dysphagia (Fuccio et al. 2017).

Simple dilation can provide relief for 2–4 weeks. Expandable metal stents can provide durable relief for patients who are not candidates for other therapies, but about 30 percent of patients develop complications related to the placement (e.g., aspiration) or the stent (e.g., esophageal perforation, stent migration). Tumor growth into the stent can cause occlusion. Patients cannot return to normal eating, unfortunately, after an esophageal stent is placed. They must remain on a liquid or low-residue soft diet (Johnson et al. 2018), which can be difficult for them to accept.

Nausea and Vomiting Unrelated to Treatment

Etiology. Causes of nausea and vomiting include chemotherapy and radiation therapy, disorders of the eighth nerve or vestibular apparatus, constipation, opioids, anxiety, disease of the CNS, hepatic or renal failure, gastritis or gastric ulcer disease, gastric outlet or bowel obstruction, hyponatremia, or hypercalcemia. Those interested in learning more about the physiology of nausea and vomiting can review the paper by Wickham (2020).

Therapy. Reversal of the underlying causes, whenever possible, is recommended. Constipation is a particularly common cause of nausea that can be overlooked because patients assume that they should not have many bowel movements if they are not eating much. Management of constipation, including that induced by opioids, is reviewed above and in Chapter 7. For patients with other underlying causes, both nonpharmacologic and pharmacologic methods can be employed.

Practice Points: Nonpharmacologic Therapy for Nausea

- Provide frequent, small feedings of cold foods.
- Remove foods with unpleasant smell or visual appearance, even if they were prepared for other family members.
- Serve meals in pleasant, comfortable surroundings.
- Refer the patient for progressive relaxation training, hypnosis, or acupuncture.

Families can provide frequent, small feedings of cold foods (which have less odor than warm foods) and remove foods whose sight or smell is unpleasant for the patient. Acupuncture, hypnosis, and progressive relaxation techniques have all shown some effectiveness, especially when the cause is anxiety. Inhaled cannabis can help nausea, or paradoxically, can cause a severe hyperemesis syndrome (Howard 2019; Monte et al. 2019)

Therapy can often be customized to treat the cause of the nausea (Table 10.2; https://pinkbook.dfci.org). Prochlorperazine (Compazine) and ondansetron (Zofran) prevent nausea that commonly occurs during the first few days of opioid therapy. Hyoscyamine (Levsin), scopolamine (Transdermal Scōp), or meclizine (Bonine, Antivert) are helpful for patients with persistent nausea due to vertigo, position change, or noninfectious inner ear problems; patients with these problems describe symptoms of motion sickness or may complain that the room is spinning (LeGrand and Walsh 2010). For nausea caused by gastric irritation from excess acid, a proton pump inhibitor (e.g., esomeprazole 20 mg p.o. daily or b.i.d.), an H2 blocker (e.g., famotidine 300 mg b.i.d.) for patients on capecitabine, or a TKI will help. For gastroparesis not due to opioids, metoclopramide is effective orally or intravenously (5 to 10 mg b.i.d. to q.i.d.) or by continuous subcutaneous or intravenous infusion (1 to 3 mg/hr). If patients develop akathisia from metoclopramide, discontinue it and start a beta-blocker: oral propranolol (40 mg orally t.i.d.) or intravenous metoprolol at an equivalent dose (Avital et al. 2009). Zolmitriptan (7.5 mg p.o. daily), in a double-blind comparative study (Avital et al. 2009), and mirtazapine (15 mg p.o. daily), in a double-blind placebo- and propranolol-controlled trial (Poyurovsky 2006), have also shown efficacy comparable to propranolol in reversing the akathisia, but patients in the Poyurovsky study were given only 40 to 80 mg of propranolol daily.

For patients with uremia or liver metastases, try haloperidol (Haldol) (0.5 to 1 mg t.i.d.), prochlorperazine (Compazine) (5 to 10 mg every 6 to 8 hours p.o. or 25 mg every 12 hours p.r.), or olanzapine (2.5 to 5 mg p.o. or sublingual b.i.d. to q.i.d.). For those with brain metastases, try dexamethasone (4 to 6 mg b.i.d. to q.i.d.); and for those with anxiety, lorazepam (Ativan) (0.5 to 1 mg every 4 to 6 hours p.o. or sublingual) or hydroxyzine (Vistaril) (25 to 100 mg t.i.d. or q.i.d.).

Gels are *ineffective*: lorazepam (Ativan), diphenhydramine (Benadryl), and haloperidol (Haldol) in gels do not reach therapeutic levels after being rubbed into the skin (Smith et al. 2012). If patients receiving gels report decreased nausea, it is likely because of decreased anxiety and the soothing nature of rubbing the gel into the skin. Do not substitute a gel for an oral, intravenous, or rectal formulation of any of these agents.

Treatment-Induced Nausea and Vomiting

While chemotherapy-induced vomiting comes under control in at least 75 percent of patients when the guidelines are followed, chemotherapy-induced nausea (CIN) continues to plague patients with cancer. Younger patients and those receiving high emetogenicity chemotherapy (HEC) are at most risk for severe CIN, and if they develop it, they have a higher incidence of sleep disturbance, depression, morning fatigue, and intrusive thoughts than do those with lower levels of CIN (Singh et al. 2020). While the guidelines I describe below for HEC have been widely available for many years, and a neurokinin (NK-1) inhibitor has been included since 2006, they are underused (Mahendraratnam et al. 2019; Roeland et al. 2020). Only 51 percent of patients have received guideline concurrent care; the NK-1 inhibitor prescription is omitted most often (Mahendraratnam et al. 2019).

Patients at highest risk of developing both nausea and vomiting when they receive chemotherapy are women and those younger than 50 years of age (NCCN 2020). Other risk factors are previous history of CIN, anxiety or high pretreatment expectation of nausea, low alcohol intake, being prone to motion sickness, or having a history of nausea during pregnancy (NCCN 2020a; Mosa et al. 2020).

Pathophysiology. The most likely mechanism for acute and delayed chemotherapy-induced nausea and vomiting (CINV) is stimulation of a neural network in the medulla oblongata called the *central pattern generator.* Several neurotransmitters are thought to be involved, including serotonin, dopamine, and substance P. Drugs that block type 3 serotonin (5-HT3) (e.g., ondansetron), D-2 (e.g., olanzapine), 5HT2C and D2 (e.g. olanzapine), and NK-1 receptors (e.g., aprepitant), if used along with dexamethasone, are able to prevent most CINV (Hesketh et al. 2020; Einhorn et al. 2017). How dexamethasone works remains a mystery, but when it is not included in the antiemetic regimen, patients experience significantly more delayed nausea and vomiting (Roscoe et al. 2012). Vomiting that occurs within a day of receiving chemotherapy is considered *acute,* and that occurring from the second to the fifth day after treatment is considered *delayed.*

The efficacy of cannabinoids is controversial. If they are helpful, it may be because endocannabinoid receptors are in the same area of the brain that contains the 5-HT3, dopamine, and substance P receptors (NASEM 2017). NCCN guidelines (2020a) include the synthetic oral cannabinoids dronabinol (Marinol) and nabilone (Cesamet) for breakthrough nausea or vomiting. The ASCO guidelines, however, did not find the evidence strong enough to include them as a recommended therapy (Hesketh et al. 2020).

Patients can also develop *anticipatory* nausea and vomiting as a classic conditioned response. Those who develop nausea from chemotherapy learn to pair the office sights, smells, and sounds with the nausea and vomiting they experience there or shortly thereafter and experience nausea and vomiting before their scheduled treatment or even at a routine office visit. Having motion sickness (Leventhal et al. 1988), being aware of tastes or odors during infusions, being generally anxious, and having acute or delayed CINV—all increase the odds of developing anticipatory nausea and vomiting (Cohen et al. 1986; Roscoe et al. 2011).

Unfortunately, patients with anticipatory nausea and vomiting can become ill by simply being in your office or seeing people whom they associate with it. Imagine the scene as I greeted a former patient I encountered unexpectedly at an airport. I watched her smile turn to distress as the conditioned reflex took over! I felt nearly as bad as she did.

Therapy. The best way to prevent both anticipatory and delayed CINV is to eliminate the acute symptoms by giving aggressive preventive antiemetic therapy before and after the chemotherapy infusion. Fewer than 15 percent of patients who do not experience acute nausea and vomiting will go on to develop delayed nausea or vomiting; 50 percent of those who do have acute problems will develop delayed vomiting, and 75 percent will have delayed nausea (Roila et al. 2002).

Both nonpharmacologic and pharmacologic approaches are effective for patients with anticipatory nausea and vomiting. Nonpharmacologic therapies include hypnosis (NCCN 2020a; Roscoe et al. 2011), progressive muscle relaxation with guided imagery (NCCN 2020a), systemic desensitization (NCCN 2020a; Morrow and Morrell 1982), distraction techniques (Roscoe et al. 2011), music therapy, yoga, and acupuncture or acupressure (NCCN 2020a). Acupressure was not helpful, however, in reducing acute or delayed nausea (Molassiotis et al. 2013). Lorazepam (0.5 to 2 mg on the night before and the morning of treatment) or alprazolam (0.5 to 2 mg p.o. t.i.d. beginning on the night before treatment) are particularly useful agents for these patients (NCCN 2020a). They cause amnesia for the events surrounding the chemotherapy and decrease anxiety (Laszlo et al. 1985).

Using the ASCO consensus guidelines, Dana-Farber Cancer Institute (DFCI) clinicians created antiemetic therapy order sets (e.g., Hesketh et al. 2020) matched to the emetogenicity of the agents; clinicians are therefore prompted to order the appropriate antiemetics when they order the chemotherapy. The guidelines recommend basing the choice of antiemetic agent(s) on the emetogenic potential of the chemotherapy or radiotherapy regimen (Hesketh et al. 2020; NCCN 2020a), the side-effect profile of the antiemetic agent(s), and patient preferences and characteristics. For patients without prescription programs, unfortunately, cost differences may dictate the outpatient regimen for the days following chemotherapy and therefore the effectiveness of the regimen used.

The side effects of the drugs often vary by age. Younger patients have a higher incidence of CINV. Therefore, even when they are receiving only moderately emetogenic therapy, they may need the multidrug regimen normally prescribed to prevent symptoms in patients receiving drugs of high emetogenicity (Johnson, Moroney, and Gay 1997).

5-HT3 Receptor Antagonists. The 5-HT3 receptor antagonists (e.g. ondansetron, granisetron, dolasetron, and palonosetron) are extremely effective for patients with acute nausea and vomiting from chemotherapy or radiation. They are given orally or intravenously, usually along with dexamethasone, to patients receiving moderate or highly emetogenic chemotherapy (Einhorn et al. 2017; Hesketh et al.

Risk Factors for Chemotherapy-Induced Nausea and Vomiting

- History of acute chemotherapy-related nausea or vomiting
- Emetogenicity of drug
- Age <50
- Female sex
- Low alcohol intake
- Generalized anxiety / high pretreatment expectation of nausea
- Prone to motion sickness / history of nausea/morning sickness during pregnancy

---

2020). When these agents are given along with dexamethasone, 75 percent of patients have no acute vomiting. Palonosetron blocks the 5-HT3 receptor for as long as 40 hours (NCCN 2020).

Patients receiving ondansetron or the other 5-HT3 receptor antagonists often develop constipation and may develop mild headache and elevations in transaminases. QTc prolongations occur at higher doses of ondansetron, and the recommendations therefore suggest that the maximum daily dose be 24 mg/day. Palonosetron has shown minimal prolongation of the QTc in limited studies.

Corticosteroids. We still do not understand how corticosteroids prevent CINV. Some have suggested that they relieve the cerebral edema induced by chemotherapeutic agents, such as cisplatin (Roila et al. 2002). Corticosteroids can be used either alone, when the chemotherapy has only low or moderate potential to cause vomiting, or as part of a regimen with a 5-HT3 antagonist, olanzapine, or an NK-1 inhibitor (Einhorn et al. 2017; Hesketh et al. 2020). Dexamethasone and methylprednisolone are the best-studied agents, but no trials have demonstrated the superiority of one corticosteroid over another. In patients with severe liver impairment, use prednisolone or methylprednisolone rather than prednisone, which the liver converts to prednisolone.

NK-1 Inhibitors. Substance P, a neurotransmitter that plays a key role in the transmission of the pain signal, can also cause vomiting, and it appears to play a role in CINV and radiation-related nausea and vomiting. Its effects are mediated through NK-1 receptors. Agents that cross the blood-brain barrier and act as NK-1 inhibitors (e.g., aprepitant, fosaprepitant, rolapitant, netupitant-palonosetron, fosnetupitant-palonosetron) are particularly effective in decreasing the delayed nausea and vomiting occurring after cisplatin chemotherapy (Einhorn et al. 2017; Hesketh et al. 2020).

Aprepitant itself has few side effects, but it is an inhibitor of CYP3A4 and therefore may elevate levels of dexamethasone and chemotherapeutic agents primarily metabolized by this route. Aprepitant can also cause significant decreases in the prolongation of the international normalized ratio (INR) induced by warfarin.

Patients will have less nausea and vomiting if they take aprepitant as part of the antiemetic regimen both on the day of chemotherapy and for two days after their last dose of chemotherapy for each cycle (Einhorn et al. 2017; Hesketh et al. 2020). Fosaprepitant is given intravenously on Day 1 and has not been found to be inferior to aprepitant in preventing the nausea and vomiting of patients treated with cisplatin (Grunberg et al. 2011). Similarly, netupitant in combination with palonosetron or fosnetupitant with palonosetron are taken orally on Day 1 and provide equivalent protection (Einhorn et al. 2017; Hesketh et al. 2020).

Olanzapine. Olanzapine is an atypical antipsychotic that increases appetite and weight in patients not receiving chemotherapy. It binds a number of CNS receptors and is now part of the standard antiemetic regimen for patients receiving some forms of highly emetogenic chemotherapy. It is also a useful rescue agent for patients whose nausea hasn't responded to the agents discussed above. Olanzapine usually has few side effects, but it does lower the seizure threshold, can cause dystonic reactions, and has been reported (rarely) to cause neuroleptic malignant syndrome or insulin-resistant diabetes.

Ginger. Pretreatment with ginger, which is known to bind 5-HT3 receptors, may be an effective adjuvant antiemetic, but there was insufficient evidence of its efficacy for it to be included in the ASCO 2017 antiemetic guidelines (Hesketh et al. 2020). Ginger may be useful for acute (Day 1) CINV related to carboplatin/paclitaxel (Uthaipaisanwong, Oranratanaphan, and Musigavong 2020) or for nausea, dysmotility, and reflux-like symptoms unrelated to chemotherapy (Bhargava et al. 2020).

Prevention of Nausea and Vomiting from Chemotherapy		
Emetogenic Risk	**Day 1 Therapy**	**Day 2 to Day 4**
High	Dex + 5-HT3 RA + NK-1 inhibitor + olanzapine	Dex d 2–4 + NK-1 + olanzapine
AC	Dex + 5-HT3 RA + NK-1 inhibitor	Olanzapine
Carboplatin	Dex + 5-HT3 RA + NK-1 inhibitor	
Moderate	Dex + 5-HT3 RA	
Low	Dex or 5-HT3	

Note: Level of risk is based on emetogenicity of the drug. AC = Adriamycin + cyclophosphamide therapy.

(From Hesketh et al. 2020)

Prevention of Nausea and Vomiting from Radiation Therapy

Emetogenic Risk	Day 1 Pretherapy	Pretherapy Day 2 to Day following end of XRT
High	5-HT3 RA + dex	5-HT3 RA + dex
Moderate	5-HT3 RA ± dex	5-HT3 RA ± dex (next 4 fractions)
Brain Rescue	Dex	Rescue dex
H&N, thorax, pelvis rescue	5-HT3 RA + Dex or dopamine antagonist	
Low	Dex or 5-HT3	

Note: Level of risk is based on emetogenicity of the radiation therapy.

(From Hesketh et al. 2020)

Other agents. For patients who are not responding to these drugs alone, adding haloperidol, droperidol, prochlorperazine, scopolamine, or oral cannabinoids may be helpful (NCCN 2020a). Many of these agents, however, have significant side effects. Haloperidol and droperidol can produce dystonic reactions, akathisia, QTc prolongation, and occasionally hypotension. Transdermal scopolamine causes dry eyes and a xerostomia that can be intolerable.

Combination antiemetic therapy. Prophylactic and breakthrough antiemetic recommendations for chemotherapeutic drugs and radiation regimens with low to high emetogenic potential are listed above (Einhorn et al. 2017; Hesketh et al. 2020). Radiation of the GI tract is particularly problematic because it releases significant amounts of both serotonin and substance P from the gut, which contains 80 percent of the body's stores of these neurotransmitters.

Malignant Bowel Obstruction–Induced Nausea and Vomiting

The extent of the evaluation of a patient with a malignant bowel obstruction (MBO) depends on the presumed etiology of the obstruction, the likely responsiveness of the cancer to specific antineoplastic therapy, and the patient's nutritional status, prognosis, and wishes for aggressive therapies. Soriano and Davis (2011) provide an excellent review of the evaluation and therapeutic options for patients with advanced disease. Consultation with a surgeon (Englert et al. 2012) or gastroenterologist who specializes in treating patients with malignant bowel obstruction is often indicated. Surgeons can, in selected patients, resect the obstruction and anastomose the remaining bowel, bypass a gastric or small bowel obstruction with a gastrojejunal bypass, or leave the obstructed bowel itself untreated but create ileostomies or colostomies to decompress the bowel and allow patients to eat normally again.

Stents. Patients who are not candidates for surgery or who do not wish to undergo it may benefit from insertion of a self-expanding metal stent to relieve gastric outlet or proximal small bowel obstruction (SBO) (Katsanos, Sabharwal, and Adam 2010). Stents most often are successful in patients who are not elderly and do not have ascites, peritoneal carcinomatosis, previous radiation to the pelvis, or evidence of multiple sites of obstruction (Ripamonti, Easson, and Gerdes 2008). Pyloric or duodenal stenting was found to provide symptomatic relief in 80 percent of patients (Johnson et al. 2018). Patients are limited, however, to a low-residue diet. These stents can, of course, migrate, perforate the bowel, or cause bleeding, but the incidence is low, 0 to 4 percent (Johnson et al. 2018).

Colonic stents can usually be placed endoscopically (success rate of 90 to 93 percent) but are not recommended when the blockage is less than 5 cm from the anal verge, because of the accompanying incontinence, rectal pain, and risk of migration (Johnson et al. 2018). Whether or not stenting the colon is a helpful bridge to surgery remains controversial, but the evidence seems to suggest that stents are not helpful in this role (Allievi et al. 2017; NIHCE 2011).

Before surgery, stenting, or medical therapy provide more definitive relief, nasogastric (NG) intubation is often required as a temporary measure. Patients with only a partial bowel obstruction or an ileus often respond to a corticosteroid (I often use dexamethasone 2 to 4 mg daily or twice daily) and metoclopramide (5 to 10 mg IV every 6 hours or 1 to 2 mg/hr). Metoclopramide's procholinergic activity enhances gastric motility and, to a lesser extent, motility in the jejunum, ileum, and colon. If cramping increases, however, the obstruction may be worsening; the metoclopramide should be discontinued and anticholinergic agents added if the cramping persists.

When the small bowel is obstructed, intestinal cells produce increased amounts of serotonin, substance P, nitric oxide, acetylcholine, somatomedin, and VIP (Bozzetti 2019). Medical treatment therefore includes, in addition to decompression with an NG tube and opioids, dexamethasone, anticholinergic agents, and for refractory patients, somatostatin. Glycopyrrolate, hyoscyamine, or scopolamine can be helpful for patients who have a great deal of cramping abdominal pain. The anticholinergic activity decreases motility and therefore abdominal colic, so that opioids can be minimized. Anticholinergics also activate muscarinic receptors, and thus decrease the secretion of water, sodium, and chloride. Scopolamine, however, often produces excessively dry mouth and eyes as well as mydriasis, and because it crosses the blood-brain barrier, it can increase the chance of the patient becoming delirious.

For patients who cannot tolerate anticholinergic agents, or whose obstruction does not respond to the combination of these agents, stop the anticholinergic agents, consider adding intravenous olanzapine for nausea (2.5–5 mg IV q6h PRN), and add octreotide. If the obstruction is not complete, octreotide is often very effective. It is a synthetic analogue of somatostatin, and as such, it inhibits

---

**Practice Points: Treating Bowel Obstruction in Patients
Who Are Not Candidates for Surgery**

- Gastric outlet obstruction:
  - NG tube; evaluate for a self-expanding metal stent or venting gastrostomy (PEG)
  - Medical therapy: dexamethasone + octreotide + analgesics (± metoclopramide)
  - Consider duodenal stent
- Small intestinal obstruction:
  - Initial: dexamethasone + opioids; consider glycopyrrolate or scopolamine patch for persistent nausea, vomiting, and cramping abdominal pain
  - If only a partial bowel obstruction or an ileus, add metoclopramide (5–10 mg IV q6h or 1 to 2 mg/hr) rather than glycopyrrolate or scopolamine
  - Persistent obstruction: NG tube if not already in place; discontinue scopolamine or glycopyrrolate (if complete obstruction, discontinue metoclopramide) and add octreotide 300 to 600 µg/24 hr SQ in divided doses (b.i.d. or t.i.d.). Consider adding olanzapine 2.5 to 5 mg IV q6h for nausea
  - For responders to octreotide: administer depot version (e.g., LAR octreotide) monthly, 20–30 mg deep IM; continue SQ octreotide for ≈14 days after depot is given

---

secretion of growth hormone, gastrin, secretin, VIP, pancreatic polypeptide, insulin, and glucagon, as well as blocking the secretion of gastric acid, pepsin, pancreatic enzymes, bicarbonate, and, probably most important for these patients, intestinal epithelial water and electrolytes.

A typical patient who would benefit from octreotide is someone with advanced ovarian cancer whose symptoms are due to recurrent partial bowel obstructions by tumor implants or adhesions. At doses of 150 to 300 µg subcutaneously, twice daily (or 300 to 600 µg/24 hr continuous SQ infusion), octreotide has produced major improvements in these patients' lives. In about three days (range of one to six days), it can eliminate the nausea and vomiting in the majority of patients for whom it is tried and, in patients who are able to minimize oral fluid intake, dramatically decrease the volume of nasogastric drainage enough to allow removal of the NG tube (if the secretions fall to <1 L/day) (Mercadante and Porzio 2012; Bozzetti 2019).

Patients who respond to SQ octreotide and are expected to have persistent bowel obstruction should be given an intramuscular injection of the LAR form of octreotide or lanreotide microparticles monthly. The agents are released from a microsphere polymer matrix, and it takes two to three weeks for therapeutic blood levels to be achieved. Patients need to continue taking their SQ octreotide, therefore, for two to three weeks after either LAR injection (Mariani et al. 2012; Prommer 2008).

In 2006, Laval and colleagues published the results of their prospective study of patients who required medical therapy for a malignant bowel obstruction (Laval et al. 2006). In 2019, a study of a pilot interprofessional program for patients with gynecologic cancer was published (Lee et al. 2019), but as of 2021, no randomized controlled trials have appeared, and the Laval study is the largest prospective study of patients with malignant bowel obstruction from any type of cancer reported to date. This study followed 75 consecutive patients with peritoneal carcinomatosis (80 obstructive episodes). The largest group had cancer of the ovary (21 patients) or colorectal cancer (19 patients); 10 had pancreatic, and 9 had esophageal or stomach cancer.

For the first five days, patients had an NG tube placed and received a corticosteroid (Solumedrol 1–4 mg/kg), an antiemetic (haloperidol 1–5 mg/8 hr, or chlorpromazine 25–50 mg/8 hr, or continuous IV or SQ pump), an anticholinergic agent (scopolamine), and analgesics as needed. If their bowel obstruction resolved, the corticosteroids and antisecretory drugs were tapered off. If they were still obstructed, or the NG tube was putting out more than 1 L/24 hours, they received octreotide 200 µg every 8 hours or 600 µg/day by continuous infusion. If the patient was still refractory to therapy three days later, when possible, a venting gastrostomy tube or a stent was placed.

This protocol was very effective. In general, 92 percent of patients who improve on medical therapy will do it by Day 7 (Bozzetti 2019). In this study, the median time to controlled symptoms was 5 days. Fifty of 80 obstructive episodes improved in the first five days. In 25 of those 50, the obstruction was relieved. It was most effective in corticosteroid-naive patients: 20 of 25 whose obstruction was relieved had not received previous corticosteroids. The obstruction resolved in only 30 of 55 who had received previous steroids ($p < .03$). Of the remaining 30 patients, the addition of octreotide relieved the obstruction in 4 patients, and an additional 7 achieved symptom control.

Nutrition. Some patients with partial bowel obstruction can maintain intake of a low to minimal fiber diet, or, if the symptoms are severe, a liquid or blenderized diet, especially if they have had a stent placed successfully. Dieticians can provide definitions of the foods in each category and recipes to maximize nutrition within these limitations. Enteral nutrition is not recommended.

It is not clear which patients benefit from total parenteral nutrition (TPN), because no randomized trials have been done, and systematic reviews are inconclusive. Overall, patients with inoperable MBO have a median survival of 1–9 months after diagnosis (Bozzetti 2019). Careful consideration must be given to the goals of TPN supplementation, the prognosis using parenteral fluids alone without TPN, the ability of the family to manage the infusions safely, and the likelihood of improved length and quality of life.

Nausea and Vomiting of Unclear Etiology

Symptomatic therapy is used for patients with nausea of unclear etiology. A systematic review of the studies on nausea or vomiting not caused by radiation or chemotherapy concluded that the studies were inadequate to provide definitive recommendations (Davis and Hallerberg 2010).

Most of the available guidelines are based on expert opinion. What follows, therefore, is my "expert opinion." For someone with nausea or vomiting of unknown etiology, start with a proton pump inhibitor to minimize stomach acid; patients may not complain of burning or have bleeding, but their gastritis is presenting as nausea. Omeprazole 20 mg by mouth once or twice daily is often helpful, except for patients who are taking capecitabine or a tyrosine kinase inhibitor (TKI). Those patients should be given an H2 blocker, such as famotidine, instead, 300 mg by mouth daily to twice a day. For patients who feel "full up to here" (gesturing at the top of their necks), I use metoclopramide (Reglan) (5 to 10 mg p.o., SQ, or IV every 6 hours or 1 hour before meals). Give it "standing" not as needed for several days and reassess. At this dose, metoclopramide is associated with few side effects, but monitor for increased anxiety and akathisia. If nausea persists, discontinue the metoclopramide and add olanzapine.

Olanzapine is an atypical antipsychotic agent that blocks the receptors of several neurotransmitters, including dopamine and serotonin. It is not surprising, then, that a series of case reports indicate that it is effective against nausea of unclear etiologies in patients with cancer. It rarely causes extrapyramidal side effects. Doses start at 2.5 mg at bedtime and can be increased to 5 mg four times a day as needed. Weight gain is a serious problem for patients without cancer who take olanzapine, but this can be a helpful side effect for many with cancer.

If olanzapine is not effective, discontinue the olanzapine and try dexamethasone (4 mg daily or b.i.d at 8 a.m. and 2 p.m.), ondansetron (Zofran) (4 to 8 mg p.o. b.i.d. to t.i.d.), lorazepam (0.5 to 1 mg p.o. b.i.d. to t.i.d.), or haloperidol (Haldol) (1 to 2 mg p.o. b.i.d. to q.i.d.). For patients who do not mind the associated alterations in mental status, dronabinol (synthetic tetrahydrocannabinol) (Marinol) (2.5 to 10 mg p.o. b.i.d. to t.i.d., or higher as needed and tolerated) or medical marijuana can be an effective oral antiemetic. Unfortunately, its oral absorption is somewhat variable. Data on the ideal ratio of tetrahydrocannabinol:cannabidiol (THC:CBD) are not available for nausea. Inhaled cannabis is absorbed quickly, and the peak effect is reached within 30 minutes. It has much the same side-effect profile as dronabinol, although the higher the CBD content, the more the psychoactive effects of the THC may be tempered. The integrative therapies for nausea, such as hypnosis, acupuncture, and mindfulness-based stress reduction, are discussed in Chapter 8.

RESPIRATORY PROBLEMS
Dyspnea

Dyspnea is frightening to patients with advanced cancer and to their families, who fear they will die of suffocation. You may not realize that a patient is experiencing dyspnea if you rely solely on observing tachypnea. In one study of hospice patients, 77 percent of patients reported dyspnea, but only 39 percent were recorded as having dyspnea (Thomas and von Gunten 2003).

Pathophysiology. Dyspnea is mediated by (1) J-receptors at the junction of capillaries and alveoli, which respond to alveolar fluid or to microemboli; (2) mechanoreceptors in the lungs, airways, and chest wall that respond to stretch; (3) peripheral chemoreceptors in the aorta and carotid bodies that respond to hypoxemia; and (4) central chemoreceptors that respond to increases in carbon dioxide. When the CO_2 rises to 75 mm Hg, endorphins are released centrally, causing the dyspnea to abate and the patient to become somnolent.

Patients experience dyspnea in one of three situations: when breathing requires more work (e.g., with interstitial lung disease or pleural effusions); when the patient is hypercapnic; and when the brain perceives less ventilation than it "expects" from the amount of work being done to provide the ventilation. The brain receives input on the work the muscles are doing, and "expects" a certain amount of return on the investment in terms of flow rate of air. When there is less airflow than expected, the patient experiences dyspnea. Patients who are not hypoxemic, therefore, can still be dyspneic. But oxygen therapy is no better than nasal air for them (Clemens, Quednau, and Klaschik 2009). The nasal air infusion "tricks" the mechanoreceptors into thinking the muscles are doing more work than they are. This "tricking" of the mechanoreceptors also likely explains the efficacy of a bedside fan or open window.

Etiology. In 25 percent of patients with dyspnea, no specific cause will be identified, but muscle weakness or anxiety may contribute. In the other 75 percent, a thorough physical exam and a few simple tests (e.g., chest x-ray, electrolytes, complete blood count, and pulse oximetry) are likely to reveal the cause of the dyspnea. The most common etiologies are pulmonary or cardiac pathology, ascites, anemia, and superior vena cava syndrome.

Pleural effusions are a frequent cause of dyspnea in patients with lung or breast cancer but also occur in patients with other kinds of cancer.

Pericardial effusions and tamponade are particularly subtle causes of dyspnea in cancer patients. A tumor infiltrating the pericardium causes it to become thick and rigid, and even a small amount of fluid can significantly impair cardiac filling. Because of the rigidity of the invaded pericardium, chest films may show a normal heart size even when tamponade is present. Have a high index of suspicion when a patient with known mediastinal disease or, more commonly, a left-sided pleural effusion which has already been drained remains anxious and dyspneic.

. *Superior vena cava syndrome* is most often seen in patients with lung cancer, though lymphoma and other cancers each cause about 10 percent of cases, with a smaller contribution from clotted indwelling central venous catheters. In addition to dyspnea, patients may have headache or blurred vision and appear plethoric, with facial, neck, and upper extremity edema in advanced cases. Chest films reveal disease in the right upper mediastinum, and radionuclide or MRI studies show compression of the superior vena cava with decreased flow.

Procedures to Reverse the Cause

When possible, and as appropriate, reverse the specific medical cause of the dyspnea. Because dyspnea can be so distressing, it is reasonable to consider somewhat aggressive attempts to reverse obstruction of bronchi, blood vessels, or lymphatics to decrease the dyspnea. External beam or endobronchial radiation therapy, laser treatments, cryotherapy, and stents all can reopen blocked airways. For some patients whose bronchial obstruction is not relieved, radiation therapy still relieves the dyspnea, possibly by decreasing compression of the surrounding blood vessels and lymphatics.

Pleural effusions. Many patients experience relief only when their pleural effusions are drained. Because the effusion reaccumulates within one month in 97 percent of treated patients, most patients with malignant effusions will need more than a simple thoracentesis. Sclerotherapy has been done with bleomycin (Barbetakis et al. 2004) and doxycycline, but talc slurries inserted via thoracoscopy have been shown to be most effective (Shaw and Agrawal 2004; Dresler et al. 2005). The chemotherapeutic drug mitoxantrone (40 mg) is another effective sclerosing agent, infused after chest tube drainage (Barbetakis et al. 2004).

Some patients have such extensive effusions or such a high rate of fluid production that the pleural space cannot be drained enough for a sclerosing agent to be effective; in others, despite adequate drainage, the lung will not re-expand. The quality of life of such patients may be severely impaired by the effusions or the collapsed lung. For those with a reasonable life expectancy (e.g., patients with breast cancer or lymphoma), a surgical procedure may be helpful.

Some surgeons believe that for patients who can tolerate general anesthesia, an open procedure is indicated; they can decide at surgery whether to use talc pleurodesis or to insert a pleural catheter. If, after the fluid is drained, the lung re-expands fully, the surgeon uses talc as an irritant. This procedure has been successful in preventing recurrent effusions in more than 90 percent of those undergoing it. If, however, the lung does not re-expand, the surgeon inserts a pleural catheter (e.g., PleurX). Patients drain the pleural fluid at home, and spontaneous pleurodesis often occurs.

Symptomatic therapy, however, is appropriate for very debilitated patients whose prognosis is so short that they are not candidates for surgical drainage of pleural effusions. In one study, patients with malignant pleural effusions who had leukocytosis, hypoxemia, and hypoalbuminemia had a median survival of only 42 days, compared with those with none of those factors who lived a median of 702 days ($p < .00001$) (Pilling et al. 2010).

Superior vena cava syndrome. About 70 percent of patients with superior vena cava syndrome will respond to radiation therapy for a median of about 3 months. High-dose corticosteroids are also usually included; they are tapered after a week if no benefit is observed or after the end of radiation treatments.

Anemia. Blood transfusion may be tried for hypoxia due to anemia.

Pericardial effusion. Some patients' effusions stop after pericardiocentesis followed by drainage with a pigtail catheter. Other patients may need a pericardial window draining into the left or right hemithorax. If both sides of the chest are already sclerosed, the window is placed through the diaphragm into the abdomen to provide ongoing drainage of the effusion.

Pharmacologic-Specific Therapies

Anxiety. Anxious patients are likely to benefit from both pharmacologic and non-pharmacologic therapies. Lorazepam (0.5 to 2 mg every 4 to 6 hours p.o. or sublingual), clonazepam (0.5 to 1 mg p.o. at bedtime or b.i.d.), or the other agents listed in Table 10.3 are helpful to decrease anxiety in the average patient. For very anxious patients or patients in an uncontrolled panic due to a perceived inability to breathe, give midazolam (0.2 to 0.5 mg IV very slowly); morphine (2 to 5 mg IV), or another opioid at an equivalent dose; or chlorpromazine (12.5 to 25 mg p.o. or IV). Morphine and midazolam (Kloke and Cherny 2015) or lorazepam (Clemens and Klaschik 2011; Kloke and Cherny 2015) have been given together without inducing respiratory depression.

Relaxation techniques or formal hypnotic imagery may be effective adjuncts that skilled practitioners can teach to anxious patients and their families. Medical practitioners of hypnosis are listed in the directory of members of the American Society of Clinical Hypnosis (www.asch.net).

Hypoxia. Oxygen is indicated even for patients who retain CO_2 to maintain an oxygen saturation of 88 to 90 percent (pO_2 of 55 to 60 mm Hg). Oxygen is helpful both in hypoxemic patients (Swan et al. 2019) and those with normal oxygenation but increased work of breathing. As noted above, the flow of oxygen through the nares will trick the mechanoreceptors, and the dyspnea will decrease. In fact, "medical air" via nasal cannula is helpful for patients who are dyspneic (Swan et al. 2019). Both high-flow oxygen and high-flow air relieved dyspnea in hospitalized cancer patients (Hui et al. 2020).

High-flow nasal cannula (HFNC) oxygen therapy has become more commonly used to support hypoxemic patients to avoid intubation and to provide extra time for patients near the end of life who do not want to be intubated. It is more comfortable than other forms of noninvasive ventilation, causes less skin breakdown, and provides better reduction in dyspnea and respiratory rate (Shah, Mehta, and

Mehta 2018). Flows of 50–60 L can be delivered at oxygen concentrations up to 100 percent. It is contraindicated in patients with hypercapnic respiratory failure.

The use of HFNC can prevent patients from coming home, however, since the high flows they need cannot be delivered outside a hospital setting. Staff may find that while ethically they are identical, they have more moral distress weaning the HFNC in someone who no longer wants it for life prolongation than they would extubating the same patient. They benefit from support and discussion of the ethical issues, as well as an ethics consultation, if requested.

Lymphangitic tumor. High-dose corticosteroids alone (e.g., 80 mg solumedrol IV t.i.d. for 3 days) can ameliorate dyspnea in patients with lymphangitic tumor spread, possibly by inhibiting the inflammatory reaction to the tumor and lessening alveolar capillary fluid leak (Kloke and Cherny 2015).

Symptomatic Therapy

For the 25 percent of patients for whom no specific cause of dyspnea can be identified, symptomatic treatment is still possible. For these patients and for those in whom we cannot reverse the underlying cause, various nonpharmacologic and pharmacologic (Table 10.3) therapies will significantly relieve their distress.

Nonpharmacologic. Pulmonary rehabilitation has been shown to be an effective quality-of-life intervention for lung cancer patients recovering from surgery (Cavalheri et al. 2019), undergoing active cancer therapy (Tiep et al. 2015), or with COPD or advanced cancer (Peddle-McIntyre et al. 2019), but the 2021 ASCO guideline found insufficient evidence to recommend for or against it (Hui et al. 2021). And something as simple as sitting in front of an open window or having a fan blowing air softly onto the face provides significant relief for some (Qian et al. 2019; Swan et al. 2019). Counseling alone, or with relaxation-breathing training, music therapy, relaxation training, and psychotherapy have all been shown to be effective (Bausewein et al. 2008). Other validated therapies include vibration of the patient's chest wall, electrical stimulation of leg muscles, walking aids, and breathing training; results for acupuncture and acupressure are mixed (Bausewein et al. 2008).

Opioids. The most useful treatment, even for cancer patients taking high doses of systemic opioids, is an oral, subcutaneous, or intravenous opioid (Barnes et al. 2016; Benítez-Rosario et al. 2019; Viola et al. 2008). A 2017 *Cochrane Review* found no clinically relevant adverse effects from their use in patients with chronic breathlessness (Verberkt et al. 2017). Nebulized opioids are not recommended (Barnes et al. 2016; Viola et al. 2008). In patients who are acidotic with compensatory tachypnea, opioids will not decrease the tachypnea and should not be escalated for that purpose.

Typical starting doses for dyspnea may be less than what is required for pain. In an opioid-naive patient, 2.5 to 5 mg of morphine may be given orally every 4 hours as needed, or fentanyl 10–25 mcg every 1–2 hours by IV or subcutaneously.

For opioid-tolerant patients, the usual rescue dose is used initially, and then increased by 30–50 percent as needed until the dyspnea is relieved, though sedation may occur at higher doses. The 2021 ASCO guideline supported the use of continuous palliative sedation for refractory dyspnea in patients with a life expectancy of days (Hui et al. 2021). Palliative sedation is discussed in Chapter 12.

Fentanyl (in a spray delivered sublingually) used prophylactically was found in a small double-blind randomized trial of opioid-tolerant cancer patients to decrease exertional dyspnea and improve walking distance (Hui et al. 2019). Fixed-dose controlled-release oxycodone (5 mg q8h), however, was not more effective than placebo in essentially opioid-naive patients with chronic breathlessness (Ferreira et al. 2020), but it is hard to conclude that the agent, rather than the dose, was ineffective.

Cough

Etiology. Cough, present in about 40 percent of patients with advanced cancer, is caused by many of the same disorders that cause dyspnea. It is mediated by stimulation of the vagus nerve by receptors in the pharynx, larynx, and upper airways and by airway opiate receptors.

Cough can occur in patients with postnasal drip, infection, heart failure, asthma, chronic obstructive lung disease, esophageal reflux, or those taking ACE inhibitors. Specific cancer-related causes include both obstruction of the airway and disorders of swallowing. Swallowing disorders can be due to ischemic vascular disease or brain metastases, injuries of the ninth and tenth cranial nerves from local or metastatic tumor invasion or carcinomatous meningitis, impairment of the recurrent laryngeal nerve by tumor in the left hilar area, or tumor of the head and neck or esophagus. Such patients can aspirate their routine secretions, and cough can be their most troubling symptom.

Therapy. Specific therapies are used for the causes listed above. Laser or radiation therapy may resolve a distressing cough due to an airway obstruction. For those without an obstruction whose cough is productive, chest physical therapy, humidity, and suctioning can help.

Various pharmacologic agents for symptomatic treatment of cough are listed in Table 10.3. Benzonatate (Tessalon Perles) (one or two p.o. t.i.d.) has an anesthetic action that numbs the stretch sensors in the lower airways and lung and thus prevents the coughs induced by deep breathing. Relief starts within 15 minutes, and the effect of each dose can last for several hours. Hyoscyamine (Levsin) or scopolamine (Transderm Scōp) can decrease excessive secretions. For patients who cough because of tenacious mucus, nebulized saline, albuterol (0.5 mg in 2.5 mg of normal saline), or terbutaline have been helpful, while expectorants such as guaifenesin and mucolytics have not. Since ipratropium worsens this problem, discontinue it when possible.

When specific therapy is unavailable or ineffective, oral opioids are the most effective nonspecific therapies for cough. Initially, try sweet elixirs containing dextromethorphan or one of the opioids used for mild pain; methadone syrup, if available, can also be useful.

For more resistant coughs, higher doses of oral opioids (see "Dyspnea," above) may be needed. In addition, nebulized anesthetics (e.g., 2 ml of 2% lidocaine in 1 ml of normal saline for 10 minutes) can be given up to three times a day. Unfortunately, the anesthetics cause patients to lose their gag reflex temporarily. To avoid aspiration, ask patients to fast for about one hour after a nebulized anesthetic treatment. Since some patients develop bronchospasm after nebulized anesthetics, the first dose should be taken under close observation.

Hemoptysis

Although 50 to 70 percent of patients with lung cancer complain of hemoptysis, it is a problem for only about 25 percent of those admitted to hospice programs. Despite its relative rarity, however, hemoptysis is one of the most frightening symptoms that patients experience. Letting the family know what to do should the hemoptysis worsen and advising them to use red or dark-colored bedding and towels, on which the blood is less apparent, may lessen their anxiety. (For a discussion of managing patients with massive hemoptysis at the end of life, see Chapter 12.)

As in patients without cancer, hemoptysis in cancer patients may be due to bronchitis, pneumonia, or a pulmonary embolism. In patients with cancer of the head and neck or lung, however, it is often due to cancer recurrence. Even for patients who have previously received radiation treatment, small amounts of additional radiation can control the bleeding in almost 90 percent. Tranexamic acid is an antifibrinolytic available for inhalation. In one well-done double-blind randomized placebo-controlled trial of patients with <200 mL/24 hours of expectorated blood, 96 percent of patients who received tranexamic acid resolved their bleeding within 5 days, as opposed to 50 percent of those receiving placebo ($p < 0.0005$); no patients in the tranexamic acid arm required an interventional procedure, versus 18 percent in the placebo group. At one year, the treated group had a 4 percent recurrence rate, compared with 22.7 percent in the placebo group (Wand et al. 2018).

Bronchial lavage with iced saline, topical epinephrine, topical fibrinogen-thrombin solutions, balloon tamponade, and laser therapy may also be helpful. Embolization of the portions of the bronchial artery involved has been found to be particularly effective for patients with bronchiectasis and inflammation. In patients with lung cancer, more than three-quarters of the patients embolized stopped bleeding (Marcelin et al. 2018). The optimal therapy for a given patient, therefore, may depend both on the site of bleeding and on the radiation, pulmonary, and angiographic expertise available.

Hiccups

Hiccups are embarrassing and exhausting, and they interfere with a patient's ability to eat, drink, and sleep.

Etiology. Although hiccups can occur in patients with any of one hundred different diseases, the most common causes are gastroesophageal reflux disease (GERD) or gastric distension, problems in the chest or lung, or problems in the central nervous system (Calsina-Berna et al. 2012). Eighty percent of the time, hiccups are caused by a unilateral contraction of the left hemidiaphragm, and the problem is almost always (91 to 99 percent of the time) self-limited (Calsina-Berna et al. 2012).

Hiccups may occur in patients whose vagus or phrenic nerves are injured (anywhere in their course) or who have certain metabolic derangements (especially uremia, but also hyponatremia or hypocalcemia). Patients can develop hiccups as a side effect of benzodiazepines, barbiturates, progesterone, anabolic steroids, intravenous corticosteroids, or, more rarely, chemotherapy (e.g., cisplatin) or hydrocodone. Occasionally, you will find a previously unidentified ear infection, pharyngitis, or esophagitis, which, if treated effectively, may end the hiccups, as may treating ascites, pneumonia, pleuritis, or pericarditis. The systematic review by Calsina-Berna and colleagues (2012) offers an exhaustive list of potential causes.

Therapy. The nonpharmacologic treatments are those we've all used: granulated sugar, drinking from the far side of a glass, rubbing the back of the neck with a cool cloth, holding one's breath, or doing a Valsalva maneuver while breath holding. Acupuncture was effective in one retrospective series. For selected patients with intractable hiccups, phrenic nerve block (e.g., with bupivacaine) or lysis may be required, but these treatments are rarely needed.

Some pharmacologic treatments are listed in Table 10.3. Baclofen, gabapentin, and metoclopramide (5 to 10 mg p.o. q.i.d) are the best studied. Metoclopramide and baclofen are the only ones studied in RCTs (Polito and Fellows 2017). Baclofen is started at 5 to 10 mg orally three times a day and may be increased as needed; concomitant alcohol use should be avoided to prevent excessive sedation. Gabapentin, which blocks calcium channels, improved hiccups in 83 percent of patients in one retrospective chart review, at a dose of 300 mg initially, increasing to 1200 mg if needed; and pregabalin is equally effective. Metoclopramide is started at 5 to 10 mg by mouth or IV every 6 hours as needed. Chlorpromazine (Thorazine) (25 to 50 mg IV, then p.o. or p.r. t.i.d.) is the only FDA-approved drug for hiccups. It is effective, but it causes significant postural hypotension (Howard et al. 2011) and sedation. Haloperidol (Haldol) (2 to 5 mg p.o. or p.r. or 0.5 to 2 mg IV) is probably equally effective but safer in older patients; amantadine worked in a patient with Parkinson's disease (Hernandez et al. 2015), perhaps by improving the disease-associated gastroparesis. Hiccups due to GERD respond to proton pump inhibitors, but they cannot be used in patients who are on capecitabine or a TKI. Midazolam, nifedipine (10 to 20 mg p.o. t.i.d.), sertraline (50 to 100 mg/day p.o.), benztropine (Cunningham 2002), nefopam (Bilotta and Rosa 2000), and valproic acid (Polito and Fellows 2017) have all been reported to be effective.

IMMUNOTHERAPY TOXICITIES

As of this writing (2021) the most common immunotherapies used to treat cancer patients include (1) checkpoint inhibitors (anti-CTLA-4 and anti-PD-1 -*mabs*) and (2) cell-based therapies (e.g., CAR T-cells).

Immune Checkpoint Inhibitors

Immune checkpoint inhibitors allow immune cells to activate and kill tumor cells by blocking the receptors on T, B, and/or natural killer cells that render the tumor "invisible" to them. In doing so, however, they also enable immune cells to target certain of the patient's normal cells. Both the tumor destruction and the side effects related to these therapies therefore arise from newly activated immune cells.

Mechanism. Anti-CTLA-4 targets a receptor that appears only on T cells; anti PD-1 targets the PD-1 protein present on T, B, and natural killer cells and allows what is called *programmed cell death* of tumor cells that express PD-Ligand 1 (PD-L1). If PD-1 is allowed to bind the PD-L1 receptor on the tumor, it will prevent the tumor cell from dying. Blocking either PD-1 or PD-L1 with monoclonal antibodies, therefore, allows the tumor cell to die (Hansen et al. 2018).

Ipilimumab blocks CTLA-4; pembrolizumab and nivolumab block PD-1; and atezolizumab, avelumab, and durvalumab block PD-L1. They have delivered amazing results in a variety of tumors, including melanoma, non–small cell lung cancer, renal cell carcinoma, and lymphomas, with less dramatic responses in other tumor types. Ongoing studies are likely to make this list incomplete by the time this book is published. Using a combination of these agents leads to better clinical tumor responses but markedly enhanced toxicity, as I review below.

Pseudoprogression. Because the agents induce an inflammatory response as they kill the tumors, the time to response and the criteria for it differ from those of chemotherapy or radiation. Responses take longer to appear and a paradoxical increase in the size of the tumor may precede the response, so-called pseudoprogression.

Toxicities. The skin, gastrointestinal tract, lung, and endocrine system are most commonly involved (in that order) in the inflammatory reactions, along with the liver and central nervous system. More rarely, the kidneys, uvea, joints, and muscles, including the heart muscle, are involved. The inflammation can be transient or can cause permanent tissue destruction (Hansen et al. 2018; Weisenthal et al. 2018). In 2020, the Multinational Association of Supportive Care in Cancer (MASCC) published its clinical practice recommendations of the management of adverse events induced by immune checkpoint inhibitors (Rapoport and Anderson 2020), including severe toxicity to skin (Choi et al. 2020) and gastrointestinal tract and liver (Dougan et al. 2020), as well as adverse events to lung (Shannon et al. 2020); heart, bone/muscle, and kidney (Suarez-Almazor et al. 2020); and endocrine glands (Cooksley et al. 2020).

Immune reactions are more frequent with anti-CTLA-4 therapy, but in general, they occur earlier, and are more frequent and more severe, when anti-CTLA-4 and anti-PD-1/anti-PD L1 therapy are given together (Hansen et al. 2018). Skin lesions usually arise no sooner than 4–7 weeks after the immunotherapy has begun. Colitis, hepatitis, and pneumonitis do not appear before 5 weeks after the second dose, usually 10–12 weeks. Endocrine abnormalities appear during the second month of therapy or later. Nephritis occurs after 14–42 weeks on immunotherapy. The onset, manifestations, and time to resolution of each of the most common toxicities are found in Table 10.4.

Therapy. Mild rashes are managed with topical corticosteroids and oral antihistamines; and mild pruritus with oral antihistamines, gabapentin or pregabalin, moisturizing creams and ointments, oatmeal baths, low-dose topical steroids, or urea topical cream. Moderate rashes require high-dose and sometimes systemic corticosteroids and a consideration of discontinuing the therapy, while for severe rashes the therapy is held and dermatology is consulted (Lacouture et al. 2021). Grade 1 diarrhea is managed with usual antidiarrheal medications and avoidance of lactose and caffeine-containing products, alcohol, and high osmolar supplements; if the stools increase to more than 4 a day, patients are instructed to call their clinicians, who generally recommend adding extensive oral fluid support and a combination of antidiarrheal medications (e.g., diphenoxylate/atropine [Lomotil], loperamide [Imodium], and deodorized tincture of opium [DTO]) and consultation with a registered dietician for additional dietary recommendations (Hansen et al. 2018; Matts and Beck 2019; NCCN 2020a; Wiesenthal et al. 2018).

In general, for moderate (grade 2) toxicity, the agent is held and resumed when the toxicity deceases to grade 1 or less. Corticosteroids can be added (prednisone 0.5–1 mg/kg/day or equivalent) if the symptoms continue for more than a week after the agent is stopped. For grade 3 or 4, the agent is stopped and not used again, and prednisone 1–2 mg/kg/day for 4–6 weeks is given, followed by a slow taper after the symptoms decrease to grade 1 or resolve. Patients who do not respond are given more intense immunosuppressive agents such as infliximab, mycophenolate mofetil, or cyclophosphamide.

Dermatologic toxicities generally resolve in 3 to 12 weeks, diarrhea and hepatitis in 2 to 4 weeks, lung toxicities in 5 to 6 weeks, and neurologic toxicities in 8 weeks. Only half of the renal toxicities resolve, and that takes about 10 weeks. The endocrinopathies, which are not limited to but include hypothyroidism, hypophysitis, and autoimmune diabetes, resolve in only about half of patients, and that takes 11 to 54 weeks. Many patients require prolonged or permanent replacement therapy.

While oncologists may want to avoid corticosteroids in these patients, they will not withhold them when they are needed to manage toxicities. Most allow for oral prednisone up to 10 mg daily (or the equivalent) along with the immunotherapy (Weisenthal et al. 2018).

CAR T-Cell Therapy Toxicity

Chimeric antigen receptor T cells (CAR T cells) are raised against the patient's specific tumor antigens, as, for example, CD19 found in cells of B-cell lymphomas, and can induce durable remissions even when the lymphoma has been refractory to other therapies. CAR T-cells, however, induce two distinct adverse reactions: cytokine release syndrome and neurologic toxicity/encephalopathy (Neelapu 2019).

The cytokine release syndrome is mediated by elevated levels of several cytokines, including IL-6. If an infusion of the anti-IL-6 antibody tocilizumab doesn't reverse the syndrome, systemic corticosteroids are often effective (Neelapu 2019). The encephalopathy, associated with confusion, word-finding difficulties, and aphasia, is also reversible. Patients with the lower grades of toxicity receive supportive care, and corticosteroids are used for patients with more severe encephalopathies (Neelapu 2019).

SKIN PROBLEMS

Patients with cancer can have skin problems caused by the cancer or its treatment. A comprehensive treatment guide for these conditions is beyond the scope of this volume. Dr. Mario Lacouture, however, has written an excellent book for patients and their families (Lacouture 2012). There is also an excellent review article in the *2020 ASCO Educational Book* on dermatologic syndromes caused by antineoplastic therapies (Deutsch et al. 2020); the ESMO guidelines for skin toxicities were published in 2021 (Lacouture et al. 2021). In this section, I review hand-foot syndrome, immune checkpoint inhibitor skin toxicity, epidermal growth factor receptor (EGFR) inhibitor-associated toxicities, fungating skin lesions, pressure ulcers, and pruritis.

Hand-Foot Syndrome

There are two types of cancer treatment-related disorders of the hand and foot skin, one related to infusional chemotherapy and the other to the tyrosine kinase inhibitors. The hand-foot syndrome (plantar-palmar erythrodysesthesia) related to chemotherapy was first described 30 years ago. It is a dose-limiting toxicity of infusional fluorouracil, capecitabine, and liposomal doxorubicin (Wolf et al. 2010). Patients experience toxicities that range from erythema without pain to peeling, blisters, bleeding, edema, or pain, to a limitation of function due to worsening of those symptoms or pain. The mechanism of hand-foot syndrome is unknown.

Prevention. Topical urea-based creams, antiperspirants, and regional cooling have all shown efficacy in prevention (Miller, Gorcey, and McLellan 2014).

Treatment. If therapy can be discontinued or the dose decreased, symptoms resolve in 1 to 2 weeks (Miller, Gorcey, and McLellan 2014). Low-level laser therapy decreased pain in half the patients compared with sham treatment, and no adverse reactions were seen (Latifyan et al. 2020). Celecoxib decreased capecitabine-induced lesions (Miller, Gorcey, and McLellan 2014). Symptomatic therapy includes potent topical steroids, wound care, moisturizing creams, and pain control (Lacouture et al. 2021). A urea and lactic acid–based keratolytic agent was not found to be effective in patients receiving capecitabine and may have actually worsened the symptoms in the first week of use (Wolf et al. 2010).

A different type of hand-foot skin reaction occurs in 14 to 62 percent of patients taking one or more of the tyrosine kinase inhibitors, such as sorafenib, sunitinib, lapatinib, or regorafenib (Manchen, Robert, and Porta 2011; Lacouture et al. 2021). The mechanism of this reaction is thought to be a simultaneous blockage of vascular endothelial growth factor receptors (VEGFRs) and platelet-derived growth factor receptors (PDGFRs) by these agents. In addition to the changes in the hands and feet, these patients develop facial erythema, scalp dysesthesia, alopecia, and subungual splinter hemorrhages (Manchen, Robert, and Porta 2011). As with hand-foot syndrome, the only effective treatment is decreasing the offending drug. Symptomatic therapies include using the "3 C approach": "control calluses, comfort with cushions, and cover with creams" (Manchen, Robert, and Porta 2011, p. 22), as well as 10 percent urea cream three times a day (Lacouture et al. 2021).

EGFR-Inhibitor-Associated Toxicities

EGFR inhibitors include, for example, erlotinib, afatinib, dacomitinib, osimertinib, lapatinib, and gefitinib; monoclonal antibodies such as cetuximab, necitumumab, pertuzumab, and panitumumab; and mitogen-activated protein-kinase inhibitors (MEKIs) such as trametinib, binimetinib, and cobimetinib. EGFR inhibitors commonly cause a papulopustular rash that resembles acne; increased brittleness of the hair, alopecia, or hypertrichosis of scalp hair, eyelashes, and eyebrows; xerosis so severe that the skin develops fissures; paronychia; pruritus; and mucositis (Lacouture et al. 2021). Patients on EGFR inhibitors also have worse radiation dermatitis than patients not taking them. If the toxicities are severe enough, doses of the offending agent or the radiation are reduced. Provide or refer for education and psychological support as the patient's appearance may markedly change.

To prevent the acneiform rash, the ESMO 2021 guidelines recommend avoidance of frequent washing with hot water (hand washing, shower, baths); avoidance of skin irritants, such as over-the-counter (OTC) anti-acne medications, solvents, or disinfectants; alcohol-free OTC moisturizing creams or ointment b.i.d. preferably with urea-containing (5%-10%) moisturizers to the body; avoidance of excessive sun exposure; sunscreen SPF -15 applied to exposed areas of body and every 2 hours when outside; and oral antibiotics for 6 weeks at start of therapy with or without topical low/moderate strength steroid to face and chest b.i.d. (Lacouture et al. 2021).

The rash typically presents in the first 2 to 4 weeks of treatment. Aggressive prophylactic treatment with hydrocortisone (1%) combined with moisturizer, sunscreen, and doxycycline 100 mg twice daily for 6 weeks has been shown to diminish its severity (Lacouture et al. 2021). Minocycline 100 mg daily for 8 weeks is also effective and less photosensitizing, but doxycycline has a better safety profile. If the rash worsens, high-potency topical corticosteroids and low-dose isotretinoin are recommended, though the evidence is not as good for these agents.

Minoxidil may help patients with nonscarring alopecia (Lacouture et al. 2021). Scarring alopecia may be lessened by topical hydrocortisone (0.2%), steroid shampoos, class 1 steroid lotions, bath oils, or mild shampoo followed by an antibiotic spray (Lacouture et al. 2021). Excess facial hair can be treated by eflornithine cream or hair removal; to prevent corneal abrasions, treat trichomegaly by clipping the eyelashes (Lacouture et al. 2021).

Lacouture and colleagues review symptomatic treatment for oral complications, xerosis, fissures, and paronychia in their discussion of clinical guidelines for the care of patients receiving these agents (Lacouture 2012; Lacouture et al. 2021).

Fungating Skin Lesions

Fungating lesions from cancers growing out through the skin can cause embarrassment, shame, and profound loss of self-esteem. Not only are the lesions painful, but the associated discharge and odor can be so offensive that even family members find it hard to remain near the patient.

Primary skin cancers, breast cancers, and cancers of the head and neck that become refractory to chemotherapy and radiation can cause fungating skin lesions, as can metastases. Patients with breast cancer are particularly prone to developing skin metastases on the chest wall or scalp, but they also occur in about 10 percent of those with renal cancer and 5 percent of those with other cancers. Chemotherapy and radiation can be effective, especially in reducing bleeding. Surgery should also be considered as a palliative measure, especially in recurrent breast cancer and extensive melanoma metastases.

Symptomatic treatment. Although these wounds rarely heal completely, symptomatic treatment is often effective for tumors that are refractory to specific modalities. Skin care protocols and tables of wound care products are included in the *Oxford Textbook of Palliative Medicine: Principles and Practice of Supportive Care in Oncology* (Cherny et al. 2015), and *Handbook of Palliative Care in Cancer* (Waller 2000; see General References in this chapter's online bibliography). Hospitals and visiting nurse associations have policies and guidelines as well. Specially trained advanced practice nurses are also valuable resources in caring for patients with decubitus ulcers, tumor metastases, skin infections, and other chronic skin wounds. Sarah Kagan, MSN, CRNP, a colleague of mine who is a geriatric nurse practitioner and wound care expert, and Ilene Fleisher and Diane Bryant, certified enterostomal therapy nurses, have generously contributed material for the recommendations that follow. For additional questions, use your visiting nurse association as a resource.

Practice Points: Care of Fungating Skin Lesions and Pressure Ulcers

- Keep the wound clean.
- Control odor.
- Gently debride it.
- Relieve pain (e.g., consider topical intrasite gel with 1% morphine with each dressing change for open skin areas).
- Use antibiotics and antifungals.
- Apply the correct, layered dressing.
- Control bleeding.
- For pressure ulcers: minimize shear forces and the time spent in one position; provide the correct mattress.

Wound cleaning. Keep the wound clean by irrigating it with sterile saline, lactated Ringer's, or homemade saline solution (1 tsp. of salt dissolved in 1 pint of boiled water), or by showering. For wounds that are colonized with anaerobic organisms, consider sprinkling with metronidazole powder, or apply gauze sponges soaked in metronidazole gel.

Debridement. Debride the wound gently, using continuous moist saline dressings. For dry but purulent tissue, use an enzymatic debriding ointment (e.g., collagenase, Accuzyme) or a gel such as Debrisan. Debrisan is composed of polysaccharide dextranomer granules, which can be poured in a clean, moist wound and covered with a semi-occlusive dressing. The granules will draw the bacteria and dead cells out of the wound.

For wet, heavily exudative wounds, with or without colonization or obvious infectious findings, use absorptive dressings, which include hydrofibers, collagen, and calcium alginates; hydrophilic foams; and polymers such as cadexomers.

These are widely available under many trade names, including Aquacel, Hydro-fiber wound dressing, Kaltostat, Sorbsan, Iodosorb, and Allevyn. Avoid hypertonic saline dressings, which would literally put salt in the wound. To prevent the exudate from macerating the tissue, providing a medium for infection, and embarrassing the patient, use absorbent foam topped by a thick gauze pad and an alginate dressing. The alginate dressings do not have to be removed; they wash off during bathing.

Antibiotics. Consider adding topical or systemic antibiotics. Aerobic bacteria can easily superinfect fungating tumors. *Staphylococcus aureus* and other common pathogens often respond to topical antibiotics such as triple antibiotic ointment or mupirocin. Gram-negative organisms may be more prominent in anogenital areas, and you may need to recommend silver sulphadiazine cream and potassium permanganate sitz baths to prevent recurrent infection. Anaerobes respond to topical metronidazole; fungus to Nizoral or other ketoconazole creams; and painful viral lesions to acyclovir ointment.

Control of bleeding. Widespread oozing can be controlled with a sucralfate paste, made by mashing a 1-gram tablet in a small amount of water-soluble gel. Gauze soaked in 1:1000 epinephrine solution, Gelfoam soaked in thrombin, Avitene, topical thromboplastin (100 μg/ml), or Surgicell can also be used. Silver nitrate sticks should be reserved for isolated bleeding points. Nonadherent, moist dressings can often decrease oozing by diminishing the trauma associated with dressing changes.

Control of odor. Eliminate the bacteria that are causing the odor, which are mostly anaerobic. Despite its toxicity to the skin and newly budding capillaries, you may consider using a disinfectant solution such as quarter-strength Dakin's or 1 percent chlorhexidine gluconate as a first measure. Unfortunately, although these solutions are not expensive, they can cause discomfort and are not always effective. Most cases also require more expensive therapies: metronidazole gel (0.75%) applied to or the oral medication sprinkled on the lesion, along with oral metronidazole (200 to 400 mg p.o. t.i.d.) if needed. Metronidazole has been shown to be totally effective in 50 percent and reasonably effective in an additional 45 percent of patients for whom it was used. Rice bran sheets, placed over the gauze after daily dressing changes, significantly decreased wound odor in all 15 patients treated (Hayashida et al. 2020). No side effects were observed.

Topical aromatherapeutics can be mixed into a bland base (e.g., vitamin A and D ointment) to provide odor control and a sense of well-being. Essential oils for first-line, nontoxic use include lavender (soothing, deodorizing); tea tree oil (antimicrobial, cleansing); and peppermint (deodorizing, cleansing). These should be added to the base at 10 to 30 drops per ounce.

If cost is an issue or metronidazole gel is not available, try applying Maalox, which may also relieve burning. Oral chlorophyll tablets can decrease the odor because the chlorophyll will be included in all secretions. Natural remedies such as applying yogurt or buttermilk, which prevent growth of odor-forming bacteria, or powdered sugar or honey, which compete with the bacteria for water, have also been effective in controlling odor. The yogurt can also relieve burning. One-quarter percent menthol may be added to a bland base for topical antipruritic use on intact skin.

Pain relief. Topical morphine is often helpful (Zeppetella and Ribeiro 2003). Morphine-infused IntraSite gel (0.1 w/w solution or 1 mg morphine/1 ml IntraSite gel) is spread on a clean ulcer, then covered by a 4 by 4 inch gauze dressing; or the gel is placed on the dressing, which is then applied to the wound to cover the entire ulcerated wound surface. New gel is applied when dressings are changed (usually twice a day). In a pilot randomized study, no side effects were noted.

Wound dressing. Wound dressings serve a number of purposes. They allow the removal of excess exudate, bacterial toxins, and dead skin cells; maintain a moist, clean environment; are relatively impermeable to bacteria; and provide comfort and protection from further injury. Unless the patient is neutropenic or there is a reason to use sterile technique, clean technique can be used, including clean gloves, for dressing changes at home.

For a dressing to accomplish all this, it must be made up of layers with different functions. The material closest to the skin should be sterile, should allow exudates to pass through it, and should not stick to the skin. Hydrocolloid dressings (Duoderm, Tegaderm, Granulex, hydrogel, Xeroform) are particularly useful if there is little exudate, because they are nonadherent and provide pain relief; alginate dressings (Kaltostat, Aquacel hydrofiber, Tegaderm alginate dressings) are better for a large amount of exudate. The middle layer should be absorbent, and the outer layer should be a charcoal dressing (e.g., Carboflex) to absorb odor. To minimize trauma to the lesion, ask the family and the nurses to change the dressings only when they are no longer absorbent or are not controlling the odor. The best way to remove them is to soak them off.

Pressure Ulcers

Pressure ulcers in terminally ill cancer patients have the same causes as those in other bed-bound patients: pressure leads to ischemia of the skin due to injury to the vascular, lymphatic, and other interstitial transportation structures. Friction, maceration, and shear forces contribute to vulnerability to pressure injury. Pressure ulcers occur most often in areas of bony prominence, especially the ischium and sacrum.

Prevention. Prevention of pressure ulcers is often possible, and your staff can educate the family in how it is done. Many visiting nurse associations and hospice programs include a physical therapist who can teach the health aides and family to provide the physical care the patient will need.

The goal is to minimize the time the patient lies or sits in one position, being particularly careful to relieve pressure over bony prominences. Multiple bed pillows can be used for the frequent repositioning. Bed cradles, elbow and heel pads, and wheelchair cushions are all useful in an individualized plan of care. Maintaining adequate nutrition and hydration are of course helpful but not always possible in this population. Multivitamin and mineral tablets or supplemental vitamin C (1000 mg/day) and zinc (220 mg/day) can be added to the diet of those unlikely to obtain enough from food.

Of course, the chair or mattress on which the patient lies is of particular importance, especially if the patient is very old, thin, or immobile and therefore at high risk for developing pressure ulcers. It may be worthwhile to have a consultant evaluate the need for a pressure-relieving mattress. Some devices, for example, have air cells that alternately inflate and deflate. The choice of mattress will depend on the patient's needs and what the patient can afford. The 2015 Wound Healing Society guidelines on prevention and treatment of pressure ulcers categorize the available options by efficacy (Gould et al. 2015). Medicare will pay for category 1 products for patients who have stage 2 to 3 ulcers and category 2 products for those with stage 4 ulcers.

Therapy. As with fungating wound lesions, nursing protocols are available for the treatment of all stages of pressure ulcers; sources, including the 2015 Wound Healing Society guideline on pressure ulcers, are given in the online bibliography (see Gould et al. 2015). Some general treatment principles are outlined below. Local care should be directed toward prevention and comfort. Topical care techniques described for fungating skin lesions can also be used for pressure ulcers in palliative care. A 2003 study reported dramatic healing of grade 3 to grade 4 pressure ulcers of the foot by nerve growth factor applied directly to the ulcer (Landi et al. 2003). Terminally ill patients were excluded from this study, however, and there have been no more recent studies commenting on its efficacy.

Preventing contamination and minimizing shear forces. Polyurethane films or hydrocolloid dressings (e.g., Tegaderm, Duoderm) can be used as dressings for pressure ulcers that are neither necrotic nor infected and need only a moist environment to heal. As with dressings over fungating lesions, the caregiver or nurse should change these only when necessary.

Protecting the wound and promoting healing. If the pressure ulcers are infected or have necrotic tissue, sterile normal saline irrigation is needed, and enzymatic agents (Elase, Travase, Accuzyme, Santyl [collagenase], streptokinase) can remove the eschar. As with fungating lesions, hydrocolloid dressings (Duoderm, hydrogel xeroform, Granuflex) are used if there is little exudate; alginate dressings (Kaltocarb, Kaltostat, Aquacel hydrofibers) are used if there is a large amount.

Eliminating or controlling infection; debridement. Polysaccharide dextranomer granules (Debrisan) can be poured in a clean, moist wound and covered with a semi-occlusive dressing. They will draw the bacteria and dead cells out of the wound. Unlike the other dressings, this should be cleaned and reapplied daily until the wound is clean and appears to be healing. If odor is a problem, a charcoal dressing (Carboflex) will be needed.

Pruritus

Etiology. It was formerly thought that itch and pain were mediated by the same receptors. This turns out not to be the case. Itch-specific nerves have been found in the peripheral and central nervous systems (Oaklander et al. 2003). Injury to these nerves, such as occurs in herpes zoster infections—especially those of the face—can cause a pathologic itch rather than pain. Anecdotal reports of the efficacy of aprepitant offer the intriguing idea that the same NK-1 inhibitors involved in pain transmission may be involved in mediating pruritis. Patients taking aprepitant, an NK-1 inhibitor, as part of an antiemetic regimen noted marked decrease in their pruritis (Duval and Dubertret 2009; Vincenzi, Tonini, and Santini 2010). Aprepitant has also been used effectively to treat a patient with pruritis as a paraneoplastic syndrome (Song et al. 2018). Chemical mediators of pruritus include histamine (H1, not H2, receptors) and serotonin (5-HT2 and 5-HT3 receptors).

Why scratching relieves an itch is still not entirely understood, but inducing pain in the area of the itch eliminates the itching sensation. Scratching does activate myelinated A-delta sensory fibers, which temporarily stops the pruritus. Additionally, the common itching that accompanies epidural opioids arises because the opioids inhibit only the pain, not the itch, pathways. The pruritus that accompanies cholestatic liver failure may be mediated by a similar selective blockade by endogenous opiates, because it responds to naloxone, naltrexone, and nalmefene. A central neuronal circuit for the itch sensation has been identified and may be a target for blockade in the future (Mu et al. 2017).

Pruritus and rash can be induced by EGFR inhibitors; prevention and treatment for these are discussed earlier in this chapter. Immune checkpoint inhibitors such as nivolumab, cemiplimab, atezolizumab, avelumab, durvalumab, and ipilimumab may cause pruritus without rash (Lacouture et al. 2021). If the pruritus is mild or localized, the therapy can be continued and the pruritus treated with antihistamines, topical steroids, or lidocaine patches. If it does not respond to these measures, or is moderate on presentation, immunotherapy is sometimes continued along with higher potency steroids and in some cases gabapentin or pregabalin. If the patient doesn't respond or presents with severe pruritus, consult dermatology and hold the immunotherapy.

But the vast majority of pruritus in advanced-cancer patients is not due to injury of the "itch" nerves, or EGFR or immune checkpoint inhibitor therapy. Rather, it is caused by the same conditions and illnesses that occur in people without cancer: dry skin, allergic reactions to drugs, uremia (Ragazzo et al. 2020), cholestasis, or psychological stress. In addition, pruritus can be caused by opioids, skin involvement with cancer, or a paraneoplastic process, such as is seen in patients with Hodgkin's disease, cutaneous lymphomas, myeloproliferative disorders, and some solid tumors (Song et al. 2018; Vallely et al. 2019).

Practice Points: Relieving Pruritus

- Patients should bathe with lukewarm water and avoid bath products containing deodorants or perfumes.
- Skin should be kept moist and fingernails short.
- Cooling or anesthetic creams may be applied.
- Oral antihistamines or NSAIDs may be needed.
- Cholestyramine, paroxetine, mirtazapine, sertraline, low-dose naloxone, naltrexone, nalmefene, or methyltestosterone may be effective for cholestatic pruritus.
- Naloxone and mirtazapine may help pruritus from other causes as well, such as PD-1-induced or paraneoplastic pruritus.

Patients with pruritus should keep the skin moist by frequent lubrication, cut fingernails short, and avoid all bath products that contain perfumes or deodorants. The baths themselves should be lukewarm, or oatmeal baths can be tried. Cooling the skin with menthol-containing creams (0.25% menthol), camphor, peppermint, colloidal oatmeal lotions, or ice packs can provide symptomatic relief, as can calamine lotion or Caladryl (a combination of calamine lotion and Benadryl) and topical anesthetics (benzocaine, ELA-Max, EMLA). TENS machines have been used by some patients to good effect.

Biliary obstruction. If the pruritus results from biliary obstruction, internal stenting (Dy et al. 2012) or radiation to obstructing nodes in the porta hepatis often relieves the pruritus in responding patients for as long as the patient lives. If the obstruction cannot be relieved, cholestyramine (Questran), the SSRI paroxetine (Paxil), or methyltestosterone may be effective. Sertraline reduced pruritis within days in two small trials of patients with cholestatic pruritis (Dull and Kremer 2019). A very low-dose naloxone infusion titrated to 0.2 mcg/kg/min. followed, if no opioid withdrawal effect was noted, by oral naltrexone 12.5 to 25 mg two to three times daily (Jones and Zylicz 2005) or nalmefene 5 mg orally (Bergasa et al. 1999) was effective in reducing scratching activity in patients with intractable pruritis from cholestasis. Mirtazapine, which is an H1, 5-HT2, and 5-HT3 receptor antagonist, has also been reported to relieve pruritus in patients with cholestasis, advanced Hodgkin's and non-Hodgkin's lymphomas, and renal failure (Fawaz, Chamseddin, and Griffin 2021).

Other causes. Antihistamines (e.g., diphenhydramine [Benadryl]) will help when the cause of the itching is histamine release. Paroxetine and mirtazapine are helpful for patients with paraneoplastic or opioid-induced pruritus. Naloxone is helpful for immunotherapy-induced (Kwatra, Ständer, and Kang 2018; Singh et al. 2019) and paraneoplastic pruritus (Song et al. 2018). Ondansetron, a 5-HT3 receptor antagonist, is effective for neuraxial opioid-induced pruritus (Wang, Zhou, and Sun 2017) and pruritis from myeloproliferative diseases such as polycythemia vera, but a systematic review did not find that it had significant benefit in relieving pruritis from cholestasis or uremia (To et al. 2012). As noted above, aprepitant, an NK-1 inhibitor, has anecdotal reports of efficacy.

Practice Points: Symptomatic Therapy of Pruritus

Etiology	Therapy
Histamine release	Diphenhydramine
Cholestasis	Cholestyramine, sertraline, methyltestosterone, naloxone, naltrexone, nalmefene
Paraneoplastic process	Paroxetine, mirtazapine
Neuraxial opioids	Paroxetine, ondansetron, naloxone, naltrexone, mirtazapine
Myeloproliferative process	Ondansetron
Renal failure	Gabapentin, pregabalin (first line); paroxetine, sertraline, amitriptyline, doxepin, naltrexone, antihistamines (second line)

Doses: Diphenhydramine 25 to 50 mg p.o. every 8 hours; paroxetine 10 to 20 mg/day p.o.; sertraline 50 to 200 mg p.o. daily; mirtazapine 15 mg p.o. h.s.; methyltestosterone 25 mg sublingual b.i.d. for 7 to 10 days; naloxone, naltrexone, nalmefene: see text; ondansetron 8 mg p.o. b.i.d. to t.i.d.

(Kouwenhoven, van de Kerkhof, and Kamsteeg 2017; Ragazzo et al. 2020)

Oral antihistamines are probably the best nonspecific relievers of pruritus, but they may cause excessive daytime sedation. NSAIDs are occasionally useful because prostaglandins at least partially mediate pruritus. Opioids, on the other hand, are not: as discussed above, they may induce pruritus. Paroxetine (Paxil), an antidepressant that is an SSRI (like fluoxetine [Prozac]), was effective in five patients with pruritus arising from various etiologies. Dosing ranged from 5 to 30 mg/day (Zylicz, Smits, and Krajnik 1998).

INSOMNIA

Sleep disturbances occur in 30 percent to 75 percent of cancer patients (Berger, Matthews, and Kenkel 2017; Guzman-Marin and Aidan 2015). Fifty-nine percent of patients who underwent curative surgery for various cancer types had insomnia when first studied prior to the surgery, and 36 percent had persistent insomnia at the time of the last follow-up, 18 months later (Savard, Ivers, and Villa 2011). No specific type of cancer appears to have the highest rates of sleep disturbances, but less well-educated and young patients report symptoms more often; other factors reliably related to insomnia included comorbid medical conditions, less physical activity, current use of tobacco, and more depression and fatigue (Phillips, Jim, and Donovan 2012).

Schutte-Rodin and colleagues (2008), in their clinical guideline for chronic insomnia, offer a set of questions that can help you obtain a comprehensive sleep history. To meet the official criteria for insomnia, a patient must have either difficulty falling asleep (i.e., taking more than 30 minutes) or difficulty staying asleep (when in bed trying to sleep, actually asleep less than 85 percent of the time). This problem must occur at least three times a week and must affect the patient's function in the daytime. Patients may have transient insomnia (lasting a month or less), short-term insomnia (1 to 6 months), or chronic insomnia (longer than 6 months). Insomnia occurs in one-third to one-half of people with advanced cancer. These patients usually do not report difficulty falling asleep, but they have trouble staying asleep.

The sleeplessness can often be more troublesome to the patient's family than to the patient, but whether or not patients recognize it, lack of sleep can be contributing to their distress in many ways. At a minimum, they will feel much as we did when, as residents, many of us were up all night on call. But in addition, sleep deprivation may exacerbate pain and increase a patient's chance of becoming depressed.

Etiology. Patients with cancer have numerous reasons for sleepless nights. Among them are many of the problems I have already discussed—pain, depression, anxiety, delirium, dyspnea, nocturnal hypoxia, nausea and vomiting, pruritus, or hot flashes from estrogen or androgen deficiency (discussed in the next section). Medications that can cause insomnia include corticosteroids and antiemetics (prochlorperazine, metoclopramide, 5-HT3 receptor antagonists).

Patients' sleep-wake cycle may be somewhat reversed, because they are inactive and napping much of the day and then not sleepy at night. If they are severely iron deficient or uremic, are taking tricyclic antidepressants, or have a peripheral neuropathy, they may also be wakened by restless leg syndrome. Consider obstructive sleep apnea and have the patient evaluated for that if they snore frequently or have been told they stop breathing during sleep. For some people, very small doses of caffeine or alcohol may be enough to keep them awake at night.

Therapy. Patients with obstructive sleep apnea should be referred to a specialist for therapy. Insomnia may be treated either nonpharmacologically or with medications. When appropriate, I ask patients to consider professional counseling to explore some of the psychological, financial, and spiritual implications of their illness that are contributing to their insomnia, and to get help in resolving them. A visit from the lawyer to finalize a will, from the hospice team to reassure the patient that his family will be supported through his final days, or from the rabbi or parish priest can often solve the problem and end the sleepless nights.

Encourage patients not to nap during the day and to remain out of bed as long as possible. Suggest that they go to bed and get up at a set time, no matter how tired they are, and if they do not fall asleep within 30 minutes, that they engage in some relaxing activity, either out of or in bed.

Practice Points: Nonpharmacologic Therapy for Insomnia

- Psychological, legal, or spiritual counseling for concerns contributing to insomnia
- Eliminating daytime naps
- Going to bed at a set time
- If awake 30 minutes later, doing some relaxing activity in or out of bed
- Instruction in biofeedback, relaxation therapy, or hypnosis

---

If these efforts are not sufficient, techniques developed by sleep experts for patients without cancer may be. The most effective therapy for insomnia is cognitive-behavioral therapy for insomnia (CBTi) (Brasure et al. 2016). For patients able to participate, suggest training in tai chi chih, which was noninferior to CBTi (Irwin et al. 2017), or aerobic exercise 30 minutes a day. Mindfulness-based stress reduction, progressive muscle relaxation or other forms of relaxation therapy, biofeedback, and hypnosis using imagery have been shown to be helpful as a component of short-term management, particularly for patients who cannot get to sleep or cannot regain sleep after they've awakened in the night. Medications can alleviate insomnia when these other approaches are ineffective (Table 10.5).

Ideally, choose an agent that specifically addresses the cause of the insomnia, such as agents for pain, anxiety, and depression discussed in Chapters 7 and 9 and earlier in this chapter. Patients with restless leg syndrome may benefit from the anti-parkinsonian agents pramipexole, ropinirole, and rotigotine patch, as well as gabapentin, all of which are approved to treat this syndrome (Muth 2017). Pregabalin can also be tried.

For patients who develop nighttime delirium that is keeping them and their families awake, oral quetiapine (Seroquel) is useful. For older patients, start with 25 mg at bedtime and titrate as needed. Patients with organic brain syndromes causing *sun-downing* may need doses up to 200 mg given either at bedtime or an hour after sunset to prevent agitation. Younger patients can tolerate initial doses of 50 mg at bedtime. Olanzapine (e.g. Zyprexa) (2.5 to 5 mg p.o. at bedtime) or haloperidol (e.g., Haldol) (beginning at 0.5 to 2 mg p.o. and increasing as needed to 5 mg), given before the onset of the agitation and repeated if needed during the night, is also usually effective.

When you cannot determine the cause of the insomnia, data from controlled trials indicate that nonbenzodiazepine hypnotics such as zolpidem (e.g. Ambien), zaleplon (e.g. Sonata), or eszopiclone (e.g. Lunesta); the antidepressant doxepin; the orexin receptor antagonist suvorexant (Belsomra); and the melatonin receptor agonist ramelteon (e.g. Rozerem) are effective agents (Denlinger et al. 2020). Melatonin itself is not. Benzodiazepines are *not* recommended.

HOT FLASHES

Hot flashes are intermittent feelings of heat, profound sweating, and flushing of the face and chest; anxiety and palpitations may also occur (Morrow, Mattair, and Hortobagyi 2011). Episodes last 3 to 10 minutes.

Etiology. Women and men with either estrogen or androgen deprivation induced by cancer treatments suffer from hot flashes. Tamoxifen causes more frequent hot flash symptoms than the aromatase inhibitors. Premenopausal women receiving cytotoxic therapy are likely to experience hot flashes because the therapy causes an early menopause. Up to 75 percent of men who undergo androgen-deprivation therapy experience hot flashes.

Therapy. Patients with mild hot flashes can try dressing in layers and using a fan. Yoga has not been convincingly shown to be helpful (Buchanan et al. 2017), and exercise exacerbates hot flashes, especially in overweight women in whom it increases the core body temperature. In contrast, relaxation therapy may decrease overall symptoms, especially when used in conjunction with pharmacologic therapy (Tremblay, Sheeran, and Aranda 2008).

Although estrogen and progestational agent oral therapies are effective, they are no longer used even for women without cancer because of the excessive associated risk of inducing cancer. Vitamin E, soy phytoestrogen, and black cohosh are *not* effective therapies for hot flashes. Both venlafaxine and gabapentin are effective. In a head-to-head trial, most patients preferred venlafaxine (37.5 mg daily for 7 days, then 75 mg daily for 21 days) to gabapentin (300 mg daily for 3 days, then 300 mg b.i.d. for 3 days, then 300 mg t.i.d. for 22 days) (Bordeleau et al. 2010). Oxybutynin (5 mg p.o. b.i.d.) can be effective for both men (Smith, Loprinzi, and Deville 2018) and women (Simon, Gaines, and LaGuadia 2016).

WEAKNESS AND FATIGUE

Fatigue is even more prevalent than pain in patients with metastatic cancer, but much less research has been done to define its pathophysiology, etiology, or effective therapy. The 2020 NCCN cancer-related fatigue treatment guidelines define fatigue as a "distressing persistent, subjective sense of physical, emotional and/

or cognitive tiredness or exhaustion related to cancer or cancer treatment that is not proportional to recent activity and interferes with usual functioning" (2020b, p. FT-1). Those doing research on the epidemiology, etiology, and therapy of fatigue use multiple fatigue assessment tools. These researchers documented that half of the patients being treated for acute leukemia or non-Hodgkin's lymphoma have severe fatigue, and almost all patients receiving chemotherapy or radiotherapy (96 percent) or in the terminal phases of cancer suffer from fatigue.

The treatment guidelines include recommended screening and evaluation protocols, as well as separate intervention guidelines for patients under active treatment, undergoing long-term follow-up, or at the end of life. The screening guidelines are similar to those for patients with pain, which is also a subjective experience that can be validly quantified. The guidelines recommend, as for pain, assessment on a 0 to 10 scale (0 = no fatigue to 10 = worst fatigue imaginable), expert multidisciplinary evaluation, and education and training of professionals and family members. Patients who scored greater than 7 were found to have a "dramatic decrease in physical functioning" (NCCN 2020b, p. MS-5). The NCCN guidelines recommend further evaluation for any patient with a fatigue level greater than 4.

Identifiable, and sometimes even reversible, causes of fatigue can be found for some patients (Table 10.6), though the mechanisms by which they produce fatigue are not known. Pain, anxiety, depression, and insomnia are important causes of generalized weakness and fatigue. Drug side effects; pulmonary, renal, hepatic, or cardiac failure; infection; under- or overactive adrenal or thyroid function; hypogonadism (Fleishman et al. 2010; Strasser et al. 2006); and certain neurologic problems—all can present as generalized weakness, and the weakness may resolve if the causes can be reversed. Anemia (see below), poor nutrition, and alcohol or other substance use disorder may also contribute, and, depending on the patient's stage of disease, may be reversible.

For patients on active treatment and post-treatment, category 1 recommendations include exercise programs with both cardiovascular endurance and weight training, yoga, massage, and cognitive-behavioral and psychoeducational therapies (NCCN 2020b) Although data on their effectiveness in patients with advanced disease are limited, there is no reason to think they shouldn't be tried.

If no specific cause of fatigue is identified, or the therapy is ineffective, the NCCN 2020 fatigue guidelines support using the psychostimulant methylphenidate. Long-acting methylphenidate was effective for patients with advanced disease and severe fatigue (Moraska et al. 2010), and short-acting methylphenidate is also effective (Pedersen et al. 2020). One study explored the effect of titration (Kerr et al. 2012). The most effective methylphenidate doses were a mean of 10 mg by Day 3 of therapy, rising to 20 mg by Day 14, with a range of 10 to 40 mg.

Also, a "placebo effect" was clearly demonstrated in 40 female cancer survivors (Zhou et al. 2019). Though the survivors knew they were taking a pill that did not contain any active ingredients, they reported significantly decreased fatigue at 8 and 22 days after taking the placebos compared with the control group of survivors not taking any pills! In a phase III randomized, double-blind placebo controlled study, armodafinil (150 or 250 mg daily) failed to reduce moderate to severe fatigue more than placebo in patients with high-grade glioma (Porter et al. 2020).

Lambert-Eaton Syndrome

Lambert-Eaton syndrome is a very rare autoimmune complication of lung cancer that can cause weakness, most prominent in the proximal muscles, which sometimes remits when the cancer remits. Antibody-mediated inhibition of transmission of acetylcholine at the neuromuscular junction causes the weakness and fatigue (Kesner et al. 2018). Patients with this syndrome experience a sort of *reverse myasthenia*: they get stronger, instead of weaker, as the day progresses. Amifampridine (Firdapse) is the treatment of choice, demonstrating in two phase III trials significant improvement in symptoms with minimal adverse effects (Yoon et al. 2020).

Myositis

Myositis can be a painful, debilitating cause of weakness. Gemcitabine has been reported most often to cause radiation-recall myositis, which can occur 3–8 months after the radiation therapy is completed (Ravishankar et al. 2018). Irinotecan, capecitabine, and a combination of carboplatin and docetaxel have each been reported to cause it. Treatment with corticosteroids and hyperbaric oxygen is suggested, with mixed results.

Anemia

Patients whose anemia is caused only by renal insufficiency respond to erythropoiesis-stimulating agents (ESAs) (50 to 150 U/kg t.i.w.) and oral iron supplementation. Some patients with cancer or a diseased marrow (e.g., myelodysplasia) will respond to ESAs, but they are not indicated for patients undergoing myelosuppressive chemotherapies with curative intent because of the possible risk of increased mortality and disease progression (NCCN 2020c). Those patients should receive transfusions as needed.

Blood transfusion can ameliorate fatigue in patients whose hemoglobin is less than 10 g/dL (Mitchell et al. 2007). Because blood is such a scarce resource, NCCN guidelines recommend a transfusion when hemoglobin levels fall to 7 g/dL for asymptomatic patients with chronic anemia who do not have acute coronary syndrome (NCCN 2020c, p. MS-22).

ESAs did not improve the fatigue or weakness of patients with progressive disease, but patients who are receiving palliative therapies for stable or responsive disease may experience an improved quality of life for each gram/deciliter of increase, with the maximum effect being between 11 and 12 g/dL. The regimen is expensive and requires subcutaneous injections weekly, or every 2 to 3 weeks, of ESA dosed according to a fixed or weight-based dosing regimen, along with supplemental oral iron for optimal response, even if total body iron stores are increased.

All ESA use is associated with a significantly increased absolute risk of venous thromboembolism: 7.5 percent in treated patients versus 4.9 percent in controls (NCCN 2020c, p. MS-25); and the risk is greater for patients with hemoglobin levels greater than 10 g/dL. Patients are also at risk of developing pure red cell aplasia (NCCN 2020c). Because of these increased risks, all clinicians prescribing ESAs for any indication must be registered in a REMS program and prescribe only using the REMS guidelines; patients must give their informed consent.

Metabolic Abnormalities

Cancer-related metabolic abnormalities that can present as weakness include hypercalcemia, hypomagnesemia, hyponatremia, hypokalemia, hyperglycemia, and hypoglycemia (Table 10.6).

Hypercalcemia. Hypercalcemia is a common complication of cancer. Prior to the widespread use of bisphosphonates and RANK-L inhibitors to slow the development of skeletal-related events, it was reported in 10 to 40 percent of cancer patients at some time in the course of their illness.

Subtle personality changes, fatigue, anorexia, polyuria, or increased constipation may be the only presenting features, but many patients or their families will, on close questioning, report nausea, increased sedation, difficulty concentrating, or symptoms typical of delirium. The severity of symptoms correlates more closely with the speed with which the hypercalcemia developed than with the absolute level of serum calcium. Mental status changes may not resolve for several weeks following normalization of serum calcium.

In studies published in 1990 and 2005, hypercalcemia of malignancy had a reported median survival of only a month (Wright et al. 2015). But in those years, hydration, calcitonin, and corticosteroids for corticosteroid-responsive tumors were the only symptomatic therapies. There are no survival data reported for outpatients with hypercalcemia of malignancy who are treated with bisphosphonates or RANK-L inhibitors that can prevent a hypercalcemic death; the in-hospital mortality rate, before denosumab was used for this indication, was reported to be 6.8 percent (Wright et al. 2015). Recurrent hypercalcemia despite therapy with bisphosphonates or denosumab does portend a grim prognosis; hospice care should be offered, if this has not yet been done.

> ### Practice Points: Cancer-Related Hypercalcemia
>
> - Patients should be monitored for subtle signs and symptoms, especially nausea, increased constipation, and mental status changes.
> - Severity of symptoms correlates with speed of development of hypercalcemia, not absolute level of calcium.
> - Mental status changes may not resolve for several weeks following normalization of serum calcium.
> - Adequate hydration and weight-bearing activity should be encouraged.
> - Initial therapy is hydration and intravenous bisphosphonate, and for severe hypercalcemia, calcitonin; add furosemide only after the patient is fully rehydrated. RANK-L inhibitors (e.g., denosumab) are second-line therapy. Discontinue hydrochlorothiazide and, when possible, lithium.
> - Patients with refractory tumors or those who do not wish to receive tumor-directed therapy should be referred to hospice programs. Median survival is 30 days.

Bony metastases may cause mild hypercalcemia, which can sometimes be reversed by hydrating the patient well and making sure she stays out of bed and takes in adequate amounts of salt. Activity is helpful because bone resorption from the metastases is increased when the patient is recumbent and minimally mobile, and hypercalcemia can result. Thiazide diuretics contribute to hypercalcemia and should be discontinued, as should lithium, if possible.

In 80 percent of cancer patients with hypercalcemia, however, parathyroid hormone–related peptide is the cause. Specific pharmacologic therapy is usually required in addition to rehydration and furosemide diuresis. Pamidronate (Aredia) (60 to 90 mg IV over 2 hours) or zoledronic acid (Zometa) (4 mg IV over 15 minutes) will reverse hypercalcemia caused by tumor production of parathyroid hormone–related peptide or by bone metastases within 24 to 48 hours. Pamidronate is preferred for patients with renal insufficiency, but it cannot be given when the creatinine clearance falls below 30 mL/min. per 1.73 m². A normal calcium level is often maintained for several weeks to a few months. For patients with severe hypercalcemia, adding calcitonin (4 to 8 IU/kg SQ or IV every 6 to 12 hours or via nasal spray) speeds normalization of the calcium levels. When the calcium level is normal, additional doses of intravenous pamidronate or zoledronic acid can be given, but after several months they tend to lose their effect unless the tumor responds to therapy.

While the RANK-L inhibitor denosumab (120 mg SQ monthly) is not FDA approved for treating cancer-related hypercalcemia, it is effective and often more long lasting than that induced by bisphosphonates (Feldenzer and Sarno 2018).

Corticosteroids are effective in reversing hypercalcemia only for patients with steroid-responsive tumors, such as multiple myeloma or some lymphomas, or the very rare lymphoma that is producing 1,25-dihydroxy vitamin D.

Hypomagnesemia. This may be caused by diuretics or may persist as a residual side effect of chemotherapy with platinum derivatives. If you cannot modify the diuretic therapy, oral replacement with magnesium oxide (400 mg daily or b.i.d.) is usually effective.

Hyponatremia. In patients with lung cancer, hyponatremia is most likely due to ectopic production of antidiuretic hormone (ADH). This syndrome of inappropriate antidiuretic hormone secretion (SIADH) can be treated by fluid restriction, but for patients with advanced cancer, tolvaptan, an oral vasopressin V2 receptor antagonist, is effective palliative therapy (Gralla et al. 2017; Schrier, Gross, and Gheorghiade 2006). Begin with 15 mg/day, increasing to 30 to 60 mg daily if necessary.

Rarely, hyponatremia is due to Addison's disease. Metastases from some tumors (especially lung cancers) replace the adrenal gland and cause adrenocorticoid insufficiency manifested by hyponatremia and hyperkalemia. Patients taking therapeutic doses of megestrol acetate (400 mg p.o. b.i.d.) to increase their appetites can also develop adrenal insufficiency if the megestrol is discontinued abruptly. Addison's disease is possible but extremely rare (<1 percent) in patients receiving immunotherapy. Oral hormone replacement with hydrocortisone (20 mg p.o. every morning and 10 mg p.o. every evening) plus fludrocortisone (Florinef) (0.05 to 0.15 mg p.o.) is usually adequate.

Hypokalemia. Hypokalemia usually results from vomiting, diarrhea, renal potassium wasting caused by certain chemotherapies (e.g., cisplatin), or diuretics used to treat edema. Very rarely, the cause is ectopic production of adrenocorticotropic hormone (ACTH) (Raff and Carroll 2015), usually from a lung tumor. If pasireotide, a somatostatin receptor analogue that targets corticotroph adenoma ACTH production, is not effective, one of various agents that ablate the adrenals (i.e., aminoglutethamide, metyrapone, mitotane) can reverse the hypokalemia. Patients who undergo attempted pharmacologic adrenal ablation need careful monitoring and, if the procedure is successful, hormone replacement.

Hyperglycemia and hypoglycemia. A common complication of the high-dose corticosteroid therapy needed by patients with spinal cord or brain metastases, or of high-dose prolonged octreotide therapy, is *hyperglycemia,* which responds to standard diabetic regimens. *Hypoglycemia* resulting from insulin-producing islet cell tumors is rare, but other, non–islet cell tumors can also impair hepatic gluconeogenesis and cause hypoglycemia. One-fifth of these tumors are hepatomas, and about two-thirds are of mesenchymal origin (i.e., mesotheliomas, fibrosarcomas, leiomyosarcomas, neurofibrosarcomas, and hemangiopericytomas).

Frequent oral feedings of simple carbohydrates often help patients with insulin-producing tumors refractory to cytotoxic chemotherapy, alcohol ablation, peptide receptor radionuclide therapy, octreotide, everolimus, pasireotide, or sorafenib, but intravenous infusions of glucagon and/or glucose through indwelling central catheters or PICC lines may be required. For patients with large tumors of mesenchymal origin who require high-dose intravenous dextrose infusions to control their hypoglycemia, consider palliative debulking surgery.

Anorexia and Cachexia

Anorexia is a common complication of cancer, occurring in as many as 85 percent of patients with advanced disease. If it is part of a syndrome of depression, accompanies an infection or a gastrointestinal disturbance, is from a metabolic derangement (e.g., hypercalcemia), or is a side effect of a drug that alters the taste of food (e.g., metronidazole), the anorexia may be reversible. But in many patients with advanced cancer, anorexia and cachexia occur with no definable cause.

Cachexia (weight loss of >5 percent of body weight over the preceding 6 months in the absence of starvation; or body mass index <20 and weight loss >2 percent; or sarcopenia and weight loss >2 percent; Roeland et al. 2020) is a complex metabolic syndrome most commonly found in patients with non–small cell lung cancers and gastrointestinal malignancies. In addition to weight loss, the hallmark of cachexia is muscle loss, which contributes to weakness and fatigue. Treatment of the cancer, nutritional counseling from a licensed nutritionist, and adding fortified foods and supplements may reverse so-called precachexia (patients with <5 percent weight loss and anorexia). But cachexia is more difficult to treat and usually becomes refractory cachexia when the tumor or noncancer illness is refractory. Patients with refractory cachexia have a less than 3 months prognosis (Jozwiak and Recka 2020; Roeland et al. 2020).

Dysgeusia. Dysgeusia is a loss of taste acuity or a distortion of taste, often induced by chemotherapy (Hovan et al. 2010). It is one of the causes of anorexia and cachexia. Patients report food aversion (especially for meat or umami) and/or unpleasant changes in taste and smell. In patients with solid tumors receiving therapy, in one study, 56 percent reported dysgeusia (Frowen, Hughes, and Skeat 2020); a similar number of patients with dysgeusia was found in those with hematopoietic stem cell transplants or hematologic malignancies.

Patients report a bitter or metallic taste from changes in the oral epithelial mucosa, as well as from drugs excreted into the saliva (IJpma et al. 2015). In a small study of 5 patients with hematologic malignancies and 9 with head and neck cancer, all had lost taste for umami, which affects interest in eating and may have the strongest correlation with appetite (Epstein et al. 2019). In another study of more than 240 patients, difficulty tasting salt was most common, followed by umami and sweetness, but the severity and nature of the taste changes varied by chemotherapy regimen (Campagna et al. 2018).

Any drug can cause these alterations, but taxanes and vincristine are most problematic. Despite treatment with zinc, folic acid, alpha-lipoic acid, and

B vitamins, the dysgeusia can last up to two months after the last dose of chemotherapy. Patients should be advised to eat soft, moist, fatty foods that require little chewing. Salty foods are often better tolerated than sweet ones.

Treatments. Symptomatic treatments for patients with reversible anorexia (e.g., from chemotherapy or following mucositis) include frequent and appetizing meals, supplements, appetite enhancers, and, for carefully selected patients, parenteral or enteral feeding (Table 10.6).

Meals and supplements. Nutritionists will explore with patients and their families ways to make meals more appealing and can supply booklets containing recipes and relevant nutritional information for patients who have advanced cancer but are not in the last weeks of life; this counseling can increase caloric intake by about 500 calories a day. For example, substitutes can be offered for meat, which is often distasteful: nuts or nut butters, for example, or protein powders added to drinks such as milkshakes or blended fruit combinations containing, for example, ice, bananas, and orange juice. Patients can be advised to eat high-calorie foods and to change to a grazing style, eating several small meals a day. They can take a multivitamin pill so that they can eat what they want and not worry about maintaining a balanced diet. Some patients like nutritional supplements (e.g., Ensure, Sustacal, Resource), but others prefer the taste of some of the powdered breakfast drinks dissolved in extra-rich milk for additional calories or, for those with lactose intolerance, in lactose-reduced milk.

There is no demonstrated benefit, however, to forcing meals or intake of these high-calorie supplements. Unfortunately, within a month after dietary counseling, most patients have returned to their previous caloric intake.

Appetite Enhancers

Several medications can act as appetite enhancers.

Megestrol acetate. Megestrol acetate (Megace) (400 mg b.i.d.), which has moderate support from the ASCO guidelines, can improve appetite and cause weight gain, which may be important to patients who are concerned about their appearance (Roeland et al. 2020). It usually does not improve strength, however, because there is no increase in muscle tissue; and if the weight gain is excessive, it may even impair the patient's activity. A 2-week trial is adequate; if there is no change in appetite or weight in that time, the agent can be discontinued. Chronic use of megestrol acetate can cause subclinical and, rarely, clinically apparent adrenal suppression, which manifests as adrenal insufficiency if the drug is abruptly discontinued. Taper it over a week or more and give stress corticosteroids to patients recently withdrawn from megestrol acetate who develop a severe medical illness or are to undergo surgery. Use of megestrol acetate is also associated with an increased risk of venous thromboembolism, which is already increased in many cancer patients, particularly those with a history of venous thromboembolism.

Corticosteroids. In randomized double-blind crossover trials, corticosteroids (e.g., 0.75 to 1.5 mg of dexamethasone q.i.d., 5 mg of prednisone t.i.d., or 16 mg of methylprednisolone b.i.d.) improved patients' appetites and food intake for a month or even two, but at the cost of significant side effects and no increase in weight or change in nutritional status. Other regimens with lower doses (2–4 mg dexamethasone/day for 7 days) improved appetite in 68.5 percent of palliative care patients (Yavuzsen et al. 2005). The ASCO guideline is moderately in favor of using corticosteroids (Roeland et al. 2020).

Cannabinoids. Dronabinol (δ-9-tetrahydrocannabinol) (2.5 to 7.5 mg t.i.d.—also available by suppository) has been particularly effective in improving the appetites of patients with AIDS, but its side-effect profile limits the population that finds it useful. ASCO has a "weak against" recommendation for its use in cancer patients (Roeland et al. 2020).

Mirtazapine. Mirtazapine (Remeron) at low doses (15 mg p.o. at bedtime) improves appetite, but no data are available on whether mirtazapine produces weight gain in patients with advanced cancer. The orexic effect is lost at higher doses.

Androgens and selective androgen receptor modulators. Oxandrolone is an oral testosterone derivative that has been shown in several nonrandomized studies to increase weight in patients with HIV/AIDS. A prospective descriptive study demonstrated that in addition to increasing body weight, patients taking oxandrolone increased their body cell mass and their lean soft tissue mass. A similar improvement in patients taking oxandrolone (10 mg p.o. b.i.d.) was noted in an open-label study of 131 cancer patients who were losing weight, but no results of randomized double-blind placebo-controlled trials have appeared. Nandrolone is an androgenic anabolic steroid that has proved effective in reversing the weight loss of patients on dialysis or patients with AIDS, but there are not enough data on patients with cancer to recommend its use.

Selective androgen receptor modulators (SARMs) reversed sarcopenia and increased lean muscle mass in non–small cell lung cancer patients but caused no significant functional improvement. Ghrelin mimetics improved appetite and lean and fat body mass but also caused no functional improvement in this population (Temel et al. 2016). The ASCO guideline gave "no recommendation" about their use. There is also "no recommendation" regarding olanzapine, thalidomide, L-carnitine or other vitamins, minerals, omega-3 fatty acids, or other dietary supplements. There is a moderate recommendation against melatonin and TNF inhibitors, and a strong recommendation against hydrazine sulfate (Roeland et al. 2020).

Enteral or parenteral feeding. Enteral or parenteral feeding is most useful early in the course of cancer, when patients are undergoing surgery, chemotherapy, or radiation therapy. If a patient cannot eat because of gastrointestinal disease resulting from cancer or its treatment, invasive techniques to provide nutrition are warranted, especially if the process is expected to respond to therapy.

Enteral therapy. Enteral therapy through a J-tube is usually offered to patients along with initial therapy for esophageal or gastric cancer. Patients who are aspirating because of reversible recurrent laryngeal nerve paralysis, or whose enteral obstruction is expected to improve after specific therapy for cancer of the esophagus or the head and neck, for example, are likely to benefit from an NG feeding tube or a feeding gastrostomy or jejunostomy for several months until the paralysis or obstruction resolves. Continuous feeding (e.g., over 12 hours in the evening and while the patient sleeps) is usually well tolerated and, unlike bolus feeding, does not induce diarrhea. If diarrhea does occur, it can usually be managed by diluting the hypertonic preparations or changing to a supplement with a different formulation. The tubes are placed in the patient either in the hospital or in a short-procedure unit, and the family is taught how to use them. Often, patients can give themselves the feedings.

Parenteral nutrition. Parenteral nutrition benefits selected populations (e.g., bone marrow transplant recipients and those undergoing hepatectomy for hepatocellular carcinoma) and patients with bowel obstruction who do not have cancer cachexia but who cannot use the enteral route.

Severely malnourished patients with gastrointestinal malignancies (i.e., who have lost >10 percent of their usual body weight over the 6 months prior to diagnosis) probably benefit from perioperative parenteral nutrition. A large randomized trial in gastric and colorectal cancer patients demonstrated decreased noninfectious complications and possibly decreased mortality in patients randomized to parenteral nutrition 10 days before surgery and 9 days after (Bozzetti et al. 2000). Bozzetti and colleagues recommend attention to preoperative hydration status (to minimize pulmonary complications) and prevention of hyperglycemia (to minimize infections).

A 2020 randomized clinical trial in patients with advanced cancer cachexia showed that parenteral nutrition improved neither health-related quality of life nor survival and was associated with more serious adverse events (Bouleuc et al. 2020), and ASCO's recent clinical practice guideline recommends moderately *against* parenteral or enteral nutrition for cancer cachexia in patients with advanced cancer (Roeland et al. 2020). Though many patients having parenteral nutrition will take in more calories and gain weight, routine use of parenteral nutrition does not decrease chemotherapy-induced complications, prolong life, or reduce perioperative morbidity or postoperative mortality (Casarett, Kapo, and Caplan 2005).

Patients with far-advanced cancer are unlikely to benefit either from a feeding tube or from parenteral nutrition. They rarely complain of hunger or thirst, and small amounts of water or food satisfy them. Nevertheless, they may ask for enteral or parenteral nutrition because they associate their lack of food or water intake with their weakness or lethargy. Unfortunately, while malnutrition can contribute to weakness, reversing malnutrition does not lead to marked increase in strength or energy in patients with extensive, refractory disease. The reasons for this are unclear.

Rarely, even after I explain this, some patients or their families are still interested in enteral or parenteral nutrition. For some families, this is because they harbor one of the hidden concerns discussed earlier: feelings of personal rejection because the patient does not want to eat; a sense that the patient has given up and will abandon them when they are not ready to let her go; or a feeling that the patient does not love them enough to continue the fight.

Others may not fully understand the implications of receiving an enteral device and being fed with tube feedings. The complications that may ensue from enteral feeding via feeding tube, gastrostomy, or jejunostomy are listed below (adapted from Ahronheim 1996).

Problems Related to the Feeding Device or Its Placement

- Discomfort
- Dislodgment
- Nasal, esophageal, gastric, or intestinal erosions or perforations
- Bleeding
- Peritonitis
- Abdominal wall leakage or cellulitis
- Ileus or bowel obstruction
- Pneumothorax
- Complications of the anesthesia required for placement
- Restraints on patient mobility

Problems Related to the Solutions Infused

- Electrolyte disturbance
- Bloating
- Regurgitation
- Aspiration
- Diarrhea

When patients and their families understand both the limited benefits and the magnitude of the problems enteral feeding can cause, it can become much less attractive.

Parenteral feeding is likewise fraught with complications both during catheter insertion (e.g., pneumothorax, hemorrhage) and later (e.g., bacterial and fungal infections, catheter occlusion, and migration leading to superior vena cava syndrome). Palliative care practitioners can partner with you to help these patients and families weigh the benefits and burdens of artificial nutrition. When in doubt, a time-limited trial may be helpful to determine whether artificial nutrition remains effective in enabling patients and families to achieve their goals.

Coping Strategies

When the weakness and fatigue is not reversible, it is useful to give the patient and his family some strategies for dealing with it. Patients may mistakenly think that going to bed for a time will help them regain their normal strength, as it did in the past when they had another illness. Advise them to minimize the time they spend in bed to maximize their remaining strength. Selected patients may benefit from physical therapy consultation.

Practice Points: Helping Patients Cope with Weakness and Fatigue

- Encourage patients to spend time out of bed.
- Advise patients to obtain equipment that will help them maintain mobility.
- Encourage patients to continue the activities that are most important and to relinquish others.
- Encourage sensory, intellectual, and interpersonal stimulation.
- Provide emotional support to family members who are distressed by the patient's symptoms.

Patients can maintain mobility by renting portable equipment: walkers, wheelchairs, lift chairs, electric hospital beds, tray tables, and commodes or shower chairs. Many insurance companies cover these rentals, and eligible veterans can obtain them free of charge.

Common sense advice like planning for short rest periods during the day, limiting trips, and delegating exhausting chores can be surprisingly helpful. It is often hard for people to relinquish these tasks, especially if the tasks helped define their role in the family. You or your staff can often assist patients in identifying which of these tasks are most important to them and which they wouldn't mind delegating: cooking, for example, may be more important than shopping; reading the bedtime story may be as satisfying as giving the nighttime bath.

For those who are bedridden, sensory, intellectual, or interpersonal stimulation is still important. Listening to music, reading, or drawing can be encouraged. Or you can urge the family to play audiobooks or movies or encourage other family members or friends or hospice volunteers to drop by to reminisce, play games, or read to the patient.

A friend of mine was even more imaginative. One Saturday, she turned her mother's hospital room into a picnic site, complete with a hamper and Italian delicacies. On another occasion, for a holiday meal, she brought formal linens and tableware and arranged a Zoom call on her computer so her mother could join the rest of the family in the festivities.

It helps me to remember that, in most cases, the weakness is not troublesome to the patient, who is often living a satisfying life despite what others may see as disabling limitations. Families are much more likely to be suffering than the patient himself because of the changes in their loved one. The family members are often the most in need of our help.

SUMMARY

In this chapter I have reviewed the major problem areas affecting patients with far-advanced cancer: xerostomia, infections and other lesions of the oral cavity; ascites, diarrhea, dysphagia, nausea, vomiting, and bowel obstruction; dyspnea, cough, hemoptysis, and hiccups; therapy- or cancer-induced skin problems; sleeplessness; hot flashes; and weakness and fatigue.

Patients with far-advanced cancer can experience many of these distressing symptoms. The causes of these problems can sometimes be reversed, even in very frail patients. When we cannot reverse the cause of the problem, there is often an effective symptomatic treatment available, along with support for coping with the new reality advanced cancer creates.

Tables

TABLE 10.1 Oral Care

Problem	Therapy
Routine maintenance	Multivitamins/minerals
	Brushing, flossing
	Antibacterial rinses (sans alcohol)
Candida	Troches (miconazole, clotrimazole) q.i.d.
	Ketoconazole (Nizoral) 200 mg b.i.d. p.o.
	Fluconazole (Diflucan) 200 mg p.o. Day 1, then 100 mg/day p.o.
	Itraconazole (Sporanox) (tablet or solution) 100–200 mg/day p.o.
	Amphotericin B solution (100 mg/ml) 1 ml t.i.d. to q.i.d., rinse and spit
Treatment-induced mucositis	
Prevention	Frequent saline and antiseptic rinses daily (prevention) without chlorhexidine
	KGF-1 infusion
	Oral cryotherapy
	+/- Photobiomodulation with low-level laser therapy
Treatment	Frequent saline and antiseptic rinses daily (prevention) without chlorhexidine
	Magic mouthwash: diphenylhydramine + lidocaine + antacid; or doxepin
	Topical morphine (0.2%) q4h p.r.n.
Xerostomia	Sugar-free sour candies
	Moist gauze
	Pilocarpine (Salagen) 5–10 mg t.i.d. p.o.
	Cevimeline (Evoxac) 30 mg p.o. t.i.d.
	Acupuncture

TABLE 10.2 Pharmacologic Treatment of Nausea and Vomiting

Etiology of Nausea	Drug	Dose
Known Etiology		
Initiation of opioid therapy	Prochlorperazine (Compazine)	10 mg p.o. t.i.d or q.i.d. to 25 mg b.i.d p.r.
	Ondansetron	1–4 mg p.o. t.i.d.
Gastric acidity	Proton pump inhibitors (e.g., esomeprazole)	20 mg daily to b.i.d. p.o./IV
	H2 blockers (e.g., famotidine)	300 mg b.i.d. p.o. (may cause delirium in elderly patients)
Vertigo	Hyoscyamine (Levsin)	1–2 tsp. (elixir) or 1–2 tablets p.o./ sublingual/chewed q4h
	Scopolamine (Transderm Scōp)	1 patch q72h
	Meclizine (Bonine, Antivert)	25–50 mg t.i.d. p.o.
Delayed gastric emptying	Metoclopramide (Reglan)	5–10 mg b.i.d. to q.i.d. p.o. or 1–5 mg/hr IV or SQ
Uremia, liver metastases	Haloperidol (Haldol)	0.5–1 mg t.i.d. p.o., p.r., or SQ
	Prochlorperazine (Compazine)	5–10 mg p.o. q4-6h or 25 mg p.r. b.i.d. or t.i.d.
Brain metastases	Dexamethasone	10 mg q.i.d. or 40 mg every morning p.o., p.r., or SQ
Anxiety	Lorazepam (Ativan)	0.5 to 2 mg q4-6h p.o. or sublingual
Bowel obstruction	Dexamethasone +	10 mg IV or SQ b.i.d.
	Hyoscyamine (Levsin) or	1–2 tsp. (elixir) or 1–2 tablets p.o./ sublingual/chewed q4h
	Scopolamine (Transderm Scōp) or	1 patch q72h
	Glycopyrrolate	0.2 to 0.4 mg IV q4h
	Metoclopramide (Reglan)	10 mg p.o./SQ/IV q6h if partial bowel obstruction
Refractory bowel obstruction	Dexamethasone +	10 mg IV or SQ b.i.d.
	Octreotide (Sandostatin)	100–200 mcg SQ b.i.d to t.i.d
Unknown Etiology		
	Omeprazole	20 mg po daily or b.i.d.
	Metoclopramide (Reglan)	10 mg p.o./SQ/IV q6h or 1 hr before meals
Refractory nausea	Olanzapine (Zyprexa, Zydis)	2.5–5 mg p.o./sublingual q.h.s. to q.i.d.
Nausea still refractory	Dexamethasone	4 mg daily or b.i.d. at 8 a.m. and 2 p.m.
	Ondansetron (Zofran)	4–8 mg b.i.d. or t.i.d. p.o. or IV
	Lorazepam	1 mg b.i.d. to t.i.d. p.o. or IV
	Haloperidol (Haldol)	1–2 mg p.o. t.i.d. to q.i.d., 0.5–2 mg IV b.i.d. to q.i.d.
Other	Tetrahydrocannabinol (Marinol)	2.5–10 mg p.o. b.i.d. to t.i.d.

TABLE 10.3 Pharmacologic Treatment of Dyspnea, Cough, and Hiccups

Cause	Drug	Dose
Dyspnea from anxiety/panic	Lorazepam (Ativan)	0.5–2 mg p.o. or sublingual q4-6h
	Clonazepam (Klonopin)	0.5–1 mg p.o. h.s. or b.i.d.
	Midazolam (Versed)	0.2–0.5 mg IV slowly or 0.1-3 mg/hr SQ
	Morphine*	2–5 mg IV, p.o.
	Chlorpromazine (Thorazine)	12.5–25 mg p.o., p.r., or IV
Dyspnea—other etiology	Morphine*	2.5–5 mg q4h p.o.; titrate upward as needed
	Fentanyl	10–25 mcg q1-2h IV or SQ, titrate upward as needed
Cough	Dextromethorphan elixir	15–30 ml q6h p.o. p.r.n.
	Benzonatate (Tessalon Perles)	1–2 p.o. t.i.d
	Hyoscyamine (Levsin)	1–2 ml (drops) or 1–2 tablets p.o./ sublingual/chewed q4h
	Glycopyrrolate (Robinul)	0.1–0.2 mg IV t.i.d. to q.i.d.
	Scopolamine (Transderm Scōp)	1–3 patches q72h
	Morphine*	2.5–5 mg q4h p.o.; titrate as needed
	Albuterol	0.5 mg in 2.5 mg normal saline
	Nebulized lidocaine	2 ml of 2% lidocaine in 1 ml of normal saline, for 10 min.
Hiccups	Baclofen (Lioresal)	5–10 mg p.o. b.i.d. to 20 mg t.i.d.
	Gabapentin	100 mg p.o. t.i.d.; titrate to effect
	Pregabalin	50 mg p.o. b.i.d. to t.i.d; titrate to effect
	Metoclopramide	5–10 mg p.o. or IV q.i.d
	Chlorpromazine (Thorazine)	25–50 mg IV once; then 25–50 mg t.i.d. p.o. or p.r.
	Haloperidol (Haldol)	2–5 mg/day p.o. p.r., or 0.5-2 mg IV q4h
	Proton pump inhibitor	20 mg p.o. daily or b.i.d.
	Nifedipine	10–20 mg p.o. t.i.d.
	Sertraline	50–100 mg/day p.o.

*Other opioids may be substituted for morphine. Begin with equipotent dose of the other opioid and titrate to effect.

TABLE 10.4 Immunotherapy Toxicities

Toxicity	Onset	Time to Resolution	Manifestations
Skin	4–7 weeks	3–12 weeks	Rash, pruritus
GI tract and liver	10–12 weeks (rarely 5 wks)	2–4 weeks	Diarrhea, hepatitis
Lung	10–12 weeks (rarely 5 wks)	5–6 weeks	Diffuse pneumonitis
Central nervous system	Variable	8 weeks	Sensory and motor neuropathy; rare encephalitis; Guillain Barre; myasthenia
Endocrinopathies	2nd month of therapy	11–54 weeks (many need permanent replacement)	Endocrine deficiency from inflammation
Kidney	14–42 weeks	10 weeks (only half resolve)	Nephritis

Sources: Hansen et al. 2018; Weisenthal et al. 2018.

TABLE 10.5 Pharmacologic Treatment of Insomnia

Cause	Drug	Dose
Anxiety	Lorazepam (Ativan)	0.5–2 mg p.o. h.s.
	Clonazepam	0.5–1 mg p.o. h.s.
Delirium	Olanzapine (Zyprexa)	2.5–5 mg p.o. h.s.
	Haloperidol (Haldol)	0.5–2 mg p.o., up to 10 mg p.o. in p.m.
	Quetiapine (Seroquel)	25–50 mg p.o. h.s.; titrate p.r.n.
Menopausal symptoms	Venlafaxine (Effexor)	37.5–75 p.o. b.i.d.
	Gabapentin	100–300 mg p.o. h.s.
Restless leg syndrome		
Idiopathic	Dopamine agonists	
	Pramipexole (Mirapex)	0.125 mg/day p.o.; increase by 0.125 mg q. 2–3 days as needed
	Levodopa-carbidopa (Sinemet)	25/100 mg; 1–2 tabs. qhs
Painful	Gabapentin (Neurontin)	100–300 mg p.o. h.s.
Other	Clonazepam (Klonopin)	0.5–1 mg p.o. h.s.
Unknown	Ramelteon (Rozerem)	8 mg p.o. h.s.
	Zaleplon (Sonata)	5–10 mg p.o. h.s.
	Eszopiclone (Lunesta)	1–3 mg p.o. h.s.
	Doxepin	25–50 mg p.o. h.s.
	Suvorexant (Belsomra)	10–20 mg p.o. h.s.
	Zolpidem (Ambien)	5–10 mg p.o. h.s.

Source: Early 2003.

TABLE 10.6 Treatment of Weakness and Fatigue

Cause	Drug/Procedure	Dose
Undefined	Endurance and weight training, yoga, massage, cognitive-behavioral and psychoeducational therapies	
	Methylphenidate	5–40 mg in divided doses daily
Lambert-Eaton	Amifampridine (Firdapse)	5–10 mg p.o. t.i.d.
Anemia	Transfuse per guideline	
Renal failure	Erythropoietin (Epogen) + iron	50–150 U/kg SQ t.i.w.
Cancer/treatment related in stable or responsive patients	Erythropoietin (Procrit) + iron	40,000–60,000 U SQ q1 week (REMS required)
	Darbepoetin-α (Aranesp) + iron	200–300 μg q2 weeks SQ (REMS required)
Hypercalcemia	Pamidronate (Aredia)	60–90 mg IV over 2 hr
	Zoledronic acid (Zometa)	4 mg IV over 15 min.
	Denosumab (Xgeva)	120 mg SQ q4 weeks
	Calcitonin	4–8 IU/kg SQ or IM q6-12h or via nasal spray
Hyponatremia		
SIADH	Tolvaptan (Declomycin)	15 mg p.o. daily, increase to 30–60 mg daily if needed
Adrenal replacement with tumor	Hydrocortisone + fludrocortisone (Florinef)	20 mg every morning p.o. and 10 mg every evening p.o. + 0.05–0.15 mg/day p.o.
Hypokalemia from ectopic ACTH	Pasireotide	0.6–0.9 mg SQ b.i.d.
	Aminoglutethimide (Cytadren)	Consult with oncologist/endocrinologist
	Metyrapone	
	Mitotane (Lysodren)	
Hypoglycemia		
Insulinoma	Glucagon	Consult with endocrinologist
Mesenchymal tumors	Debulking surgery	
Anorexia		
Dysguesia	Replace zinc, B vitamins, folate; easily chewed foods	
Idiopathic	Adjust diet/supplements	
Appetite enhancers	Megestrol acetate (Megace)	400 mg b.i.d. p.o.
	Dexamethasone	0.75–1.5 mg q.i.d. p.o., IV
	Prednisone	5 mg t.i.d. p.o.
	Methylprednisolone	16 mg b.i.d. p.o.
	Mirtazapine (Remeron)	15 mg q.h.s.

PART III

End of Life and Bereavement

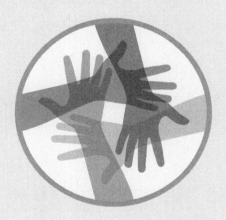

CHAPTER 11

Approaching the End

Concerns of Patients and Their Families at the End of Life

Chapters 11, 12, and 13 are about the care for and support of patients and their families at the end of life, both before and following the patient's death. In Chapters 12 and 13, we review how to provide sophisticated symptom control, as well as other aspects of the clinical management of patients in their last weeks of life, and how to care for their bereaved families. In this chapter, I discuss the components of a "good death," the tasks of dying patients, the role of hospice and palliative care teams in the communication challenges presenting at this stage of illness, and the integration of palliative care with oncology.

I also review what for me has been a very distressing matter—a patient's request that I help him take his own life or, worse, that I end his life. I examine why patients ask this of us and suggest how we can respond—whether or not we help them achieve their wishes. I discuss Medical Aid in Dying (MAiD), where it is legal, eligibility requirements, the interdisciplinary team challenges, and the ethical concerns held by many clinicians asked to consider or take part in MAiD.

COMPONENTS OF A "GOOD DEATH"

We cannot change the downhill course of some patients with far-advanced ill-nesses. We can, however, strive to provide all patients with care as they die. In 1997, the Institute of Medicine offered the following definition of a good death: "free from avoidable distress and suffering for patients, families, and caregivers; in general accord with the patients' and families' wishes; and reasonably consistent with clinical, cultural, and ethical standards." (IOM 1997). Marilyn Webb (1997), in the conclusion to her book *The Good Death: The New American Search to Reshape the End of Life*, operationalizes these in the ten components that she found to be present when someone died a "good death":

- Open, ongoing communication
- Preservation of the patient's decision-making power
- Sophisticated symptom control
- Limits on excessive treatment
- A focus on preserving the patient's quality of life
- Emotional support
- Financial support
- Family support
- Spiritual support
- The medical staff's not abandoning the patient even when curative treatment is no longer available

All of the above components of a "good death," except for "limits on treatment," have been found to be important to a majority of nonwhite as well as white pa-tients (Cain and McCleskey 2019; Ko et al. 2013; Mori et al. 2018; Tong et al. 2003). Differences have been noted, however, when the preferences of different popula-tions are examined, although of course an individual may not share the majority views of a group to which they belong. On the whole, when studied, nonwhite pa-tients and families report a greater preference for religious and spiritual care and for preservation of the family's decision-making power. This is in comparison to whites, who, on the whole, seem to prefer a focus on autonomy and the individual.

Many patients and families would add the additional domains of respect for cultural and religious traditions, including food allowed, care of the body after death, and inclusion of members of not just the nuclear family of choice but also the extended family. The latter may be of particular importance to patients who have experienced alienation from their families of origin, whether due to their identity, religious preference, or any other reason. In this book and this chapter, I want to stress the importance of cultural curiosity, of avoiding stereotyping on the basis of ethnicity or culture, and instead asking what is important (Tong et al.

2003). Both nonwhite and white U.S. clergy (77 percent Protestant) were found to associate a good death with these same factors: lack of physical suffering, being surrounded by loving persons (i.e., community), dignity (e.g., recognizing a person's unique personhood and maintaining physical appearance and function), and preparedness (spiritual, emotional, social reconciliation, and conflict resolution) (LeBaron et al. 2015).

Special concerns of LGBTQ+ cancer patients at the end of life that could interfere with experiencing a good death include whether it is safe to disclose sexual orientation or gender identity to clinicians—whether that will hamper the care they receive and the questions they can ask, and how their family and surrogates will be treated by providers (Stein et al. 2020). It is important to identify their chosen family members and informal caregivers to clinicians so all can get the support they need. Health care providers should recognize that though patients may have experienced prior discrimination or exclusion by certain religious traditions due to their identity or choices, they and their family members may still be spiritual or religious. Unless this is done, the chosen family and caregivers are at risk of being denied the spiritual assessment and support they may need as the patient is dying and in their bereavement (Cloyes, Hull, and Davis 2018; Stevens and Abrahm 2019).

Older LGBTQ+ women have specific issues and experiences, related to what was described as "vulnerability associated with isolation and poverty, women's social needs and support networks, and preferences for complementary care" (Valenti et al. 2020). They preferred to die at home, in hospice care, and relied on former partners and chosen family.

TASKS OF THE DYING

Many patients have endorsed the following goals at the end of life (adapted from Block 2001, p. 2900):

- Maintaining a sense of continuity with one's self
- Maintaining and enhancing relationships
- Making meaning of one's life and death
- Achieving a sense of control
- Confronting and preparing for death

Knowing that time is shorter than you hoped and cultivating patients' and families' prognostic awareness (see Chapter 5) can focus patients and families to work on important areas of their lives. Spiritual counselors and social workers can be effective guides and partners, as can psychological counselors and palliative care clinicians.

Psychotherapies that have proven to be effective for these patients include dignity therapy, individual meaning-centered psychotherapy, short-term life review (Ando et al. 2008), and Managing Cancer and Living Meaningfully (CALM) (Saracino et al. 2019). Dignity therapy and individual meaning-centered psychotherapy are of particular help for those patients at the end of life with existential distress; they are reviewed in detail by Saracino et al. (2019). We discuss existential distress in depth in Chapter 9. In the coming years, psychedelics, such as psilocybin, may prove helpful to some who are searching and aid patients with significant existential distress (Back 2019). Early data support the use of psilocybin for anxiety, depression, and existential distress in selected patients with life-threatening illness (Agin-Liebes et al. 2020).

In their practical and readable 2019 book, *A Beginner's Guide to the End: Practical Advice for Living Life and Facing Death*, Dr. Bruce J (B. J.) Miller and Shoshana Berger include some practical guidance in how to accomplish other "tasks" of the dying. Table 11.1 lists the tasks they discuss. B. J. is one of our former Dana-Farber Cancer Institute (DFCI) hospice and palliative care fellows and the executive director of the Zen Hospice Project in San Francisco, California from 2011 to 2016. As with the goals listed above, these tasks are not accomplished alone, but with the help of family, loved ones, and experts in each area.

TABLE 11.1 Tasks of the Dying

Planning ahead
1. Clean out your attic.
   a. Distribute family heirlooms.
   b. Sell things you don't want.
2. Now clean out your emotional attic.
   a. Secrets and lies
   b. Say the "four" things: I love you, Thank you, I forgive you, Please forgive me (Byock 2004)

Leaving a mark—your legacy
1. Bequeath money.
2. Capture your story (e.g., Storycorps.org and StoryWorth.com).
3. Write an ethical will.
4. Leave a letter.

Yes, there's paperwork
1. Prepare a will, revocable living trust, an advance directive with a health care agent, and a durable power of attorney for finances. Let them know you appointed them and discuss your wishes with them. Give them a copy of your forms.
2. Decide what to put into your "When I Die" file (for your family's easy reference).
3. Choose someone to manage your health care and finances.

Can I afford to die?
1. Add up the costs at the end of life and what's covered by insurance.
2. Determine what happens to debt.
3. What does long-term care insurance cover?
4. What does Medicaid cover?

Source: Adapted from Miller and Berger 2019.

PRIORITIZED SYMPTOM LISTS

You may find yourself wondering where to concentrate your efforts when patients and their families come with a seemingly insurmountable problem list, including physical symptoms, as well as social, spiritual, and emotional challenges. Dr. Russell Portenoy (currently professor of neurology at Albert Einstein College of Medicine, director of the MJHS Institute for Innovation in Palliative Care, and chief medical officer of MJHS Hospice and Palliative Care) and his colleagues taught me how to prioritize these complaints.

Clinicians, families, and patients first determine which symptoms are most troublesome, which are likely to respond to therapy, and what, if any, aggressive diagnostic evaluations and therapies the patient is still willing to accept. They use this information to rank the problems in order of both import to the patient and ease of reversal (RK Portenoy, personal communication, 1993). Using this *prioritized symptom list* as a guide, your efforts can be focused on controlling the most distressing and the most reversible problems. Understanding the discordance among the patient's, family's, and clinician's lists is often the key to caring for patients and families.

The Patient's List

Mr. Smith, whom we met in Chapter 5, was a patient with castrate-resistant prostate cancer. His symptom list included:

- Pain
- Dry mouth
- Constipation
- Weakness

Dr. Verna, his oncologist, reassured Mr. Smith that his pain could be relieved to a degree that would be satisfactory to him. With oral, parenteral, transmucosal, or transdermal medications, you can expect to relieve the pain of 95 percent of your patients with cancer. Constipation, whether due to hypercalcemia, inactivity, or opioids, is even more likely to be entirely relieved with appropriate medications. The mouth dryness will lessen if the patient discontinues medications with anticholinergic properties (such as diphenhydramine) or adds a wetting agent such as Biotene or agents that stimulate saliva production—pilocarpine or sour candies, for instance. (Chapters 10 and 12 provide more details on the therapies that are effective for these complaints.) Weakness, however, unless it is caused by anemia, is likely to be more difficult to reverse.

In that case, what can be done? I'd tell Mr. Smith that I was confident we could treat the first three symptoms successfully, but I'd admit that his weakness was less likely to be reversible and was an expected symptom of his advancing cancer. I would offer supportive counseling, PT, OT, and any assist devices he needed to maximize his function. I would also help him to grieve his loss of strength and the associated losses of independence and important roles, such as those he held in his church and his family. As Dr. Cassell recommends (see below, and our discussion in Chapter 1), to address his suffering, I would have to help him accommodate to the loss of these aspects of his personhood and, if possible, find other roles and activities that held meaning for him.

The Family's List

The family's list is rarely as straightforward as the patient's. Underlying the problems they report are the hidden concerns and unasked questions that are usually equally troubling and often harder to address. One family with such concerns was the Hermans.

Unspoken Family Expectations

Mr. Herman was a 65-year-old man whose metastatic lung cancer had progressed despite therapy. He had the same complaints as Mr. Smith (pain, dry mouth, constipation, weakness), but he seemed satisfied with the treatment regimen I had instituted. I looked forward to his weekly visits. But at one visit, his wife and daughters accompanied him, and they were by no means pleased with his progress. The daughters detailed their concerns:

> Dad is not eating enough and is spending most of his day in bed because he's so weak. We don't understand why you haven't given him something to increase his appetite, or maybe put a feeding tube in his stomach. If he got more food, we're sure he'd get stronger and feel much better. Also, Mom tells us that he keeps her up half the night, helping him to the bathroom or worrying that he needs something as he tosses and turns. She thinks this means he's still in pain, though he's taking the medicine you gave him. We know there's nothing that will stop the cancer, but he lies around in bed all day. We bring him his favorite foods, but he only picks at them. Can't you do something?

As I listened, I mentally created what you might call the family's priority list.

The Patient's List	The Family's List
• Pain	• Weakness
• Dry mouth	• Lack of appetite
• Constipation	• Sleeplessness
• Weakness	• Pain

As you can see, the family's priority list differs significantly from Mr. Herman's. Pain and weakness make it onto the list, but their order of importance is reversed. Mr. Herman's lack of activity was not troublesome to him, but it was severely distressing to his family, as was his sleeplessness. He had *no* complaints of hunger or thirst, and yet his family was asking me to put a feeding tube in him. I knew that feeding tubes are not helpful for patients like Mr. Herman, who can eat; for older patients with decubiti and poor oral intake; or for patients with dementia who are no longer eating (Davies et al. 2021; Teno et al. 2012). How was I to meet his family's needs without subjecting Mr. Herman to unnecessary procedures or medications?

The key was to understand the hidden concerns that led to such disparate priority lists. What were the underlying causes of the family's distress? Dr. J. Andrew Billings's *Outpatient Management of Advanced Cancer* (1985) offers useful answers in its discussion of the concept of *attribution*—what meaning the family *attributes* to the patient's actions, rather than what the patient's actions actually *mean*.

Mr. Herman did not eat because he wasn't hungry, but his family was attributing his failure to eat to a rejection of the food they prepared and, by extension, a rejection of the people preparing it. This same reaction manifests in families in which children have made food choices that differ from those of their parents. Meat-eating parents of vegan children may be outraged at their offsprings' choice of diet. Why? Not because the diet they have chosen is unhealthy but because, in rejecting their parents' food choices, the children may be rejecting their parents and their values.

Mr. Herman is simply not hungry—but his family feels rejected and left out. They also attribute his failure to eat to his "giving up." We all know that without food there is no life, so food can become tied to concerns about survival and struggles with anticipatory grief and letting go. It feels to them like the first step toward the eventual abandonment his death will bring. They want me to prevent or at least delay this. His staying in bed only reinforces their conviction that he is giving up or, in other words, that he is leaving them before they're ready for him to go. And they cannot bear that.

Once I understood these hidden concerns, I could address them, rather than just deal with the requests themselves. As a palliative care physician, I often have conversations like this with families. But as his oncologist, I could also have said:

I know it must hurt when your dad doesn't eat much of the foods you prepare especially for him. But as he's told you, he's really not hungry or thirsty. It's common for people who have as much cancer as your dad does not to feel hungry or thirsty and to get enjoyment from much less food than we need. But rejecting your food doesn't mean he's rejecting you—he loves you and wants to be with you as long as he can. He is getting weaker, but that is because his cancer is getting worse. Putting a feeding tube in him won't make him live any longer, and it's likely to make him less comfortable in the time he has left. He can already eat anything he wants, and even though he doesn't eat a lot of what you bring him, knowing you make or bring anything he asks for really makes him feel loved and special.

To families for whom *giving up* seems to be an important issue, I might also say:

I know it must seem as if he's giving up—as if he's leaving you—and that hurts, too. But he's fought this cancer a long time, and he's tired of fighting now. He loves all of you very much, and that hasn't changed just because he can't fight anymore. Let's all concentrate on helping him have what he wants and on helping him be as comfortable as possible for as long as he has left. We can help fight for him to have peace and comfort now.

In my experience, this difference between patient and family priority lists is the rule rather than the exception. It is common for me to have discussions similar to those described above. Almost always during such a talk, family members begin to acknowledge their feelings and begin to accept the seriousness of the patient's condition. Requests for medications to increase appetite or for placement of a feeding tube disappear. As we discuss in Chapter 5, sometimes just acknowledging that families have helped their loved one to "fight the good fight" and to shift "blame" to the cancer itself can help allow for this emotional transition.

It would have been quicker and simpler for me to accede to the Herman family's requests to refer him for a feeding tube, but to do so would have been a disservice to Mr. Herman—and to his family as well. I would not have discovered or helped them deal with their feelings of rejection and grief. If they never realized that these feelings were underlying their requests to me, their final days and weeks with Mr. Herman might have been marred by their unspoken anger at him misplaced from the cancer, and their grieving after his death would have been unnecessarily complicated by this anger as well. Uncovering and thereby managing these feelings optimized family members' interactions with him in his final days and improved their ability to deal with their eventual loss.

The Clinician's List

Errors of commission. As clinicians we are not immune to creating priority lists that differ from both the patient's and the family's. We have had personal experiences that make us feel we must offer or withhold certain treatments to or from patients, whether or not they express a need for them. This became clear to me when I was working with a surgical chief resident who had admitted one of my patients.

Misdirected Efforts

Mr. Jackson had colon cancer that was metastatic to his peritoneum and liver. He had been admitted to the surgical service for a possible small-bowel obstruction. The obstruction responded to conservative measures, but Mr. Jackson had to remain in the hospital while awaiting placement in a nursing home.

The surgeon complained to me about Mr. Jackson's poor oral intake. I explained to him that the patient had told me he was comfortable since the obstruction had resolved and that he was eating all he wanted. To my surprise, however, when I returned three days later from a conference, Mr. Jackson had a feeding tube in place.

I sought out the surgeon and asked why, despite my express wishes to the contrary, he had placed a feeding tube in Mr. Jackson. At first he reiterated his concerns about Mr. Jackson's poor oral intake, but finally he explained his real reason. It seems that his own grandfather was dying of esophageal cancer and was unable to swallow anything. The surgeon's father was therefore delivering medications via suppository, which the surgeon found extremely degrading. He told me vehemently, *"No other family is going to have to go through what my grandfather is going through!"*

I gently reminded him that my patient had a totally patent esophagus and could swallow perfectly well—he just had no appetite. The surgeon rather sheepishly agreed that Mr. Jackson hadn't needed the tube and that he did not realize how much his own family situation had clouded his judgment.

Errors of omission. In addition to errors of commission (such as inserting an unnecessary feeding tube), our own needs can also lead us to equally serious errors of omission. In Chapter 1, for example, we reviewed the barriers that prevent us from discussing advance care planning with patients with far-advanced disease. It is even harder for many of us to participate in the emotionally intense and often draining care of patients who are in their final months.

Eric Cassell, in *The Nature of Suffering and the Goals of Medicine* (2004), offers insights into the factors that prevent clinicians from appreciating the needs of dying patients. The initial obstacles appear during medical school, where we learn what he calls "The promise of science: to know the disease is to know the illness and its treatment" (p. 20). He notes that "many doctors—perhaps most people—still believe that different persons with the same disease will have the same sickness" (p. viii). But a disease such as pneumonia, he explains, can cause different illnesses in different people. Moreover, Cassell writes that medical science is perceived by clinicians as value-free and objective, but clinicians themselves are in the business of treating *people*, who are value-laden and, by their nature, subjective. A sick person, he says, is the subject not the object of care. There is no population for whom this is truer than the dying.

But how are you to know your patients' values? Some of you are lucky enough to have the luxury of longitudinal relationships with your patients. You may come to know their values through the choices they make as you treat their various acute medical problems or guide them through their cancer therapies. Are they risk-takers? Is quality of life of paramount importance, or quantity? How did they tolerate treatment-related side effects? Did incapacity affect their sense of self-worth? And so on.

To discover more about their hopes, worries, values, and goals, it would be useful to ask the questions in the Serious Illness Conversation Guide (Figure 11.1), even if you've asked them before, and to document the answers.

This knowledge is invaluable for anyone who seeks to understand how best to serve their dying patients and their families. You must elicit the information through careful questioning of your patients about the goals they hope to achieve and how their family functions, and you must take care not simply to substitute your values for theirs.

Serious Illness Conversation Guide

PATIENT-TESTED LANGUAGE

SET UP
"I'd like to talk about what is ahead with your illness and do some thinking in advance about what is important to you so that I can make sure we provide you with the care you want — **is this okay?**"

ASSESS
"What is **your understanding** now of where you are with your illness?"

"How much **information** about what is likely to be ahead with your illness would you like from me?"

SHARE
"I want to share with you **my understanding** of where things are with your illness..."

Uncertain: "It can be difficult to predict what will happen with your illness. I **hope** you will continue to live well for a long time but I'm **worried** that you could get sick quickly, and I think it is important to prepare for that possibility."
OR
Time: "I **wish** we were not in this situation, but I am **worried** that time may be as short as ___ (express as a range, e.g. days to weeks, weeks to months, months to a year)."
OR
Function: "I **hope** that this is not the case, but I'm **worried** that this may be as strong as you will feel, and things are likely to get more difficult."

EXPLORE
"What are your most important **goals** if your health situation worsens?"

"What are your biggest **fears and worries** about the future with your health?"

"What gives you **strength** as you think about the future with your illness?"

"What **abilities** are so critical to your life that you can't imagine living without them?"

"If you become sicker, **how much are you willing to go through** for the possibility of gaining more time?"

"How much does your **family** know about your priorities and wishes?"

CLOSE
"I've heard you say that ___ is really important to you. Keeping that in mind, and what we know about your illness, I **recommend** that we ___. This will help us make sure that your treatment plans reflect what's important to you."

"How does this plan seem to you?"

"I will do everything I can to help you through this."

© 2015 Ariadne Labs: A Joint Center for Health Systems Innovation (www.ariadnelabs.org) and Dana-Farber Cancer Institute. Revised April 2017. Licensed under the Creative Commons Attribution-NonCommercial-ShareAlike 4.0 International License, http://creativecommons.org/licenses/by-nc-sa/4.0/   SI-CG 2017-04-18   **ARIADNE LABS**

FIGURE 11.1. Serious Illness Conversation Guide. A free, well-studied communication tool that provides you with specific language for conversations with patients who have life-limiting illnesses and their families about goals, hopes, worries, fears, sources of strength, what abilities are critical to their lives having quality, and what they would trade for more time. *Source:* Ariadne Labs; reprinted with permission. https://www.ariadnelabs.org/areas-of-work/serious-illness-care/.

HOSPICE PROGRAMS

How can we help patients at the end of life, as well as their families, achieve some of their goals? Hospice programs are often the answer. A majority of cancer patients prefer to die at home (Higginson et al. 2017). Their families, who provide much of their care, often find this a particularly difficult time and need much support from the hospice team.

Families of patients dying of cancer share many needs (Cherny, Coyle, and Foley 1996):

- Comfort for the patient
- Information and communication
- Evaluation of the family's needs and resources
- Education about care
- Emergency provisions
- Review of how the family is coping
- Care of the family when the patient is unconscious
- Preparation of the family for the dying process
- Conflict resolution

In addition to the needs listed above, Billings (1985) suggests that families taking care of their dying loved ones may experience insecurity, which generally arises from a combination of factors: (1) anticipation of problems (i.e., anything they can imagine happening might indeed happen); (2) a sense of isolation combined with an overwhelming sense of responsibility; and (3) vulnerability and helplessness, which can lead to outrage and even anger.

To help a family avoid feeling insecure, Billings suggests that the medical team must (1) be available, (2) be consistent and dependable, (3) anticipate problems and rehearse responses, (4) elicit and address attributions (misinterpretations of what the patient's actions mean), and (5) offer reassurance, encouragement, and hopefulness.

The members of a hospice team can help in all these areas. They can also help you stay connected with patients and families, preventing any fears of abandonment by their oncology team. The role of the hospice team is to anticipate problems and rehearse and deliver solutions for patients' psychological, social, financial, and spiritual needs. If, for example, the patient is likely to become delirious, they include appropriate medications (e.g., haloperidol) in the *hospice comfort kit* the family has at home, teach the family how to identify delirium and how to reach the hospice nurse 24/7, and reassure them that the hospice nurses on call will tell them how to administer these medications if needed.

Hospice team members also reassure family members that they are doing a wonderful job, that they are special people for assuming this responsibility, and that by doing so, they are enabling their loved one to remain at home. They remind the family that they are not expected to be experts and that hospice personnel will be there to help, if not in person, then by phone or a virtual visit. When I (*Molly Collins*) was a child and my family cared for my grandmothers at our home on hospice, I can vividly recall how much confidence the capable hospice nurses instilled in my family that we could do this.

Hospice nurses, social workers, chaplains, and volunteers are superb problem-solvers who have developed strategies that are often effective in addressing the complex sources of distress of dying patients, including those with advanced cancer. But home hospice care is not the best solution for everyone. Patients will receive about 2 hours a day of help from a home health aide if the patient needs that help, but the family and friends are responsible for the care for the other 22 hours. Palliative care clinicians, discharge planners, and hospice liaisons can help patients and families choose the right location for care at the end of life.

Families with enough financial resources can supplement the hospice team with private home health aides, especially for the overnight hours, so the caregivers can get some much-needed sleep. But if the patient needs several hands to turn her or get her out of bed, and there is only one caregiver in the home, she may be better cared for by moving to a nursing home and having a hospice team visit her there. Patients who have numerous "ostomy" bags or tubes to empty, are incontinent and need beds changed several times a day, or have an NG tube to suction because they are obstructed also may be better served in a skilled nursing facility, where family members can visit but are not responsible for around-the-clock nursing care.

Families who do not have the means or the training may not be able to care for those patients whose comfort requires complex medical regimens, which may include parenteral delivery of fluids or opioids for those who have bowel obstructions. Those families can be helped a great deal by the clinician explaining that it is a medical decision that the patient would not be best served at home. You might say, *"I know how much you want him home. And if we could find a way where he could be comfortable there, we would send him home with you and a hospice team. But his care is just too complex to be delivered at home, as much as you'd love to do that."*

For patients whose care is less complex, all the family may need is help and education from the nurses and nursing aides that the home hospice program can provide. While you continue to approve the orders, nurses and social workers from the team make the needed assessments, and they educate the family in techniques of care and ensure that the appropriate medications, supplies, and services are obtained to provide optimal patient comfort.

Hospice services. Hospice programs are required to offer four levels of care: routine home care, continuous home care (24-hour nursing), respite care in a facility (a nursing home or inpatient hospice facility) for up to 5 days every month, and inpatient care in a hospital or inpatient hospice facility if the patient needs that level of care to control symptoms. Of these four levels, it is most difficult for hospices to provide the nursing staff for continuous home care; patients who need that level of care may instead be admitted to an inpatient hospice facility or even a hospital to ensure their comfort. The patient can stay enrolled in the hospice program at those other sites. Many hospices have their own inpatient facilities, and all contract with local hospitals and nursing homes so that they can provide continuous care at whatever site the patient requires it. The different services provided in each level of clinical care are described in Table 11.2. A helpful booklet, *Medicare Hospice Benefits,* describes who is eligible for Medicare hospice and what the benefit entails. It is free from Medicare and Medicaid services.

Routine care. Hospice nurses make routine home visits as often as needed and are a source of information and of communication from the family to you or other caregivers. For patients who are referred months before their death, these visits can provide much-needed care and support for patients and families, as well as, ideally, the chance to build rapport and trust with hospice staff. A hospice nurse will be available by phone 24 hours a day, and the program will try to provide a nurse for a home visit for emergencies that cannot be handled by phone, as staffing allows. Some patients require only weekly visits from them; others may need a nurse daily; and a few will need 24-hour nursing, though staffing concerns affect how often hospices are able to provide this level of care.

TABLE 11.2 Levels of Clinical Care Provided by Hospice Programs

	Routine	Continuous	Inpatient	Respite
24-hr on call	✓	✓	✓	✓
Home health aide	≤2 hr/day			
RN visits	≤3/wk + p.r.n.			
Social worker visits	q2wk			
Chaplain visits	q2–4 wk			
Volunteer	2–4 hr/wk			
MD	p.r.n.			
Occupational/physical/ respiratory therapy	p.r.n.			
Continuous nursing		≥8 hr RN/day		
Inpatient care			p.r.n.	
Respite care				5 days/month

Note: Continuous home care is for patients with, for example, refractory cough, dyspnea, pain, or delirium; they can receive 24-hour nursing and home health aide services.

Inpatient care is for refractory symptoms that cannot be controlled at home, even with continuous care. The referring physician admits the patient and may bill for services under Medicare Part B.

The goal of *respite care* (in a community skilled or intermediate nursing facility) is either to provide a rest for the caregiver or to remove the patient to an adequate facility when the home is temporarily inadequate to meet the patient's care needs.

For those patients who need them, the nurses will also authorize home health aide services up to 2 hours a day, typically 5 days a week, to help with bathing, dressing, and other care needs. Oxygen and all needed durable medical equipment (like hospital beds and commodes) are provided, and the hospice pharmacy delivers all symptom-related medications to the home. But because of the small amount hospices are reimbursed daily to care for each patient (see "Hospice Finances," below), patients usually will not be able to receive blood transfusions or parenteral nutrition or antibiotics when enrolled in hospice care. A limited amount of intravenous hydration may be provided if it is thought necessary for patients to complete their final goals.

The hospice team can also help patients without a *skilled need* who live in a nursing home, because the nursing home is considered a patient's place of residence. It can, however, be difficult to place hospitalized patients directly into a nursing home for the first time for hospice care, unless families have the means to pay the daily rate for care in a nursing home.

If patients have a skilled need, they will qualify for a skilled nursing facility and can receive palliative care, but not hospice care if their insurance is Medicare. Medicare patients cannot receive both skilled care and hospice care at the same time. The hospice program can provide the patients' palliative care in the skilled care facility and, as they decline, transfer them to a hospice house or a nursing home with whom they have contracts. The hospice liaisons work with the inpatient and skilled nursing facilities to help patients find the best place allowed by their insurance plans.

I often recommend that patients enter hospice programs, and I have developed my own way of explaining the benefits and limitations of hospice programs to patients and their families who may be wary of enrolling. They may hold a number of common myths and misconceptions about hospice programs, the most common of which are reviewed in the Practice Points below.

Practice Points: Hospice Myths and Misconceptions

- *"Hospice is a place I will be sent to."*
- *"They will put my loved one on a morphine drip, and then he will die quickly thereafter."*
- Hospice is only for the final hours or days of life: *"My loved one isn't dying yet, so why are you suggesting hospice?"*
- Hospice means *"We are giving up."*
- You can't be full code on hospice.

I usually ask whether the patient or family knows anyone who has been cared for by a hospice program and, if so, what their experience was. This line of questioning can be revealing for which of the myths or misconceptions I need to address in the introduction to hospice care.

I sometimes include the hospice philosophy of care and the services that are provided, while addressing or correcting common myths about hospice care. My explanation might sound something like this:

> *Now that we won't be focusing on the treatment of your cancer, we can focus on helping you make the most of the time you have. I think a home hospice program could help us do that. You would qualify, because, as we've discussed, given that your cancer has not been responding to treatment, as sad as I am to say this, you are not likely to live longer than 6 months, if the disease takes its usual course. I think you have [days to weeks, weeks to months, many months] left, and that's why I am recommending a hospice program. May I tell you a little bit about hospice care?*
>
> *Some folks know a lot about it already, and it's new for others. How about you?* [Continue for those unfamiliar with it] . . . *Hospice care is an enriched home nursing program that can provide the care you and your family need now. A lot of people think that a hospice is a place, but it's actually a set of services. For most people, it's provided at their home, and it's the most comprehensive home care we can offer. Hospice programs are there to support you and your family in the final portion of your illness, all the way to the end, so that you can stay at home and be with your family. The hospice program brings the care to you.*
>
> *I will of course continue to be your physician, but to be able to keep you as comfortable and functional as possible, I need their expert eyes and ears, letting me know how you're doing at home. I will work with them to adjust your medications as I always have.*
>
> *If you enroll in the hospice program at home, they will send a hospice nurse and can provide a home health aide if that would be useful. Most people also want to visit with the hospice social worker, and there is also a hospice chaplain who can make visits if you like. The hospice nurse will be in close touch with me, and I'll sign all your orders, as I always have. He or she will visit as often or as little as you need, typically one to two times a week initially and more often if necessary.*
>
> *Our goal is to manage your symptoms well at home and not to exhaust your family, so that you can stay at home, and be comfortable, without needing to come to the hospital. Even if your symptoms get worse, or new ones arise, we will all work together to manage those for you. And the hospice nurses and social workers will be there to help support your family as*

they care for you. Your family will need to provide the care for almost all of the day. An aide will come for only 2 hours a day, to provide personal care, so your family will need to provide care the remaining 22 hours [if you think they need/can afford private help, especially overnight, I suggest you bring this up here]. *If you need to, or want to, you of course can always be admitted to the hospital or to an inpatient hospice facility to make you more comfortable.*

 That was a lot of information—what questions do you have?

 Preventing family burnout. Family members are understandably reluctant to leave the patient alone, so to help prevent family burnout, the hospice team will urge them to allow a friend, relative, or trained hospice volunteer to stay with the patient for an hour or two each day to enable them to get the break they need. I recommend they use a two-way talk-back baby monitor system; the intercom base is in the patient's room, and one or two caregivers carry or wear the portable units. In this way, even bedridden patients can have some privacy, and the caregivers can be assured that they can pursue other tasks while still being available should the patient need them.

 Caregivers must stay mentally and physically healthy, and full-time care of a patient with advanced cancer is exhausting. Hospice programs are also required to arrange for 5 days of respite care every month for each patient enrolled in the program, if the family requests it. The patient is cared for in a nursing home or hospice house during this time, and caregivers can then go to a family reunion, graduation, or wedding or just catch up on some much-needed sleep.

 The hospice team also tries to ensure that families are comfortable with the choices they have made about the patient's care so that they will have no guilt about these choices when the patient dies. In *Dying Well,* Dr. Ira Byock (1997) shares an important technique he uses to help families explore these issues. For example, when asking a family to consider discontinuation of tube feedings, he says to them, "This is wrenching stuff, so take as much time as you need. None of us, in the months to come, and especially after [the patient] has died, wants to look back and wonder whether we did the right thing" (p. 180). This contains two helpful notions. The first is to treat this transition in an unharried, unpressured manner if the clinical situation allows, and the second is to ask families to look to the future and try to avoid decisions that my lead to regret.

 I have begun using this approach each time I ask for family input in a significant decision, such as *"Should a feeding tube be placed?"; "Should we change the focus to comfort care?";* or *"Will you be able to keep him here at home when he is dying?"* I ask the family to imagine that it is now several months since the patient has died, and they are looking back at the choices I am asking them to make now: *"How do you feel about this decision? Do you still think we did the right thing? Was everything we did in agreement with* [the patient's] *values and goals, and with yours?"* If they are able to answer yes to these questions, they are much more likely to remain at peace with their decisions after their loved one dies.

As patients near death, hospice nurses can bring emergency provisions, prepare the family for the dying process, and help support the family if the patient becomes unconscious. Hospice nurses can also serve the important role of being with the family at the bedside as the patient dies, adjusting the patient's medications, and reassuring the family that everything possible is being done; they will also talk with the family immediately after the death to offer comfort and to assess and attempt to alleviate any persistent concerns. Hospice nurses pronounce patients' death and provide immediate bereavement support in the aftermath of death.

Hospice financing. The Medicare hospice benefit (and the other hospice benefit plans modeled after the Medicare program) pays for all these services: personnel, medications, durable medical equipment, supplies, and any other authorized services needed to provide patient comfort (e.g., a surgical consultation to debride a wound, thoracentesis for pleural effusion, sometimes radiation if necessary to treat painful bony metastases).

Some people are reluctant to elect this benefit because they misunderstand several of its provisions. For example, patients may think they have to give up their private physician and other clinicians who have been caring for them. That is not true: patients can continue to see you; you are allowed to bill for professional services separately under Medicare Part B, as before. And patients can be hospitalized if they develop a problem requiring an inpatient stay for management of a symptom, such as rapidly escalating pain or severe delirium. They do not have to agree to be DNR/DNI. The hospice nurses will not perform the resuscitation themselves, but they will call 911.

Hospice services are also available to patients without the Medicare hospice benefit. Private insurance, managed care plans, and Medicaid programs offer various hospice benefits, and the indigent can sometimes be enrolled for free. Your local hospice agencies, some of which are nonprofit, others for-profit, will be happy to inform patients and families of the range of services they can provide. Patients and families can review websites, visit inpatient facilities, and talk with their nursing liaisons. Hospital or outpatient social workers or discharge planners are often excellent sources of information. Families can also compare markers of quality and caregivers' experiences on a Medicare website (www.medicare.gov /care-compare). If they have other questions, they can contact the National Hospice and Palliative Care Organization (NHPCO, www.nhpco.org).

In sum, even when further life extension and cancer-directed treatment becomes impossible or too risky, there is still much more we can do to support patients and families at the end of life. It is important that we understand and describe the hospice program and its services accurately and avoid thinking, *We can do nothing.* Hospice programs provide a critical extra layer of support, with robust evidence supporting their benefits for patients and families.

Practice Points: Benefits of Hospice Care

- The hospice philosophy is to ensure the best quality of life for patients with terminal illnesses.
- Patients are eligible for the hospice benefit if two doctors (i.e., the patient's doctor and the medical director of the hospice program) certify they are expected to live for 6 months or less with the disease taking its usual course.
- Multidisciplinary team care usually takes place in the patient's home. The team includes nurses, social workers, nursing aides, chaplains, volunteers, nurse practitioners, and physicians (including the patient's physician).
- Care is centered on the goals and values of patients and their families.
- Attention is paid to the physical, psychological, social, financial, spiritual, and existential causes of distress.
- All medications, equipment, and supplies related to the diagnosis for which the patient entered hospice, which are needed to maintain patient comfort, are provided.
- If needed, 24-hour home nursing or hospitalization of the patient for uncontrollable symptoms is available.
- Respite care for the patient in a nursing or inpatient hospice facility is available for about 5 days every month, if needed by the family.
- The patient does not have to request DNR to enroll, although some inpatient hospices and hospice houses do require this.

Hospice Care Isn't Right for Everyone

Lack of provision of transfusions. Patients with hematologic malignancies or refractory cytopenias from nonmalignant marrow disease or as a result of cancer-directed therapies may need transfusions to maintain quality of life and in some cases life itself. They and their caregivers value what hospice programs provide but consider transfusion a key service that the vast majority of hospice programs can't afford to offer. When insurance providers other than Medicare *carve out* (i.e., pay for) transfusions and hospice care, caregivers have reported being very satisfied with the hospice services provided (Henckel et al. 2020).

Lack of nonwhite enrollment. Adult patients make up the bulk of patients in hospice care in the United States, and nonwhite patients enroll in hospice services much less often than their numbers would predict (Fishman et al. 2009). The reasons are complex, including provider behavior, patient preferences, and systemic barriers. Providers reported that barriers to hospice referral for nonwhite patients included the provider's difficulty in conducting end-of-life goals of care conversations and lack of knowledge about hospice eligibility criteria; language barriers without adequate access to skilled interpreters; lack of comfort in caring for people of diverse cultures; and perceived lack of trust in the health care system by nonwhite patients (Cicolello and Anandarajah 2019).

As with all other areas of medicine, systemic racism and bias infiltrates the care that is provided, especially to and for Black and Latinx patients. An ongoing desire for cancer-directed and other life-prolonging therapies would exclude patients from the hospice benefit, and Black patients have been found to have a stronger preference for continuing cancer treatment than white patients, although Black patients would have enrolled in hospice if they could continue cancer treatment while receiving hospice services.

A specific barrier to the enrollment of Hispanic and Latinx patients is that the Spanish cognate for hospice, *hospicio*, is a term that actually refers to an "orphanage" or "a place for poor people." For Central and South American Latinx patients, many barriers to hospice enrollment and care have been identified (Kreling et al. 2010). These include language barriers, both of those referring and the hospice caregivers; lack of insurance; legal status; direct rather than indirect communication about prognosis; lack of appreciation for the family decision-making style; hospice referrals made during hospitalization crises with no familiarity with those making the referral; and the focus of hospice teams on preparing patients for death (Kreling et al. 2010).

A survey of Queens County, New York, Hispanic and Asian adults (Chinese, Korean) in their preferred language revealed that patients had little experience with or information about hospice services but were open to learning more (Pan et al. 2015), findings that are similar to the findings of others studying these nonwhite populations.

Some of these barriers were present when I (*Molly Collins*) referred Jade Markman, whose story I shared in Chapter 1, to a hospice program. Jade was a 30-year-old mother of two with triple-negative breast cancer who had brain metastases, leptomeningeal disease, and no further options for cancer-directed treatment. Jade initially agreed that hospice care at home would be most appropriate, stating, "*I want to stay home on hospice care as long as I can do for myself. Once self-care is not possible, I would like to be transferred to the hospice facility. In the event I am unable to speak for myself, my doctors know to do as much as they can and then just keep me comfortable.*" Jade had completed a POLST consistent with her stated wishes, that she only be rehospitalized for comfort, and as required in our state, an out-of-hospital DNR form. Dr. Mehta, Jade's social worker Janice, and I breathed a sigh of relief, knowing that Jade would be comfortable at the end, and she would not receive futile care in an ER if she landed there after hours.

But things don't always go as we hope. Jade and her family did not feel reassured by the hospice agency's presentation of their palliative philosophy of care, in which the dying process was treated as imminent and expected. They, like many other patients and families, didn't want to be reminded of her demise; while they were aware it would come sooner than they wished, they wanted professional and personal caregivers to focus on what Jade could still accomplish, and keep Jade as comfortable as possible while allowing her enough alertness to complete important tasks.

When Jade called the hospice agency after hours with questions about why she felt short of breath, she was told by a nurse whom she did not know to take liquid morphine from the comfort kit. But the nurse was not able to review her record and recommended too low a dose for her, given her opioid tolerance. Jade had for years gotten frequent attentive care focused on addressing each issue and symptom with a medicalized approach, and it had served her well. Dr. Mehta, Janice, and I were not surprised, therefore, when Jade disenrolled from the hospice program two weeks after enrolling, feeling dissatisfied with their services.

Just as important, Jade and her family really had not come to terms with her prognosis. They still had faith that Jade's life could be prolonged indefinitely and that a miracle would occur. Jade's reluctance to discuss her anticipated death and prepare her children for this made it less likely that the hospice philosophy would meet her needs. While Jade was clear that she wanted to maximize her time at home with family, she also wanted any reversible problems causing symptoms reversed and was willing to undergo straightforward procedures (e.g., pleural catheter insertions) or abbreviated hospitalizations to enable her to live as long as possible.

Our health system struggled to bend itself to provide care exactly matched to Jade's goals. She was hospitalized several times in the ensuing months as her disease progressed to help her deal with progressive neurologic deficits, pain, and third-spacing due to malnutrition. The hospitalists caring for her each admission wondered aloud why Dr. Mehta and I couldn't "get her on hospice already" when it was clear she was dying, though slowly.

Her heart was young and strong, and Jade was still alive four months after her initial decision to enroll in hospice care. When COVID-19 hit, Dr. Mehta and I were suddenly crystal clear that further hospitalization would be far more dangerous than helpful to Jade. We initiated weekly telehealth family meetings with Jade, her caregivers, Dr. Mehta, her social worker Janice, and me.

We also convinced her to accept home palliative care services with one of the more robust hospice and home care agencies in our geographic region. Arising from a local academic medical center, this hospice program provided more services than some of the others. Team members understood that many patients hold on to the hope of life prolongation while still benefiting from maximal home care services short of hospice care. Unfortunately, we do not have any *open access* hospice programs in our region, which share the same philosophy that patients may benefit from hospice services while still pursuing life-prolonging care.

I was surprised by the amount of work we were able to do with our telehealth visits with Jade in the final months of her life. This was a labor of love and a substantial weekly time commitment that Dr. Mehta, Janice, and I made to Jade and her family. Given Jade's and her family's difficulty accepting that her death was closer every day, we needed to do this work if we had any hope of preventing a catastrophic full-court-press admission at the end of her life—lines, tubes, and all.

At each marathon telehealth visit, we carefully addressed each of Jade's symptoms, worked with her on her coping, encouraged continued conversations with her family about her imminent death, and ended with, *"You know, Jade, a hospice program would make a lot of sense for you right now."* We framed this with our hopes that hospice care would provide additional support in the event of a crisis and prevent hospitalization.

Only when the end came for Jade did we understand the depths to which her mother was never on board with a purely palliative approach to her care. One morning, Jade developed sudden severe shortness of breath, and her mother called 911, panicked. Jade had had a respiratory arrest at home, and though there was an out-of-hospital DNR form and a POLST we had all discussed many times, her mother asked that the EMTs attempt resuscitation. This was unsuccessful, and Jade died at home. Dr. Mehta, Janice, and I spoke to her mother that day, who told us she had been encouraging Jade to forgo hospice care, hoping beyond hope for a miracle. She was still in shock at how short Jade's time on this earth had been.

Dr. Mehta, Janice, and I weren't surprised by what happened at the end of Jade's life, recalling, *"She wouldn't have wanted it any other way, telling us she wanted to 'fight until I flatline.'"* I knew in my heart that we could not have given Jade more attention or better goal-directed care. There are some families and patients whom I cannot help to accept that death is near, no matter what. And for these families, hospice care may always represent death.

BRIDGE PROGRAMS

If a hospice program does not fit the family's needs, a *bridge to hospice* program can help by arranging for home care nurses and health aides and limited visits from social workers. This is often called *home palliative care* and is typically provided by a hospice agency, but it may be provided by a palliative home care team associated with visiting nurse services.

The services are more limited than what can be provided under the hospice benefit, but they nonetheless provide additional support. They can also provide physical therapy, hospital beds, commodes, and oxygen if the patient qualifies and insurance approves. Sometimes 24/7 phone support is offered by these services but not always. That support may be crucial when patients have a crisis but prefer not to be hospitalized. Home palliative care can typically be converted to hospice care with just a phone call. The agency may already be in the home, familiar with the family, and sometimes the same staff can then provide hospice care.

ROLE OF THE PALLIATIVE CARE TEAM

A comprehensive palliative care program includes both hospice and palliative care services. It provides safe passage for patients with life-threatening illnesses and their families during the course of active therapy and, when the burdens of therapy outweigh the benefits, as they die, and their families become bereaved. Hospice and palliative care services should be available at home, in the outpatient setting, and in the hospital, wherever the patient's need can best be served (Figure 11.2).

Unlike hospice teams, palliative care teams can help patients and families from the onset of the cancer diagnosis. Palliative care is an extra layer of support, available throughout the course of a life-threatening illness (Figure 11.3). Palliative care teams address all the domains of distress of patients with cancer and their families, as do hospice teams. Figure 11.4 illustrates the similarities and differences between what palliative care and hospice services provide to patients and families.

As the Center to Advance Palliative Care (CAPC 2021) explains,

> Palliative care is specialized medical care for people with serious illnesses. This type of care is focused on providing patients with relief from the symptoms, pain, and stress of a serious illness. The goal is to improve quality of life for both the patient and the family.
>
> Palliative care is provided by a team of doctors, nurses, social workers, chaplains, and other specialists who work with a patient's other clinicians to provide an extra layer of support. Palliative care is appropriate at any age and at any stage in a serious illness and can be provided together with curative treatment.

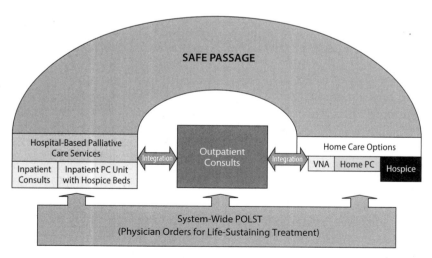

FIGURE 11.2. Elements of a Comprehensive Palliative Care Program. A comprehensive palliative care program can ensure "safe passage" for its patients and families with life-limiting illnesses when it includes integrated home, outpatient, and hospital-based services, including palliative care and hospice programs, and is supported by system-wide communication of resuscitation choices, such as a POLST form, readily accessible in a shared electronic health record.

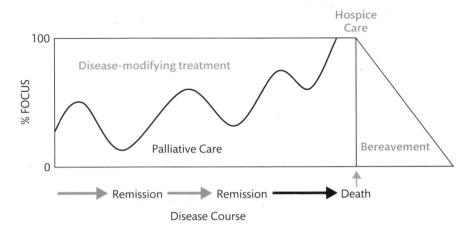

FIGURE 11.3. Concomitant Disease-Modifying Treatment and Palliative Care. Palliative care starts at diagnosis of a life-limiting illness and supplements disease-modifying therapy, even when the main focus of care is on that therapy. Hospice programs are accessed when disease-modifying therapy ends, and the patient has 6 months to live if the disease takes its usual course. Hospice programs support the bereaved family for at least a year after the patient's death.

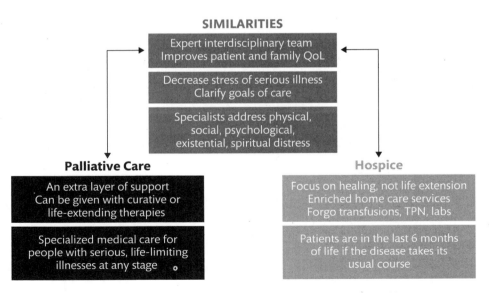

FIGURE 11.4. Functions of Palliative Care versus Hospice Programs. Palliative care and hospice programs have both similar and unique foci and functions.

Palliative care teams usually include nurses (usually nurse practitioners) and physicians, and some also include social workers, chaplains, pharmacists, bereavement counselors, and volunteers. These multidisciplinary or interdisciplinary teams offer assessment and management of physical, psychological, social, and spiritual causes of distress; patient and family education; and counseling, problem solving, and support for the family and often for the referring clinicians. If you don't have an oncology social worker as part of your team, the palliative care team's social worker can be of particular help to you.

Most patients do not require specialty-level palliative care, which is lucky because there certainly are not enough palliative care specialists to care for all who have life-threatening illnesses. The vast majority of patients can receive *primary* palliative care from you, their clinicians, provided you have been trained in the basics of symptom management and effective communication (which is the goal of this book); in the future, individualized symptom management may even be available to clinicians in the electronic medical record, when patient-reported outcomes are integrated with clinical decision support to generate recommendations for symptom assessment and management (Back, Friedman, and Abrahm 2020).

There are, of course, important roles for specialty palliative care teams. They can help educate their colleagues and assist in the care of patients with more complex issues (Quill and Abernethy 2013). Meta-analyses of the efficacy of palliative care teams from randomized controlled studies (RCTs) indicate positive effects on patients' physical symptoms, mood, and quality of life, as well as improved family satisfaction, while decreasing hospital costs and resource utilization (Hui et al. 2018).

Integration of Oncology and Palliative Care

Oncology and palliative care clinicians are increasingly collaborating in the care of cancer patients and their families (Abernathy and Currow 2011; Abrahm 2012; Gilligan 2003). The 2017 ASCO guideline endorses the integration of palliative care into routine oncology care (Ferrell et al. 2017, 2020), and there was a call in 2020 for an integrated fellowship pathway that would lead to dual certification in oncology and palliative care (Sedhom, Gupta, and Kamal 2020).

Patients in phase I trials would appear to be an ideal target for palliative care intervention, but qualitative studies have indicated a lack of interest in palliative care by and for these patients because of misunderstandings about the role of palliative care or a perceived antagonism on the part of the clinicians running the trials to concomitant palliative care (Bellhouse et al. 2020; Cassel et al. 2016). A pilot randomized study found that patients with solid tumors enrolled in phase I trials who had a palliative care intervention had less psychological distress and a trend toward improved quality of life, but more studies are needed (Smith et al. 2020).

Concurrent palliative care is especially important for those patients who have advanced disease and are undergoing treatment, as well as patients who would qualify for a hospice program but do not feel ready for one, or who have become accustomed to an intensity of supportive care (e.g., total parenteral nutrition or transfusions) that they or their family feel contributes significantly to their quality of life (see Figure 11.4). These services may not be available from local hospice programs because those programs receive about $200 per day per patient (as of 2020) to provide all the services, medications, and equipment described in Table 11.2 (see the NHPCO website, www.NHPCO.org). (N.B. the daily per diem rate provided to hospices has not risen proportionally with the rise in health care costs.)

Cancer itself and its treatments cause significant impairments in the quality of life of patients and their families, including their physical, psychological, social, financial, existential, and spiritual selves. In the first year after diagnosis, patients with cancer of many sites carry a heavy symptom burden, with moderate to severe symptom scores, worse in the first month after diagnosis (Bubis et al. 2018).

Palliative care teams can work with these patients, as well as cancer patients at any point along their disease trajectory (diagnosis, relapse, or terminal care). They can provide both consultation and primary clinical care. Teams can be hospital based, outpatient in the cancer center, or make home visits, sometimes as part of an organization that also runs a hospice program (see the discussion of home palliative care, or bridge programs, above). Some insurance companies are now staffing palliative care teams that visit patients in their homes and can improve quality of life and prevent unnecessary hospitalizations (Back, Friedman, and Abrahm 2020).

Strategies for building outpatient palliative care services that provide excellent clinical quality and are financially viable are available (Finlay, Rabow, and Buss 2018; Finlay et al. 2019). In some institutions, patients receiving palliative radiotherapy are cared for by a dedicated supportive and palliative radiation oncology team; these teams have demonstrated improvement in the quality of care, communication with patients and families, and clinician rating of their department's palliative care service (Tseng et al. 2014).

Benefits of early integration of palliative care to patients. Early palliative care is of benefit to patients with advanced cancer who are undergoing active therapy (Bakitas et al. 2015; El-Jawahri et al. 2016, 2017; Schneiter et al. 2019; Temel et al. 2010, 2017; Zimmermann et al. 2014). In the 2010 Temel RCT, integrating palliative care from diagnosis of an incurable malignancy (advanced non–small cell lung cancer) into oncology care resulted in life prolongation of 2.7 months compared with patients who were referred to palliative care consultants only at the discretion of the medical oncologist.

In the 2017 study that replicated and expanded on Temel's 2010 results, lung cancer patients again reported improved quality of life and depression, whereas those receiving usual care deteriorated. There was no change, however, in patients with GI malignancies. Elements of the palliative care intervention that were significantly associated with improved outcomes included a focus on "coping, treatment decisions, and advance care planning" (Hoerger et al. 2018, p. 1096). Patients receiving the intervention showed an increased use of *approach-oriented* coping, which included active coping, positive reframing, and acceptance, as well as a reduction in *avoidant* coping, which included self-blame and denial (Greer et al. 2018).

Even patients undergoing therapy for acute myeloid leukemia (El-Jawahri et al. 2021) or curative hematopoietic stem-cell transplant benefit from early palliative care intervention (El-Jawahri et al. 2016, 2017; Loggers et al. 2016). The stem-cell transplant patients had a stable or improved sense of hope, without negative effects, less decline in quality of life, less increase in depression symptoms and symptom burden, and decline in anxiety symptoms from baseline to Week 2 (El-Jawahri et al. 2016). At 6 months, they had less depression and fewer PTSD symptoms than the patients not receiving the palliative care intervention (El-Jawahri et al. 2017).

Patients with hematologic malignancies, however, rarely use palliative care services, though they have many unmet palliative care needs (LeBlanc and El-Jawahri 2015). Misconceptions about the role of palliative care clinicians and the reaction of the patient to being referred to a palliative care clinician (e.g., taking away hope, giving up), along with the natural reluctance to add yet another team to the care of these complex patients ("I do my own palliative care") can pose significant barriers to providing the most comprehensive care to patients and their families (LeBlanc and El-Jawahri 2015). Financing of palliative care teams is another important limitation. While palliative care has been shown to save money, this care often receives poor reimbursement in a medical system that rewards procedures and volume over care that takes time (Smith and Cassel 2009).

Benefits of integration of palliative care to the oncology team. The NCCN guideline for palliative care (2020) and the ASCO 2017 clinical practice guideline update (Ferrell et al. 2017) both recommend increased integration and early consults for selected cancer patients. By collaborating with board-certified hospice and palliative care physicians or nurse practitioners, oncologists and oncology nurse practitioners can improve prognostication and communication (LeBlanc et al. 2019) and offer the most comprehensive care to patients and their families (Bruera and Hui 2012; Ferrell et al. 2017). Such collaborations have markedly improved patients' ability to discuss their prognosis and other topics of concern with their oncologists (Rodenbach et al. 2017).

Oncology clinicians are trained to learn about the disease and its treatments, but typically not to be expert communicators (Gilligan 2018). During encounters with patients and families, they primarily discuss symptom management, medical updates, and treatment decisions. Palliative care clinicians supplement these conversations by assessing the extent of relief of the patients' symptoms, along with the patients' understanding of both the process of treatment and their prognosis, as well as their hopes, worries, and fears and the congruence of the care plan with what they value (e.g., longevity, quality of life).

More often than oncologists, palliative care clinicians work with the patient and family on coping, supporting the needs of the caregiver, and discussing advance care planning (Thomas et al. 2019). To assist oncologists in improving their skills in these areas, an ASCO multidisciplinary team including both oncology and palliative care experts developed a Patient-Clinician Communication Guideline (Gilligan et al. 2017; Gilligan, Salmi, and Enzinger 2018), which will be of great help to current oncology clinicians as well as future trainees.

The palliative care team remains a useful partner to your team in both the inpatient and the outpatient setting. If you bring them in to help you manage a difficult symptom, members of the team can get to know your patients and their families early in the course of their disease. After working with your patients over months to years, the palliative care team members will more easily assist your team during difficult family meetings. They can remain in the room after you have left to answer questions that the patient or family may have forgotten to or may be reluctant to ask you.

Palliative care team members can be there, as well, to support you when you break really bad news, recommend stopping chemotherapy, discuss hospice care, explore goals and values, and help your patients and their families determine their wishes regarding resuscitation. The palliative care team can offer you and your staff support in dealing with the emotional toll these situations exact. The team can even arrange services of remembrance to help families and oncology team members acknowledge and process the grief associated with this work (see Chapter 13).

Institutional benefits. Finally, palliative care teams benefit the institutions within which they work, helping to increase staff morale, decrease staff turnover, and enhance staff expertise in palliative and end-of-life care. Palliative care teams based in academic medical centers and in teaching hospitals affiliated with these centers also provide training and perform research in palliative medicine (von Gunten 2002). Through consultations and through formal and informal teaching sessions, palliative care teams offer education about the palliative care needs of patients undergoing active therapies, as well as offering insight into the stresses of patients and families as they make the transition to care without chemotherapy (Abrahm 2000; von Gunten et al. 1995).

Many specialties, such as emergency medicine, surgery, hematology-oncology, and pulmonary and critical care medicine, are now including palliative care competencies in their training. For other clinicians, palliative care teaching rounds and seminars offer medical students, residents, and fellows strategies for working within an interdisciplinary group and providing comprehensive care across care sites (inpatient, outpatient, home). Clinicians collaborate in joint, team-based problem solving to arrive at integrated solutions, a practice not often observed in standard medical training (Beninghof and Singer 1992; Billings and Block 1997; Boaden and Leaviss 2000). This instruction can supplement the deficits of medical education and training that leaves clinicians ill-prepared to alleviate the suffering of patients with advanced disease or of their families (Abrahm 2012; Block 2002; Rabow et al. 2000).

MEDICAL AID IN DYING

As I write this in 2021, Medical Aid in Dying (MAiD) (formerly referred to as physician-assisted suicide) is legal in Europe (Belgium, Germany, Luxembourg, The Netherlands, and Switzerland), Colombia, Canada, and the United States. Canada has less clear and broader eligibility requirements than those in the United States' laws: the patient must have "a grievous and irremediable condition, referring to incurable illness causing decline in functioning, reasonably foreseeable natural death, and intolerable physical or psychological suffering which cannot be relieved by means acceptable to the patient. Natural death must be reasonably forseeable" (Isenberg-Grzeda et al. 2020, p. 158).

As of November 2021, MAiD is legal in the District of Columbia and ten states (California, Colorado, Hawaii, Maine, Montana, New Jersey, New Mexico, Oregon, Vermont, and Washington). All states model their eligibility requirements on those of Oregon.

In 33 states (Alaska, Arizona, Arkansas, Connecticut, Delaware, Florida, Georgia, Idaho, Illinois, Indiana, Iowa, Kansas, Kentucky, Louisiana, Maryland, Michigan, Minnesota, Mississippi, Missouri, Nebraska, New Hampshire, New York, North Dakota, Ohio, Oklahoma, Pennsylvania, Rhode Island, South Carolina, South Dakota, Tennessee, Texas, Virginia, Wisconsin), there are statutes that expressly forbid MAiD. Three states criminalize assisted suicide through common law: Alabama, Massachusetts, West Virginia; and Nevada, North Carolina, Utah, and Wyoming have no specific laws or unclear laws in this area.

Euthanasia is currently legal in Canada, Colombia, Belgium, Luxembourg, and The Netherlands. Euthanasia, however, is *illegal* throughout the United States. Webster defines *euthanasia* as "the act or practice of killing or permitting the death of hopelessly sick or injured individuals (such as persons or domestic animals) in a relatively painless way for reasons of mercy." In practice, the clinician administers a fatal dose of an appropriate drug with the goal of ending that patient's suffering. Patients who wish MAiD, in contrast, must take the medications themselves; they are not administered by a clinician. By definition, MAiD is "a physician providing, at the patient's request, a prescription for a lethal dose of medication that the patient can self-administer by ingestion, with the explicit intention of ending life" (AAHPM 2020).

Practice Points: Eligibility in the United States for MAiD

- 18 years of age or older
- Able to prove current (state) residency
- Capable of making and communicating health care decisions for him/herself (psychiatric evaluation may be needed)
- Diagnosed with a terminal illness that will lead to death within 6 months

---

Since 1997, when Oregon passed the first Aid in Dying legislation, much has been learned about why patients request MAiD, how clinicians can respond, and how clinicians (physicians, nurses, nurse practitioners, physician assistants, social workers, and pharmacists) feel about participating.

Responding to Requests for Hastened Death

I (*Janet Abrahm*) have been asked many times either to hasten someone's death or to assist patients who want to end their own lives. The first request I had was from an unexpected source.

The Patient Who Seeks Help in Dying

I was caring for Mr. D'Angelo, a 55-year-old man with Waldenström's macroglobulinemia. Plasmapheresis controlled his blood viscosity, but he had anemia, massive splenomegaly, and an acquired coagulation inhibitor that had caused a von Willebrand's–like disease that was refractory to clotting factor replacement. His only symptoms were weakness and shortness of breath when the anemia became too severe. Splenectomy might have helped, but his coagulopathy made the operation impossible.

Mr. D, as he asked us to call him, was an active gardener and had often brought me homegrown vegetables and herbs. Now, however, even with transfusions, he noted he was getting weaker, and one day, even using his walker, he felt too weak to ambulate. He asked whether he would ever get out of his wheelchair again, and I told him that I didn't think he would. He replied, *"Fine, doc. Then I guess it's about time for you to help me to 'get out' permanently. Life in a wheelchair is not for me."*

I was taken aback. Other than being in a wheelchair, he did not seem to me to have a life that was not worth living. Except for his weakness, his symptoms were easily controlled, and his mind was working well. At the time, projecting my standards of an acceptable quality of life onto Mr. D, it seemed inconceivable that someone would want to die just because he had to use a wheelchair to get around. If he had been closer to bedridden or in severe pain, I could have understood his request. But for Mr. D, the wheelchair created limitations that were simply not acceptable; his quality of life was unsatisfactory, and he wanted to die.

I did not act on his request, and I was unable to comfort him. He refused psychological help but said he would allow a visit from his parish priest. A week later his wife found him dead in his wheelchair. The autopsy, which she requested, revealed a massive myocardial infarction.

Causes of requests for physician-assisted death. Mr. D'Angelo was the first, but since then, like many other physicians, I have had other patients ask me to kill them or to help them end their lives. Studies indicate a number of reasons that patients make such requests (Block and Billings 1994; Quill, Back, and Block 2016).

In Block and Billings's 1994 paper on this subject, they suggest that patients ask us to kill them because they expect us "to be a guide, companion, and caretaker in their final passage. Patients, in fact, lack the technical knowledge to kill themselves quickly and comfortably" (p. 2040). Since we have been managing their care throughout the treatment phase of their illness, they expect us now to provide the expertise to help them die.

Block and Billings also list several reasons that patients who seem to have a lot to live for, like Mr. D, want to end their lives. Some may be concerned that as they get sicker, we will not provide effective control of their symptoms. They may have had bad experiences with the health care system in the past, feel that their symptoms were inadequately treated, and fear a prolonged period of unalleviated suffering. In my experience, a few questions can often unearth these as the main reasons for the request.

They may also fear that their family will fail them. The diagnosis of cancer and the side effects of the treatments may have stressed the family's emotional and financial resources already. Patients may feel their family is overwhelmed or even resentful. Patients who are well cared for may feel that in the future, they will become too great a burden. They cannot risk putting it to the test: failure would be too painful.

When I was their oncologist, I knew that they might also fear that I would abandon them. I would let my patients know almost from their first visit that I would be there "for the duration." I half-jokingly said, *"You know, once you're in my care, there's nothing you can do to lose me. You can take or reject my suggestions for treatment, but you can't get rid of me. You're stuck with me until the end."* Often just my willingness to listen and to give them the security that I would not abandon them offered enough comfort.

I am convinced that for patients who know and accept they are dying, there may be unique opportunities for growth (sometimes called *post-traumatic growth*) that they would miss if they ended their lives prematurely. In my current role as a palliative care physician, I encourage patients to search for new meaning in altered life roles, to accept borrowed strength, and to pursue transcendence (Cassell 1991). I suggest they try to replace some of the losses caused by their illness by

> ### Why Patients Request Medical Aid in Dying
>
> - Patients lack the technical expertise to end their lives themselves.
> - The physician is expected to serve as "guide, companion, and caretaker."
> - Patients worry about adequate symptom control now and in the future.
> - Patients worry that the family will be unable to care for them.
> - Patients do not wish to burden their family.
> - Patients experience loss of personhood, dignity, sense of worth, autonomy, and meaning in life.
> - The physician's attention to the patient's concerns is felt to be inadequate.

finding new roles for themselves in their communities and within their families (Byock 1997). For the many patients so used to being the caregiver, I can help them to see what a gift it can be to let others care for them in the ways they have always done for others.

In Byock's *Dying Well*, for example, Mayor Burke came to understand that by accepting help from a hospice program, his neighbors, and his family, he was filling an important community role and bringing satisfaction to many people. It was his final gift to them. As he said, "I guess it's time to be on the receiving end" (1997, p. 97). The dignity that he sought lay not in his physical condition (he was dying of amyotrophic lateral sclerosis [ALS]) but in something larger, which had, if anything, grown as his health had worsened.

Finally, there are patients who do not know another way to have their concerns addressed, and they use the request for MAiD to shock us into paying attention. While we were concentrating on their physical problems, we may have overlooked their psychological, spiritual, or even financial concerns. Requests for euthanasia or assisted death suggest that the patient harbors such worries and that they are very serious. Asking us to end their lives may be the only way patients feel they can enlist our aid in ending their suffering.

Contributing factors include physical or psychological disorders and the patient's personal values. Patients suffering from existential distress, uncontrolled pain, depression, anxiety, organic brain disorders (such as delirium or brain metastases), or personality disorders are more likely to want to die. And unfortunately, both inadequately controlled pain and psychiatric disorders are common in the terminally ill patient population. In addition, patients who are grieving the many losses associated with their illness (loss of personhood as well as physical, social, financial, and spiritual losses) may feel that death offers the best answer.

When you encounter patients in this kind of despair, you should, in addition to evaluating them for reversible causes, have a low threshold for referring them to professionals skilled in treating psychological, social, and spiritual problems. You or these other professionals may be able to reduce the suffering of these patients, and they will no longer want to hasten their death. Chapter 9 includes a discussion of existential distress, which may be present in patients asking us to help end their lives.

Patients' personal values may also lead to requests for euthanasia or MAiD. Such requests from people with personality disorders may be among the hardest to handle (Block and Billings 1994). Some, for whom remaining in control is especially important, may feel that relinquishing control or their independence is worse than dying. Those who have always been self-reliant, who have had trouble accepting help from others, or who have never been comfortable with the disabilities of others may find it intolerable to imagine becoming dependent on anyone. That is what they are asking you to prevent. In retrospect, I think Mr. D may have been such a person.

Interdisciplinary Team Challenges

Clinicians who receive the request. Clinicians' personal responses to requests to assist in a death vary widely (Block and Billings 1994). Some of us avoid the subject and deny to ourselves that it was even raised. Others feel guilty or depressed about forcing the patient to continue an unwanted, suffering-filled existence. From time to time, a few of us, especially those of us who know the patient well, comply.

There are several ways to deal with such a request other than rejecting or acceding to it outright (Block and Billings 1994). First, acknowledge it and encourage the patient to talk about what has prompted it. Then offer a compassionate, consistent presence to the patient and his family. Next, be clear about what you will and won't do. Although you might be willing, for example, to provide medications to control symptoms, the patient should not expect that you will actually administer a bolus of drug intended to kill him.

Quill and colleagues (2016) suggest how we might address two common patient concerns: worry about future suffering and intolerable current quality of life (Quill, Back, and Block 2016, p. 246). For the former, they suggest asking, "What are you most worried about? Tell me more about exactly what frightens you. What kinds of deaths have you seen in your family? How are you hoping I can help you?" For the latter, "What makes your situation most intolerable right now? Tell me more about the worst part. How do you think your family feels or would feel about your wish? Exactly how are you hoping I can help you?"

Finally, address the change in your relationship with the patient that results from a request for euthanasia or assisted death. Ask how she will feel about you if you cannot fulfill her request—how it will affect future requests of other kinds, and whether it diminishes her trust. Reiterate your offer of help, short of killing her, and let her know that if she now feels she needs to see another clinician, you will understand.

Concerns of clinicians involved in implementing the request. Implementing MAiD involves a team of clinicians to provide care and support for the patient and family members. A scoping review of studies of clinicians who practice MAiD or euthanasia or both indicated several clinician concerns that are likely to be relevant not only for those writing the prescriptions, but also for those who help implement MAiD. Addressing these concerns in preparation to implementing a program of MAiD may help the team function smoothly without developing burnout or moral distress.

The clinicians studied included nurses, mental health providers, physicians, pharmacists, social workers, and medical examiners (Fujioka et al. 2018). Challenges were numerous. Role ambiguity was a particular concern for all the clinicians, but especially for the nurses, who were unclear about the scope of their practice and legal liability (especially when they participated in euthanasia). In MAiD, mental health clinicians were unclear about their role, and pharmacists were unclear about their ability to decline to dispense the medications if they had conscientious objections. While physician practice guidelines were also unclear, there were no reports of their struggle with the role, likely because they chose to opt in to participate in MAiD.

Physicians, nurses, and pharmacists all complained of the lack of interprofessional collaboration, and they and mental health and social workers noted the lack of clarity about conscientious objection. Lack of assurance of safety for those providing MAiD and legal ambiguity in how to evaluate eligibility, capacity, and consent were also areas of major concern. In Canada, for example, what does the law mean by "irremediable" or "intolerable suffering" criteria, and who should decide? All professionals (except pharmacists) wanted more training in end-of-life matters and MAiD.

In countries and states where MAiD is legal, therefore, clinicians who may be asked by patients or family members about the practice need support and education. Just as hospice and palliative care teams are interdisciplinary, efforts to establish interdisciplinary MAiD teams at the state or province level can serve as important resources and support for clinicians implementing MAiD in their practices (Fujioka et al. 2018). Fujioka and colleagues work at the University Health Network, a Toronto-based teaching hospital, but the challenges they identified may apply more broadly. They ask for clarification in regulations and guidelines that stipulate each professional's role: clear "'criteria,' checklists, guidelines for capacity and consent, special considerations for vulnerable populations, processes of consultation and secondary opinion, a clear referral system in the case of conscientious objection, mandatory notification procedures, recommendations to handle conflicting family requests and available resources to further support decision making. In addition, improved education on end-of-life options and MAiD should be integrated into all professional education curricula" (Fujioka et al. 2018, p. 1573).

> **Practice Points: Challenges**
>
> - Absence of clear professional and/or legal guidelines and role ambiguity
> - Lack of interprofessional collaboration
> - Conscientious objection
> - Lack of safeguard assurance
> - Legal ambiguity regarding eligibility, capacity, and consent
> - Lack of knowledge and training in end-of-life matters and MAiD

Clinicians' Ethical Concerns about Medical Aid in Dying

Clinicians in 2021 understand that ethically and legally, patients have the right to refuse to have their lives prolonged artificially. They have the choice to refuse nutrition via oral, IV, G- or J-tube routes; hydration of any type; and cardiac and pulmonary support. Withholding or withdrawing of life-prolonging treatment is ethical and *legal*, even if it means that the patient will die as a result. Nearly all religious leaders as well as legal experts and ethicists agree that withholding or withdrawing such therapy should be distinguished from euthanasia and from MAiD.

Let us be clear: this means that if people want to end their lives, they can choose to forgo water and food and expect death within a few weeks. Voluntarily stopping eating and drinking (VSED) is completely legal and ethically acceptable but often requires a clinician's assistance for management of problems such as dry mouth or delirium that can occur before the person becomes somnolent (Quill, Lo, and Brock 1997; Quill, Truog, and Pope 2018).

Clinician organizations in the United States and elsewhere are divided in their opinions on MAiD. Some, like the American Academy of Hospice and Palliative Medicine, the American Academy of Neurology, the British Medical Association (revised position in 2021), and the American Nursing Association, take a position of "studied neutrality," noting, "morally conscientious individuals adhere to a broad range of positions on this issue." The American Medical Women's Association is in favor. But in 2017 the American College of Physicians reaffirmed its opposition, as did the American Medical Association in 2019, the National Hospice and Palliative Care Organization in 2020, and the American Academy of Pediatrics in 2021.

Pain, palliative care, and hospice experts are divided as well. Dr. Timothy Quill (the Georgia and Thomas Gosness Distinguished Professor of Palliative Care, and professor of medicine, psychiatry, medical humanities, and nursing at the University of Rochester School of Medicine), who was the plaintiff in *Vacco vs. Quill* in 1997, was an early advocate, while Dr. Kathleen Foley (professor of neurology, neurosciences, and clinical pharmacology at Weill Cornell Medical College; the founder and the former chief of the Pain Service at Memorial Sloan-Kettering Cancer Center; and the former medical director of the International Palliative Care Initiative of Open Society Foundations) opposed legalizing either MAiD or euthanasia (Foley and Hendin 2004), as have Dr. Daniel Sulmasy and others (2018).

Those in favor of MAiD argue on the basis of patient autonomy and nonabandonment that MAiD is the "ultimate, merciful medical means of ending suffering the patients deem intolerable" and that not allowing MAiD denies patients who do not rely on life support (which can be ethically discontinued) medical assistance in dying (Sulmasy et al. 2018). Organizations and clinicians who are opposed to MAiD argue that autonomy does not include the right to "demand" a procedure from a clinician, that clinicians do not have the tools to assess what patients (even imminently terminal patients) report as intolerable suffering that has been refractory to medical therapies, and that MAiD is in opposition to the primary medical directives to do no harm and to heal, if not cure, patients (Sulmasy et al. 2018).

Further, some are concerned that with legalization, MAiD would replace other, more appropriate treatment of a patient's distress. It remains true that most health professionals have inadequate training in the symptom management skills of palliative care, such as treating uncontrolled pain; they also lack the training to recognize and therefore to address the reasons for requests for MAiD discussed above, including depression or existential suffering (Foley 1991, 1995, 1997; Foley and Hendin 2004). Clinicians who remain unaware of what expert palliation can offer may find MAiD an attractive solution.

It is clear that now, more than ever in the past, clinician education in how to recognize and relieve suffering, education of the public about the efficacy of currently available treatments for suffering, and enhanced provision of hospice services and palliative care consultations must accompany any legislation that makes MAiD more readily available. The Oregon example is one that can be followed.

Palliative care availability in Oregon is the best of all 50 states, and Oregon has by far the highest percentage of the population that is able to die at home. In the 21 years since 1998, when the Death with Dignity Act went into effect, as of 2019, only 2,518 people received lethal prescriptions, and only 1,657 (66 percent) used them (Oregon Public Health Division 2019). It seems there was no "slippery slope." Less than 1 percent of deaths in Oregon involve MAiD. In 2019, only 290 prescriptions were written, and only 188 (65 percent) were used.

The concerns that uncontrolled symptoms or fear of being a burden on families would lead people to choose MAiD were unfounded. Patients who chose to take the lethal prescription, both in Oregon and in Washington, where physician-assisted death became legal in 2009 (Loggers et al. 2013), did so for three main reasons: loss of autonomy (93.5 to 97 percent), inability to participate in activities that make life enjoyable (88.9 to 92.2 percent), and loss of dignity (75 to 77.9 percent).

As of 2019, 90 percent of the people died at home; 90 percent were enrolled in a hospice program; and 99 percent had some form of health insurance (Oregon Public Health Division 2019).

While we can already achieve symptom control for the vast majority of patients, what can be done for the others? Infusion of Precedex or palliative sedation to unconsciousness may be considered. I review the details of both techniques in Chapter 12. Some clinicians, however, consider palliative sedation to unconsciousness tantamount to MAiD. This remains a matter of individual conscience.

Many respected physicians believe that they should have the legal option to assist someone who asks for help ending his life and for whom all available expert palliative care has not led to a satisfactory quality of life. They do not disagree with the need for better education in the provision of care. But when that care has not produced a satisfactory outcome, they do not think it morally wrong to help patients end their lives. Regardless of your opinion, we can acknowledge that educated, compassionate clinicians may have very different beliefs about MAiD.

This debate has raised the level of public discussion about the importance of striving for an acceptable quality of life for patients with advanced cancer. I am hopeful that as the availability of comprehensive palliative care for patients improves, requests for euthanasia and MAiD will decrease. But I also recognize that there may be some patients who find the loss of autonomy, function, and dignity intolerable and seek to end their lives.

SUMMARY

Collaborating with palliative care teams and hospice programs can enhance your ability to provide comfort and quality of life to your patients and their families at the beginning of treatment and when disease advances. Together, you can aim to help them achieve a "good death" and complete the tasks of dying patients. Palliative care teams can also help you understand and deal with patients' requests for MAiD and cope with the challenges to you and your team that such requests may present.

CHAPTER 12

The Last Days

THE DYING PATIENT

The last few days of life pose special problems for cancer patients, their families, and the clinicians caring for them. In fact, taking care of dying patients has been found to be a major contributor to burnout among medical oncologists (Whippen and Canellos 1991; Jackson et al. 2008). Oncologists who saw both a biomedical and psychosocial role for themselves, however, who felt skilled in communicating with dying patients, and who obtained support from colleagues were more satisfied with the care they delivered and seemed to be protected from burnout. Significantly, they were the more experienced clinicians (Jackson et al. 2008) (We discuss burnout more extensively in Chapter 13.)

If you are a younger clinician, you may not realize that you can get the support you need to help these patients and their families from your oncology mentors or from a palliative care or hospice team member. You might feel you have nothing to offer. But that is far from the truth. Both the patients, if awake, and their families will welcome your calls or visits and your ongoing involvement in their care. Don't worry about being blamed for what is happening, and let your instincts guide you in offering the patient and the family the respect and comfort you want to give them.

Dr. Ned Cassem, a talented psychiatrist and teacher who worked extensively with dying patients, articulated nine components essential to care of the dying that are still relevant today (Cassem 1991).

COMPONENTS OF CARE OF THE DYING

- Clinical competence
- Comfort
- Compassion
- Consistency and perseverance
- Cheerfulness
- Equanimity
- Visits from children
- Family cohesion and integration
- Communication

Of these components, the keys for me (*Janet Abrahm*) have been acquiring the *clinical competence* to relieve a patient's physical and psychological distress, the communication skills to help him as he struggles with questions about his goals of care, and the equanimity to remain present with him. I collaborate routinely with nursing, social work, and spiritual care colleagues in this work. When I know we have decreased a patient's distress to a tolerable level, I find I can, with compassion, hold his hand, talk with him, and be cheerful. As we clarify his and his family's goals and values, I find I increasingly connect with all of them, am able to manifest an equanimity that I truly feel, and to offer my presence. When a patient is lucky enough to experience increased physical, psychological, and spiritual comfort, it becomes much easier for his family to be near and, if they wish, to be present at the time of death.

CARING FOR A DYING PHYSICIAN

There are special challenges when our patients are themselves physicians. Fromme and Billings described these well in their 2003 article: "Care of the Dying Doctor: On the Other End of the Stethoscope." They report that physicians may have greater anxiety about death than do members of the general population, and while physicians understand more about what is happening to them, they have no more emotional resources to deal with their dying than other people do. The oncology team who is caring for a physician may feel an extra sense of obligation, along with a heightened sense of vulnerability, since this is happening to "one of us."

Fromme and Billings caution us not to succumb to VIP syndrome, during which we give the patient too much control and we lose our usual boundaries; this often results in patients getting worse care from us. We can help our physician patients by being aware of and compassionate about their attempts to self-doctor and to retain control and self-respect, and by trying to maintain our equanimity. At the same time, we need to remain open to our connection with them, allowing them the same space to grieve, to share their distress, hopes, values, and goals as we do any other patient.

Fromme and Billings end by offering several strategies, including a detailed table describing how to negotiate the relationship, and helpful insights into how the physician patient is both "like all patients" and "different." These challenges can extend to caring for other health care providers as well, or for family members who are clinicians. I typically address this by saying that although circumstances may demand we clinicians put on the patient or caregiver "hat," we can never take off the clinician "hat." We have to find a way to wear both hats, awkward as it may sometimes be. As providers for clinician patients and their families, we can honor both these identities and help negotiate them.

SUPPORTING THE FAMILY

The dying patient presents an increased burden for an already stressed family, especially when the patient is dying at home. But families who have been able to care for a dying loved one at home often express their profound satisfaction that they did everything they could. Even those who need to bring the patient to the hospital or an inpatient hospice for the final few days or hours may feel an appropriate sense of pride and accomplishment.

Most family members have never seen anyone die and, while willing to do whatever is necessary to allow the patient to die at home, they are totally unprepared for the reality of that death. When I was still practicing oncology, as a patient entered his final weeks to months, I met with or talked on the phone with the patient and his family whenever possible to review the implications of dying at home. Along with the nurses and social workers on my team, I found I needed to validate caregivers' requests for additional home care resources or, if the patient and caregiver preferred, to move the patient to an inpatient hospice or nursing facility in which he could receive hospice services.

Enrolling patients in hospice programs is one of the most important things you can do to enhance the bereavement of those they will leave behind; the bereaved will be less likely to develop a major depressive disorder, prolonged grief disorder (Chapter 13), or post-traumatic stress disorder. They will even be less likely to die themselves (Bradley et al. 2004; Christakis and Iwashyna 2003; Wright et al. 2010).

Caregivers are particularly prone to becoming exhausted and frustrated if they are trying to provide this care alone, and we must validate their need for help.

When the patient was likely to die in a matter of weeks, I talked with caregivers about how their roles in the care of their loved one now needed to change. Before, they were the eyes and ears of the oncology team, monitoring the patient for early warning signs as he rode the roller coaster typical of chemotherapy treatments.

Families may not even realize that this monitoring of blood counts and being hypervigilant for any signs of deterioration have become second nature to them. They need to know that they can now relinquish those tasks without exposing the patient to danger, and that they have equally important tasks to work on in the time that remains. Patients have stories to tell, meaning to make, legacies to leave—and likely need help with these and with maintaining a sense of purpose. We also encouraged patients and their families to work with their spiritual care providers, social workers, and hospice caregivers to aid them in these tasks.

When a patient who was not enrolled in a hospice program was dying at home, I made every effort to call the patient and the family two or three times a week, increasing the frequency for the last few weeks. I think that the calls were particularly helpful for the caregivers. I answered their questions, provided emotional support, praised their efforts, and demonstrated my continuing concern. I also had the opportunity to modify the patient's treatment regimen frequently to ensure the best possible control of symptoms during those last days.

Practice Points: Communication during the Last Days

- Have a family meeting to discuss what is likely to happen next.
- Call frequently to give support and adjust the medical regimen.
- Mention that patients often need family permission to let go and reassurance that the survivors will be OK.
- Tell the family Dr. Byock's "Five Things" (Byock 1997): I forgive you; forgive me; I love you; thank you; and good-bye.
- Provide written reminders: "Don't call 911"; "Signs and symptoms of dying"; "Who to call for help"; "What to do when death occurs."
- Assuage ethical or religious concerns about symptom management.
- Revisit the benefits of hospice care.

Family members often want to know how they will recognize that the last days are approaching. I always provide anticipatory guidance about the signs they may see as their loved one approaches and enters the final days. Some want to know how to focus their care. Over the course of the patient's illness, after all, they have frequently needed to be enthusiastic coaches; without their urging, the patient would not have bounced back as readily from what proved to be temporary setbacks. But if the patient is dying this time, it is important to let them know so that their goals as caregivers can change. For some who would like to be at home with the patient, vacation, sick, and even family leave days are limited, as is the time for which another person can assume that person's other obligations. Caregivers need to know when to take that time and when to call in extra help, so that they can feel free to be present full time with the patient during the important last few weeks.

What are the signs of what Doyle-Brown (2000) has termed "the transitional phase" (i.e., as the patient becomes bed-bound), and what effects do they have on the family? Characteristics that denote the beginning of this phase include increased sleep, almost total loss of appetite, and then weakness. If I am with a patient and family member as a patient is transitioning, I will point out and describe "from head to toe" the normal parts of the dying process that I am seeing. I will also point out the reassuring signs I see (a calm face and body, no guarding or furrowed brow) that show me their loved one is comfortable, or, if needed, describe how we will try to increase the patient's comfort.

Some caregivers mistakenly believe that the patient has some control over this phase, and they may be angry at the patient, thinking, "He's giving up!" As I discuss in Chapter 11, repeated rejection of specially prepared food is particularly distressing. Caregivers may have great difficulty allowing confused patients to remain as independent as they think they can still be. Some patients are not fully convinced that they need help until they have fallen or become incontinent.

> **Practice Points: The Transitional Phase**
>
> - Increased somnolence
> - Loss of appetite
> - Weakness
> - Confusion
> - Falls
> - Incontinence
>
> *(From Doyle-Brown 2000)*

When it seems appropriate, remind caregivers and clinicians that it is important to give the patient "permission" to die. I learned this many years ago from one of my residents. One day on rounds, John gently told me that a patient of mine, Mr. Garabaldi, was "holding on" because he didn't want to let me down—that I was the only one Mr. Garabaldi hadn't told that he wanted to die. I felt chastened and went to visit Mr. Garabaldi that afternoon. During our visit, I reassured him that he would not be disappointing me, that I knew he had been fighting for a long time, and that I understood his need to rest. His relief was obvious, and he died within the week.

Up until that point, I had no idea how important it was to tell someone explicitly that he can let go. It does not matter whether the patient can respond verbally or indicate in any way that he has heard you; it still needs to be said. Share this insight with family members and urge them to give this kind of permission to their loved one. And ask them to tell the dying person not to worry about them, that they will be OK. A phrase I often say to the patient is: *"Your work is done; your family will take care of each other; you can rest now."*

Dr. Ira Byock, in *Dying Well*, lists an additional "Five Things" that both the dying patient and the family members need to say and, when possible, discuss. The "Things" are not just sentences to be said but emotions to be explored. They are *I forgive you; Forgive me; Thank you; I love you;* and *Good-bye.* Some families can talk about these feelings and the stories that underly them more easily than others, but almost all eventually can say or discuss one or more of these with their dying loved one. When they do, both family members and patients seem much more at peace.

Written reminders. If the patient is enrolled in a hospice program, the nurses or social workers give the families written reminders of how to reach them. They suggest that the family put these somewhere they will be easily found in an emergency, such as on the refrigerator or stuck onto a coffee maker. Someone from the hospice program can be reached 24 hours a day, 7 days a week.

Some states have out-of-hospital DNR forms or the POLST forms that we describe in Chapter 1. These also should be put in a prominent place, like on the refrigerator. In addition, encourage someone in the family to inform the local ambulance company that the patient has an advance directive and does not want to be resuscitated. You can even send the ambulance company a copy of the directive to keep in its files. Then, if 911 is called by mistake when the patient dies, the paramedics will know not to institute cardiopulmonary resuscitation.

It's also helpful to reiterate in the written reminders how to reach you or your covering clinicians in an emergency. If the patient is not followed in a hospice program, ask the family members to call you when the patient dies and to tell the funeral director that you will be responsible for completing the death certificate.

The family's ethical concerns about pain management. Despite many reassurances to the contrary, a major source of concern for family members is giving pain medicine to someone who is dying. They fear that in trying to relieve pain, they might inadvertently be hastening death. Even though they cannot relieve the person's suffering in any other way, they may have religious concerns—often because they are not aware of the writings of their religious leaders on this subject.

I discuss in Chapter 7, and it is worth reiterating here, that Catholicism, Orthodox Judaism, and Islam all encourage the relief of suffering, even if there is a chance that, as a secondary effect, the person may die sooner than if the pain medicine were withheld. This is the so-called doctrine of double effect (Bradley 2009). The Catechism is very clear on this point: intent is the key. Unlike Roman

Catholicism, Islam and Orthodox Judaism do not have one spokesperson, but in recent writings, the majority of opinions from clerics of both faiths are identical to that of the Roman Catholic hierarchy: if the intent of the caregiver or the clinician is to relieve the patient's pain, the caregiver should give whatever medication is required.

These three religions are generally also in concert about the right of the patient to refuse artificial means of prolonging life (e.g., ventilators, dialysis, high-flow oxygen, continuous positive airway pressure [CPAP], or other therapies that delay a natural death), but some orthodox theologians, such as some ultra-orthodox rabbis, do not agree. Artificial nutrition or hydration can also be withheld if they are only prolonging the dying process. But Roman Catholic patients have been advised not to sign an advance directive or living will "that invites patients to remove food and water provided by artificial means should they become incapacitated . . . A better alternative is the designation of a health care agent, who can, case by case, make a determination of the morality of medical interventions consistent with the will of the patient and the teaching of the Church" (Bradley 2009, p. 376).

Referral to a hospice program. Even if the patient or the family has previously resisted accepting the referral, make every effort to engage hospice services for dying patients, including those dying in hospitals or in long-term care facilities. In Chapter 11, we offer a full description of the services provided by hospice programs and of the ongoing role for the oncology team. The hospice clinicians may have useful suggestions for improving the patient's symptoms and will also address psychological, social, and spiritual sources of distress of the patient and family. Hospice personnel begin to prepare the family for their loss and offer continued assistance through bereavement programs that continue for more than a year after the death. Chapter 13 includes a more extensive discussion of bereavement programs.

In a period as short as the few days or week before death, hospice care can be an enormous source of comfort to families and professional caregivers, particularly when they have never witnessed a "natural" death. The team members have "been there," can explain what is likely to happen, and can provide expert symptom management during the last hours or days. For patients at home, hospice staff will provide practical instruction in how the family can help with toileting, daily care, feeding, massage, and giving medications. As dying approaches, hospice personnel provide suggestions for answering the patient's questions and written materials that explain how the family or the staff in the inpatient or long-term care facility can determine that death is imminent.

WHEN PATIENTS DIE IN THE HOSPITAL

Supporting the Inpatient Team

When one of the patients we are following is dying in the hospital, we feel the additional obligation of helping the primary and oncology teams, the house staff, physician assistants, and the ward staff (social workers, nurses, patient aides, the environmental services staff, and ward clerks) cope not only with the patient's and family's needs but with their own feelings of distress. The dying process often brings ward staff closer to patients and their families, even if this is the patient's first admission to that ward.

To allay feelings of guilt and anxiety, we review with all team members the history of the illness, the limits of the treatments that remain, the burdens of those treatments, and, when appropriate, the limits the patient has placed on further supportive measures. We also remind them that, despite our best efforts, patients still die and that it is no one's fault. This can be very comforting. Even more helpful is suggesting things they can do that will enhance the patient's last days and further the healing process of the survivors. One simple thing is to have the team ask the electrophysiology service or cardiology staff to adjust the rate of the ICD or pacemaker to the lowest response settings for those patients who have one. Believe it or not, 65 percent of patients with DNR orders still had the defibrillators active the day before they died, and 24 percent of them received one or more shocks (Kelly, Kabir, and Keshvani 2020).

Not uncommonly, however, the primary team are the undeserving target of a patient's or a family's anger, as was the case for Mr. Champion's team.

Mr. Champion

Mr. Champion underwent definitive therapy for lung cancer, but 6 months later he was admitted for bilateral malignant pleural effusions. He required bilateral chest tubes and sclerosis, was febrile from resistant pneumonia, and was significantly malnourished. Despite control of his pain, Mr. Champion was unable to clear his numerous secretions, was severely tachypneic, and became recurrently hypoxic. No pulmonary emboli or clots were present in his upper or lower extremities.

Although Mr. Champion had told his oncologist, Dr. Rydell, that he did not wish to be intubated electively or resuscitated if that meant he would have to be on a ventilator, no advance directive was completed. Because of Mr. Champion's rapidly deteriorating pulmonary status, I asked Dr. Rydell to confirm and document that Mr. Champion did not wish to be electively intubated.

The next morning, nurses on the unit told me of the conversation they had overheard between a furious Mrs. Champion and the house staff. It went something like, "Why did you have to ask Dr. Rydell to talk about those things with my husband? Look what you've done to him. You took away all his hope! He was fine until you made us have that talk—now look at him!" She went on in this vein for some time, and the next day she would not speak with the physician assistants whom she blamed for her husband's ongoing deterioration.

After Dr. Rydell confirmed that Mr. Champion did not wish to be intubated, the team treated his progressive dyspnea symptomatically with pulmonary toilet, suctioning, oxygen, antibiotics, anxiolytics, and opioids. He died two days later, in no apparent distress. As we gathered around him, his wife asked for forgiveness from the physician assistants, "for what I said out there in the hall." She included them in the prayers she led, and in the thank-you gift she sent to all the floor staff later in the week.

Not all medical teams are so lucky. Mr. Champion's wife was able to understand that her anger had been misplaced and to apologize to the staff. Many families don't, and the interns, residents, students, physician assistants, and nurses caring for the patient add the family's unjust accusations to their own unwarranted feelings of guilt about the patient's death.

Be sure to support the team through these stressful situations. Explain that they are often the lightning rod for the family's or patient's helplessness, despair, and anger. Encourage them not to take family attacks personally, to continue their exertions on the patient's behalf, and to work with the palliative care team to eliminate or minimize sources of distress. During hospitalizations that lead to death, and after the death itself, dispel any misconceptions the staff may have about their fault for the death and praise the work they did to make the dying person as comfortable as possible. Praise coming from nurses who have shared in the care of the patient can be particularly healing to house staff or physician assistants. In turn, you can encourage the team to praise the nurses for the care they have delivered. This kind of support goes a long way toward enabling young clinicians and ward staff to recover from the pain they experience when a patient dies and to allow themselves a feeling of satisfaction for a job well done.

Resuscitation status. In Mr. Champion's case, as the crisis neared, Dr. Rydell simply needed to confirm that Mr. Champion's wishes had not changed. Later, when intubation would have been needed to support him (his pH was 7.24, pCO2 80 mm Hg, and pO2 55 mm Hg with maximum oxygen support), we all felt confident that in not intubating him, we were caring for Mr. Champion within the limits he had set.

Unfortunately, the 1995 SUPPORT study (of patients dying in teaching hospitals) indicated that physicians often do not know the wishes of their hospitalized patients suffering from life-threatening illnesses—only 47 percent were aware that their patients did not wish to be resuscitated. One-third of outpatients had not even told their physicians that they had an advance directive.

Practice Points: Supporting the Inpatient Ward Team

- Remind the team of medicine's limitations in the face of illness that is refractory to treatment.
- Relieve anxiety and unwarranted guilt; explain patient/family anger.
- Develop a plan of care through which they can minimize patient and family suffering.
- Dispel misconceptions and praise their efforts.
- Record/update advance directives regarding elective intubation and resuscitation.
- To enable a truly informed choice, give realistic prognoses and realistic descriptions of the burdens and benefits of any remaining therapeutic options, including mechanical ventilation.

We still have a long way to go in this area. A 2011 review concluded, "The persistent problems with DNR suggest that physician behaviors toward communication with patients about goals of care and resuscitation decisions have not measurably changed in the past 20 years" (Yuen, Reid, and Fetters 2011). They cite one study, for example, of 500 patients who had a cardiac arrest during a hospitalization. When these patients were admitted, 89 percent would have been able to participate in a DNR discussion, but by the time the DNR discussion actually occurred, only 24 percent were able to do so.

I hope that the work of the Serious Illness Care Program (Bernacki et al. 2019), described in Chapters 1 and 11, and other national efforts such as the Conversation Project will soon improve documentation of patients' wishes about attempts at resuscitation. In 2013, a survey of Americans by the Conversation Project (https://theconversationproject.org) indicated that while 90 percent thought it was important to have the conversation, only 27 percent actually had it. In a similar survey in 2018, 32 percent had had the conversation.

We should do all we can to inform ourselves of the wishes of patients with far-advanced disease while they are still well enough to make rational decisions, and we should communicate these directives to all members of their health care teams in and out of the hospital. If you are realistic when you inform your patients of the extent of their disease, the likelihood that the remaining treatments will add meaningfully to the time they have left, the realities of mechanical ventilation, and the odds of ever being weaned from it, you enable them to make informed decisions about resuscitation and preventive intubation. Difficult discussions will then not have to be initiated in crisis situations, and you will avoid resuscitating patients whose disease is essentially untreatable and who might have been able to die comfortably, saving both them and their families needless suffering. We discuss communication strategies for these conversations in Chapters 1, 5, and 11.

Supporting the Families of Inpatients

Despite our best efforts to enable those who wish to die at home to do so, many patients who have cancer require such complex care that they must remain in the hospital until they die. Our palliative care team is often consulted to help care for these patients and their families. The families may have promised to take the patient home and are feeling distraught at what they see as their failure to fulfill the patient's last wish.

I cared for Elmo, a 45-year-old man who required significant respiratory support, more than could be delivered in any other setting. Some hospitals have one or two rooms they have redecorated as comfort suites for these patients; they look something like a nice hotel room, or home, with ample space for friends and family to stay overnight, but they also include the technology and nursing care the patients need to remain comfortable as they die.

Our hospital does not have rooms like these, but we were able to do several things to assuage his family's feeling that they had let him down, and to support them. We were clear that it was a medical decision that was keeping him in the hospital, that as much as they loved him, even with the help of a home hospice program, they simply could not provide the care he needed at home. We said that while we, too, had wished we could ensure his comfort at home, we just couldn't; he needed a hospital level of care.

Then, we asked them to make Elmo's hospital room look, sound, and smell like his room at home, and encouraged them to bring bed covers, pictures, one of his son's favorite stuffed animals, music, whatever would make it feel more familiar. We were able to allow them unlimited visiting hours, and for his last day, the hospital provided drinks and snacks (a "bereavement tray"), so they would not have to leave his room.

Elmo was unstable enough that we successfully enrolled him in a hospice program at the inpatient level of care in our hospital, and the hospice team came daily to provide him and his family extra support, which they appreciated. When Elmo died, he was completely surrounded by his family members. We let them know that the last faces he saw, the last voices he heard, the last touch he felt was that of his family, and that they had done everything any family could do to help him have his wish: home, after all, is the place where you are with those whom you love and who love you, and they created that in the hospital for him. It is my hope that as they told the story of Elmo's death, pride at what they had been able to do for him would replace any regret that he had to die in the hospital.

For all patients coming to the end of their lives in the hospital, involve social work, spiritual care services, psychiatry, palliative care, and interpreter services to address spiritual, social, cultural, and psychological aspects of patient or family distress. Identify important cultural or spiritual practices at the end of life that may inform patient's choices for their care and identify whose presence the patient considers important as a source of support, whether or not these are family members.

Family members and staff should all be involved in the decision-making and have an opportunity to express their concerns with the plan of care. In discussions, you can discover from the patient or family how you can help them personalize their good-byes, for example, which rituals, music, or other things should occur; who should be present (in person or by video or telephone); and whether clergy are important. Inform them that procedures such as taking vital signs, drawing lab tests, doing x-rays, hemodialysis, or CVVH will also be stopped because they do not contribute to the patient's comfort. Some families find the monitors helpful, so they do not always need to be turned off, but the alarms do.

Collaborate with professional medical interpreters, not family members or untrained staff who happen to speak that language, for all communication with patients who have limited English proficiency or use ASL as their language of choice. Consider working with medical interpreters for improving communication across cultural barriers (cultural mediation) even when language interpretation may not be needed, especially when you have had difficulty communicating with a patient or family from a cultural background different from your own.

COVID-19. In the first year of the 2020 COVID-19 epidemic, family members were not able to be present in the hospital, and this was an additional source of anguish. We used video communications whenever possible, bringing at least the sight and sound of their loved ones to the patients, but this was a poor substitute for their presence. When someone was actively dying, one family member was allowed to be present, and sometimes, with special nursing agreement, a few more could come. The staff served as surrogate family, and at our hospital, Brigham and Women's Hospital in Boston, as I imagine was true in many hospitals, I am honored to report that the nursing staff never let anyone die alone. We were also able to provide enhanced bereavement services.

SYMPTOM MANAGEMENT GUIDE

Symptom management in patients' last days can be challenging. The SUPPORT study also revealed that family members often felt the patient's symptoms were not adequately controlled. Researchers found that among the conscious patients, family members thought that 40 percent had unrelieved severe pain and, of those with lung cancer or an underlying malignant condition with superimposed multi-system organ failure, that 70 percent had severe dyspnea and 25 percent had moderate anxiety or dysphoria (Lynn et al. 1997). These tragic findings were one of the major catalysts for the growth of our field of specialty palliative care.

Symptoms change rapidly during these last days. If possible, when the patient is dying in the hospital, be present for at least 5 to 10 minutes several times a day. Sit at the bedside and observe the patient for any signs of pain, delirium, excessive upper airway secretions ("death rattle"), or myoclonus. If you find them, correct them as suggested in the following pages. Ask family or friends who are there what they have observed and answer their questions. Let them know they can touch and speak to the patient, as they may be afraid to do so if the patient is attached to multiple machines or intravenous lines.

Symptom complex of dying patients. Data on the frequency of the various symptoms that occur in the last days to week before death are somewhat conflicting. Patients usually have multiple symptoms, with combinations of those listed below varying with the underlying disease process:

- Pain
- Noisy or moist breathing
- Urinary incontinence or retention
- Restlessness, agitation
- Dyspnea, cough
- Nausea and vomiting, anorexia, dysphagia, xerostomia
- Delirium
- Fatigue
- Existential or spiritual distress
- Cooling of extremities
- Fecal incontinence

Up to 70 percent of patients with advanced cancer have pain, and this pain requires ongoing therapy until death. Noisy or moist breathing, urinary incontinence or retention, and restlessness and agitation are seen in almost half of patients who are actively dying.

Manifestations of Active Dying: The Last 10 to 14 Days

- Dehydration, tachycardia, followed by decrease in heart rate and blood pressure
- Perspiration, clammy skin, cool extremities; just before death, mottling
- Diminished breath sounds, irregular breathing pattern with periods of apnea or full Cheyne-Stokes respiration; grunt or moan with exhale
- Mouth droop; difficulty swallowing; loss of gag reflex with pooling of secretions, causing "death rattle"
- Incontinence of bladder or rectum
- Agitation ± hallucinations; stillness; difficult to arouse

(From Pitorak 2003)

One in 5 patients will be short of breath, and about 1 in 10 will have nausea and vomiting. The incidence of delirium in patients dying of advanced cancer is 88 percent (Lawlor et al. 2000). Manifestations of delirium are described in Chapter 9.

Patients lose the ability to swallow and become much less interactive. It is as though they are living in a large mansion in which they gradually move to rooms that are farther and farther from the front door. Responding to voice or touch takes them much longer, and they may stop showing any response. Most families seem to understand that the patient is not personally rejecting them. I often say that it just takes too much energy for the patient to "come to the front door, although they are still there, and can hear you."

Some patients may experience existential or spiritual distress, but others articulate visions of spiritual peace. One night at midnight, a patient from the north of India whom I cared for asked her husband for "water from the Ganges." Until then, he had seemed not to understand how ill she was. But after the request, he realized she was dying. They were able to grieve together, talk, and say their last good-byes. She died the next morning. And a patient from Ireland spoke glowingly to me of "going to the Isle to meet my people." She could see them waving at her. Could I? Her eyes were closed as she added, "My job is to get there. They're waiting for me." She continued to speak, but in Gaelic. As I got ready to leave, I wished her a peaceful journey. To my surprise, without opening her eyes, she said, in English, "Thank you."

Commonly required medications. Most of the problems experienced by dying patients can be controlled by a limited number of medications given by the oral, rectal, transdermal, or, if necessary, parenteral route (Table 12.1) (McPherson, Kim, and Walker 2012). Patients who previously appeared comfortable may at some point need medications for discomfort, rattling secretions, and terminal anxiety, agitation, or delirium. Some patients need treatment for dyspnea or various other miscellaneous problems.

While it would be wonderful if patients who were no longer able to take oral medications could absorb medications through their intact skin in gel form, *this does not work.* While compounding pharmacies commonly make gels with antiemetics or antianxiety agents in them, there is no evidence that these are absorbed through intact skin (Smith et al. 2012). Haloperidol, diphenhydramine, metoclopramide, and lorazepam can be absorbed through the rectal mucosa, as I describe below, but they are not absorbed from intact skin, and recurrence of symptoms is likely to follow if needed oral medications are given in a gel format.

Liquid oral concentrates, subcutaneous infusions, and, if needed, intravenous infusions will ensure symptomatic relief for most patients. Liquid preparations of many medications can be administered through a rectal Macy catheter if this is acceptable to the patient and family. For those very few patients whose extreme distress cannot be controlled in any other way, the palliative care team is likely to recommend dexmedetomidine or palliative sedation to unconsciousness (see below).

TABLE 12.1 Treatment of Common Problems in the Final Days

Problem	Agent	Route; Dose
Baseline pain	Concentrated oxycodone or morphine solution	p.o.; SQ q4h around the clock; individualized
	Fentanyl	Transdermal; individualized
	Methadone liquid	p.o.; individualized
	IR Morphine/hydromorphone suppositories	p.r. q4h
	SR opioids put in gel capsules into the rectal vault	p.r. q8 to 24 hr depending on the preparation's usual oral schedule
	NSAIDs: acetaminophen, naproxen	p.r. t.i.d. to q.i.d.
	Dexamethasone (requires compounding)	p.r. daily to b.i.d.
Breakthrough pain	Concentrated oxycodone or morphine solution	Sublingual, SQ q4h; individualized
	Fentanyl	Transmucosal* (buccal, sublingual); individualized
Death rattle	Scopolamine	Transderm Scōp, 1–3 patches q3d; 0.1–2.4 mg/24 hr SQ, IV
	Hyoscyamine (Levsin SL)	0.125–0.25 mg sublingual q4h (discontinue when renal function declines significantly)
	Glycopyrrolate (Robinul)	0.2–0.4 mg SQ, IV t.i.d. to q.i.d. or 1–2 mg p.o. b.i.d. to t.i.d.
	Atropine	0.4 mg sublingual, SQ, IV q4-6h
	Atropine 1% opth solution	1–2 gtt sublingual, p.o. q4h
Anxiety	Lorazepam (Ativan)	1 mg p.o., IV, or sublingual q2h
	Diazepam suppository	5 to 10 mg p.r. daily
Delirium	Haloperidol (Haldol)	2–4 mg p.o., SQ, IV q60min p.r.n. to total 20 mg/24 hr
	Olanzapine (Zyprexa, Zydis)	2.5–5 mg p.o./sublingual/IV qhs to b.i.d. plus p.r.n. q4h
	Chlorpromazine (Thorazine)	25–50 mg p.o. q4-8h or 25 mg p.r. q4-12h; preferred for dyspnea
Dyspnea due to anxiety/panic	Lorazepam (Ativan)	1 mg p.o., IV, or sublingual q2h
	Morphine	5–10 mg sublingual, IV, or by nebulizer
	Chlorpromazine (Thorazine)	25 mg p.o., p.r. q4-12h; or 12.5 mg IV q4-8h

Note: Medications compounded into gels are *not* absorbed through intact skin (Smith 2012). All liquid p.o. medications can be given per G-tube.

*Only for opioid-tolerant patients.

Pain control. You will be able to relieve most patients' pain at the end of life if you use the WHO guidelines for cancer pain relief (see Chapter 7). Patients require close monitoring, and both opioids and nonopioid adjuvants are usually required.

If the patient is unable to take pills, transmucosal, sublingual, rectal, or transdermal opioids are usually effective. In some cases, however, subcutaneous or, when intravenous access is available, intravenous infusions will be needed. Concentrated morphine or oxycodone solutions (20 to 40 mg/ml) can be given sublingually every 1 to 2 hours and are often satisfactory. Rectal administration of sustained-release opioid preparations is not approved by the FDA, but studies indicate that morphine absorption from a sustained-release preparation placed in the rectal vault is equivalent to that from oral administration, and oxycodone levels from rectal administration are higher than those achieved when the patient takes the pills by mouth.

Practice Points: Medication for Pain Control When Pills Cannot Be Swallowed

- Concentrated morphine/oxycodone (20 to 40 mg/ml), buccal or sublingual
- Sustained-release preparations, p.r.
- Adjuvants, p.r. (e.g., NSAIDs, acetaminophen, doxepin)
- Opioids and dexamethasone, subcutaneous injection or infusion
- Liquid preparations of opioids (including methadone), anxiolytics, antiemetics through a feeding tube (when present) or a rectal (Macy) catheter

---

As many as 50 percent of dying patients need an increase in opioid dose during their last days. If the calculated opioid dose is too large to be delivered by sublingual, transdermal, or rectal routes; if pain relief does not seem satisfactory using any of these routes; or if the routes are unacceptable to the patient or the caregiver, give the opioid by subcutaneous infusion or, if intravenous access is available, by intravenous infusion. Both types of infusion can be delivered in the home with the aid of hospice or other home nurses working with nurses from infusion services. The starting opioid dose for a patient whose pain is well controlled should be the intravenous equivalent of the oral dose (see Table 7.4); if the pain is not under control, give a dose that is slightly higher than the equivalent dose.

Other symptom management medications should be continued. When the patient is no longer able to take oral medications, they can be given rectally (Samala and Davis 2012) or subcutaneously. Patients previously benefiting from oral NSAIDs can receive rectal aspirin, naproxen, ibuprofen, or diclofenac, and suppositories of indomethacin and acetaminophen are commercially available;

patients taking a stable glucocorticoid dose for bone or nerve pain can receive subcutaneous dexamethasone or specially compounded dexamethasone suppositories. Rectal doxepin can replace oral tricyclic antidepressants.

Dexmedetomidine. In select inpatients with uncontrolled symptoms, addition of a dexmedetomidine (Precedex) infusion can improve the patients' pain control and help reverse opioid-induced hyperalgesia and delirium (Hofherr, Abrahm, and Rickerson 2020). Dexmedetomidine is a selective alpha-2 agonist traditionally used for perioperative anesthesia and sedation of mechanically ventilated patients. But it also acts synergistically with opioids and can produce pain relief with a low risk of impairing breathing or alertness at the low doses needed in these patients. It can also be used to lower opioid doses in patients with opioid-induced hyperalgesia or delirium and delay or prevent altogether the need for palliative sedation.

Our protocol at BWH requires that patients reside on our intensive palliative care unit, a specialty oncology floor staffed by expert palliative care clinicians (MDs, PAs, SWs, pharmacists, social worker, chaplain, and nurses) who are knowledgeable about dexmedetomidine. Patients receiving dexmedetomidine must have refractory symptoms, be DNR/I, and have chosen comfort as their goal; they do not want to be admitted or readmitted to the ICU. We do not require monitoring of vital signs. We use a continuous dexmedetomidine infusion of 0.1–1.5 mcg/kg/hr and an optional IV bolus of 0.4–1 mcg/kg over 10–30 minutes (administered by a physician). There is no limit on duration (days) of infusion. In all eight patients we reported who received a dexmedetomidine infusion, the drug decreased their distress and provided comfort to the end of life (Hofherr, Abrahm, and Rickerson 2020).

Oral/respiratory secretions. Excess oral secretions occur in 60 to 90 percent of dying patients. The sound of excess oral secretions is often referred to as the "death rattle" among staff, though I recommend you avoid using it, as families can overhear you. The sounds are often distressing to families, so it is important to let them know that they are not distressing to the patients, who are unaware of them. Sometimes, simply repositioning patients is helpful because they may breathe more easily in a lateral recumbent position than supine. Most patients benefit from an antihistamine, such as oral hyoscyamine (Levsin SL), scopolamine in a transdermal patch, intravenous or oral glycopyrrolate, or intravenous or oral atropine (via 1% ophthalmic drops).

None of these anticholinergic agents has been shown to be better than the others in controlling secretions of dying patients. Scopolamine and atropine, however, cross the blood-brain barrier, so I use glycopyrrolate or hyoscyamine if I am worried about increasing the patient's confusion or causing or exacerbating delirium. I also take into account the routes that are available and that the patient prefers. All these agents cause xerostomia, and patients will need to have their mouths moistened periodically.

> ### Practice Points: Treatment of "Death Rattle"
>
> • Place the patient in the lateral recumbent position.
> • Administer one of the following antihistamines:
>   – Glycopyrrolate (Robinul) 0.2–0.4 mg SQ, IV q 2-4h p.r.n. or
>   1–2 mg p.o. q4h p.r.n.
>   – Hyoscyamine (Levsin SL), 0.125–0.25 mg sublingual q4h
>   – Scopolamine patch q72h*
>   – Atropine 0.4 mg sublingual, SQ, IV q4-6h; 1–2 gtt 1 percent
>   ophthalmic solution p.o. q4h*
>
> *Do not use if delirium is a concern.

Terminal restlessness. Almost half of the patients who are actively dying of cancer show signs of restlessness and agitation. They may toss and turn, moan, have muscle twitching or spasm, and only intermittently awaken. Even though patients may appear to be out of contact with the external world, they often seem to be reassured by familiar voices or by being touched.

The agitation is sometimes due to reversible physical problems, such as a full bladder, fecal impaction, pain, nausea, or trouble breathing due to hypoxia or poorly cleared secretions. In other patients, unresolved spiritual, psychological, or social problems induce the distress. All members of the hospice or inpatient palliative care team will reevaluate the patient with these issues in mind. They often can detect the cause of the problem and offer workable solutions.

Patients may need a mild sedative such as lorazepam (e.g., Ativan) suppositories or diazepam (e.g., Valium) gel if they are unable to take oral medications; consider spiritual reassurance, a visit from an estranged family member or friend, or just permission to let go. When it is possible to arrange these, the anxiety often disappears entirely, and the patient will appear calm and peaceful.

Other patients, however, are agitated because they are delirious. Some patients may have developed delirium either as an opioid side effect or in response to increasing blood levels of opioid as renal or hepatic function deteriorates. If the patient is expected to live for several more days, try lowering the opioid dose or changing the opioid. Rehydrating the patient won't improve delirium, agitation, or myoclonus in these patients (Good et al. 2014).

No matter what the underlying etiology of the delirium is, if it is distressing to the patient, try to control it with haloperidol (e.g., Haldol), olanzapine (Zyprexa, Zydis) or chlorpromazine (Thorazine). A small double-blind randomized trial of patients with terminal delirium suggested that for patients refractory to initial doses of haloperidol (2 mg IV), chlorpromazine (25 mg), or a combination (1 mg of haloperidol and 12.5 mg of chlorpromazine), escalation of haloperidol doses, rotation to chlorpromazine, or a combination of the two agents all provides rapid control of the restlessness without extrapyramidal side effects (Hui et al. 2020). For patients with dyspnea, chlorpromazine, which is effective for both delirium and dyspnea, may be used as first-line therapy. Chlorpromazine is also more sedating than haloperidol, and this extra sedation may be beneficial at this time. Lorazepam (oral) or diazepam (rectal) can alleviate myoclonus; if the myoclonus is refractory to these agents, and the IV route is available, use midazolam (titrated to effect).

Practice Points: Treatment of Terminal Agitation

- Evaluate the patient for reversible physical problems: full bladder, fecal impaction, pain, nausea, hypoxia, secretions, opioid side effects (especially if there is decreased urine output), marked dehydration.
- Consider the need to change opioid, opioid dose, or opioid preparation (i.e., from sustained to immediate release given as needed).
- Consider the need for psychological or spiritual counseling (e.g., for resolution of family estrangements or for permission to let go).
- Medicate for anxiety.
  - Lorazepam (e.g., Ativan), 1 mg p.o. or sublingual every 2 hours.
- Medicate for mild agitated delirium (see also Chapter 9).
  - Haloperidol (e.g., Haldol), 2 mg p.o., SQ, or IV, repeated at 60 minutes p.r.n. After an additional 60 minutes, double the dose, if needed, to a total of 20 mg/24 hr.
  - Olanzapine (Zyprexa, Zydis), 2.5 to 5 mg p.o./SL/IV b.i.d. to q.i.d.; may give an additional 2.5 to 5 mg q4h p.r.n.
  - Chlorpromazine (Thorazine), 25 to 50 mg p.o. or p.r. or 12.5 mg IV every 4 to 8 hours; preferred for dyspneic patients or for those who would benefit from sedation.

Dyspnea. Dying patients with dyspnea benefit from the same symptomatic therapies recommended for patients with less advanced disease (see Table 12.1). Aggressive treatment of panic due to perceived breathlessness is particularly important for these patients, and hospice nurses often instruct families in how to administer the necessary opioid, chlorpromazine, or, for refractory panic, lorazepam.

Practice Points: Treatment of Dyspnea that Is Causing Panic

- In opioid-naive patients, morphine, 5 to 10 mg liquid sublingual or p.o., IV; double the usual rescue dose in opioid-tolerant patients
- Chlorpromazine, 25 mg p.o. or p.r., or 12.5 mg IV
- Lorazepam 1 mg sublingual, p.o., or IV; Midazolam, 0.5 to 1 mg IV very slowly

---

Hydration. While patients are unlikely to be thirsty or hungry, they may have a dry mouth. A prospective study at St. Christopher's Hospice in London found no difference in the reports of thirst or dry mouth between dehydrated and normally hydrated dying patients (Ellershaw, Sutcliffe, and Saunders 1995). More than 90 percent of all patients with these complaints were receiving opioids. In a report from Oregon, most hospice patients who voluntarily refused food and fluids to hasten their deaths seemed to their hospice nurses to have had a "good death," and they did not complain of hunger or thirst (Ganzini et al. 2003). A systematic literature review on hydration in the last weeks of life found mixed results: two studies found less nausea and fewer physical signs of dehydration; two found adverse effects, such as increased ascites; and four showed no effect on problems such as delirium, thirst, or chronic nausea (Raijmakers et al. 2011).

Practice Points: Hydration in Dying Patients

- Remember: dry mouth ≠ dehydration.
- Moisten lips with mouth swabs, gauze soaked in ice water, or offer sips of ice water or plain or fruit-flavored ice chips.
- If parenteral hydration is chosen, do not exceed 1 liter 2 to 3 times a week to avoid increasing distress (e.g., increasing urine output, pulmonary secretions, nausea and vomiting, ascites, or pulmonary or peripheral edema).

Parenteral hydration can cause increased distress by increasing urine output, inducing pulmonary or peripheral edema, increasing pulmonary secretions and cough, and causing nausea and vomiting from increased gastric secretions. If you think parenteral hydration is indicated to allow the patient time to finish last goals, try to limit replacement to a liter two or three times a week. Moistening the mouth with mouth swabs or gauze soaked in ice water or offering sips of water, ice chips, mouth swab sponges, or fruit-flavored Italian ice is usually all that is needed for the sensation of a dry mouth. The colder the water, it turns out, the quicker the brain turns off the "thirst signal" (Zimmerman 2020). Parenthetically, when family members need to feel that they are "doing something" while sitting vigil with a dying loved one, I often recommend moistening the mouth as a regular comfort measure that they can perform. You can also reassure them that because the brain's thirst signals are triggered by ingested food, by not eating, their loved ones who are no longer eating are also decreasing their thirst (Zimmerman 2020).

Massive hemoptysis (or gastrointestinal bleeding). Massive hemoptysis is relatively rare, in one report occurring in 7 percent of about 500 patients hospitalized in a cancer hospital. In a dying patient, it will usually have been preceded by less extensive hemoptysis, giving you and the home care or hospice team the opportunity to prepare the patient and family. If you think the patient is likely to develop either a massive gastrointestinal bleed (e.g., from a colonic tumor) or massive hemoptysis, suggest the family get dark-colored sheets, towels, and blankets to mask the blood. Because emergency intravenous access may be needed for patient sedation, consider insertion of a PICC line in patients without an indwelling venous access device.

Practice Points: Treatment of Massive Hemoptysis or Exsanguinating Bleeding

- Ask the family to purchase dark-colored towels, blankets, or sheets to mask the blood.
- When appropriate, insert a PICC line for emergency IV access.
- Teach the family how to place the patient bleeding side down in the Trendelenburg position when bleeding occurs.
- Ascertain whether the family feels comfortable giving medications IV, SQ, or p.r. and instruct them as appropriate in administering the following:
  - Rectal diazepam gel (10 mg), rectal lorazepam (2 mg), or IV midazolam (1 to 5 mg) from prefilled syringes
  - Morphine IV from prefilled syringes

    Dose for opioid-naive patient: 10 mg morphine

    Dose for patient on opioids: the intravenous equivalent of the "rescue" opioid dose

    Example. For a patient taking 300 mg SR morphine every 24 hours:

      Oral rescue: 30 mg; IV rescue: 10 mg (i.e., 30 mg/3 hours)

      Opioid dose for the emergency: 10 mg IV morphine

If the family feels capable of giving an intravenous injection, the hospice nurse can leave a kit in the home that contains prefilled syringes of appropriate medications for a patient likely to develop massive hemoptysis or an exsanguinating bleed. It includes morphine, to be given intravenously, and a benzodiazepine.

Midazolam (Versed) can be given intravenously; diazepam gel (e.g., Valium) can be given rectally. When the event occurs, the patient is placed bleeding side down, in the Trendelenburg position, and the medications noted above are given. If the nurses arrive in time, they can position the patient and administer these medications or start continuous infusions of morphine and/or midazolam, if necessary.

Miscellaneous. For patients with catheters who are experiencing dysuria, lidocaine can be added to saline bladder irrigation. For patients with nausea or vomiting due to bowel obstruction, add dexamethasone and a scopolamine patch for cramping if delirium is not a concern or continue octreotide and dexamethasone if the patient is already receiving these; for nausea or vomiting from other causes, sublingual lorazepam (e.g., Ativan) or haloperidol (e.g., Haldol) liquid can be effective, as can specially compounded dexamethasone suppositories, commercial prochlorperazine or lorazepam suppositories, or haloperidol liquid through a Macy rectal catheter. All these medications can be given in the home by the caregivers or by home care or hospice nurses.

Practice Points: Treatment of Other Distressing Problems

- Catheter-induced dysuria: lidocaine bladder irrigation
- Nausea/vomiting
  - Due to bowel obstruction: continue dexamethasone and octreotide if previously prescribed; if not, add dexamethasone and, if delirium is not a concern, a scopolamine patch.
  - Due to other causes: haloperidol or lorazepam p.o. or p.r.; prochlorperazine p.r.; haloperidol liquid 5 mg (2mg/ml solution through Macy Catheter) q6h p.r.n.
- Myoclonus due to opioid toxicity or liver failure: lorazepam 1 mg sublingual, p.o., IV q4h p.r.n.; diazepam gel 5 mg p.r. daily; midazolam 5 mg loading dose (2 mg for patients over 60), then 10 to 100 mg/24 hr IV infusion.

Sedation as a side effect. Unfortunately, the doses of opioid, neuroleptic, or benzodiazepine that will control pain, cough, dyspnea, seizures, or agitation in a dying patient may sedate the patient so profoundly that unconsciousness ensues. Some ethicists have invoked the doctrine of double effect, discussed above, to support the use of medications to the point of sedation with the intent of relieving symptoms. They argue that while harm is foreseen, no harm is intended by the sedation-induced unconsciousness; on the contrary, the clinician has an obligation to help the patient, and no alternative ways remain to provide that help. Since the action meets both these conditions (i.e., no harm is intended, and benefit will accrue), such sedation may be considered ethical.

Some have gone as far as suggesting that "death-hastening or death-causing palliative analgesic administration" is obligatory in such settings (Cavanaugh 1996, p. 248). Situations may occur, Cavanaugh suggests, when our obligation to relieve the patient's pain or suffering is greater than our obligation to avoid hastening or causing death. In such instances, he says, the use of opioids or other agents to induce sedation would become obligatory.

Palliative sedation to unconsciousness. Palliative care experts consider using palliative sedation to unconsciousness when, despite their ongoing evaluation and management, a patient who is near death continues to experience intolerable physical, psychological, or spiritual/existential distress. In palliative sedation, the sedation is not a side effect of a medication given to relieve a symptom, such as the sedation induced by high doses of opioids for pain or dyspnea, or that induced by chlorpromazine for delirium. Here, sedation is the desired effect, and medications designed to induce sedation (e.g., midazolam, pentobarbital, or propofol) are used.

In 2020, the Japanese Society for Palliative Medicine published the results of their consensus process creating initial recommendations for clinical palliative sedation therapy (Imai et al. 2020), in which they offer the possibilities of respite sedation (i.e., sedation limited to several days, after which the patient is reawakened), continuous proportional sedation (tailored to the patient's distress), and continuous deep sedation. Their guidelines include refractory existential suffering among the indications for the sedation, though when it is the only cause of the suffering, they write: "the appropriateness of continuous sedation for psycho-existential suffering should be very carefully addressed" (p. 1188), and they recommend consulting a psychiatrist, psychologist, and pastoral care worker for these patients.

Clinicians throughout Europe continue to struggle to define palliative sedation, indications for ethical palliative sedation (e.g., whether they should include patients without refractory physical symptom or delirium), and appropriate methods of providing palliative sedation (Payne and Hasselaar 2020). In 2019 they began a 5-year project, Palliative Sedation, to explore practices of what they termed "proportional palliative sedation" across countries. They plan to present their findings in various venues, revise and update the current framework (Cherny and Radbruch 2009), and provide free educational resources, including an e-book, to highlight best practices in symptom management and palliative sedation.

In the United States, there is legal and professional support for palliative sedation to unconsciousness. The U.S. Supreme Court (in *Vacco vs. Quill* 521 U.S. 793 (1997)) recognized the right of patients to receive palliative sedation to unconsciousness if that is what is required to relieve their suffering at the end of life. The codes of ethics of the national professional societies of medicine, nursing, and pharmacy all have determined that the provision of palliative sedation to unconsciousness is consistent with ethical practice. When used in appropriate terminally ill patients and carefully dosed, the sedation itself does not hasten death beyond what would occur due to the dying process itself, or if artificial nutrition or hydration are not provided (Maltoni et al. 2012).

In 2020, the main area of controversy is the use of palliative sedation in an imminently dying patient suffering from intractable existential distress alone (i.e., in the absence of refractory physical symptoms or delirium). Most professional clinical organizations in the United States (e.g., the American Medical Association, the American Nurses Association, and the Hospice and Palliative Care Nursing Association) exclude existential distress alone as a valid reason to give a dying patient palliative sedation to unconsciousness. The American Academy of Hospice and Palliative Medicine, however, does not specifically exclude palliative sedation for existential distress alone, and the Ethics Committee of the National Hospice and Palliative Care Organization was unable to reach consensus on whether it should be included (Kirk and Mahon 2010). Some noted ethicists, however, such as Dr. Eric Cassell, have argued that it should be allowed (Cassell and Rich 2010).

How would you recognize a patient suffering from existential distress alone? Consider the situation of Glen Smith, an 85-year-old man with refractory leukemia and profound pancytopenia. He decided to discontinue blood product support and all antimicrobials. His oncologist expected him to die in a matter of days. Glen asked to be sedated: "I don't want to watch myself die." Glen had long ago said his good-byes to his family and friends, who supported his request. He had consulted with his pastor and knew that his spiritual beliefs did not preclude sedation prior to or at the time of death. But the hospital policy that allowed palliative sedation for refractory symptoms or delirium in imminently dying patients would not apply to Glen. So, we discharged him home with hospice support, and his family told us that they were able to sedate him to his satisfaction using the lorazepam supplied in the hospice kit. He died peacefully three days later.

Most often, however, the consideration for palliative sedation to unconsciousness arises when a patient is suffering from refractory pain or other physical problem or from refractory delirium. In our facility, the palliative care team must be consulted, and if the refractory problem is delirium, psychiatry must be consulted. If chaplains or social workers are not already seeing the patient, and we feel that would be helpful, we ask the team to consult them as well.

It is especially important to inquire whether the patient practices a faith that has specific rituals associated with the end of life, so that the patient can engage in them before the sedation begins (the same applies to the discussion of terminal extubation, below). Catholic priests will anoint the patient and administer the Sacrament of the Sick; patients of the Muslim faith will say the tahlil (*laa ilaaha illallaah*), or declaration of faith ("None has the right to be rightfully worshipped but Allah the Exalted") before they lose consciousness, so that they can be guaranteed *jannah* (paradise) (Chakraborty et al. 2017); those of the Jewish faith will want to say the "Vidui," a final confession. As discussed in Chapter 3, "if one cannot say the Vidui audibly, one can say it in their heart . . . someone near the person can lead them in the Vidui, they can say it, and the dying person can repeat it" (Shulchan Aruch Y.D. 338:1 [Yachter 2007]).

When clinicians have been doing their best, often for weeks, to bring the patient's suffering under control, they feel terrible when the suffering continues. Feelings of helplessness at being unable to lessen the patient's suffering may influence our choices about how to respond to a patient's request for hastened death or for sedation (Kelly, Varghese, and Pelusi 2003; Schuman-Olivier et al. 2008). When we are considering instituting palliative sedation to unconsciousness, therefore, we always have a second palliative care physician evaluate the patient; is there something that is contributing to the suffering that could be reversed?

Whenever possible, we ask a senior, experienced physician for this second opinion. Both palliative care physicians must document their assessment of the patient, that sedation is the only means to relieve the patient's suffering, that the nurse manager of the unit agrees, and that the patient and family have given informed consent to the sedation. See Figure 12.1 for an algorithm that describes the assessment and management that should precede consideration of palliative sedation to unconsciousness.

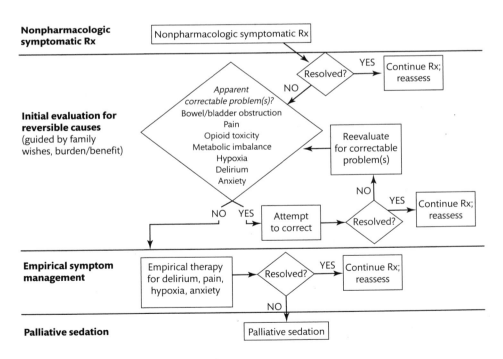

FIGURE 12.1. Patient Evaluation and Management Preceding Consideration of Palliative Sedation

Discussions among the health care team, the patient, and family members usually achieve consensus on the need for and acceptability of sedation to unconsciousness as a means of achieving symptom control. We explain to the family that the patient is not likely to regain consciousness before death. Patients must be DNR/DNI, and if the patient has an implanted defibrillator, we ask the electrophysiology service or cardiology staff to adjust the rate to the lowest response settings. We turn off the monitor alarms, and in most circumstances, turn off the monitors themselves and measure only respiratory rate, as a proxy of distress (except in patients with tachypnea from acidosis). We continue medications that helped to provide comfort or manage delirium.

While no good evidence suggests that the sedation to unconsciousness itself hastens death (Beller et al. 2015; Maltoni et al. 2012), there is also no uniformity on whether artificial nutrition or hydration should be continued (Claessens et al.

Practice Points: Palliative Sedation

- Indications: The patient is imminently dying and is experiencing suffering (physical, psychological, or spiritual/existential) that is refractory to expert attempts at management, including palliative care and psychiatric and spiritual consultation.
- Family counseling:
  - Obtain informed consent from the patient and family or from the health care proxy. Explain that the patient is not likely to regain consciousness before death.
  - Ask, "Look ahead to a few months after she dies; looking back from there, do you still feel that we did the right thing today? Do you feel that anything should have been done differently?"
- If the patient has a responsive symptom that is not the indication for the palliative sedation to unconsciousness, continue the specific treatment for that problem. For example, opioids for pain, cough, or dyspnea; haloperidol for delirium.
- For distress that is refractory to specific therapies and counseling, choose one of the following initial doses and titrate to comfort. A physician must give the loading dose of phenobarbital or pentobarbital and be present when the infusion is initiated or be present when the loading doses of the other agents are given and the infusion initiated; he or she must remain continuously present until the patient appears calm. Either a nurse or physician can do the subsequent monitoring.

Midazolam	Bolus 0.5 mg; then 0.5–1.5 mg/hr
Phenobarbital	130 mg q30 min p.r. to 1000 mg/24 hr
Pentobarbital	3 mg/kg load, then 1–2 mg/kg/hr
Thiopental	3–5 mg/kg/hr
Propofol	Up to 5 mcg/kg/min

2008). Retrospective reports indicate that 34 percent of patients died within 24 hours after initiation of palliative sedation to unconsciousness, and 96 percent died within one week, so discontinuing the hydration was not likely to have been the cause of these patients' deaths (Claessens et al. 2008). Some ethicists argue that if the patient is expected to survive more than two weeks, the cause of death would more likely be lack of supplying artificial hydration than the malignancy or other underlying cause of the patient's condition (Berger 2010). In those cases, families or patients might choose to continue hydration. We discuss with patients or their health care proxies the burdens and benefits of continuing hydration or artificial nutrition. In my experience, no one has chosen to continue these.

In addition to the formal informed consent that we obtain either from the patient or from the health care proxy, Dr. Byock (1997) recommends that we try to ensure that families will not regret their decision after the patient dies. He asks them to imagine that, several months after the death, they are recalling the events immediately preceding it and asking themselves whether anything should have been done differently. If the answer is no, he proceeds with the agreed-on plan. He finds that families who have had these conversations do not develop subsequent guilt or regrets.

We use propofol (Moyle 1995), midazolam, or pentobarbital to induce palliative sedation to control the symptom or to unconsciousness (Schuman and Abrahm 2005). Patients are usually comfortably sedated within an hour, and adjustments to the sedation are provided as needed, which is usually only during the first 24 hours. We continue careful monitoring for comfort until the patient dies. A sample hospital guideline for palliative sedation is included in the online materials for this chapter.

LVAD WITHDRAWAL AND TERMINAL EXTUBATION OR WEAN

Intensive care staff may ask palliative care clinicians to consult when a patient's care has become focused on comfort and a left ventricular assist device (LVAD), endotracheal tube, or ventilator support are not felt to be contributing to those goals.

LVAD Withdrawal

Withdrawing an LVAD is generally agreed to be ethical, as is withdrawal of ventilatory support, and they can share similar religious objections. Palliative care clinicians can help patients, their families, and the medical team sort through ethical concerns, as well as the psychological and existential distress that can arise (Slavin et al. 2020). They provide the communication of the plan with all parties as described to ensure the patient will not suffer, determine who wishes to be present, and counsel and provide support to the bereaved survivors. If value conflicts persist, however, consult the ethics service. The LVAD team performs the actual LVAD deactivation, but the palliative care clinicians often advise on appropriate sedation with lorazepam or midazolam (IV boluses), which can also prevent or treat seizures that can occur if an embolus follows deactivation.

Cessation of Ventilatory Support

The techniques needed to achieve symptom control during cessation of ventilatory support are similar whether or not the tube is left in place. The patients receive additional sedating medications, if necessary, after which they are either extubated or weaned from ventilator support with the tube left in place. Staff and families need support prior to and after the extubation or wean, and patients need to be made as comfortable as possible. For detailed information, see von Gunten and Weissman (2003a, 2003b, 2003c).

Earlier in this volume, we review how to have discussions with patients and families about withdrawing life-sustaining therapy and moving to comfort care (Chapters 5 and 11). When terminal extubation or wean is being considered as part of a comfort care plan, remember to review with the family that medications providing comfort will all be continued, and those that don't will be stopped. Explore or reexplore any cultural or religious barriers. The family's own religious leader(s) should be involved whenever possible with these discussions, even when there are no perceived barriers. Such collaborations can reach solutions that were otherwise not apparent, as was the case for the patient presented by Pan and colleagues (2020). As they discussed, the rabbi was able to help the team find a solution that allowed terminal extubation without violating any terms of the patient's Orthodox Jewish faith.

Stopping extra hydration, pressors, and antibiotics may be enough for the patient to have a peaceful death even with the tube in place. Help the family understand why stopping any artificial nutrition, be it enteral or parenteral, will not cause added discomfort (see discussion in Chapter 11). Procedures such as taking vital signs, drawing lab tests, doing x-rays, hemodialysis, or CVVH will also be stopped. If the patient has a pacemaker or an ICD, ask the electrophysiology service or cardiology staff to adjust the rate to the lowest response settings. If the family would prefer that the patient continue to be monitored, ask that the alarms be turned off or overridden by staff. Ask the nurses to remove restraints and any other extraneous devices.

Be sure to let the family know that the patient might linger for hours or even days, if you think that possible. And carefully document all these discussions. If there is a disagreement as to whether the extubation or wean meets the patient's goals, either between members of the staff (e.g., nurses and physicians) or between staff and the family, it is often helpful to consult with the ethics team.

To extubate or to wean? In extubation, the patient is suctioned, humidified oxygen added, and the patient receives sedating medications (described below). If the patient is to be weaned with the tube left in place, the PEEP (positive end expiratory pressure), oxygen levels, and ventilatory rate are decreased over about 30 to 60 minutes. If the patient survives, a T-piece can replace the connection to the ventilator.

Some dying patient's secretions are so voluminous that leaving the tube in place and decreasing the support from the ventilator will actually provide more comfort. Patients may have had bad experiences from past extubations, and they or their families ask that the tube be left in place when ventilatory support is stopped. In the COVID-19 pandemic, the secretions themselves were so dangerous to the staff that the tubes were left in place. In other situations, especially if the patient is conscious, secretions minimal, and the airway likely to be open after the procedure, extubation may be preferred.

Practice Point: Terminal Extubation or Wean

- Initiate or continue discussion to ensure you are providing goal-concordant care.
- Consider recommending wean instead of extubation for patients with excessive secretions.
- Check that an order for DNR/DNI/comfort-focused care is placed.
- Ask the team to adjust other orders, monitors, and ICD/pacemaker settings to promote a comfortable death.
- If requested, advise ICU respiratory therapy and other staff about comfort medications.
- Adjust family expectations for timing of death after extubation or wean.
- Debrief with family; offer to debrief with staff immediately or at a later time.

Medications. If the patient was on a paralytic, the ICU team will stop it prior to the procedure, and they will confirm that the patient has a spontaneous respiratory rate before they begin the extubation or wean. They may continue midazolam or propofol, but at a dose that allows for spontaneous respirations. After the extubation, no increase in the propofol dose or rate is permissible.

You may be asked to advise on which medications to give to establish and maintain comfort during this procedure. Intensive care unit staff are usually more experienced in and more comfortable managing extubations when the patient is expected to survive; when the extubation or wean is expected to allow the patient's death, they are anxious to ensure that the patient be as comfortable as possible. They may not be familiar with the medications needed to provide that comfort at the end of life.

The palliative care clinicians will monitor the patient for evidence of distress, which may be from pain, anxiety, or air hunger, and suggest appropriate medications. If the patient has tachypnea alone, however, it is likely to be reflexive and unlikely to respond to medications. Table 12.1 describes strategies for treating dyspnea using opioids for either opioid-naive or opioid-tolerant patients and common agents and doses of anticholinergics for excessive secretions. Delirious patients who survive the procedure will require continuation of their antipsychotics.

Debriefing. You would normally spend time with the family after any death. Here, you need to spend time with the staff as well, providing support for their grief and, what may provide even more anguish, their feelings of inadequacy (*"If only someone else had been on, they might have seen something correctable that I missed"*). Identify which family members to refer to bereavement counselors and who, among the staff, may need special support as well.

IMMEDIATELY AFTER THE DEATH

Studies indicate that many house officers are not trained in what to do after a patient dies (Ferris et al. 1998; Bailey and Williams 2005). If you are present at the death, or if you have been asked to pronounce the patient dead, offer your unhurried condolences to all others present before you leave the room. Such expressions can be very comforting. If you are invited to participate in a prayer, this is perfectly appropriate if you so wish. Encourage those present to spend as much time as they need to, to say or do whatever they need to say or do, including touching the body. Answer the family's questions, and if the family was not present at the death, answer any questions about how their loved one died. Reassure them about pain control or other concerns they have about the patient's suffering.

If hugging comes naturally to you and seems to be called for now, this, and the tears that may accompany it, are also OK. Just be sure to mitigate the manifestations of your sorrow so that the family doesn't feel the need to take care of you. As one of my colleagues, Vicki Jackson, has said, "no ugly cries; don't make it about you." Also offer condolences to the nurses and other staff who have cared for the patient. If the family has shared with you praise for the care that the patient received, be sure to share this with the staff as well: *"Her family told me they were so appreciative of the wonderful care you gave her."* Those of you who work with house staff and physician assistants can help them deal with their grief by allowing them to review the circumstances of the death, their feelings for the patient, and their contributions to the care of the patient. Studies indicate that interns, in particular, need this support (Redinbaugh et al. 2003).

The nurses will be bathing and caring for the patient's body according to the patient's wishes. Some religions require special rituals after a person has died. These needs should be known prior to the death and arrangements made to have the appropriate people informed. Some Jewish patients, for example, will direct that their body be bathed and prepared for burial by a specially trained group of men or women (the Chevra Kadosha). In Chapter 13, we review what you and the team can do to help the bereaved family.

WHAT OUR INSTITUTIONS CAN DO TO SUPPORT US

Finally, I want to say a word about what the hospitals we work in and your palliative care colleagues can do to support you. A survey of oncologists who were asked how their institutions could support them was published in 2012 (Granek et al. 2012). Oncologists, of course, are already engaged in working through their feelings about their many patients each year who die. Support from their office colleagues and staff and from friends and family, participation in religious observances or other spiritual practices, a good exercise routine, hobbies, and vacations (for those with the time) are all helpful.

But not enough. The oncologists reported that the hospitals they worked in could do much more to support them. They wanted training during fellowship on how to cope with their own losses, not just how to help patients and their families. They advocated for having mentors during training who modeled for fellows how to work through the feelings that are associated with patient deaths. Grand rounds and regular opportunities to debrief could continue the education for graduate physicians. Some wanted the hospital to host regular meetings in which they could normalize their feelings and share their stories. They thought the hospital could provide a grief counselor or other mental health professional to whom they could go if more complex or painful concerns persisted.

Hospitals or other institutions that already have a palliative care team could involve them in supporting their oncology clinicians in all these areas. Palliative care teams can give talks, sponsor memorial services, and teach oncology fellows through seminars, or better, through inpatient or outpatient clinical rotations. They can host a monthly meeting and create a safe space in which oncologists can share their stories, normalize their grief, and learn how to be better role models for their junior colleagues or trainees. Through these kinds of interactions, oncologists can begin to see their palliative care colleagues as resources between the meetings, when they see each other on the wards, or when there has been a particularly troubling case that the oncologist would really like to debrief with someone. In this way, palliative care clinicians can help prevent the compassion fatigue that results from unacknowledged or unprocessed grief (Abrahm 2012). As oncology clinicians learn ways to care for themselves, they will be much more helpful to the patients and families they want to comfort. You can find a more extensive discussion of compassion fatigue and burnout in Chapter 13.

CHAPTER 13

Bereavement

with Bethany-Rose Daubman, MD

THE BEREAVED

Our responsibilities to the patient and family continue after the patient's death, as we try to help bereaved family members. The suffering of the bereaved can manifest in many ways; for example, they are often sleepless, are at increased risk of developing major depression or prolonged grief disorder, and are at higher risk of suicide (Lobb et al. 2010; Lundorff et al. 2017; Prigerson and Jacobs 2001). To anticipate their needs and to develop a suitable support program for them, it is useful to understand the many dimensions and manifestations of grief and mourning. The writings of Dr. Colin Parkes, Dr. Therese A. Rando, and Dr. Holly Prigerson are superb resources for physicians or other clinicians wanting in-depth, scholarly, and clinically useful discussions of normal and complicated mourning. Their work is based on research and practice in patients living in Western countries, and I have used their formulations as the foundation of the following discussion. References to their works, as well as to those of others working in this area, are listed in the online bibliography.

LOSS, GRIEF, AND MOURNING

Those who are bereaved are suffering from multiple losses. In addition to losing their loved one, secondary losses can occur, such as losing the medical care team

(Prigerson and Jacobs 2001), having to leave the family home, or changing one's social standing (such as from wife to widow). In addition, the death is likely to revive the pain of losses that occurred many years before. A father's death, for example, may evoke memories of a divorce or the death of a child. The bereaved also suffer from the loss of "what might have been"—a reconciliation that never happened, a father to walk with down the aisle, a twenty-first birthday party. At the time of the death, bereaved family members enter this maelstrom of loss and may need help sorting out the sources of their pain.

A bereaved person's grief is a "process of experiencing the psychological, behavioral, social, and physical reactions to the perception of loss" (Rando 1993, p. 22). The intensity of a bereaved person's grief is predicated on several factors relating to the deceased and their relationship with the deceased, characteristics of the mourner, the nature of the death, and societal and cultural factors.

For example, being very attached to or dependent on the deceased or having a great deal of ambivalence in one's feelings toward the deceased can exacerbate grief, as can a personal history of clinical depression or difficulty in handling previous losses. A sudden or accidental death, suicide, or homicide also magnifies the grief experienced, while a good support system and religious rituals can lessen it.

Differentiation between grief and depression. It can sometimes be challenging to distinguish between manifestations of grief and those of depression (Block 2001; Prigerson et al. 1996). Grief is characterized by "intense feelings of sadness, yearning for the deceased, anxiety about the future, disorganization and feelings of emptiness" (Morris and Block 2012, pp. 272–73). While there can be some overlap with acute grief and depression, the majority of grieving people do not generally express the characteristics of depressed patients, which include "generalized feelings of hopelessness, helplessness, worthlessness, guilt, lack of enjoyment and pleasure, and active suicidal thoughts" (Morris and Block 2012, p. 274). People with grief tend not to have any plans to end their lives and can still experience pleasure at times and look forward to the future.

Depression responds better to pharmacologic therapy than does grief. Methylphenidate, SSRIs, and bupropion SR (sustained-release) all have been found to improve depression without worsening grief intensity (Block 2001; Zisook et al. 2001). For patients with prolonged grief disorder (see definition and discussion below), cognitive-behavioral therapy (CBT) with a therapist skilled in working with the bereaved may be helpful (Doka and Martin 2010; Greer 2010). Unfortunately, patients suffering from prolonged grief disorder have not been shown to improve with pharmacological treatment (Kristensen, Dyregrov, and Dyregrov 2017), though some medications such as citalopram have been shown to reduce comorbid symptoms of depression (Shear et al. 2016). These patients may also respond to a type of psychotherapy called complicated grief treatment, which is discussed later in this chapter (Shear 2010; Shear et al. 2016).

Styles of grieving. Each bereaved person's loss is unique, as are the experience and manifestations of the grief and mourning. Building on the work of Drs. Therese Rando, Colin Murray Parkes, William Worden, and others, Kenneth J. Doka, PhD, MDiv (professor of gerontology at the Graduate School of the College of New Rochelle and senior consultant to the Hospice Foundation of America) and Terry Martin, PhD (professor of psychology at Hood College) have published extensively about patterns of grief and mourning. Their book (Doka and Martin 2010) sheds even more light on the causes of two distinct mourning styles, as well as on how we can recognize them in patients. The book is targeted to "grief counselors, psychologists, social workers, mental health counselors, pastoral counselors, and other therapists" (p. 4), but along with the theoretical discussions that would be of most interest to that group, we found clear descriptions of what they argue are the two most common types of functional grief and mourning, the *intuitive* and the *instrumental* styles.

People who are aware of their feelings are likely to experience and manifest grief and mourning in the intuitive style, which is different from the instrumental style of people who are less in touch with their *feelings* but very in touch with their *thoughts* about the events surrounding their loved one's death, and who normally evaluate, plan, and "do things" to decrease their pain when they are distressed. To illustrate the differences, consider Melinda and Winifred. They are stay-at-home moms in their forties, each with two teenage children, both of whom lost their husbands unexpectedly two months ago.

Melinda has an intuitive pattern of grief and mourning. When we think of a grieving person, hers is the picture that usually comes to mind: she is likely to cry often, to need to share her grief with others, and to experience "intense inner pain, helplessness, hopelessness, and loneliness" (Doka and Martin 2010, p. 58). Melinda is eager to talk about her feelings, in a group or to a therapist; she wants help with her increased anxiety and with working on the emotional problems she is experiencing that seem to overwhelm her. She is distressed by her "prolonged periods of confusion, lack of concentration, disorientation, and disorganization" (p. 63). Her sister has moved in temporarily to help care for the children, since Melinda is unable to focus on that right now. And she has not even begun to think about learning to deal with financial matters.

Winifred is an instrumental griever. Her family thinks she is uncaring and wonder if she's experiencing any grief at all. She, like Melinda, is experiencing "prolonged periods of confusion, lack of concentration, disorientation, and disorganization," which are frightening because they are completely foreign to her (p. 63). Instrumental grievers like Winifred have less intense feelings of grief and may even feel guilty and worried that they don't need to cry. Winifred has not been crying, but she does have feelings of "sadness, anxiety, loneliness and yearning" (p. 66) that are not as strong or as overwhelming as Melinda's. And unlike Melinda, Winifred's grief is triggered by *thoughts* about her lost husband and the times they shared together.

Also unlike Melinda, Winifred has been intensely concerned about the logistics and obligations that are now a part of her life. She is exhausted, partly because of the mental strain, and because she has been staying up late at night bringing order out of what she is experiencing as chaos. While her family may not recognize it, Winifred is grieving by righting her world, not by talking about her grief.

Because of the way men and women are socialized in the United States, women are expected to be like Melinda: demonstrably emotional (intuitive), and men are expected to be the strong silent types, the "doers," who usually show more of an instrumental style of grief. As oncology and palliative care clinicians, you see many people with *anticipatory grief* every day in your office. You've easily recognized the intuitive grievers. But if you and your staff are not familiar with the instrumental style of grieving, you may easily misinterpret as indifference the lack of overt emotion in a husband, wife, or partner of someone with far-advanced cancer. These instrumental grievers are grieving by providing meticulous care to their loved ones or by focusing on the tasks that need to be done for them. Harold might build a ramp for Maude's wheelchair so she can still get out of the house; Savannah might be taking care of Audrey's garden now that she cannot care for it herself. Harold and Savannah, of course, care just as much and need just as much support as people who grieve in the more easily recognized, intuitive style.

Gender is less of a determining factor in whether a person experiences and manifests the intuitive or instrumental style than are gender socialization, personality, and culture. Women are expected to show the intuitive style of grieving, but a man who grieves this way may have difficulty being supported at home or at work: he is supposed to "suck it up" and go on. Winifred, being a woman, is not supposed to grieve in the instrumental style, and her family misunderstands her actions and thinks she is even less caring than a man acting the same way would be perceived.

Most mourners express a mixture of intuitive and instrumental styles. They find ways both to express their grief emotionally and to function within their new family roles or to return to their jobs. Problems can arise, of course, in either type of person if unable to find any way to express their grief. We refer you to Doka and Martin for more in this area, including a discussion of dissonant responses to grief, and of the roles of personality, gender socialization, and culture in shaping an intuitive or an instrumental style. The book also includes a discussion of other adaptive strategies mourners use, a chapter on self-help and interventions, and a Grief Pattern Inventory and instructions on how it should be scored.

Phases of grief and mourning, and processes of mourning. Although there is no set order, many people pass through one or more identifiable phases of grief and the rebuilding of a life without the deceased (Maciejewski et al. 2007). Dr. Sue Morris, a clinical psychologist who specializes in bereavement and is the director of Bereavement Services at Dana-Farber Cancer Institute (DFCI), likens the pattern of grief to that of a wave in her 2018 book, *Overcoming Grief.* The intensity of the waves is typically greatest early in the course of the bereavement, and the amplitude generally decreases as time goes on (Morris 2018).

Dr. Therese Rando describes a useful framework for thinking about the processes of grief, which includes three phases of grief and mourning and six processes of mourning experienced by most of the bereaved, who are eventually able to reintegrate. Of course, not everyone experiences all these phases, but being familiar with them may help you understand the processes the bereaved survivors of your patients may be going through.

The phases, which include periods of overlapping manifestations, are *avoidance, confrontation,* and *accommodation,* as detailed in the box below (Rando 1993, p. 45).

During the *avoidance* phase, the bereaved person may initially appear numb, confused, or dazed, but some form of denial usually follows as the reality of the death intensifies. A wide range of behaviors can be expected, from uncontrolled shrieking to an unnerving calm.

Phases of Grief and Mourning, and the Six "R" Processes of Mourning

Avoidance Phase

1. *Recognize* the loss.
   Acknowledge the death.
   Understand the death.

Confrontation Phase

2. *React* to the separation.
   Experience the pain.
   Feel, identify, accept, and give some form of expression to all the psychological reactions to the loss.
   Identify and mourn secondary losses.
3. *Recollect* and *reexperience* the deceased and the relationship.
   Review and remember realistically.
   Revive and reexperience the feelings.
4. *Relinquish* the old attachments to the deceased and the way things were.

Accommodation Phase

5. *Readjust* to move adaptively into the new world without forgetting the old.
   Rebuild a new outlook on how the world is supposed to be.
   Develop a new relationship with the deceased.
   Adopt new ways of being in the world.
   Form a new identity.
6. *Reinvest*
   Resume old relationships and responsibilities and risk putting energy into new ones.

During the *confrontation* phase, the pain intensifies because the absence of the person who has died asserts itself repeatedly. The mourner begins to yearn for the one who is dead, and waves of intense grief occur each time the deceased is sought and not found (Morris 2018); denial dissolves, and disorganization, depression, disinterest, and despair take its place (Parkes 1987). During this phase, the bereaved person commonly experiences various feelings, behaviors, physical symptoms, spiritual concerns, and thoughts (listed in Figure 13.1; for a more complete list of psychological, behavioral, social, and physical responses, see Rando 1993; Morris 2018; Morris and Block 2012).

The family must adjust to an environment without the person who has died. The role that the deceased played in the marriage, the family, and even the community may be increasingly revealed to the bereaved as time goes on, and mourning may be needed for each loss. Ideally, the bereaved will be able to cope with the increasing responsibilities, but many may need assistance or training—for example, in household finance or taking care of children.

Accepting the reality of the loss and experiencing its pain are essential if the pain is to be overcome. It is very difficult for people to move beyond loss if they never allow themselves to feel it in some way that is appropriate for them. Family obligations and unspoken strictures against demonstrations of grief can further impair a bereaved person's ability to experience the pain of the loss adequately. Putting those feelings aside to deal with later or denying their existence altogether will only prolong or inhibit the process.

Eventually—and there is no useful timetable to determine when this will occur—most survivors reach *accommodation*. Dr. Rando chose this word carefully. It does not imply closure or return to the premorbid state. Instead, it suggests passage to a state in which life will never be the same, but in which bereaved persons tacitly acknowledge that an accommodation must be made if they are ever to resume old relationships and responsibilities. And even more difficult is the decision to try to establish new ones and risk recurrent loss, to realize that loving someone new need not mean betraying the memory of the person who has died. The bereaved person must craft a new relationship with the deceased, a new identity, and a new role in society.

Throughout the confrontation phase, and even in the accommodation phase and for years after the death, the bereaved are likely to experience what Dr. Rando calls "subsequent temporary upsurges of grief (STUGs)" (Rando 1993, p. 64). Precipitants for these recurrent pangs of grief (or "triggers" of a resurgent "wave" of grief [Morris 2018]) include anniversaries, holidays, and seasonal changes; reaching the age at which the loved one died; having a child reach the age of the child who died; favorite shared activities and personal reminders (e.g., music, smells, favorite objects); and a new personal or public trauma that resurrects the pain of old losses, especially if the one who died was the person turned to in times of crisis. The severity of the grief can match that of the initial loss and can be frightening for the bereaved, who had thought themselves beyond experiencing pain of that intensity.

WHAT TO EXPECT

Recovery from the loss of someone you love is often a long and painful process. However, if you can make it through the pain, things will get better. Most people find that their grief lasts anywhere from six months to two years. Since each person is unique, you will progress at your own pace and in your own way.

Grief is often associated with certain feelings and physical symptoms. Some of these include:

Common Feelings/Behaviors
- Fear and anxiety
- Anger and guilt
- Depression and despair
- Separation and longing
- Sudden wave of psychic pain
- Confusion and inability to concentrate or make decisions
- Tearfulness and crying
- Sighing
- Restlessness
- Yearning
- Helplessness
- Relief
- Hope

Spiritual Responses
- Faith may be strengthened, altered, or abandoned

Common Physical Symptoms
- Decreased or increased appetite
- Decreased energy; weakness of muscles
- Nausea and diarrhea
- Decrease or increase in your sex drive
- Inability to sleep or sleeping too much
- Feeling something stuck in your throat
- Tightness in chest, breathlessness
- Oversensitivity to noise
- Vivid dreams
- Dry mouth

Common Thoughts
- Disbelief
- Preoccupation with "if only" and "what if" and with memories
- Sense of his/her presence
- "Who am I now?"

WHAT TO DO

1. Give yourself permission to feel loss and to grieve over the loss.
2. Recognize that your grief is unique.
3. Expect to have some negative feelings.
4. Accept the help of others; let people know how they can help you.
5. Give yourself time alone.
6. Engage in physical activity.
7. Read books about feelings of grief and the process of recovery.
8. Talk to others about your loss.
9. Attend community support groups.
10. <u>Most important:</u> Recognize that at some point your pain will lessen.

WHAT NOT TO DO

1. Avoid making major changes.
2. Try not to withdraw from social activities.
3. Avoid excessive smoking or drinking.

WHEN TO CALL

Please call:
- If you have any questions or would like further information.
- If you feel that you would like professional counseling.

FIGURE 13.1. What to Expect—for the Bereaved. *Source:* From J. Abrahm, M. E. Cooley, and L. Ricacho, "Efficacy of an Educational Bereavement Program for Families of Veterans with Cancer," *Journal of Cancer Education* 10:207–12, 1995; reprinted with permission.

Interventions

Given this understanding of what phases bereaved people are likely to experience, clinicians and researchers have devised interventions to ameliorate their suffering and have demonstrated the value of these interventions. Some take place in anticipation of the patient's death, as described in earlier chapters. These include skillfully communicating the diagnosis and terminal prognosis; providing emotional, psychological, and spiritual support, as well as physical comfort; and helping families to resolve outstanding issues. It is also important to provide support in the final days and make the death as peaceful as possible.

Some patients may need CBT techniques to help them regain control. The bereaved can use Dr. Sue Morris's *Overcoming Grief* (2018) on their own or with the guidance of a therapist. *Overcoming Grief* is filled with straightforward explanations of what the bereaved are likely to experience and when they should seek professional help. It offers insights into how to understand and help children who are grieving, helpful tips for those in any phase of grief, and several practical, easy-to-understand exercises that can help bereaved people find their way again after a significant loss.

Many of these exercises take the form of writing in a personal journal and answering specific questions that help elucidate thoughts and feelings so that the bereaved person can, with this new knowledge, allow new feelings and new behaviors to arise. When approaching painful emotions, such as regret, for example, Dr. Morris suggests that the bereaved person create a chart with five columns, A through E. Under A, the bereaved person writes the "situation or trigger"; B—"unhelpful thoughts"; C—"feelings" (score/10) and "behavior" resulting from A; D—"helpful thoughts"; and E—"new feelings" (score/10) and "new behavior" (that results from D).

Dr. Morris gives us a sample chart written by a bereaved daughter experiencing a common cause of regret—she hadn't told her mother she loved her before leaving her that morning, and her mother died before she saw her again. In this chart (adapted from Lara's Diary Entry, Morris 2018, p. 90), the daughter completed the columns as shown in the box below.

Lara hadn't been aware that her regret, and the sobbing that accompanied it, was in response to a *thought*. The crying just seemed normal and spontaneous as she reflected about her mother's death; she wasn't aware of any intervening thought that could have triggered her feelings of regret and associated sobbing. But writing in the chart made that underlying connecting thought *visible*, and once it was there, Lara could consider whether it was true or not. She examined the *evidence* for what she first thought in column B and was able to generate alternative thoughts as shown in column D. Once she could understand what she was blaming herself for, she could "think" her way to beginning to forgive herself, and as a result, she had less regret and more acceptance, as shown in column E.

Sample Framework for Challenging Unhelpful Thoughts

A. Situation or trigger	B. Unhelpful thoughts	C. Feelings (score/10)	D. Helpful thoughts	E. New feelings (score/10)
		Behavior		*New behavior*
Thinking about mom's death	*Why didn't I tell her I loved her that last time?*	Regret (9/10) Sobbing	I did not know she was going to die. I can't predict the future.	Regret (5/10) Acceptance (5/10) Less crying

(Morris 2018, reprinted with permission from Little, Brown Book Group)

Dr. Morris's book is full of many other similarly helpful exercises for coping with grief, moving forward to address difficult relationships, having difficult conversations, keeping that connection to the person you've lost, setting future goals, and more. The book can be used with or without the help of a social worker, a therapist, or a bereavement counselor. The bibliography, available online, is also likely to be helpful for people who are bereaved.

A Sample Bereavement Program

Hospice programs must offer a formal bereavement program that takes place during the first 13 months after the patient's death; accommodation is usually well under way by the end of that time. After the formal program ends, the bereaved are welcome to continue participating in any bereavement activities that have been useful to them. Even families who are coping well benefit from support for this extended period after the patient's death. In addition, you might consider providing your own yearlong bereavement program. Various people in the office can participate, and it can be rewarding for each of them. DFCI in Boston and Boston Children's Hospital have hospital-wide bereavement programs that follow an education, guidance, and support model of care (Morris and Block 2015; Morris et al. 2017). Consider encouraging your institution to invest in a bereavement program as a model of care for your patients and families with serious illness.

At the time of death: the avoidance phase. Supporting the bereaved should begin immediately after the death (if not earlier). Family members are often in a state of shock; their moods may swing wildly, changing from moment to moment. This volatility may be frightening for them—to be detached and numb one minute and distraught the next—and we try to reassure them that this reaction is normal and that they should not worry about controlling themselves.

> ## Practice Points: Supporting the Bereaved
>
> - Reassure family members that their response to the patient's death is normal.
> - Listen empathically if they wish to review the circumstances of the patient's death.
> - Reassure the family that you will remain available to them to help them with the grieving process.
> - During the first year following the patient's death, call and write to the family at regularly scheduled intervals; don't wait for them to get in touch with you.
> - Offer to send educational materials on manifestations of grief, coping techniques, and professional resources if the family wishes.
> - Invite them to participate in a memorial service.
> - Identify family members at high risk for prolonged, intense grief and arrange a referral for professional support even before the patient dies.

When I (*Janet Abrahm*) am present at the death and meeting with the family, if I am sad, I let myself cry with them, as long as I am not seeming so distraught that the family feels the need to comfort or reassure me. If they seem to need to talk things over, I ask leading questions to help them feel free to tell me their feelings. I find that they often want to review the circumstances of the death, to assure themselves that the person was not suffering and that everything that could have been done was done. I always try to find something for which I can praise them, such as their care of the patient or their advocacy role for him and add how lucky he was to have had them there when he needed them. Even if I was not present at the death, when I call them later, I try to offer as much of this kind of reassurance and support as I can in the course of a telephone call.

Initial follow-up call. Calling the family within 24 to 48 hours of the death to offer our condolences and help can be an impactful practice. During this call, we offer comfort and provide a listener for a retelling of the story of the death and the meaning of it for the bereaved. If necessary, we again reinforce the normality of the wide emotional swings or other symptoms of acute grief they may be experiencing. We listen empathically and indicate our unconditional continued support. I (*Molly Collins*) have found that delayed calls to the bereaved (2–6 weeks after death) can reveal those who may already be in the *accommodation* phase, as well as those at risk of complicated grief. These calls can also be a unique moment to reflect on the work you and the bereaved did to care for the deceased during their illness and can provide a glimpse into how the bereaved move on from the pain of such a profound loss.

Institutional education, guidance, and support model. Drs. Morris and Block outline a comprehensive model for structuring an institutional bereavement program (Morris and Block 2015) that goes beyond the initial steps immediately surrounding the death. First, this includes acknowledgement of the death of the patient by the institution and clinicians. Sending a condolence letter (from the institution, as well as individual letters from staff) is one way to do this. A sample of a condolence letter is given in Figure 13.2. You can find a full discussion of the principles that underlie the writing of a good condolence letter in Fast Facts #022, 3rd edition, on the Palliative Care Network of Wisconsin Fast Facts and Concepts website (https://www.mypcnow.org/fast-facts/). As Drs. Morris and Block emphasize, disseminating guidance for writing condolences and sympathy cards to staff may be helpful for those of us who have a difficult time knowing what to say. Many institutions also have memorial services that bereaved family members are invited to attend.

Letter sent one week after death

Dear _____ :

We share your sadness about your loss of _____ . We realize how hard it is when death occurs and want to let you know how important it is to be with family and friends at this time. If we can help you in any way, please call us at _____ . Again, all of us in the Hematology/Oncology department send our deepest sympathy.

Sincerely,

Letter sent three to six weeks after death and repeated at six months

Dear _____ :

When we spoke on the phone, you said you would like more information to help you understand what you have been going through since _____ died. We have therefore enclosed information describing common feelings many people experience at the loss of a loved one as well as a list of books you could read that discuss these issues and a list of groups in your area that you could try for more support.

We realize that this is a hard time for you and we offer this information in the hope that it may be of some help. If you have any questions or want to talk with someone, please feel free to call us at _____ and ask for me.

Sincerely,

Holiday letter

Dear _____ :

We were thinking of you because we know that this time of year may be difficult, since this is the first time without _____ . Others around you may also be thinking of _____ at this time. We want you to know that it is OK to talk about your loved one, of your memories of those special times together.

Remember to take one day at a time. If you find yourself feeling anxious, depressed or lonely, please feel free to call. We all hope you find comfort and peace at this time. If there's anything we can do to help, please call.

Sincerely,

FIGURE 13.2. Letters to the Bereaved. *Source:* From J. Abrahm, M. E. Cooley, and L. Ricacho, "Efficacy of an Educational Bereavement Program for Families of Veterans with Cancer," *Journal of Cancer Education* 10:207–12, 1995; reprinted with permission.

Drs. Morris and Block also emphasize the importance of providing the bereaved with information and education about grieving, as well as support services, if available. This may include mailed pamphlets or handouts, access to a website with information on bereavement, or seminars/support groups on coping with grief. Figure 13.1 is one such example of materials that could be sent to provide a list of readings, a description of grief, a list of feelings and physical signs commonly experienced by those who are grieving, and what to do or not do about them. Consider including a list of support groups in their area (including those hosted by your institution as well as the hospice). Bereavement support groups can help in recovery by encouraging talking about loss with skilled bereavement counselors and finding connection with others who have suffered similar losses. Groups such as Widow-to-Widow and, for parents who have lost a child, Compassionate Friends or Candlelighters (www.candle.org) can provide much-needed understanding and help with rebuilding a life. The support services provided through Drs. Morris and Block's bereavement program also include risk screening and referral information, individual assessment and short-term support, and an online bereavement community.

Being mindful that we as clinicians also experience grief when our patients die, which may be compounded if we aren't sure how to reach out to families, Drs. Morris and Block also suggest staff support and education as an essential component of a bereavement program. This may include grief and remembrance rounds, as described later in this chapter. Last, they suggest evaluation of the bereavement program and risk screening.

I think you and your staff will also find the process of supporting bereaved family members rewarding. You may find that as you speak to them at longer and longer intervals and begin to remember patients as they were before the terminal stages of their illness, it may help you to achieve closure and make it easier for you to move on.

Prolonged Grief Disorder

After the initial period of intense grieving, 80 to 90 percent of families do well (Morris and Block 2012), but the remainder do not. For these families, the bereavement process is severe and prolonged, and many are unable to reach any kind of accommodation with their loss. Even though they have been bereaved for 6 months or longer, they experience daily or disabling intense yearning or searching for the deceased (Prigerson et al. 2009). In addition, they have several cognitive, emotional, and behavioral symptoms that cause significant impairments in their ability to function in, for example, the social, occupational, or domestic spheres.

These bereaved survivors have developed what is now termed *prolonged grief disorder* (Prigerson et al. 2009), an entity different from depression (major depressive disorder), post-traumatic stress disorder, and generalized anxiety disorders. Prolonged grief disorder is now included in ICD-11 and the *DSM5* as a disorder specifically associated with stress following the death of a loved one characterized by a state of intense yearning and sadness, typically accompanied by persistent thoughts of the deceased and intense emotional pain such as guilt, anger, denial, emotional numbness, and difficulty engaging in social activities (ICD 2021). This grief response persists for a minimum of 6 months (Prigerson et al. 2009), though symptoms of prolonged grief disorder can last for several years (Prigerson and Jacobs 2001). Also noted in ICD-11 is that, while each individual has different expected social, cultural, and religious norms for grieving, a diagnosis of prolonged grief disorder is made when a grief response persists for an atypically long period that exceeds the social, cultural, or religious norms for that individual's unique context and culture. These persons are at increased risk for social dysfunction and various adverse health consequences, such as cardiac events, hypertension, and cancer (Prigerson et al. 2009).

Who is at risk? Several characteristics of the death itself, of the bereaved, and of their relationship with the deceased can predict whether a survivor is likely to remain reasonably functional or is at high risk for severe psychological distress (Kissane and Zaider 2015; Lobb et al. 2010; Lundorff et al. 2017; Rando 1993; Stroebe, Schut, and Stroebe 2007; Wright et al. 2010; Zhang, El-Jawahri, and Prigerson 2006). Personal characteristics of bereaved survivors who are likely to be at high risk include having had a psychiatric disorder or separation anxiety as a child; poor social supports (or thinking that their support network is poor); abuse or neglect as a child; other stresses happening at the same time as the death; previous losses; having a very dependent relationship with the person who died or having conflict or unresolved issues at the time of the death; being present during a death that was apparently filled with suffering for the patient; and having a high level of distress immediately following the death (Morris and Block 2012).

Bereavement risk assessment tool. A tool, such as the Bereavement Risk Assessment Tool developed at St. Christopher's Hospice in London, can help you identify people who might be at high risk for a more troubled bereavement period (Figure 13.3). Families at high risk are those who score 15 or higher on this scale or those whom, for whatever reason, the evaluator suspects are likely to cope either badly (requiring special help) or very badly (requiring urgent help). For example, people who have many young children at home, who are burdened by feelings of anger and self-reproach, who do not work outside the home, or who are clingy or pining could easily score above 15 on this assessment tool.

Detecting prolonged grief disorder. Some of the bereaved who did not appear to be at high risk before the patient died will nevertheless manifest signs of prolonged grief disorder long after the death. Some people, for example, may remain in denial, having failed even to begin grieving. They may have never seemed sad and may even have avoided the funeral. Others are unable to make decisions; they lose initiative; they are filled with guilt and self-reproach, exhibit self-destructive behaviors, and may ultimately develop a major depression beginning at the time of the death and recurring at important anniversaries (Block 1985).

PATIENT NAME_____ S/O NAME _____ DATE _____

A. Children <14 @ Home:	B. Occupation of Principal Wage Earner:	C. Anticipated Employment of Key Person:	D. Clinging or Pining:
0 None 1 One 2 Two 3 Three 4 Four 5 Five or more	1 Professional and executive 2 Semiprofessional 3 Office and clerical 4 Skilled manual 5 Semiskilled manual 6 Unskilled manual	0 Works full time 1 Works part time 2 Retired 3 Housewife 4 Unemployed	1 Never 2 Seldom 3 Moderate 4 Frequent 5 Constant 6 Constant, intense
E. Anger:	**F. Self-reproach:**	**G. Relationship Now:**	**H. How Person Will Cope:**
1 None (or normal) 2 Mild irritation 3 Moderate occasional outburst 4 Severe; spoils relationships 5 Extreme; bitter	1 None 2 Mild vague 3 Moderate 4 Severe 5 Extreme; major problem	1 Close, intimate 2 Warm supportive family 3 Family supportive but live a distance 4 Doubtful 5 None of these	1 Well; normal grief and recovery without special help 2 Fair; may need no special help 3 Doubtful; may need special help 4 Badly; requires special help 5 Very badly; requires urgent help

FIGURE 13.3. Bereavement Risk Assessment Tool. Total score >15 = high risk; score 4 or 5 on item H = urgent need. *Source:* From C. Parkes and R. Weiss, *Recovery from Bereavement*, copyright © 1983 by Colin Murray Parkes and Robert S. Weiss; with permission of Basic Books, a member of Perseus Books, LLC.

Still others are unwilling to let go, refusing to allow any of the deceased's personal effects to be moved. They cannot discuss their lost relative without becoming very upset; but they repeatedly talk about their bereavement and feel it acutely, even if months have elapsed. Finally, some may be intensely angry—at the deceased, at the physicians, or at others who cared for the person who died.

I (*Bethany-Rose Daubman*) first encountered prolonged grief disorder during my palliative medicine fellowship. I was caring for Annette, a patient recently diagnosed with widely metastatic ovarian cancer, and had also grown close with her daughter, Jillian, who became her mother's primary caretaker in her last months. Though a difficult decision given how recently she was diagnosed, Annette was clear in her desire to forgo further chemotherapy and enroll in a hospice program in a nursing facility. Jillian had wanted to move in with her mother and father to care for her mother, but her father felt that Annette's caregiving needs were too high and preferred her to receive her end-of-life care in a nursing facility. Jillian accepted her father's decision, but I could tell she felt she was letting her mother down. On the day of Annette's discharge, Jillian made me promise that her mother would be comfortable when she passed. We reviewed the plan for medications, hospice involvement, and spiritual support, and I reminded Jillian that she could always call me as well if she had concerns.

One week later, I heard from the hospice team that Annette had died peacefully that morning. I reached out to Jillian for a bereavement call, and she answered the phone by screaming, "You promised! You promised me that she wouldn't be in pain when she died!" It took some time to piece together from the hospice nurse and Annette's husband (who were both also present at the time of death) that although they perceived a comfortable passing, Jillian felt that her mother's eyes appeared wild and distressed and believed she (and I) had let her mother down.

Throughout the next few weeks and months, I would check in on Jillian for bereavement calls. She had taken a leave of absence from work and then ultimately been let go when she was unable to return. She had withdrawn from her father and brother, feeling they were callous to "move on ahead with their lives when Mom will never get that chance!" She continued to tell me she thought I had let her mother down in her last moments, and that Annette's oncologist had abandoned them. I felt overwhelmed and helpless during these calls with Jillian.

I reached out to her oncologist to see if he had spoken with Jillian since Annette's death, and he relayed that he had actually met with Jillian several times when she would show up at the hospital and have him paged. He, too, was struggling with how best to support her. He and I had both recommended grief support groups through Annette's hospice, but Jillian felt that her mother's traumatic passing was something that other hospice families would not understand. Finally, I realized (far too late) that this was beyond my professional capabilities, and referred Jillian to Dr. Sue Morris, the author and bereavement expert mentioned earlier in this chapter. The last I spoke with Jillian, she was pleased to be working with Dr. Morris, someone whom she felt was much better able to understand the trauma she was experiencing. She had recently returned to part-time work. I was glad to have access to bereavement experts and vowed to incorporate Dr. Morris earlier when I was worried about prolonged grief disorder.

Treatment of patients with prolonged grief disorder. Clinicians and researchers who have done extensive work in this area recommend that to minimize psychological morbidity, we begin psychological support for family members who are at high risk even before the patient dies. For those at less risk, we should maintain close contact after the death and institute intensive support as soon as they manifest a need.

Patients suffering from prolonged grief disorder are unlikely to respond, however, to standard antidepressant medications or to standard psychotherapy for depression, also referred to as interpersonal psychotherapy. One treatment that has been proposed is called *complicated grief therapy* (Shear 2010). Interpersonal psychotherapy focuses on grief and may also deal with the transition in roles the grieving person is experiencing or with disputes the bereaved had with the person

> ### Practice Points: Deaths that Prolong or Distort Normal Grief and Mourning
>
> - Unexpected and sudden death, even in a patient with advanced disease
> - Random, traumatic, violent, or mutilating death
> - Death following a prolonged illness
> - Death that seemed to be preventable
> - Death of a child

who died. The hope of interpersonal psychotherapy is to help people develop a nuanced view of their relationship with the person who died, including both the positive and the negative aspects of that relationship.

Complicated grief therapy, in contrast, is based on the idea that the bereaved must focus on the loss itself, while creating new life goals that accommodate that loss. People receiving complicated grief therapy are asked to retell the story of the death, listen to themselves telling that story, and identify feelings of stress as they learn to confront and not avoid their feelings. The therapist asks the patient to have imagined conversations with the deceased and to revive both positive and negative memories.

Shear and colleagues (2005) compared interpersonal psychotherapy to complicated grief therapy in a randomized controlled trial. An equal number of patients (about 27 percent in each arm of the study) was not able to complete the trial, but for different reasons. About half of those dropping out of the interpersonal psychotherapy arm were dissatisfied about its effectiveness, while half of those leaving the complicated grief therapy arm felt that telling the very distressing story would not be helpful to them. Therapists other than those delivering the interpersonal psychotherapy or complicated grief therapy assessed whether patients improved.

In this study, complicated grief therapy led to a significantly improved response rate ($p < .02$), with 51 percent of patients treated with complicated grief therapy responding (95 percent confidence intervals, 37–65 percent) compared with 28 percent of patients treated with interpersonal psychotherapy (95 percent confidence intervals, 15–41 percent). Among those in each group who completed the trial, the findings were even more significant ($p < .006$), with 66 percent (95 percent confidence intervals, 50–82 percent) of those receiving complicated grief therapy versus 32 percent (95 percent confidence intervals, 16–48 percent) of those receiving interpersonal psychotherapy responding.

Unresolved grief. For some bereaved—for example, those with unresolved anger, crises of faith, or guilt—ongoing spiritual counseling is helpful. For the unfortunate remainder, however, the grief seems never to lessen. These men and women are inconsolable. We must remember that their feelings are not their "fault." It may well be that the chemistry of their brains has changed, and their world is now radically different. They are heartbroken, and over time, some of them may find wisdom, if not ease, in their heartbreak.

To these people, we offer our continuing support and sympathetic ear. As well as we can, we bear witness. We listen to the stories they need to tell, try to understand their despair and the anger they need to express, and offer what small solace our attention can bring them. We understand that we are in a special position for them: we knew the person for whom they are grieving, and we may be the only ones to whom they feel free to talk about their feelings. We neither judge them nor presume to urge them to "get over it." But if at some point they feel trapped by their grief or overwhelmed by it, and if, on their own, they begin to look for ways to find some balance in their lives, they may feel less inhibition about turning to us for the help they will then need.

WOUNDED HEALERS

Self-Care

Now, we turn our attention to the grief we experience and the compassion we can show ourselves as caregivers engaged in this rewarding and challenging work. The *wounded healer*, a term coined by psychologist Henri Nouwen, embraces the notion that helpers are often compelled to care for others because they themselves are wounded (Nouwen 1979). Awareness of our own fragility, stressors, and traumatic experiences is integral to our ongoing ability to compassionately care for our patients and their families.

Caring for even one patient who is dying with advanced cancer can be intellectually and emotionally exhausting. Like the families you work with, you may need to develop some self-care techniques. In the course of trying to help residents maintain their emotional equilibrium as they work with increasingly large numbers of extremely sick patients, I (*Janet Abrahm*) needed to analyze how I managed not to burn out or develop compassion fatigue. As I thought back, I realized that my initial self-care strategy was a disaster.

The first time I recall needing a strategy for self-care was in 1971, when I was a second-year medical student on my first clinical rotation: pediatrics. But this pediatrics was not in an outpatient office or even community hospital setting. The children I saw had been admitted to a tertiary care hospital to be treated for leukemia, which at that time was almost invariably fatal, or for illnesses of similar severity and complexity. The general pediatrics ward was filled with children with cystic fibrosis. Women were scarce in medicine back then, so I instinctively knew that crying in response to what I was dealing with was "not an option."

But a great deal of what I saw called for tears. I eventually found a place to shed them in private, when I was relaxed, and I could take my time to review the emotionally charged events. Sometimes I found myself crying silently during a concert and feeling better when the concert ended. That safety valve seemed to work so well that I used it throughout pediatrics.

But many years later, when I was in the midst of my first year of clinical training in oncology, an odd thing started to happen. I found myself dreading attending concerts. Both my husband and I had looked forward to summer evenings spent at an outdoor orchestral performance, but I began to find reasons not to go. Finally, one evening, I said, "I'm just not up to that tonight!"

My husband, quite puzzled, replied, "Up to what? Why would anyone not be 'up to' hearing Mozart?" It was only then that I realized what had happened. To deal with the troubling feelings aroused by the tragic stories of the cancer patients I was caring for, I had automatically reactivated my earlier mechanism: grieve them in private, usually during the slow moments of symphonies. What I wasn't "up to" was a mental review of the patients I'd seen recently or the full experience of the grief I had suppressed so that I could get through the work. I had developed compassion fatigue.

Compassion Fatigue and Burnout

Compassion fatigue is the detachment and depersonalization that develops in therapists who care for people who have experienced extreme suffering (e.g., torture or rape) and in clinicians like emergency department, oncology, and palliative care clinicians, who are emotionally affected by the trauma their patients experience. It develops in clinicians whose patients have prolonged downhill courses, who suffer severely, and about whom clinicians feel "guilty, insecure, frustrated, or inadequate" (Meier, Back, and Morrison 2001, p. 3009; Nouwen 1979). It is no wonder, then, that medical students (Dyrbye et al. 2008), residents (Thomas 2004), intensive care staff, oncologists (Vachon 2010), and palliative care practitioners are particularly prone to developing compassion fatigue (Kearney et al. 2009).

Those of us who develop compassion fatigue are more likely to have stress-related medical disorders, anxiety, depression, substance abuse, and family disruption (Meier, Back, and Morrison 2001; Shanafelt and Dyrbye 2012). Some of us begin to resemble a patient with post-traumatic stress disorder: we develop (1) hyperarousal, (2) reexperiencing, and (3) avoidance (Wright 2004). Manifestations of our hyperarousal can be anger at our own staff, colleagues, or even patients with refractory disease or their families. Having dreams or nightmares about conversations with patients whose disease is relentlessly progressive is a clinician's way of "reexperiencing." If you know someone who is too detached or depersonalizes her patients, makes fewer or no visits to patients who are doing badly, or does rounds when they are likely to be asleep and the family not there, that's avoidance. They're doing that because it is too painful for them to be there; they may even take more and more time off work. If any of this seems familiar to you or is a pretty good description of a colleague's recent behavior, you or she may be suffering from compassion fatigue.

Practice Points: Compassion Fatigue

- Feeling "guilty, insecure, frustrated, or inadequate" when caring for patients with persistent downhill courses
- Experiencing detachment and depersonalization
- Undergoing PTSD-like manifestations: hyperarousal, reexperiencing, and avoidance
- Having stress-related medical disorders, anxiety, depression, substance abuse, and family disruption
- Avoiding timely discussion of prognosis and true burdens and benefits of therapy
- Experiencing burnout (from cumulative grief and compassion fatigue)

I believe that unrecognized compassion fatigue among oncologists inhibits the timely discussion of prognosis and of the true burdens and benefits of therapy, as well as the collaboration between oncologists and palliative care clinicians who can help share the burden of these difficult conversations. Oncologists with compassion fatigue may even recoil from reaching out to palliative care colleagues, not recognizing that they do this because of often unconscious painful memories of the many tough meetings they have had together. One oncology fellow, for example, responded to my greeting in the elevator with, "I can't talk to you now; I don't have time to cry." When I hear, "He's not ready for palliative care," I sometimes wonder, "Who isn't ready?"

Palliative care clinicians also suffer from compassion fatigue for the same reasons oncologists do. They strive to cure suffering with the same energy and commitment as oncologists apply to curing their patients, or to prolonging their patients' quality of life as long as possible. Caring for a patient for whom we cannot relieve or even ameliorate suffering is therefore incredibly painful for us. Palliative care clinicians are often overworked, with little control of their schedules, and they feel a moral mandate to see all the patients who need them. In some settings, they practice alone, without the support of an effective team to help them process the emotions the work engenders. It is no surprise, then, that palliative care clinicians also develop compassion fatigue.

In both oncology and palliative care clinicians, cumulative grief and compassion fatigue may lead to burnout (Shanafelt and Dyrbye 2012). Those who cannot bear to sit and talk with patients, because they see their patients' impending deaths or intense suffering and feel helpless in the face of that prospect, cannot offer the presence these patients need. Without an opportunity to express those griefs and diminish their power, the clinician has less and less "room" for emotional engagement with patients, or even with her own family. For an oncologist suffering from compassion fatigue, even making a referral to palliative care may open doors that the oncologist may not be emotionally ready to go through.

Dr. McFarland and colleagues wrote an article specifically addressing burnout (as well as depression and suicide) in oncology physicians (McFarland et al. 2019). The article thoroughly addresses medicine's long history of stoicism, self-sacrifice, and hidden agendas, which can be taken too far and lead to neglected self-care. The oncology work environment and patient population may contribute to the higher levels of burnout that are seen in oncologists compared to other medical specialists in the United States (Shanafelt and Dyrbye 2012) and throughout the world (Raphael et al. 2019).

I appreciate Dr. McFarland and colleagues' focus on a need for interventions at the individual level, system level, and a combined approach (and indeed, the section at the end of Chapter 12, "What Our Institutions Can Do to Support Us" is relevant here as well). Several studies have shown that individual, structural, and organizational strategies combined can reduce physician burnout (West, Dyrbye, and Shanafelt 2018), including that of oncologists and palliative care clinicians. So, while I wouldn't want the take-home message for those suffering from or at risk for burnout or compassion fatigue to be simply, "physician, heal thyself," individual strategies may be a worthwhile focus in partnership with structural and organizational strategies.

Practice Points: Reducing Clinician Burnout

- Acknowledge and assess the problem.
- Harness the power of leadership.
- Develop and implement targeted interventions.
- Cultivate community at work.
- Use rewards and incentives wisely.
- Align values and strengthen culture.
- Promote flexibility and work-life integration.
- Provide resources to promote resilience and self-care.
- Facilitate and fund organizational science.

(Adapted from Murali et al. 2018, p. 866)

Strategies. Once I understood what I'd been doing, that waiting until I was at a symphony to let myself experience my grief was not a good solution, I was able to devise other strategies for dealing with my grief in a much more timely fashion.

After someone died, I cried if I needed to and even found a few minutes to give full vent to my sadness. I found private places around the hospital or confided in colleagues who then felt free to share their stories with me. These resources served me well throughout my career as an oncologist.

When I began doing full-time palliative care, I again found myself challenged by the almost incessant suffering I saw. Each of us needs to identify a way to process the intense emotions the work entails. Some meditate, others exercise, but all recognize that unless we grieve our losses, we will no longer be able to remain present in the face of suffering, or to offer compassion. We need to be attentive to our own emotional and spiritual needs.

My meditation practice improved my ability to connect with my patients and to relieve some of their distress. And thanks to the wonderful clinicians I am privileged to work with on our team, I have not succumbed again to compassion fatigue. My social work colleagues on the team have been particularly helpful, but all of us look out for each other. Our motto is "never worry alone." Most recently, our palliative care team members sought training together in mindfulness meditation, using a course adapted from the work of Jon Kabat-Zinn (Stahl and Goldstein 2010; see also Chapter 8 in this book). Self-awareness and mindfulness training have both been demonstrated to help prevent burnout (Kearney et al. 2009; Stahl and Goldstein 2010). I use the exercises I've learned to prepare for or to recover from emotionally charged situations.

Recognizing triggers. After my (*Bethany-Rose Daubman*) sister was diagnosed with ovarian cancer, our team's triage nurse told me that she would try to avoid assigning me consults on young women with terminal ovarian cancer, worrying that that would be triggering, given what I was going through in my family. Indeed, some members of our team found patients with diagnoses similar to personal losses they'd experienced to be particularly challenging to care for. I appreciated her concern, and it caused me to reflect on the types of cases I found most challenging.

What I found was that it wasn't necessarily patients in the same demographic as loved ones whom I had lost or who were sick, or patients who were my own age or at similar life stages who were most challenging for me to care for. But reflecting back over the past few years, I realized there were particular patients who had touched me deeply, and that the common theme was patients who coped in ways similar to how I would aspire to cope if I developed a serious illness. An older woman whose sarcastic humor belied a deep, enduring love for her partner that reminded me of my own relationship and banter with my husband; a young man whose quiet faith and deep contemplations about the meaning of suffering reflected how I might hope to grapple with illness.

It wasn't their exact diagnoses that affected me most, but more intrinsic personality traits, coping styles, and beliefs. Others might find that patients at similar ages and life stages might be most challenging. Taking the time to realize that my triggers might be different from those of others was beneficial and, moving forward, helped me to identify cases where I may need to lean on my social work colleagues for psychosocial support more readily if I found myself at risk of countertransference. I also was able to identify a trusted colleague who shared my sense of boundaries; we engaged in peer supervision, and I encouraged her to call me on it if she saw me getting enmeshed.

Professional boundaries. Another matter I have learned to factor into my own risk for burnout is the professional-personal boundaries that can so often become blurred in fields such as oncology and palliative care. As I write this, another close family member is undergoing cancer treatment. I am her health care proxy, and her oncologist is a colleague. He had been directly texting me with updates or questions about her care until I asked him not to.

The father of a medical student I mentor was recently admitted to the palliative care unit of a nearby hospital, and the student has been calling and texting me every few days with questions about his dad's care at end of life and asking if I am able to help liaise with the palliative care team there, many of whom are close friends. I am also pregnant in the middle of the COVID-19 pandemic, wondering every day if I, too, will contract COVID through the course of my daily patient care, each night "doomscrolling" through the latest research on the likelihood of a stillbirth if that were to occur.

As Jane deLima Thomas points out in her excellent article, "Breaching the Professional-Personal Boundary—An Unrecognized Risk for Burnout" (Thomas 2019), these types of calls from family members, friends, and colleagues are common in our field and at times lead to situations where we are providing clinical care for those with whom we have close personal connections. It is important to recognize the increased emotional intensity that can occur when caring for those inside our professional boundaries. In the case of my COVID doomscrolling, working on the precipice between life and death is a reminder that I am not protected from loss myself.

While we may not be able to prevent these blurred boundaries completely, it may be helpful to have guidelines and plans in place for when they occur. As Dr. Thomas suggests, have your team come to a consensus that you will care for patients you know personally only if you have the clinical expertise required, if the patients wouldn't be better served by other specialists; that a particular member of the team will not care for his or her own close relatives or friends; and that the team should follow the usual clinical procedures rather than making special allowances. Normalize talking about the unique challenges of these cases, engage in self-reflection, and expect that you will need additional psychosocial support from members of your team; consider seeking external counseling or psychotherapy, and ramp up your self-care.

Training. We teach our palliative care and oncology fellows about the importance of self-care and of recognizing the stresses that their choice of profession will entail. For them and for you, the first thing to do is to acquire the core skills of conducting difficult conversations through mentoring from palliative care clinicians or oncology communication experts. In addition to having a positive effect on patients, communication skills training has been found to reduce job-related distress for oncology clinicians (Penberthy et al. 2018). Gaining additional skill and comfort with serious illness conversations may, in fact, be a form of resilience building.

Second, identify dysfunctional beliefs, such as "Limitations in knowledge is a personal failing; responsibility is to be borne by physicians alone; altruistic devotion to work and denial of self is desirable; it is 'professional' to keep one's uncertainties and emotions to oneself" (Novak et al. 1997, p. 503).

Third, forgive yourself, accept your limitations, and accept praise; recognize and let go of mistakes, opportunities lost or mishandled; search for sources of pain and get help to learn to live with them, or do what needs to be done to help diminish them (Novak et al. 1997). Other strategies are listed in the Practice Points below.

Practice Points: Clues for Self-Preservation

- Recognize how stressful caring for dying patients can be.
- Give yourself credit for the work you are doing.
- Learn how to work with a team; delegate and thereby diffuse responsibilities; let other team members help you.
- Cultivate relationships with trusted colleagues with whom you can engage in self-reflection, discuss issues of countertransference, and clarify personal expectations and boundaries.
- Monitor your emotional reactions and take time for yourself when you need it.
- Set appropriate goals; acknowledge medicine's and your own limitations.
- Collaborate with a palliative care team.
- Incorporate structured opportunities to debrief difficult cases and the deaths of patients.

(Morris et al. 2019)

Balint groups for palliative care and oncology fellows facilitated by skilled psychologists, palliative care clinicians, or trained oncologists can also serve as a forum for discussion and exploration of grief-inducing clinical encounters, as well as for normalizing these feelings. We should train fellows in how it feels to say good-bye, and why it is important to do so, both for patients and for clinicians, as well as how useful it is to write bereavement letters and make bereavement phone calls.

Kearney et al. (2009) also offers strategies (supported by variable strength of evidence) that can prevent or treat compassion fatigue. These include "mindfulness meditation; reflective writing; adequate supervision and mentoring; sustainable workload; promotion of feelings of choice and control; appropriate recognition and reward; supportive work community; promotion of fairness and justice in the workplace; training in communication skills; development of self-awareness skills; practice of self-care activities; continuing educational activities; participation in research; mindfulness-based stress reduction for team; meaning-centered intervention for team" (p. 1159). They also offer both self-care and self-awareness practices that can be done at work.

Rachel Naomi Remen, MD, clinical professor of family and community medicine at the University of California, San Francisco, teaches undergraduates, graduates, and practicing physicians about the emotional, psychological, and spiritual aspects of care for the dying. She notes that our problems in this area may arise from our lack of experience in recovering from our own losses. We are not often shown how to process feelings associated with loss and are encouraged to develop defenses designed to deflect them. Rarely are such shields effective; more often, we succeed only in repressing painful feelings. These feelings then become even more powerful, evading our consciousness, resisting cognitive understanding, and yet directing our behavior. Because we avoid opening a wound of our own that we do not know how to heal, we risk becoming blind to the needs of our patients.

Dr. Remen's writings (1996), workshops, and courses at the Remen Institute for the Study of Health and Illness (RISHI; www.rishiprograms.org) help physicians experience the consequences of losses in their own clinical practices and teach them how to heal themselves. They learn to feel the pain of past losses and to mourn them effectively. At the end of the process, they often find they have regained their equanimity and joy in being physicians. Those who have gone through such experiences are also more likely to be sensitive to the needs of their dying patients. They understand that they need not have guilt or shame contemplating their patients' deaths, and they truly understand that while they cannot always cure, they can always help.

In some cases, just collaborating with a palliative care team will make the process bearable. They can help your team conduct those tough conversations (Gilligan 2003; von Roenn and Temel 2011) and later process the grief, leaving all of you better able to support and be empathic with your patients; more aware that the limitations are medicine's, not yours; and proud of what you can offer them.

Grief and Remembrance Rounds

Palliative care clinicians can also help trainees process their grief and prevent compassion fatigue. At Brigham and Women's Hospital, where I (*Janet Abrahm*) currently work, many years ago the chief medical residents asked Dr. Susan Block and me to support the house staff on the oncology and bone marrow transplant teams. Dr. Block had completed an intensive study of the reactions of house staff to the deaths of their patients, finding that members of the house staff often had unresolved feelings of grief, guilt, or anger about these deaths. The attending rounds in ICUs and in oncology were not able to make room for a discussion of the events surrounding a death, for airing house staff's concerns, and for education about the grief and bereavement not only of families but also of professional caregivers, such as nurses and physicians.

We therefore began to conduct grief rounds every other week, to which the interns were invited. The discussions were confidential, and, of course, food and drink were provided. The chief residents, who arranged for the food, also reminded the busy interns to come to the rounds, instructing them to sign out their beepers to their residents for the hour.

These rounds were well attended. Interns shared their concerns, learned that many of their colleagues had the same concerns, and worked out ways to interact more comfortably with patients who are dying and with their families. Later, when these rounds had ceased, our palliative care team hosted weekly rounds with the physician assistants, medical students, and house staff on the oncology and transplant teams. We found that these weekly palliative care rounds provided another forum for discussing troubling issues when they arose. I am hopeful that the rounds prevented these young clinicians from developing the kind of dysfunctional mechanism I had used to protect myself from the grief I was feeling.

Our palliative care team now uses a similar technique to care for ourselves. Dr. Sue Morris and our team chaplain, John Kearns, hold weekly "Remembrance rounds" (Morris et al. 2019). A clinician from the Palliative Care Division or one of our colleagues at BWH or DFCI leads the rounds by first offering the group something for reflection (e.g., a poem, piece of music, or snippet from a video), and explaining why he or she chose it. The leader then reads the names of each person on the remembrance list (i.e., those we cared for who died in the previous weeks), and then all who attend are encouraged to share memories or thoughts about any of them. Even via Zoom, in COVID times, this weekly one-hour gathering has proved to be healing and a way to demonstrate the power of connection.

The wounded healer. At the close of this chapter, we turn again to the model of the wounded healer. I (*Bethany-Rose Daubman*) am reminded of kintsukuroi, the Japanese art of repairing pottery with gold, understanding that the pottery is made more beautiful having been broken. In caring for the dying and their loved ones, we have undoubtedly been wounded in ways that inform the rest of our practice of medicine and healing. With self-reflection, attention to self-care, and strategies to reduce our risk of compassion fatigue and burnout, we are hopeful that we can continue to care for ourselves and for others as we navigate loss and grief.

Appendix

Wisconsin Brief Pain Inventory

Date _____   Time _____

Name _____ _____ _____
    Last   First   Middle Initial

1. Throughout our lives, most of us have had pain from time to time (such as minor headaches, sprains, and toothaches). Have you had pain other than these everyday kinds of pain today?

    Yes   No

2. On the diagram, shade in the areas where you feel pain. Put an X on the area that hurts the most.

Right ⌐ Left   Left ⌐ Right

3. Please rate your pain by circling the one number that best describes your pain at its **worst** in the last 24 hours.

    0   1   2   3   4   5   6   7   8   9   10
  No pain   Pain as bad as
                                                        you can imagine

4. Please rate your pain by circling the one number that best describes your pain at its **least** in the last 24 hours.

    0   1   2   3   4   5   6   7   8   9   10
  No pain   Pain as bad as
                                                        you can imagine

5. Please rate your pain by circling the one number that best describes your pain on the **average**.

    0   1   2   3   4   5   6   7   8   9   10
  No pain   Pain as bad as
                                                        you can imagine

6. Please rate your pain by circling the one number that best describes how much pain you have **right now**.

    0   1   2   3   4   5   6   7   8   9   10
  No pain   Pain as bad as
                                                        you can imagine

587

7. What treatments or medications are you receiving for your pain?

_____

_____

8. In the last 24 hours, how much relief have pain treatments or medications provided? Please circle the one percentage that most shows how much **relief** you have received.

0%   10%   20%   30%   40%   50%   60%   70%   80%   90%   100%

No Relief   Complete Relief

9. Circle the one number that best describes how, during the past 24 hours, pain has interfered with your:

A. General Activity

0   1   2   3   4   5   6   7   8   9   10

Does not
Interfere   Completely
                                                       Interferes

B. Mood

0   1   2   3   4   5   6   7   8   9   10

Does not
Interfere   Completely
                                                       Interferes

C. Walking Ability

0   1   2   3   4   5   6   7   8   9   10

Does not
Interfere   Completely
                                                       Interferes

D. Normal Work (includes both work outside the home and housework)

0   1   2   3   4   5   6   7   8   9   10

Does not
Interfere   Completely
                                                       Interferes

E. Relations with other people

0   1   2   3   4   5   6   7   8   9   10

Does not
Interfere   Completely
                                                       Interferes

F. Sleep

0   1   2   3   4   5   6   7   8   9   10

Does not
Interfere   Completely
                                                       Interferes

G. Enjoyment of life

0   1   2   3   4   5   6   7   8   9   10

Does not
Interfere   Completely
                                                       Interferes

Source: University of Texas M. D. Anderson Cancer Center; reprinted with permission.

Enhancements

The following audio and video recordings were created or curated, or are planned, by the Dana-Farber Cancer Institute (DFCI) Department of Psychosocial Oncology and Palliative Care.* They can be found at www.press.jhu.edu; www.janetabrahm .com; or https://www.dana-farber.org/research/departments-centers-and-labs /departments-and-centers/department-of-psychosocial-oncology-and-palliative -care/education/.

Audio Recordings

Three audio recordings of Dr. Janet Abrahm doing hypnotic induction for patients with dyspnea, dysphagia, or pain

Video Recordings

Four videos produced by the DFCI Department of Psychosocial Oncology and Palliative Care that illustrate key communication techniques: SPIKES, NURSE, REMAP, and Serious Illness Conversation Guide

Dr. Janet Abrahm interviewing Soltan Bryce regarding LGBTQ+ issues in palliative care

Three videos featuring Dr. Molly Collins (1) demonstrating how to bring "The 5 Things" into the conversation, (2) reviewing what the family can expect in the last days, and (3) providing anticipatory guidance for a patient's death

Links provided by Amanda Moment, LICSW, to videos on sexuality in cancer patients

Rev. Gloria White-Hammond, MD, discussing how to approach changing hope for patients with deep faith and how to work with patients and families who are hoping for a miracle

Detecting aberrant substance use (planned)

Using the Confusion Assessment Method to diagnose delirium (planned)

Hospice program services and team members (planned)

Detecting spiritual causes of pain (e.g., guilt) and how to respond (planned)

Detecting existential distress and how to respond (planned)

---

*With the exception of the links provided by Amanda Moment, LICSW, these materials were used with the permission of the DFCI Department of Psychosocial Oncology and Palliative Care, which has sole ownership.

Index